a LANGE medical book

Examination & Board Review

Pharmacology

fifth edition

a LANGE medical book

Examination & Board Review
Pharmacology

fifth edition

Bertram G. Katzung, MD, PhD
Professor of Pharmacology
Department of Cellular & Molecular Pharmacology
University of California, San Francisco

Anthony J. Trevor, PhD
Professor of Pharmacology and Toxicology
Department of Cellular & Molecular Pharmacology
University of California, San Francisco

Appleton & Lange
Stamford, Connecticut

Copyright © 1998, 1995 by Appleton & Lange
A Simon & Schuster Company
Copyright © 1993, 1990 by Appleton & Lange

www.appletonlange.com

98 99 00 01 02 / 10 9 8 7 6 5 4 3 2 1

Prentice Hall International (UK) Limited, *London*
Prentice Hall of Australia Pty. Limited, *Sydney*
Prentice Hall Canada, Inc., *Toronto*
Prentice Hall Hispanoamericana, S.A., *Mexico*
Prentice Hall of India Private Limited, *New Delhi*
Prentice Hall of Japan, Inc., *Tokyo*
Simon & Schuster Asia Pte. Ltd., *Singapore*
Editora Prentice Hall do Brasil Ltda., *Rio de Janeiro*
Prentice Hall, *Upper Saddle River, New Jersey*

ISBN: 0-8385-7708-3
ISSN: 1063-8636

Acquisitions Editor: David A. Barnes
Development Editor: Jim Ransom
Production Service: Rainbow Graphics, LLC
Production Editor: Sondra Greenfield
Designer: Libby Schmitz
Associate Art Manager: Maggie Belis Darrow
Art Coordinator: Becky Hainz-Baxter
Illustrators: Teshin Associates
              Linda F. Harris

ISBN 0-8385-7708-3

90000

9 780838 577080

PRINTED IN THE UNITED STATES OF AMERICA

Contents

VIII. CHEMOTHERAPEUTIC DRUGS

IX. TOXICOLOGY

X. SPECIAL TOPICS

Preface

This book is designed to help students review pharmacology and to prepare for regular course exams and board exams. The fifth edition has been extensively revised to make such preparation as efficient as possible. New tables and figures have been added and color has been used to further clarify difficult concepts. As with earlier editions, the most rigorous standards of accuracy and currency have been maintained, in keeping with the book's status as companion to the textbook *Basic & Clinical Pharmacology*.

Several strategies are employed to make reviewing effective and efficient:

First, the book breaks pharmacology down into the topics used in most courses and textbooks, rather than combining them into larger, unwieldy groups. Major introductory chapters (eg, autonomic pharmacology and CNS pharmacology) are included so that students can integrate their review of pharmacology with a review of relevant physiology and biochemistry. This chapter-based approach also encourages students to use the *Review* in conjunction with their course notes or with a larger text.

Second, each chapter explicitly lists a set of objectives, providing students with a checklist against which they can challenge themselves as they progress through the book.

Third, each chapter provides an expanded but still concise review of the core subject matter. The determination of what is core is based on a careful analysis of the content of actual board examinations in past years as well as the content of major medical school courses. Tables of definitions and diagrams illustrating the major subdivisions of drugs within each group are provided.

Fourth, a table of important drug names is provided in every chapter dealing with specific drug groups. Recognition of drug names is an important part of board exams. We make the process more efficient by distinguishing between those drugs important as prototypes, those recognized as major variants on the prototypes, and those that should simply be recognized as belonging to a particular drug group.

Fifth, each chapter ends with practice questions followed by a list of answers and explanations. Because each area of pharmacology is represented by a separate chapter, students are assured of having practice questions in every important area. Questions that require analysis of graphic or tabular data are included. Appendices II and III comprise two complete examinations, each covering the entire field of pharmacology. In keeping with the format adopted for the United States Medical Licensure Examination (USMLE), the questions are of the "A" (single best answer) and "R" (matching, including *extended* matching) types. Many of the questions are set in the "clinical vignette" format currently favored on USMLE examinations. More than 1000 questions, with answers, are provided in this book.

Sixth, Appendix I provides a list of key drugs that appear frequently in board exam questions with concise keyword descriptions. This unique learning aid provides an efficient "flashcard" list of the drugs and drug properties most likely to appear on an examination.

The book provides several additional sections of value to the student preparing for a board exam: (1) a set of 17 case histories, with questions and answers, providing additional review and testing of the student's preparation for questions about clinical pharmacology, and (2) a short appendix on test strategies, which summarizes time-saving devices for approaching specific types of questions used on most "objective" exams.

We recommend that this book be used with a regular text. *Basic & Clinical Pharmacology*, 7th edition (Appleton & Lange, 1998), follows the chapter sequence used here. However, this *Review* is designed to complement any standard medical pharmacology text. The student who completes and understands this *Review* will greatly improve his or her performance on examinations and will have an excellent command of pharmacology.

Because it was developed in parallel with the textbook *Basic & Clinical Pharmacology*, the *Review* represents the author's interpretations of chapters written by contributors to that text.

We are very grateful to these contributors, to our other faculty colleagues, and to our students—who have taught us most of what we know about teaching.

Suggestions and criticisms regarding this study guide should be mailed to us at the following address:

Department of Cellular & Molecular Pharmacology
Box 0450
University of California
San Francisco, CA 94143-0450, USA

Bertram G. Katzung, MD, PhD
Anthony J. Trevor, PhD
San Francisco
March 1998

Part I: Basic Principles

Introduction

1

OBJECTIVES

You should be able to:

- Predict the relative ease of permeation of a weak acid or base from a knowledge of its pK_a and the pH of the medium.
- List and discuss the common routes of drug administration and excretion.
- Draw graphs of the blood level versus time for drugs subject to zero-order elimination and for drugs subject to first-order elimination.

Learn the definitions that follow.

Table 1–1. Definitions.

Term	Definition
Pharmacology	The study of the interaction of chemicals with living systems
Drugs	Substances that act on living systems at the chemical (molecular) level
Drug receptors	The molecular components of the body with which a drug interacts to bring about its effects
Medical pharmacology	The study of drugs used for the diagnosis, prevention, and treatment of disease
Toxicology	The study of the undesirable effects of chemical agents on living systems; considered an area of pharmacology. In addition to the adverse effects of therapeutic agents on individuals, toxicology deals with the actions of industrial pollutants, natural organic and inorganic poisons, and other chemicals on species and ecosystems as well
Pharmacodynamics	The actions of a drug on the body, including receptor interactions, dose-response phenomena, and mechanisms of therapeutic and toxic action
Pharmacokinetics	The actions of the body on the drug, including absorption, distribution, metabolism, and excretion. **Elimination** of a drug may be achieved by metabolism or by excretion. **Biodisposition** is a term sometimes used to describe the processes of metabolism and excretion

CONCEPTS

A. **The Nature of Drugs:**
   1. **Size and molecular weight (MW):** Drugs in common use vary in size from MW 7 (lithium) to over MW 50,000 (thrombolytic enzymes). The majority of drugs, however, have molecular weights between 100 and 1000.
   2. **Drug-receptor bonds:** Drugs bind to receptors with a variety of chemical bonds. These include very strong covalent bonds (which usually result in irreversible action), somewhat weaker electrostatic bonds (eg, between a cation and an anion), and much weaker interactions (eg, hydrogen, van der Waals, and hydrophobic bonds).

B. **The Movement of Drugs in the Body:** In order to reach its receptors and bring about a biologic effect, a drug molecule must travel from the site of administration (eg, the gastrointestinal tract) to the site of action (eg, the brain).

1. **Permeation:** Permeation is the movement of drug molecules into and within the biologic environment. It involves several processes, of which the following are the most important:

    a. **Aqueous diffusion:** Aqueous diffusion is the movement of molecules through the watery extracellular and intracellular spaces. The membranes of most capillaries have small water-filled pores that permit the aqueous diffusion of molecules up to the size of small proteins between the blood and the extravascular space. This is a passive process governed by Fick's law (see below).

    b. **Lipid diffusion:** Lipid diffusion is the movement of molecules through membranes and other lipid structures. Like aqueous diffusion, this is a passive process governed by Fick's law (see below).

    c. **Transport by special carriers:** Drugs may be transported across barriers by mechanisms that carry similar endogenous substances, eg, the amino acid carriers in the blood-brain barrier and the weak acid carriers in the renal tubule. Unlike aqueous and lipid diffusion, carrier transport is not governed by Fick's law and is capacity-limited. Selective inhibitors for these carriers may have clinical value; eg, probenecid, which inhibits transport of uric acid, penicillin, and other weak acids, is used to increase the excretion of uric acid in gout.

    d. **Endocytosis, pinocytosis:** Endocytosis occurs through binding to specialized components (receptors) of cell membranes, with subsequent internalization by infolding of that area of the membrane. The contents of the resulting vesicle are subsequently released into the cytoplasm of the cell. Endocytosis permits very large or very lipid-insoluble chemicals to enter cells. For example, large molecules such as peptides may enter cells by this mechanism. Smaller, polar substances such as vitamin B_{12} and iron combine with special proteins (B_{12} with intrinsic factor and iron with transferrin), and the complexes enter cells by this mechanism. Exocytosis is the reverse process, ie, the expulsion of membrane-encapsulated material from cells.

2. **Fick's law of diffusion:** Fick's law predicts the rate of movement of molecules across a barrier; the concentration gradient and permeability coefficient for the drug and the area and thickness of the barrier membrane are used to compute the rate, as follows:

$$\textbf{Rate} = (\textbf{C}_1 - \textbf{C}_2) \times \frac{\textbf{Permeability Coefficient}}{\textbf{Thickness}} \times \textbf{Area} \qquad (1)$$

This relationship demonstrates that drug absorption is faster from organs with large surface areas, eg, the small intestine, than from organs with small absorbing areas, eg, the stomach. Furthermore, drug absorption is faster from organs with thin membrane barriers, eg, the lung, than from those with thick barriers, eg, the skin.

3. **Water and lipid solubility of drugs:**

    a. **Aqueous diffusion:** The aqueous solubility of a drug is often a function of the electrostatic charge (degree of ionization, polarity) of the molecule, because water molecules behave as dipoles and are attracted to charged drug molecules, forming an aqueous shell around them. Conversely, the lipid solubility of a molecule is inversely proportionate to its charge.

    b. **Lipid diffusion:** Many drugs are weak bases or weak acids. For such molecules, the *pH of the medium* determines the fraction of molecules that are charged (ionized) versus those that are uncharged (nonionized). If the pK_a of the drug and the pH of the medium are known, the fraction of molecules in the ionized state can be predicted by means of the Henderson-Hasselbalch equation:

$$\log\left(\frac{\textbf{Protonated form}}{\textbf{Unprotonated form}}\right) = \textbf{pK}_a - \textbf{pH} \qquad (2)$$

"Protonated" means *associated with a proton* (a hydrogen ion); this form of the equation applies to both acids and bases.

c. Ionization of weak acids and bases: Weak bases are ionized—and therefore more polar and more water-soluble—when they are protonated; weak acids are not ionized—and so are less water-soluble—when they are protonated.

The following equations summarize these points:

$$RNH_3^+ \rightleftharpoons RNH_2 + H^+ \tag{3}$$

protonated weak base (charged, more water-soluble) · unprotonated weak base (uncharged, more lipid-soluble) · proton

$$RCOOH \rightleftharpoons RCOO^- + H^+ \tag{4}$$

protonated weak acid (uncharged, more lipid-soluble) · unprotonated weak acid (charged, more water-soluble) · proton

The Henderson-Hasselbalch relationship is clinically important when it is necessary to accelerate the excretion of drugs by the kidney, eg, in the case of an overdose. Most drugs are freely filtered at the glomerulus, but lipid-soluble drugs can be rapidly reabsorbed from the tubular urine. When a patient takes an overdose of a weak acid drug, its excretion may be accelerated by alkalinizing the urine, eg, by giving bicarbonate. This is because a drug that is a weak acid dissociates to its charged, polar form in alkaline solution, and this form cannot readily diffuse from the renal tubule back into the blood. Conversely, excretion of a weak base may be accelerated by acidifying the urine, eg, by administering ammonium chloride (Figure 1–1).

C. Absorption of Drugs:

1. Routes of administration: Drugs usually enter the body at sites remote from the target tissue or organ and thus require transport by the circulation to the intended site of action. To enter the bloodstream, a drug must be absorbed from its site of administration (unless the drug has been injected directly into the bloodstream). The rate and efficiency of absorption differ depending on a drug's route of administration. In fact, for some drugs, the amount absorbed into the circulation may be only a small fraction of the dose administered when given by certain routes. The amount absorbed divided by the amount administered constitutes its **bioavailability.** Common routes of administration and some of their features include the following:

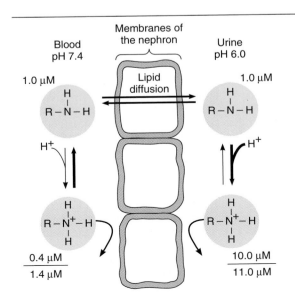

Figure 1–1. "Trapping" is a method for accelerating excretion of drugs. Because the nonionized form diffuses readily across the lipid barriers of the nephron, this form will equilibrate and may reach equal concentrations in the blood and urine; the ionized form will not. Protonation will occur within the blood and the urine according to the Henderson-Hasselbalch equation. Pyrimethamine, a weak base of pK_a 7.0, is used in this example. At blood pH, only 0.4 µmol of the protonated species will be present for each 1.0 µmol of the unprotonated form. The total concentration in the blood will thus be 1.4 µmol/L. In the urine at pH 6.0, 10 µmol of the nondiffusible ionized form will be present for each 1.0 µmol of the unprotonated, diffusible form. Therefore, the total urine concentration (11 µmol/L) may be almost eight times higher than the blood concentration.

a. **Oral (swallowed):** The oral route offers maximum convenience, but absorption may be slower and less complete than when parenteral routes are used. Ingested drugs are subject to the **first-pass effect,** in which a significant amount of the agent is metabolized in the gut wall and the liver before it reaches the systemic circulation. Thus, some drugs have low bioavailability when given orally.

b. **Intravenous:** The intravenous route offers instantaneous and complete absorption (by definition, bioavailability is 100%). This route is potentially more dangerous, however, because of the high blood levels that are produced if administration is too rapid.

c. **Intramuscular:** Absorption from an intramuscular injection site is often (not always) faster and more complete (higher bioavailability) than with oral administration. Large volumes (eg, > 5 mL into each buttock) may be given.

d. **Subcutaneous:** The subcutaneous route offers slower absorption than the intramuscular route. Large-volume bolus doses are less feasible.

e. **Buccal and sublingual:** The buccal route (in the pouch between gums and cheek) permits direct absorption into the systemic venous circulation, bypassing the hepatic portal circuit and first-pass metabolism. This process may be fast or slow depending on the physical formulation of the product. The sublingual route (under the tongue) offers the same features as the buccal route.

f. **Rectal (suppository):** The rectal route offers partial avoidance of the first-pass effect (though avoidance is not as complete as with the sublingual route). Larger amounts of a drug and drugs with an unpleasant taste are better administered rectally than by the buccal or sublingual routes. Some drugs administered rectally may cause significant irritation.

g. **Inhalation:** In the case of respiratory diseases, the inhalation route offers delivery closest to the target tissue. This route often provides rapid absorption because of the large alveolar surface area available.

h. **Topical:** The topical route includes application to the skin or to the mucous membranes of the eye, nose, throat, airway, or vagina for *local* effect. The rate of absorption varies with the area of application and the drug formulation but is usually slower than any of the routes listed above.

i. **Transdermal:** The transdermal route involves application to the skin for *systemic* effect. Absorption usually occurs very slowly, but the first-pass effect is avoided.

D. **Distribution of Drugs:**
1. **Determinants of distribution:** The distribution of drugs to the tissues depends upon the following:

a. **Size of the organ:** The size of the organ determines the concentration gradient between blood and the organ. For example, skeletal muscle can take up a large amount of drug because the concentration in the muscle tissue remains low (and the blood-tissue gradient high) even after relatively large amounts of drug have been transferred; this occurs because skeletal muscle is a very large organ. In contrast, because the brain is smaller, distribution of a smaller amount of drug into it will raise the tissue concentration and reduce to zero the blood-tissue concentration gradient, preventing further uptake of drug.

b. **Blood flow:** Blood flow to the tissue is an important determinant of the *rate* of uptake, though blood flow may not affect the steady state amount of drug in the tissue. As a result, well-perfused tissues (eg, brain, heart, kidneys, splanchnic organs) will often achieve high tissue concentrations sooner than poorly perfused tissues (eg, fat, bone). If the drug is rapidly eliminated, the concentration in poorly perfused tissues may never rise significantly.

c. **Solubility:** The solubility of a drug in tissue influences the concentration of the drug in the extracellular fluid surrounding the blood vessels. If the drug is very soluble in the cells, the concentration in the perivascular extracellular space will be lower and diffusion from the vessel into the extravascular tissue space will be facilitated. For example, some organs (including the brain) have a high lipid content and thus dissolve a high concentration of lipid-soluble agents. As a result, a very lipid-soluble anesthetic will transfer out of the blood and into the brain tissue more rapidly and to a greater extent than a drug with low lipid solubility.

d. **Binding:** Binding of a drug to macromolecules in the blood or a tissue compartment will tend to increase the drug's concentration in that compartment. For example, warfarin is strongly bound to plasma albumin, which restricts warfarin's diffusion out of the vascular compartment. Conversely, chloroquine is strongly bound to tissue proteins, which results in a marked reduction in the plasma concentration of chloroquine.

    2. **Apparent volume of distribution:** The apparent volume of distribution (V_d) is an important pharmacokinetic parameter that reflects the above determinants of drug distribution in the body. V_d relates the amount of drug in the body to the concentration in the plasma. (See Chapter 3.)

E. **Metabolism of Drugs:** Metabolism of a drug sometimes terminates its action, but other effects of drug metabolism are also important. Some drugs, when given orally, are metabolized before they enter the systemic circulation. This **first-pass metabolism** was referred to above as one cause of low bioavailability. Other drugs are administered as inactive **prodrugs** and must be metabolized to active agents. Some drugs are not metabolized at all—their action must be terminated by excretion.

    1. **Drug metabolism as a mechanism of termination of drug action:** The action of many drugs (eg, phenothiazines) is terminated before they are excreted because they are metabolized to biologically inactive derivatives.

    2. **Drug metabolism as a mechanism of drug activation:** Prodrugs (eg, levodopa, methyldopa, parathion) are inactive as administered and must be metabolized in the body to become active. Many drugs are active as administered and have active metabolites as well, eg, many benzodiazepines.

    3. **Drug elimination without metabolism:** Some drugs (eg, lithium) are not modified by the body; they continue to act until they are excreted.

F. **Elimination of Drugs:** Along with the dosage, the rate of elimination (disappearance of the active molecule from the bloodstream or body) determines the duration of action for most drugs. Therefore, knowledge of the time course of concentration in plasma is important in predicting the intensity and duration of effect for most drugs. *Note:* Drug *elimination* is not the same as drug *excretion:* A drug may be eliminated by metabolism long before the modified molecules are excreted from the body. Furthermore, for drugs with active metabolites (eg, diazepam), elimination of the parent molecule by metabolism is not synonymous with termination of action. For drugs that are not metabolized, excretion is the mode of elimination. A small number of drugs combine irreversibly with their receptors, so that disappearance from the bloodstream is not equivalent to cessation of drug action, and these drugs may have a very prolonged action. For example, phenoxybenzamine, an irreversible inhibitor of alpha adrenoceptors, is eliminated from the bloodstream in an hour or less after administration. The drug's action, however, lasts for 48 hours.

    1. **First-order elimination:** The term *first-order elimination* implies that the rate of elimination is proportionate to the concentration, ie, the higher the concentration, the greater the amount of drug eliminated per unit time. The result is that the drug's concentration in plasma decreases exponentially with time (Figure 1–2, left). Drugs with first-order elimina-

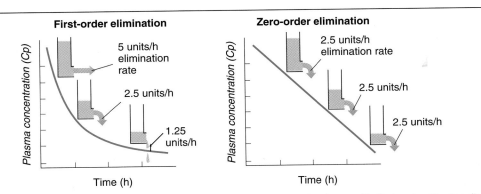

Figure 1–2. Comparison of first-order and zero-order elimination. In drugs with first-order kinetics (left panel), rate of elimination is proportionate to plasma concentration (Cp); in the case of zero-order elimination (right panel), the rate is constant and independent of concentration.

tion have a characteristic **half-life of elimination** that is constant regardless of the amount of drug in the body. The concentration of such a drug in the blood will decrease by 50% for every half-life. Most drugs in clinical use demonstrate first-order kinetics.

2. **Zero-order elimination:** The term *zero-order elimination* implies that the rate of elimination is constant regardless of concentration (Figure 1–2, right panel). A few drugs saturate their elimination mechanisms even at low concentrations. As a result, the drug's concentration in plasma decreases in a linear fashion over time. This is typical of ethanol (over most of its plasma concentration range) and of phenytoin and aspirin at high therapeutic or toxic concentrations.

G. Pharmacokinetic Models:

1. **Multicompartment distribution:** After absorption, many drugs undergo an early distribution phase followed by a slower elimination phase. Mathematically, this behavior can be modeled by means of a "two-compartment model" as shown in Figure 1–3. (Note that each phase is associated with a characteristic half-life: $t_{1/2\alpha}$ for the first phase, $t_{1/2\beta}$ for the second phase.)

2. **Single-compartment distribution:** A few drugs may behave as if they are distributed to only one compartment (eg, if they are restricted to the vascular compartment). Others have more complex distributions that require more than two compartments for construction of accurate mathematical models.

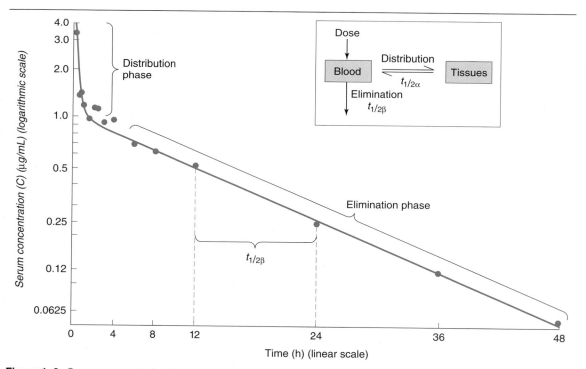

Figure 1–3. Serum concentration-time curve after administration of chlordiazepoxide as an intravenous bolus. The experimental data are plotted on a semilogarithmic scale as filled circles. This drug follows first-order kinetics and appears to occupy two compartments. The initial curvilinear portion of the data represents the distribution phase, with drug equilibrating between the blood compartment and the tissue compartment. The linear portion of the curve represents drug elimination. The elimination half-life ($t_{1/2\beta}$) can be extracted graphically as shown by measuring the time between any two plasma concentration points that differ by twofold. (See Chapter 3 for additional details.) (Modified and reproduced, with permission, from Greenblatt DJ, Koch-Weser J: Clinical pharmacokinetics. N Engl J Med 1975; 293:702.)

QUESTIONS

DIRECTIONS: Each of the numbered items or incomplete statements in this section is followed by answers or by completions of the statement. Select the ONE lettered answer or completion that is BEST in each case.

Items 1–2: Johnny, a 3-year-old, is brought to the emergency department, having just ingested a large overdose of promethazine, an antihistaminic drug. Promethazine is a weak base with a pK_a of 9.1. It is capable of entering most tissues, including the brain. On physical examination, the heart rate is 100/min, blood pressure 110/60 mm Hg, and respiratory rate 20/min.

1. All of the following are general mechanisms of drug permeation EXCEPT
   (A) Aqueous diffusion
   (B) Aqueous hydrolysis
   (C) Lipid diffusion
   (D) Pinocytosis or endocytosis
   (E) Special carrier transport

2. In this case of promethazine overdose,
   (A) Urinary excretion would be accelerated by administration of NH_4Cl
   (B) Urinary excretion would be accelerated by giving $NaHCO_3$
   (C) More of the drug would be ionized at blood pH than at stomach pH
   (D) Absorption of the drug would be faster from the stomach than from the small intestine
   (E) Hemodialysis is the only effective therapy

3. A patient with a history of episodic attacks of coughing, wheezing, and shortness of breath is being evaluated in the asthma clinic. Several drug treatments with different routes of administration are under consideration. All of the following statements about routes of administration are correct EXCEPT
   (A) Blood levels often rise faster after intramuscular injection than after oral dosing
   (B) The "first-pass" effect is the result of metabolism of a drug after administration and before it enters the systemic circulation
   (C) Administration of antiasthmatic drugs by inhaled aerosol is usually associated with more adverse effects than is administration of these drugs by mouth
   (D) Bioavailability of most drugs is less with rectal (suppository) administration than with intravenous administration
   (E) Onset of drug effect is often slower after administration by transdermal patch than after oral administration, but the transdermal route is associated with less first-pass metabolism

4. Aspirin is a weak organic acid with a pK_a of 3.5. What percentage of a given dose will be in the lipid-soluble form at a stomach pH of 2.5?
   (A) About 1%
   (B) About 10%
   (C) About 50%
   (D) About 90%
   (E) About 99%

5. If the plasma concentration of a drug declines with "first-order kinetics," this means that
   (A) There is only one metabolic path for drug disposition
   (B) The half-life is the same regardless of the plasma concentration
   (C) The drug is largely metabolized in the liver after oral administration and has low bioavailability
   (D) The rate of elimination is proportionate to the rate of administration at all times
   (E) The drug is not distributed outside the vascular system

6. Regarding termination of drug action, it could be said that
   (A) Drugs must be excreted from the body to terminate their action
   (B) Metabolism of drugs always increases their water solubility
   (C) Metabolism of drugs always abolishes their pharmacologic activity
   (D) Hepatic metabolism and renal excretion are the two most important mechanisms involved
   (E) Distribution of a drug out of the bloodstream terminates the drug's effects

7. Distribution of drugs to specific tissues
   (A) Is independent of blood flow to the organ
   (B) Is independent of the solubility of the drug in that tissue
   (C) Depends on the unbound drug concentration gradient between blood and the tissue
   (D) Is increased for drugs that are strongly bound to plasma proteins
   (E) Has no effect on the half-life of the drug

8. Pilocarpine is being considered for the treatment of glaucoma in a 58-year-old patient. Except for elevated intraocular pressure, the patient's history and physical examination are unremarkable. Pilocarpine is a weak base of pK_a 6.9. Which of the following statements is FALSE?

  (A) After parenteral administration, the concentration of pilocarpine in the aqueous humor (pH 7.8) will be lower than the concentration in the duodenum (pH 5.5)
  (B) When pilocarpine is administered as eyedrops, absorption into the eye will be faster if the drops are alkaline (pH 8.0) than if they are acidic (pH 5.0)
  (C) Excretion in the urine will be faster if urine pH is alkaline (pH 8.0) than if the urine pH is acidic (pH 5.8)
  (D) The proportion of pilocarpine in the protonated form will be approximately 90% at pH 5.9
  (E) The percentage of pilocarpine in the more lipid-soluble form will be approximately 99% at pH 8.9

DIRECTIONS (Items 9–15): Each set of matching questions in this section consists of a list of three to twenty-six lettered options (some of which may be figures) followed by several numbered items. For each numbered item, select the ONE lettered option that is most closely associated with it. Each lettered option may be selected once, more than once, or not at all.

Item 9:
  (A) Weak acid with pK_a of 5.5
  (B) Weak base with pK_a of 3.5
  (C) Weak acid with pK_a of 7.5
  (D) Weak base with pK_a of 6.5

9. Excretion will be most significantly accelerated by acidification of the urine

Items 10–15:
  (A) Distribution
  (B) Elimination
  (C) Endocytosis
  (D) First-pass effect
  (E) First-order kinetics
  (F) Lipid solubility
  (G) Permeation
  (H) Pharmacodynamics
  (I) Pharmacokinetics
  (J) Protonation
  (K) Volume of distribution
  (L) Zero-order kinetics

10. Process by which a weak acid becomes less water-soluble and more lipid-soluble
11. Properties that characterize the effects of a drug on the body
12. Properties that describe the effects of the body on a drug
13. Process by which the amount of active drug in the body is reduced after absorption into the systemic circulation
14. Process by which a drug in the body is reduced after administration but before entering the systemic circulation
15. Kinetics that are characteristic of the excretion of ethanol and high doses of phenytoin and aspirin.

ANSWERS

1. Hydrolysis has nothing to do with the mechanisms of permeation; rather, hydrolysis is one mechanism of drug metabolism. The answer is **(B)**.
2. Questions that deal with acid-base (Henderson-Hasselbalch) manipulations are common. Since absorption involves permeation across lipid membranes, we can treat an overdose by decreasing absorption from the gut and reabsorption from the tubular urine by making the drug *less lipid-soluble*. Ionization attracts water molecules and decreases lipid solubility. Promethazine is a weak base—which means that it will be more ionized (protonated) at acid

pH than at basic pH. Choice **(C)** suggests that the drug would be more ionized at pH 7.4 than at pH 2: clearly wrong. **(D)** says (in effect) that the more ionized form will be absorbed faster, and that is wrong. **(A)** and **(B)** are opposites, since NH_4Cl is an acidifying salt and sodium bicarbonate an alkalinizing one. From the point of view of test strategy, opposites always deserve careful attention and, in this case, encourage us to exclude **(E)**, a distracter. Since an acid environment favors ionization of a weak base, we should give NH_4Cl. The answer is **(A)**.

3. **(A)**, **(B)**, **(D)**, and **(E)** are correct. **(C)** is wrong: delivering the drug directly to the target organ usually reduces adverse effects because the required total dose is smaller and the concentration reaching other organs is lower. The answer is **(C)**.

4. Aspirin is an acid, so it will be more ionized at alkaline pH and less ionized at acidic pH. The Henderson-Hasselbalch equation predicts that the ratio will change from 50/50 at the pH equal to the pK_a to 10/1 (protonated/unprotonated) at 1 pH unit more acidic than the pK_a. For acids, the protonated form is the nonionized, more lipid-soluble form. The answer is **(D)**.

5. See **Definitions** on the first page of this chapter. "First-order" means that the elimination rate is proportionate to the concentration perfusing the organ of elimination. One result of this proportionality is that a plot of the logarithm of the plasma concentration on the vertical axis versus time on the horizontal axis is a straight line. The half-life is a constant. The rate of elimination is proportionate to the rate of administration only at steady state. ("Zero-order elimination" means that a constant number of moles or grams are eliminated per unit time regardless of the plasma concentration. The half-life will then be concentration-dependent and is not a useful parameter. Ethanol is the most common drug with zero-order elimination.) The answer is **(B)**.

6. Note the "trigger" words ("must," "always") in choices **(A)**, **(B)**, and **(C)**. All drugs that affect tissues other than the blood or vascular endothelium act outside of the "bloodstream." The answer is **(D)**.

7. This is a straightforward question of distribution concepts. There are no trigger words to give the answer away, but it can be deduced without much trouble. From the list of determinants of drug distribution given previously, choice **(C)** is correct.

8. More Henderson-Hasselbalch concepts. Weak bases are more protonated in an acidic environment because more protons (hydrogen ions) are available. In the protonated state, weak bases are ionized, polar, and less lipid-soluble. Therefore, less pilocarpine is lipid-soluble and thus able to diffuse through the duodenum (pH 5.5) than is able to diffuse through the surface of the eye (pH 7.8). By the same reasoning, the drug diffuses faster if the eyedrops are alkaline than if they are acidic. Less drug diffuses back into the body from the urine if the urine pH is acidic than if it is alkaline, so excretion will be faster in acidic urine. The answer is **(C)**.

9. The excretion of weak bases is accelerated by acidification of the urine. Which of the weak bases listed would be more responsive to acidification? Consider that urine pH can be modified over the range of 5.5–8.0. The weak base with a pK_a of 6.5 would shift from 90% nonionized at pH 7.5 to 90% ionized at pH 5.5. A major increase in excretion might be expected. On the other hand, the weak base of pK_a 3.5 would be 99.99% ionized at pH 7.5 and still 99% ionized at pH 5.5. This would not result in a major change in excretion. The answer is **(D)**.

10. Protonation (combination with a proton, H^+) causes a weak acid to lose its negative electrical charge and become less polar and more lipid-soluble. The answer is **(J)**.

11. More definitions. Pharmacodynamics is the term given to the properties of drug action on the body. The answer is **(H)**.

12. "Pharmacokinetics" is the general term that describes all of the body's actions on the drug. The answer is **(I)**.

13. The amount of active drug is reduced by excretion and metabolism, processes that are included in the term "elimination." The answer is **(B)**.

14. "First-pass effect" is the term given to elimination of a drug before it enters the systemic circulation, ie, on its first pass through the liver. The answer is **(D)**.

15. The excretion of most drugs is determined by first-order kinetics. However, ethanol—and, in higher doses, aspirin and phenytoin—follow zero-order kinetics, ie, their elimination rates are constant regardless of blood concentration. The answer is **(L)**.

2   Pharmacodynamics

OBJECTIVES

You should be able to:

- Compare the efficacy and the potency of two drugs on the basis of their dose-response curves.
- Predict the effect of a partial agonist in a patient in the presence and in the absence of a full agonist.
- Name two proteins in blood that have important inert drug-binding sites.
- Predict the effect of adding drug B when a barely subtoxic dose of drug A is present—if drug A and drug B both bind to the same inert binding sites.
- Specify whether an antagonist is competitive or irreversible based on its effect on the dose-response curve of an agonist.
- Give examples of partial agonists, competitive and irreversible pharmacologic antagonists, and physiologic and chemical antagonists.
- Name the coupling and effector proteins activated by muscarinic (M_1, M_3), alpha, and beta receptors.
- Name five transmembrane signaling methods by which drug-receptor interactions exert their effects.

Learn the definitions that follow.

Table 2–1. Definitions.

Term	Definition
Receptor	A component of the biologic system to which a drug binds to bring about a change in function of the system
Inert binding site	A component of the biologic system to which a drug binds without changing any function
Receptor site	A specific region of the receptor molecule at which the drug binds
Agonist	A drug that activates its receptor upon binding
Effector	A component of the biologic system that accomplishes the biologic effect after being activated by the receptor; often a channel or enzyme
Pharmacologic antagonist	A drug that binds to its receptor without activating it
Competitive antagonist	A pharmacologic antagonist that can be overcome by increasing the dose of agonist
Irreversible antagonist	A pharmacologic antagonist that cannot be overcome by increasing the dose of agonist
Physiologic antagonist	A drug that counters the effects of another by binding to a different receptor and causing opposing effects
Chemical antagonist	A drug that counters the effects of another by binding the drug and blocking its action
Partial agonist	A drug that binds to its receptor but produces a smaller effect at full dosage than a full agonist
Graded dose-response curve	A graph of the increasing responses to increasing doses of a drug
Quantal dose-response curve	A graph of the fraction of a population that shows a specified response to increasing doses of a drug
EC50	In graded dose-response curves, the concentration or dose that produces 50% of the maximum possible response; in quantal dose response curves, the dose that causes the specified response in 50% of the population
K_d	The concentration of drug that results in binding to 50% of the receptors
Efficacy	The maximum effect a drug can bring about, regardless of dose
Potency	The dose or concentration required to bring about 50% of a drug's maximum effect
Spare receptors	Receptors that do not have to bind drug in order for the maximum effect to be produced; ie, K_d greater than the EC50

PHARMACODYNAMIC CONCEPTS

Pharmacodynamics (this chapter) deals with the effects of drugs on biologic systems, while pharmacokinetics (Chapter 3) deals with actions of the biologic system on the drug. The principles of pharmacodynamics apply to all biologic systems, from isolated receptors in the test tube to patients with specific diseases. The most important principles are discussed below.

A. **Receptors:** Receptors are the specific molecular components of a biologic system with which drugs interact to produce changes in the function of the system. Receptors must be selective in their ligand-binding characteristics (so as to respond to the proper chemical signal and not to meaningless ones). Receptors must also be modified as a result of binding an agonist molecule (so as to bring about the functional change). Many receptors have been identified, purified, chemically characterized, and cloned. The majority of the receptors characterized to date are proteins; a few are other macromolecules such as DNA. The **receptor site** or **recognition site** for a drug is the specific binding region of the macromolecule and has a high and selective affinity for the drug molecule. The interaction of a drug with its receptor is the fundamental event that initiates the action of the drug.

B. **Effectors:** Effectors are molecules that translate the drug-receptor interaction into a change in cellular activity. The best examples of effectors are enzymes such as adenylyl cyclase. Some receptors are also effectors in that a single molecule may incorporate both the drug-binding site and the effector mechanism, eg, the tyrosine kinase effector of the insulin receptor and the sodium-potassium channel of the nicotinic acetylcholine receptor.

C. **Graded Dose-Response Relationships:** When the response of a particular receptor-effector system is measured against increasing concentrations of a drug, the graph of the response versus the drug concentration or dose is called a graded dose-response curve (Figure 2–1, panel A). Plotting the same data on semilogarithmic axes usually results in a sigmoid curve, which simplifies the mathematical manipulation of the dose-response data (Figure 2–1, panel B). The efficacy (E_{max}) and potency **(EC50)** parameters are derived from these data. The *smaller* the EC50, the *greater* the potency of the drug.

D. **Graded Dose Drug Binding Relationship and Binding Affinity:** It is possible to measure the fraction of receptors bound by drug and by plotting this fraction against the log of the concentration of drug, a graph similar to the dose-response curve is obtained (Figure 2–1, panel C). The concentration of drug required to bind 50% of the receptor sites is denoted the K_d and is a useful measure of the affinity of a drug molecule for its binding site on the receptor molecule. The smaller the K_d, the greater the affinity of the drug for its receptor. If the number of binding

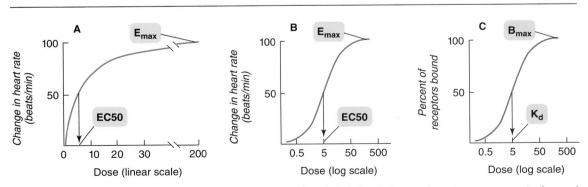

Figure 2–1. Graded dose-response and dose-binding graphs. **A.** Relation between drug dose or concentration and drug effect. When the dose axis is linear, a hyperbolic curve is commonly obtained. **B.** Same data, logarithmic dose axis. The dose or concentration at which effect is half-maximal is denoted EC50, while the maximal effect is E_{max}. **C.** If the percentage of receptors that bind drug is plotted against drug concentration, a similar curve is obtained, and the concentration at which 50% of the receptors are bound is denoted K_d and the maximum number of receptors bound is termed B_{max}.

sites on each receptor molecule is known, it is possible to determine the total number of receptors in the system from $\mathbf{B}_{\mathbf{max}}$ (Figure 2–1).

E. Quantal Dose-Response Relationships: When the minimum dose required to produce a specified response is determined in each member of a population, the quantal dose-response relationship is defined (Figure 2–2). When plotted as the fraction of the population that responds at each dose versus the log of the dose administered, a cumulative quantal dose-response curve, usually sigmoid in shape, is obtained. The **median effective (ED50), median toxic (TD50),** and **median lethal doses (LD50)** are extracted from experiments carried out in this manner.

F. Efficacy: Efficacy, often called maximal efficacy, is the maximal effect (E_{max}) an agonist can produce if the dose is taken to very high levels. Efficacy is determined mainly by the nature of the receptor and its associated effector system. It can be measured with a graded dose-response curve (Figure 2–1) but not with a quantal dose-response curve. By definition, partial agonists have lower maximal efficacy than full agonists (see below).

G. Potency: Potency denotes the amount of a drug needed to produce a given effect. In graded dose-response measurements, the effect usually chosen is 50% of the maximal effect, and the dose causing this effect is called the **EC50** (Figure 2–1, panels A and B). Potency is determined mainly by the affinity of the receptor for the drug. In quantal dose-response measurements, **ED50, TD50,** and **LD50** are typical potency variables (median effective, toxic, and lethal doses, respectively, in 50% of the population studied). Thus, potency can be determined from either graded or quantal dose-response curves (eg, Figures 2–1, 2–2), but the numbers obtained are not identical.

H. Spare Receptors: Spare receptors are said to exist if the maximal drug response is obtained at less than maximal occupation of the receptors. In practice, the determination is usually made by comparing the concentration for 50% of maximal effect (EC50) with the concentration for 50% of maximal binding (K_d). If the EC50 is less than the K_d, spare receptors are said to exist (Figure 2–3). This might result from one of several mechanisms. First, the effect of the drug-receptor interaction may persist for a much longer time than the interaction itself. Second, the actual number of **receptors** may exceed the number of **effector** molecules available. The presence of spare receptors increases sensitivity to the agonist because the likelihood of a drug-receptor interaction increases in proportion to the number of receptors available. (For contrast, the system depicted in Figure 2–1, panels B and C, does not have spare receptors, since the EC50 and the K_d are equal.)

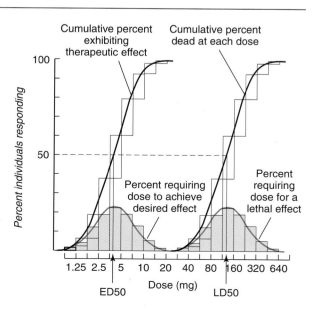

Figure 2–2. Quantal dose-response plots from a study of the therapeutic and lethal effects of a new drug in mice. Shaded boxes (and the accompanying curves) indicate the frequency distribution of doses of drug required to produce a specified effect, ie, the percentage of animals that required a particular dose to exhibit the effect. The open boxes (and corresponding curves) indicate the cumulative frequency distribution of responses, which are lognormally distributed. (Reproduced, with permission, from Katzung BG [editor]: *Basic & Clinical Pharmacology,* 7th ed. Appleton & Lange, 1998.)

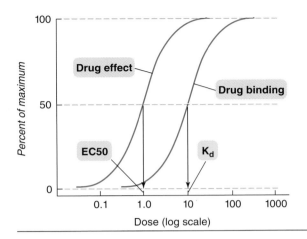

Figure 2–3. In a system with spare receptors, the EC50 is lower than the K_d, indicating that to achieve 50% of maximum effect, fewer than 50% of the receptors must be activated. Explanations for this phenomenon are discussed in the text.

I. **Inert Binding Sites:** Inert binding sites are components of endogenous molecules that bind a drug without initiating events leading to any of the drug's effects. In some compartments of the body (eg, the plasma), inert binding sites play an important role in buffering the concentration of a drug because bound drug does not contribute directly to the concentration gradient that drives diffusion. The two most important plasma proteins with significant binding capacity are **albumin** and **orosomucoid (α_1-acid glycoprotein).**

J. **Agonists and Partial Agonists:** An agonist is a drug capable of fully activating the effector system when it binds to the receptor. A partial agonist produces less than the full effect even when it has saturated the receptors (Figure 2–4). In the presence of a full agonist, a partial agonist acts as an inhibitor.

K. **Competitive and Irreversible Pharmacologic Antagonists:** Competitive antagonists are drugs that bind to the receptor in a reversible way without activating the effector system for that receptor. In the presence of a competitive antagonist, the log dose-response curve for an agonist is shifted to higher doses (ie, horizontally and to the right on the dose axis) but the same maximal effect is reached (Figure 2–5A). In contrast, an irreversible antagonist causes a downward shift of the maximum agonist effect, with no shift of the curve on the dose axis unless spare receptors are present (Figure 2–5B). The effects of competitive antagonists can be overcome by adding more agonist. Irreversible antagonists cannot be overcome by adding more agonist.

L. **Physiologic Antagonists:** A physiologic antagonist is a drug that binds to a different receptor, producing an effect opposite to that produced by the drug it is antagonizing. Thus it differs

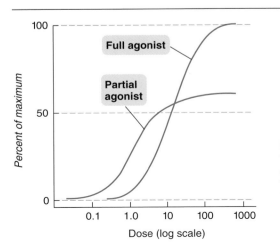

Figure 2–4. Comparison of dose-response curves for a full agonist and a partial agonist. The partial agonist acts on the same receptor system as the full agonist but cannot produce as large an effect (it has lower maximal efficacy), no matter how much the dose is increased. A partial agonist may be more potent (as in the figure), less potent, or equally potent; potency is an independent factor.

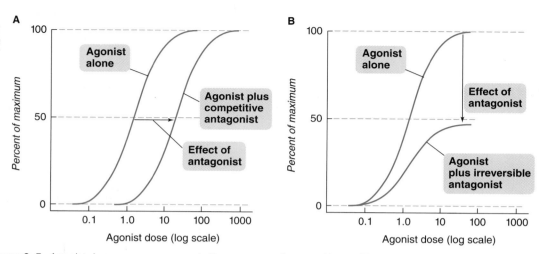

Figure 2–5. Agonist dose-response curves in the presence of competitive and irreversible antagonists. Note the use of a logarithmic scale for drug concentration. **A.** A competitive antagonist has an effect illustrated by the shift of the agonist curve to the right. **B.** A noncompetitive antagonist shifts the agonist curve downward.

from a pharmacologic antagonist, which interacts with the same receptor as the drug it is inhibiting. A common example is the antagonism of the bronchoconstrictor action of histamine (mediated at histamine receptors) by epinephrine's bronchodilator action (mediated at beta adrenoceptors).

M. Chemical Antagonists: A chemical antagonist is a drug that interacts directly with the drug being antagonized to remove it or to prevent it from reaching its target. A chemical antagonist does not depend on interaction with the agonist's receptor (although such interaction may occur). A common example of a chemical antagonist is dimercaprol, a chelator of lead and some other toxic metals. Pralidoxime, which combines avidly with the phosphorus in organophosphate cholinesterase inhibitors, is another type of chemical antagonist.

N. Therapeutic Index, Therapeutic Window: The therapeutic index is the ratio of the TD50 (or LD50) to the ED50, determined from quantal dose-response curves. The therapeutic index represents an estimate of the safety of a drug, since a very safe drug might be expected to have a very large toxic dose and a small effective dose. For example, in Figure 2–2, the ED50 is approximately 3 mg and the LD50 is approximately 150 mg. The therapeutic index is therefore approximately 50 (150/3). Unfortunately, factors such as the varying slopes of dose-response curves make this estimate a poor safety index. The therapeutic window, a more clinically relevant index of safety, is the dosage range between the minimum effective therapeutic concentration or dose and the minimum toxic concentration or dose. For example, if the average minimum therapeutic plasma concentration of theophylline is 8 mg/L and toxic effects are observed at 18 mg/L, the therapeutic window is 8–18 mg/L.

O. Signaling Mechanisms: Once an agonist drug has bound to its receptor, some effector mechanism is activated. For most useful drug-receptor interactions, the drug is present in the extracellular space while the effector mechanism resides inside the cell and modifies some intracellular process. Thus, signaling across the membrane must occur. Five major types of transmembrane signaling mechanisms for receptor-effector systems have been defined (Figure 2–6).
1. Receptors that are intracellular: Some drugs, especially more lipid-soluble or diffusible agents (eg, steroid hormones, nitric oxide) may cross the membrane and combine with an intracellular receptor that affects an intracellular effector molecule. No specialized transmembrane signaling device is required.
2. Receptors located on membrane-spanning enzymes: Drugs that affect membrane-spanning enzymes combine with a receptor on the extracellular portion of enzymes and modify their intracellular activity. For example, insulin acts on a tyrosine kinase that is lo-

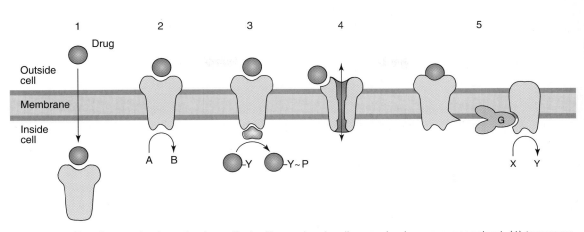

Figure 2–6. Signaling mechanisms for drug effects. Five major signaling mechanisms are recognized: (1) transmembrane diffusion of the drug to bind to an intracellular receptor; (2) transmembrane enzyme receptors, whose outer domain provides the receptor function and inner domain provides the effector mechanism; (3) transmembrane receptors that, after activation by an appropriate ligand, activate separate mobile protein tyrosine kinase molecules (JAK), which phosphorylate STAT molecules that regulate transcription; (4) transmembrane channels that are gated open or closed by the binding of a drug to the receptor site; and (5) G protein-coupled receptors, which utilize a coupling protein to activate a separate effector molecule. (Reproduced, with permission, from Katzung BG [editor]: *Basic & Clinical Pharmacology,* 7th ed. Appleton & Lange, 1998.)

cated in the membrane. The insulin receptor site faces the extracellular environment, and the enzyme catalytic site is on the cytoplasmic side.

3. **Receptors located on membrane-spanning molecules that bind separate intracellular tyrosine kinase molecules:** Like receptor tyrosine kinases, these receptors have extracellular and intracellular domains and form dimers. However, after receptor activation by an appropriate drug, the tyrosine kinase molecules (called "JAK") are activated, resulting in phosphorylation of "STAT" molecules. STAT dimers then travel to the nucleus, where they regulate transcription.

4. **Receptors located on membrane ion channels:** Receptors that regulate membrane ion channels may directly cause the opening of an ion channel (eg, acetylcholine at the nicotinic receptor) or modify the ion channel's response to other agents (eg, benzodiazepines at the GABA channel). The result is a change in transmembrane electrical potential.

5. **Receptors linked to effectors via G proteins:** A very large number of drugs bind to receptors that are linked by coupling proteins to intracellular or membrane effectors. The best defined examples of this group are the sympathomimetic drugs, which activate or inhibit adenylyl cyclase by a multistep process: activation of the receptor by the drug results in activation of G proteins that either stimulate or inhibit the cyclase. More than 20 types of G proteins have been identified; three of the most important ones are listed in Table 2–2.

Table 2–2. Examples of receptors that are coupled to their effectors by G proteins.

Receptor Types	Coupling Protein	Effector	Effector Substrate	Second Messenger Response	Result
M_1, M_3, α_1	G_q	Phospholipase C	Membrane lipids	↑ IP_3 ↑ DAG	↑ Ca^{2+} ↑ Protein kinase
β, D_1	G_s	Adenylyl cyclase	ATP	↑ cAMP	↑ Ca^{2+} influx ↑ Enzyme activity
α_2, M_2	G_i	Adenylyl cyclase	ATP	↓ cAMP	↓ in Ca^{2+} influx and enzyme activity

QUESTIONS

DIRECTIONS: Each of the numbered items or incomplete statements in this section is followed by answers or by completions of the statement. Select the ONE lettered answer or completion that is BEST in each case.

1. A 55-year-old woman with congestive heart failure is to be treated with a diuretic drug. Drugs X and Y have the same mechanism of diuretic action. Drug X in a dose of 5 mg produces the same magnitude of diuresis as 500 mg of drug Y. This suggests that
   (A) Drug Y is less efficacious than drug X
   (B) Drug X is about 100 times more potent than drug Y
   (C) Toxicity of drug X is less than that of drug Y
   (D) Drug X is a safer drug than drug Y
   (E) Drug X will have a shorter duration of action than drug Y because less of drug X is present for a given effect

2. Dose-response curves are used for drug evaluation in the animal laboratory and in the clinic. *Quantal* dose-response curves are often
   (A) Used for determining the therapeutic index of a drug
   (B) Used for determining the maximal efficacy of a drug
   (C) Invalid in the presence of inhibitors of the drug being studied
   (D) Obtainable from the study of intact subjects but not from isolated tissue preparations
   (E) Used to determine the statistical variation (standard deviation) of the maximal response to the drug

3. The results shown in the graph below were obtained in a comparison of positive inotropic agents.
   (A) Drug A is most effective
   (B) Drug B is least potent
   (C) Drug C is most potent
   (D) Drug B is more potent than drug C and more effective than drug A
   (E) Drug A is more potent than drug B and more effective than drug C

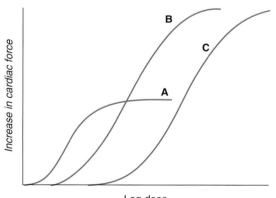

4. In the absence of other drugs, pindolol causes an increase in heart rate by activating beta adrenoceptors. In the presence of highly effective beta stimulants, however, pindolol causes a dose-dependent, reversible decrease in heart rate. Therefore, pindolol is probably
   (A) An irreversible antagonist
   (B) A physiologic antagonist
   (C) A chemical antagonist
   (D) A partial agonist
   (E) A spare receptor agonist

5. All of the following statements about spare receptors are correct EXCEPT
   (A) Spare receptors, in the absence of drug, are identical to nonspare receptors
   (B) Spare receptors will be detected if the intracellular effect of drug-receptor interaction lasts longer than the drug-receptor interaction itself
   (C) Spare receptors influence the sensitivity of the receptor system to the drug
   (D) Spare receptors activate the effector machinery of the cell without the need for a drug
   (E) Spare receptors may be detected by the finding that the EC50 is less than the K_d for the agonist

6. Two drugs, A and B, were studied in a large group of patients; the percentages of the population showing therapeutic and toxic effects were graphed as shown below. Based on the graph, it may be concluded that:
   (A) Drug A is safer than drug B
   (B) Drug B is less effective than drug A
   (C) The two drugs act on the same receptors
   (D) The therapeutic index of drug A is 10.
   (E) The therapeutic index of drug B is 10.

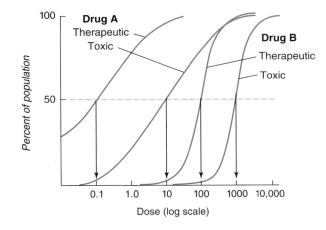

DIRECTIONS (Items 7–15): Each set of matching questions in this section consists of a list of three to twenty-six lettered options (some of which may be figures) followed by several numbered items. For each numbered item, select the ONE lettered option that is most closely associated with it. Each lettered option may be selected once, more than once, or not at all.

Items 7–9:
   (A) Pharmacologic antagonist
   (B) Partial agonist
   (C) Physiologic antagonist
   (D) Chemical antagonist
   (E) Noncompetitive antagonist

7. This term refers to the antagonism of leukotriene's bronchoconstrictor effect (mediated at leukotriene receptors) by terbutaline (acting at adrenoceptors) in a patient with asthma
8. An antagonist that interacts directly with the agonist and not at all, or only incidentally, with the receptor
9. A drug that blocks the action of epinephrine at its receptors by occupying those receptors without activating them

Items 10–12:
   (A) Maximal efficacy
   (B) Therapeutic index

(C) Drug potency
(D) Graded dose-response curve
(E) Quantal dose-response curve

10. Provides information about the variation in sensitivity to the drug within the population studied
11. Provides information about the potency and the maximum efficacy of a drug
12. The largest response a drug can produce, regardless of dose

Items 13–15: Each of the curves in the graph below may be considered a concentration-effect curve or a concentration-binding curve.

(A) Curve 1
(B) Curve 2
(C) Curve 3
(D) Curve 4
(E) Curve 5

13. Reflects the percentage *binding* of a full agonist to its receptors as the concentration of a partial agonist is increased from low to very high levels
14. Describes the percentage *effect* when a full agonist is present throughout the experiment, and the concentration of a partial agonist is increased from low to very high levels
15. Describes the percentage *binding* of the partial agonist whose *effect* is shown by curve 4, if the system has many spare receptors

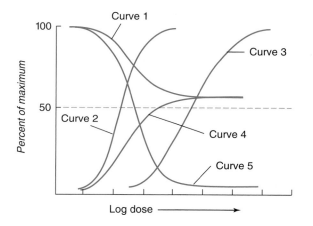

ANSWERS

1. No information is given regarding the magnitude of the maximum diuretic response to either drug. Similarly, no information about toxicity is available. The fact that a given response is achieved with a smaller dose of drug X only indicates that X is more potent than Y in the ratio of 500/5. The answer is **(B).**

2. Graded dose-response curves must be used to determine maximum efficacy (maximum response). Quantal dose-response curves show only the frequency of occurrence of a specified response, which may be therapeutic (ED) or toxic (TD). Dividing the TD50 by the ED50 gives the therapeutic index. The answer is **(A).**

3. These are straightforward graded dose-response curves. Drug A is the most potent, drug C the least. Drug A is less efficacious than drugs B and C. The answer is **(D).**

4. **(B)** and **(C)** are clearly incorrect, since pindolol is said to act at beta receptors and to block beta stimulants. The drug effect is reversible, so **(A)** is incorrect. "Spare receptor agonist" is a nonsense distracter. The answer is **(D).**

5. There is no difference between "spare" and other receptors. Spare receptors may be defined as those receptors that are not needed for binding drug to achieve the maximum effect. Spare receptors influence the sensitivity of the system to an agonist, since the statistical probability of a drug-receptor interaction increases with the total number of receptors. If they do not bind an agonist molecule, spare receptors do not activate an effector molecule. EC50 less than K_d is one indication of the presence of spare receptors. The answer is (D).

6. Note that the therapeutic index of drug A is approximately 100 while that of drug B is approximately 10. Because drug A has a flatter slope, however, patients who require a higher dose of A have a high risk of toxicity; because drug B has a steeper slope, even patients who require the highest dose of B have a low probability of toxicity. These dose-response curves illustrate the danger in assuming that a drug with a larger therapeutic index must be safer than a drug with a smaller one. The answer is (E).

7. Because terbutaline interacts with adrenoceptors and leukotriene with leukotriene receptors, terbutaline cannot be a pharmacologic antagonist of leukotriene. Because the results of adrenoceptor activation oppose the effects of leukotriene receptor activation, terbutaline must be a physiologic antagonist. The answer is (C).

8. A chemical antagonist interacts directly (chemically) with the agonist drug and not with a receptor. The answer is (D).

9. A pharmacologic antagonist occupies the receptors without activating them. The answer is (A).

10. Quantal dose-response curves provide information about the statistical distribution of sensitivity to a drug. The answer is (E).

11. Only a graded dose-response curve provides information about the maximal efficacy as well as the potency. See question 2. The answer is (D).

12. Maximal efficacy represents the largest response a drug can produce. The answer is (A).

13. The binding of a full agonist will *decrease* as the concentration of a partial agonist is increased to very high levels. As the partial agonist displaces more and more of the full agonist, the percentage of receptors that bind the full agonist will drop to zero, ie, curve 5. The answer is (E).

14. Curve 1 describes the *effect* of combining a large fixed concentration of full agonist and increasing concentrations of partial agonist, since the increasing percentage of receptors binding the partial agonist will finally produce the maximum effect typical of the partial agonist. The answer is (A).

15. Partial agonists, like full agonists, bind 100% of their receptors when present in high enough concentration. Therefore, the curve will go to 100%. If the effect curve is curve 4 and many spare receptors are present, the binding curve must be displaced to the right of curve 4 ($K_d >$ EC50). Therefore, curve 3 fits the description better than curve 2. The answer is (C).

Pharmacokinetics

3

OBJECTIVES

You should be able to:

- Compute the half-life of a drug based on its clearance and volume of distribution.
- Calculate loading and maintenance dosage regimens for oral or intravenous administration of a drug when given the following information: minimum effective concentration, bioavailability, clearance, and volume of distribution.
- Calculate the dosage adjustment required for a patient with impaired renal function.

Learn the definitions that follow.

Table 3–1. Definitions.

Term	Definition
Volume of distribution (apparent)	The ratio of the amount of a drug in the body to its concentration in the plasma or blood
Clearance	The ratio of the rate of elimination of a drug to its concentration in plasma or blood
Half-life	The time it takes for the amount or concentration of a drug to fall to 50% of an earlier measurement; this number is a constant, regardless of concentration, for drugs eliminated by first-order kinetics (the great majority of drugs). See Chapter 1. Half-life is not a constant and therefore not particularly useful for drugs eliminated by zero-order kinetics (eg, ethanol)
Bioavailability	The fraction (or percentage) of the administered dose of a drug that reaches the systemic circulation
Area under the curve (AUC)	The graphic area under a plot of drug concentration in plasma versus time, after a single dose of a drug or during a single dosing interval; the AUC is important for calculating the bioavailability of a drug given by any route other than intravenous
Peak and trough concentrations	The maximum and minimum drug concentrations—in plasma or blood—measured during cycles of repeated dosing
Minimum Effective Concentration (MEC)	The plasma concentration below which a patient's response is too small for therapeutic benefit
First-pass effect	The elimination of drug that occurs after administration but before it reaches the systemic circulation, eg, during passage through the gut wall, portal blood, and liver for an orally administered drug
Extraction	The fraction of a drug in the plasma that is removed by an organ as it passes through that organ
Bioequivalence	The equivalence of blood concentrations of two preparations of the same drug measured over time. If the concentration-time plots for the two preparations are nearly superimposable (within certain statistical limits), the preparations are said to be bioequivalent—one preparation may be safely substituted for the other
Biodisposition	Often used as a synonym for pharmacokinetics: the processes of drug absorption, distribution, and elimination

CONCEPTS

A. **Effective Drug Concentration:** The effective drug concentration is the concentration of a drug at the receptor site (in contrast to drug concentrations that are more readily measured, eg, in blood). Except for topically applied agents, this concentration is often proportionate to the drug's concentration in the plasma. The plasma concentration is a function of the rate of input of the drug (by absorption) into the plasma, the rate of distribution to the peripheral tissues (including the target organ), and the rate of elimination, or loss, from the body. These are all functions of time, but if the rate of input is known the remaining processes are well described by two primary parameters: volume of distribution and clearance. These parameters are unique for a particular drug in a particular patient but have average values in large populations that can be used to predict drug concentrations.

B. **Volume of Distribution (V_d):** The volume of distribution relates the amount of drug in the body to the plasma concentration (Figure 3–1) according to the following equation:

$$V_d = \frac{\text{Amount of drug in the body}}{\text{Plasma drug concentration}} \qquad (1)$$

(Units = volume)

The calculated value for the apparent volume of distribution has no direct physical equivalent. If a drug is avidly bound in peripheral tissues, its concentration in plasma may drop to very low

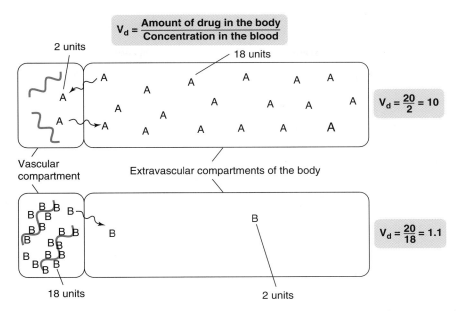

$$V_d = \frac{\text{Amount of drug in the body}}{\text{Concentration in the blood}}$$

2 units

18 units

$$V_d = \frac{20}{2} = 10$$

Vascular compartment

Extravascular compartments of the body

$$V_d = \frac{20}{18} = 1.1$$

18 units

2 units

Figure 3–1. Effect of drug binding on volume of distribution. Drug A does not bind to macromolecules (heavy wavy lines) in the vascular or the extravascular compartments of the hypothetical organism in the diagram. Drug A diffuses freely between the two compartments. With 20 units of the drug in the body, the steady state distribution leaves a blood concentration of 2. Drug B, on the other hand, binds avidly to proteins in the blood. Drug B's diffusion is much more limited. At equilibrium, only 2 units of the total have diffused into the extravascular volume, leaving 18 units still in the blood. In each case, the total amount of drug in the body is the same (20 units), but the apparent volumes of distribution are very different.

values even though the total amount in the body is large. As a result, the volume of distribution may greatly exceed the total volume of the body. For example, 50,000 L is the V_d for the drug quinacrine in a person whose physical body volume is 70 L. On the other hand, a drug that is completely retained in the plasma compartment will have a volume of distribution equal to the plasma volume (about 4% of body weight). The volume of distribution of drugs normally bound to plasma proteins such as albumin can be altered by liver disease (through reduced protein synthesis) and kidney disease (through urinary protein loss).

C. Clearance (CL): Clearance relates the rate of elimination to the plasma concentration:

$$CL = \frac{\textbf{Rate of elimination of drug}}{\textbf{Plasma drug concentration}} \qquad (2)$$

(Units = volume per unit time)

For a drug eliminated with first-order kinetics, clearance is a constant, ie, the ratio of rate of elimination to plasma concentration is the same regardless of plasma concentration (Figure 3–2). The magnitudes of clearance for different drugs range from a small fraction of the blood flow to a maximum of the total blood flow to the organ of elimination. Clearance depends upon the drug and the condition of the organs of elimination in the patient. The clearance of a particular drug by an individual organ is equivalent to the extraction capability of that organ for that drug times the rate of delivery of drug to the organ. Thus, the clearance of a drug that is very effectively extracted by an organ is often flow-limited—ie, the blood is completely cleared of the drug as it passes through the organ. For such a drug, the total clearance from the body is a function of blood flow through the eliminating organ and is limited by the blood flow to the organ. In this situation, other conditions—disease or other drugs that influence blood flow—may have more dramatic effects on clearance than disease of the organ of elimination.

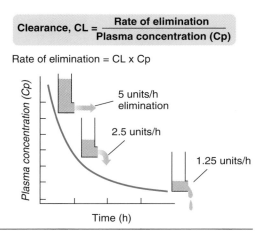

Figure 3–2. The clearance of most drugs is a constant over a broad range of plasma concentrations. Since elimination rate is equal to clearance times plasma concentration, the elimination rate will be rapid at first and slow as the concentration decreases.

D. **Half-life:** Half-life is a derived parameter, completely determined by volume of distribution and clearance. Half-life can be determined graphically from a plot of the blood level versus time (Figure 1–3) or from the following relationship:

$$t_{1/2} = \frac{0.693 \times V_d}{CL} \tag{3}$$

(Units = time)

One must know both primary variables (V_d and CL) to predict changes in half-life. Disease, age, and other variables usually alter the clearance of a drug much more than its volume of distribution. The half-life of a drug may not change, however, despite a decreased clearance, if the volume of distribution decreases at the same time. This occurs, for example, when lidocaine is administered to patients with congestive heart failure. The half-life determines the rate at which blood concentration rises during a constant infusion and falls after administration is stopped (Figure 3–3).

E. **Bioavailability:** The bioavailability of a drug is the fraction (F) of the administered dose that reaches the systemic circulation. Bioavailability is defined as unity (or 100%) in the case of intravenous administration. After administration by other routes, bioavailability is generally reduced by incomplete absorption, first-pass metabolism, and any distribution into other tissues that occurs before the drug enters the systemic circulation. To account for differing rates of absorption into the blood, the concentration appearing in the plasma must be integrated over time to obtain an integrated total **area under the plasma concentration curve** (**AUC,** Figure 3–4).

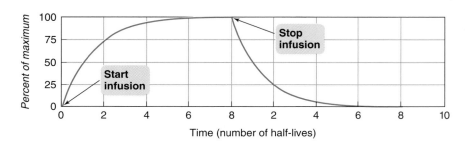

Figure 3–3. Plasma concentration (plotted as percentage of maximum) of a drug given by constant intravenous infusion for eight half-lives and then stopped. The concentration rises smoothly with time and always reaches 50% of steady state after one half-life, 75% after two half-lives, 87.5% after three half-lives, and so on. The decline in concentration after stopping drug administration follows the same type of curve: 50% is left after one half-life, 25% after two half-lives, etc. The asymptotic approach to steady state on both the increasing and the decreasing limbs of the curve is characteristic of drugs eliminated by first-order kinetics.

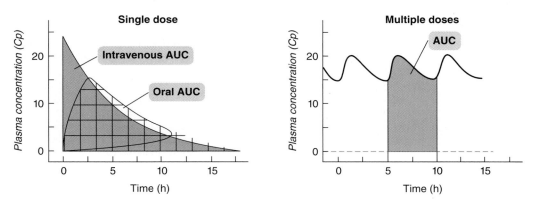

Figure 3–4. The area under the curve is used to calculate the bioavailability of a drug. The AUC can be obtained from either single-dose (left panel) or multiple-dose measurements (right panel). Bioavailability (F) is calculated from $AUC_{(route)}/AUC_{(IV)}$.

F. **Extraction:** Removal of a drug by an organ can be specified as the extraction ratio, or the fraction of the drug removed from the perfusing blood during its passage through the organ (Figure 3–5). After steady state concentration in plasma has been achieved, the extraction ratio is one measure of the elimination of the drug by that organ. Drugs that have a high hepatic extraction ratio have a large first-pass effect; the bioavailability of these drugs after oral administration will be low.

G. **Dosage Regimens:** A dosage regimen is a plan for drug administration over a period of time. An appropriate dosage regimen results in the achievement of therapeutic levels of the drug in the blood without exceeding the minimum toxic concentration. To maintain the plasma concentration within a specified range over long periods of therapy, a schedule of **maintenance doses** is used. If it is necessary to achieve the target plasma level rapidly, a **loading dose** is used to "load" the volume of distribution with the drug. Ideally, the dosing plan is based on knowledge of both the minimum therapeutic and minimum toxic concentrations for a given drug as well as its clearance and volume of distribution.
   1. **Maintenance dose:** Because the maintenance rate of drug administration is equal to the rate of elimination at steady state (this is the definition of steady state), the maintenance dosage is a function of clearance (from equation [2] above).

$$\text{Dosing rate} = \text{Clearance} \times \frac{\textbf{Desired plasma concentration}}{\textbf{Bioavailability}} \qquad (4)$$

Note that volume of distribution is not directly involved in the above calculation. The dosing rate computed for maintenance dosage is the average dose per unit time. When carrying out

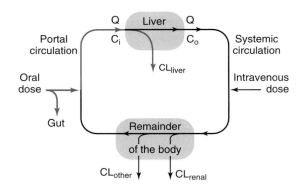

Figure 3–5. The principles of organ extraction and first-pass effect are illustrated. Part of the administered oral dose (color) is lost to metabolism in the gut and the liver before it enters the systemic circulation: this is the first-pass effect. The extraction of drug from the circulation by the liver is equal to blood flow times the difference between entering and leaving drug concentration, ie, $Q \times (C_i - C_o)$. (Reproduced, with permission, from Katzung BG [editor]: *Basic & Clinical Pharmacology*, 7th ed. Appleton & Lange, 1998.)

such calculations, make certain that the units are in agreement throughout. For example, if clearance is given in milliliters per minute, the resulting dosing rate is a "per minute" rate. For chronic therapy, oral administration is desirable; thus, doses should be given only once or a few times per day. The size of the daily dose (dose per minute × 60 minutes per hour × 24 hours per day) is a simple extension of the above information. The number of doses to be given per day is usually determined by the half-life of the drug and the difference between the minimum therapeutic and toxic concentrations (see Therapeutic Window, below).

If it is important to maintain a concentration above the minimum therapeutic level at all times, either a larger dose may be given at long intervals or smaller doses at more frequent intervals. If the difference between the toxic and therapeutic concentrations is small, then smaller, more frequent doses must be administered to avoid toxicity.

2. **Loading dosage:** If the therapeutic concentration must be achieved rapidly and the volume of distribution is large, a large loading dose may be needed at the onset of therapy. This is calculated from the following equation:

$$\text{Loading dose} = \text{Volume of distribution} \times \frac{\textbf{Desired plasma concentration}}{\textbf{Bioavailability}} \tag{5}$$

Note that clearance does not enter into this computation. If the loading dose is very large (V_d much larger than blood volume), the dose should be given slowly to avoid excessively high peak plasma levels during the distribution phase.

H. Therapeutic Window: The therapeutic window is the useful "opening" between the minimum therapeutic concentration and the minimum toxic concentration of a drug. The concept is used to determine the range of plasma levels that is acceptable when designing a dosing regimen. Thus, the minimum effective concentration will usually determine the desired **trough** levels of a drug given intermittently, while the minimum toxic concentration determines the permissible **peak** plasma concentration. For example: The drug theophylline has a therapeutic concentration range of 7–10 mg/L and a toxic concentration range of 15–20 mg/L. The therapeutic window for a given patient might thus be fixed in the range from 8 to 17 mg/L (Figure 3–6). Unfortunately, for some drugs the therapeutic and toxic concentrations vary so greatly among patients that it is impossible to predict the therapeutic window in a given patient. Such drugs must be titrated individually in each patient.

I. Adjustment of Dosage When Elimination Is Altered by Disease: Renal disease or reduced cardiac output often reduces the clearance of drugs that depend on renal function. Alteration of clearance by liver disease or other drugs may occur. The dosage in a patient with renal disease may be corrected by multiplying the dosage estimated for a normal person times the ratio of the patient's altered creatinine clearance to normal creatinine clearance (approximately 100 mL/min or 6 L/h).

$$\text{Corrected dose} = \text{Average dose} \times \frac{\textbf{Patient's creatinine clearance}}{\textbf{100 mL/min}} \tag{6}$$

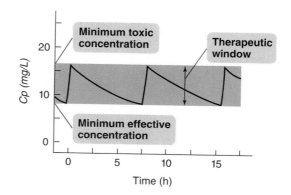

Figure 3–6. The therapeutic window for theophylline in a 13-year-old patient. The minimum effective concentration in this patient was found to be 8 mg/L; the minimum toxic concentration was found to be 16 mg/L. The therapeutic window is indicated by the colored area. In order to maintain the plasma concentration (Cp) within the window, the drug must be given at least once every half-life (7.5 hours in this patient), since the minimum effective concentration is half the minimum toxic concentration and Cp will decay by 50% in one half-life. (*Note:* This concept applies to drugs given in the ordinary, prompt-release form. Slow-release formulations can often be given at longer intervals.)

This simplified approach ignores nonrenal routes of clearance that may be significant. If a drug is cleared partly by the kidney and partly by nonrenal clearance, the above equation should be applied to that part of the dose that is eliminated by the kidney. For example, if a drug is cleared 50% by the kidney and 50% by the liver and the normal dose is 200 mg/d, the corrected dose in a patient with a creatinine clearance of 20 mL/min will be:

$$\text{Dose} = 100 \text{ mg/d} + 100 \text{ mg/d} \times \frac{20 \text{ mL/min}}{100 \text{ mL/min}} \tag{7}$$

$$\text{Dose} = 100 \text{ mg/d} + 20 \text{ mg/d} = 120 \text{ mg/d}$$

QUESTIONS

DIRECTIONS: Each of the numbered items or incomplete statements in this section is followed by answers or by completions of the statement. Select the ONE lettered answer or completion that is BEST in each case.

Items 1–2: Mr Jones is admitted to General Hospital with pneumonia due to gram-negative bacteria. The antibiotic tobramycin is ordered. The CL and V_d of tobramycin in Mr Jones are 80 mL/min and 40 L, respectively.

1. What maintenance dose should be administered intravenously every 6 hours to eventually obtain average steady state plasma concentrations of 4 mg/L?
   (A) 0.32 mg
   (B) 19.2 mg
   (C) 115 mg
   (D) 160 mg
   (E) 230 mg

2. If you wish to give Mr Jones an IV loading dose to achieve the therapeutic plasma concentration of 4 mg/L rapidly, how much should be given?
   (A) 0.1 mg
   (B) 10 mg
   (C) 115.2 mg
   (D) 160 mg
   (E) None of the above

3. Despite your careful adherence to basic pharmacokinetic principles, your patient on digoxin therapy has developed digitalis toxicity. The plasma digoxin level is 4 ng/mL. Renal function is normal, and the plasma $t_{1/2}$ for digoxin in this patient is 1.6 days. How long should you withhold digoxin in order to reach a safer yet probably therapeutic level of 1 ng/mL?
   (A) 1.6 days
   (B) 2.4 days
   (C) 3.2 days
   (D) 4.8 days
   (E) 6.4 days

4. Verapamil and phenytoin are both eliminated from the body by metabolism in the liver. Verapamil has a clearance of 1.5 L/min, approximately equal to liver blood flow, whereas phenytoin has a clearance of 0.1 L/min. When these compounds are administered along with rifampin, a drug that increases hepatic drug-metabolizing enzymes, which of the following is most likely?
   (A) The clearance of both verapamil and phenytoin will be increased
   (B) The clearance of both verapamil and phenytoin will be decreased
   (C) The clearance of verapamil will be unchanged, whereas the clearance of phenytoin will be increased
   (D) The clearance of phenytoin will be unchanged, whereas the clearance of verapamil will be increased

5. A 60-year-old man enters the hospital with myocardial infarction and a severe ventricular arrhythmia. The antiarrhythmic drug chosen has a narrow therapeutic window: the minimum toxic plasma concentration is 1.5 times the minimum therapeutic plasma concentration. The

half-life is 6 hours. It is essential to maintain the plasma concentration above the minimum therapeutic level to prevent a possibly lethal arrhythmia. Of the following, the most appropriate dosing regimen would be

(A) Once a day
(B) Twice a day
(C) Three times a day
(D) Four times a day
(E) Constant IV infusion

6. A 50-year-old woman with metastatic breast cancer has elected to participate in the trial of a new chemotherapeutic agent. It is given by constant IV infusion of 8 mg/h. Plasma concentrations (Cp) are measured with the results shown in the table.

Time After Start of Infusion (hours)	Plasma Concentration (mg/L)	Time After Start of Infusion (hours)	Plasma Concentration (mg/L)
1	0.8	16	3.7
2	1.3	20	3.84
4	2.0	25	3.95
8	3.0	30	4.0
10	3.6	40	4.0

From these data it may be concluded that

(A) Volume of distribution is 30 L
(B) Clearance is 2 L/h
(C) Elimination follows zero-order kinetics
(D) Half-life is 8 hours
(E) Doubling the rate of infusion would result in a plasma concentration of 16 mg/L at 40 hours

7. A city clinic is considering the substitution of generic drugs in order to save money. The clinical pharmacologist is asked to advise on the bioavailability of the generic products. She informs the head of the clinic that the bioavailability of drugs is

(A) Established by FDA regulation at 100% for preparations for intramuscular injection
(B) 100% for oral preparations that are not metabolized in the liver
(C) Calculated from the peak concentration of drug divided by the dose administered
(D) Important because bioavailability determines what fraction of the administered dose reaches the systemic circulation
(E) Equal to 1 (100%) only for drugs administered by any parenteral route

8. A 19-year-old woman is brought to the hospital with severe asthmatic wheezing. You decide to use IV theophylline for treatment. The pharmacokinetics of theophylline include the following average parameters: V_d 35 L; CL 48 mL/min; half-life 8 hours. If an IV infusion of theophylline is started at a rate of 0.48 mg/min, how long will it take to reach 93.75% of the final steady state?

(A) Approximately 48 minutes
(B) Approximately 5.8 hours
(C) Approximately 6 hours
(D) Approximately 8 hours
(E) Approximately 32 hours

Items 9–10: Your 74-year-old patient with myocardial infarction has a severe cardiac arrhythmia. You have decided to give lidocaine to correct the arrhythmia.

9. A continuous IV infusion of lidocaine, 1.92 mg/minute, is started at 8 AM. The average pharmacokinetic parameters of lidocaine are: V_d 77 L; CL 640 mL/min; half-life 1.8 hours. The expected steady state plasma concentration is approximately

    (A)   40 mg/L
    (B)   3.0 mg/L
    (C)   0.025 mg/L
    (D)   7.2 mg/L
    (E)   3.46 mg/L

10. Your patient has been receiving lidocaine for 8 hours and you decide to obtain a plasma concentration measurement. When the results come back, the plasma level is exactly half of what you expected. The most probable explanation is
    (A)   The patient's lidocaine volume of distribution is half the average value
    (B)   The patient's lidocaine clearance is twice the average value
    (C)   The patient's lidocaine half-life is half the average value
    (D)   The patient's infusion rate was accidentally decreased by half
    (E)   The laboratory made a mistake in the assay for lidocaine

11. A patient requires an infusion of procainamide. Its half-life is 2 hours. The infusion is begun at 9 AM. At 1 PM the same day, a blood sample is taken; the drug concentration is found to be 3 mg/L. What is the probable steady state drug concentration after 48 hours of infusion?
    (A)   3 mg/L
    (B)   4 mg/L
    (C)   6 mg/L
    (D)   9.9 mg/L
    (E)   15 mg/L

12. A narcotics addict is brought to the emergency room in a deep coma. His friends state that he took a large dose of morphine 6 hours earlier. An immediate blood analysis shows a morphine blood level of 0.25 mg/L. Assuming that the pharmacokinetics of morphine in this patient are V_d 200 L and half-life 3 hours, how much morphine did the patient inject 6 hours earlier?
    (A)   25 mg
    (B)   50 mg
    (C)   100 mg
    (D)   200 mg
    (E)   Too few data to predict

13. A normal volunteer will receive a new drug in a phase I clinical trial. The clearance and volume of distribution of the drug in this subject are 1.386 L/h and 80 L, respectively. The half-life of the drug in this subject will be approximately
    (A)   83 hours
    (B)   77 hours
    (C)   58 hours
    (D)   40 hours
    (E)   0.02 hours

14. Gentamicin is often given in intermittent IV bolus doses of 100 mg three times a day to achieve target peak plasma concentrations of about 5 mg/L. Gentamicin's clearance (normally 5.4 L/h/70 kg) is almost entirely by glomerular filtration. Your patient, however, is found to have a creatinine clearance one-third of normal. Your initial dosage regimen for this patient would probably be
    (A)   20 mg three times a day
    (B)   33 mg three times a day
    (C)   72 mg three times a day
    (D)   100 mg twice a day
    (E)   150 mg twice a day

15. Enalapril, an angiotensin-converting enzyme inhibitor, has a half-life of 3 hours but is effective and nontoxic in most patients when given once a day. Assuming IV administration, this indicates that the ratio of the minimum toxic concentration to the minimum effective concentration for enalapril is at least
    (A)   2 (ie, the toxic concentration is twice the therapeutic concentration)
    (B)   8
    (C)   21
    (D)   256
    (E)   The data are insufficient to answer

ANSWERS

1. Maintenance dosage is a function of plasma level and clearance only:

    Rate in = Rate out at steady state

    $$\text{Dosage} = \text{Plasma level}_{ss} \times \frac{\text{Clearance}}{\text{Bioavailability (F)}}$$

    $$= 4\text{ mg/L} \times \frac{0.08\text{ L/min}}{1.0}$$

    $$= 0.32\text{ mg/min}$$

    when given at 6-hour intervals:

    $$= 0.32\text{ mg/min} \times 60\text{ min/h} \times 6\text{ hours}$$

    $$= 115.2\text{ mg/dose every 6 hours}$$

    The answer is **(C)**.

2. Loading dose is a function of volume of distribution and target plasma concentration:

    $$\text{Loading dose} = V_d \times \frac{\text{Target concentration}}{\text{Bioavailability}}$$

    $$\text{Loading dose} = 40\text{ L} \times \frac{4\text{ mg/L}}{1.0} = 160\text{ mg}$$

    The answer is **(D)**.

3. Since the blood level for a drug with first-order kinetics drops by 50% during each half-life, the level will be 2 ng/mL after 1.6 days and 1 ng/mL after 3.2 days. The answer is **(C)**.

4. Verapamil is apparently metabolized so rapidly that only the rate of delivery to the liver regulates its disappearance—ie, it is blood flow-limited: further increases in liver enzymes could not increase its elimination. However, the rate of elimination of phenytoin is apparently limited by its rate of metabolism, since clearance is much less than hepatic blood flow. Therefore, the clearance of phenytoin can rise if some agent causes an increase in liver enzymes. The answer is **(C)**.

5. From the description given, if the minimum therapeutic plasma concentration of the hypothetical drug X is 100 units, the minimum toxic concentration is 150 units. If a dose is given that brings the plasma concentration to 150 units, it will fall to 75 units in one half-life (6 hours). Since 75 units is less than the minimum therapeutic concentration, this dosing interval is too long. Thus, none of the intermittent dosing schedules listed would meet the requirements of the question. For that reason, a constant IV infusion (which can be visualized as intermittent dosing at infinitely short intervals) would be more appropriate than any of the intermittent schedules. The answer is **(E)**.

6. By inspection of the data in the table, it is clear that the steady state plasma concentration is approximately 4 mg/L. Further scrutiny shows that 50% of this concentration was reached after 4 hours of infusion. According to the constant infusion principle (Figure 3–3), one half-life is required to reach one-half of the final concentration; therefore, the half-life of the drug is 4 hours. Rearranging the equation for maintenance dosing (dosing rate = CL × Cp), it can be determined that the clearance = dosing rate/Cp, or 2 L/h. The volume of distribution can be calculated from the half-life equation ($t_{1/2} = 0.693 \times V_d/CL$) and is equal to 11.5 L. This drug follows first-order kinetics, as indicated by the progressive approach to the steady state plasma concentration. The answer is **(B)**.

7. Bioavailability is calculated from the ratio of the area under the curve after oral administration ($\text{AUC}_{(PO)}$) to the AUC after intravenous administration of the same dose ($\text{AUC}_{(IV)}$; Figure 3–4), not from peak concentration measurements. Many drugs given orally are incompletely absorbed or metabolized in the lumen of the gut; they will have a bioavailability less than 1.0 even if they are not metabolized in the liver. The FDA cannot mandate bioavailability by any particular route, only that the bioavailability by that route be reasonably constant among preparations. Some drugs have a bioavailability of less than 1.0 even when given transdermally or

intramuscularly. The answer is **(D)**.

8. The approach of the drug plasma concentration to steady state concentration during continuous infusion follows a stereotypical curve (Figure 3–3) that rises rapidly at first and gradually levels off. It reaches 50% of steady state at one half-life, 75% at two half-lives, 87.5% at three, 93.75% at four, and progressively halves the difference between its current level and 100% with each half-life. The answer is **(E)**: 32 hours or four half-lives.

9. The drug is being administered continuously; the steady state concentration for a continuously administered drug is given by the equation in question 1. Thus

$$\textbf{Dosage} = \textbf{Plasma level}_{ss} \times \textbf{Clearance}$$

$$\textbf{1.92 mg/min} = \textbf{Cp}_{ss} \times \textbf{CL}$$

Rearranging:

$$\textbf{Cp}_{ss} = \frac{\textbf{1.92 mg/min}}{\textbf{CL}}$$

$$\textbf{Cp}_{ss} = \frac{\textbf{1.92 mg/min}}{\textbf{640 mL/min}}$$

$$\textbf{Cp}_{ss} = \textbf{0.003 mg/mL or 3 mg/L}$$

The answer is **(B)**.

10. If the half-life is 1.8 hours, the plasma concentration should approach steady state after 8 hours (more than four half-lives). As indicated by the equation used in question 9, the steady state concentration is a function of dosage and clearance, not volume of distribution. If the plasma level is less than predicted, the clearance in this patient must be greater than average. (In questions of this type, do not assume errors of analysis or administration as answers unless all other possible answers can be positively ruled out.) The answer is **(B)**.

11. According to the curve that relates plasma concentration to infusion time (Figure 3–3), a drug will reach 50% of its final steady state concentration in one half-life, 75% in two half-lives, etc. From 9 AM to 1 PM is 4 hours or two half-lives. Therefore, the measured concentration at 1 PM is 75% of the steady state value ($0.75 \times \text{Cp}_{ss}$). The steady state concentration will be 3 mg/L divided by 0.75, or 4 mg/L. The answer is **(B)**.

12. According to the curve that relates the decline of plasma concentration to time as the drug is eliminated (Figure 3–3), the plasma concentration of morphine was four times higher immediately after administration than at the time of the measurement, which occurred 6 hours or two half-lives later. Therefore, the initial plasma concentration was 1 mg/L. Since the amount in the body is equal to $V_d \times \text{Cp}$ (text equation [1]), the amount injected was 200 L × 1 mg/L, or 200 mg. The answer is **(D)**.

13. Half-life can be estimated from

$$t_{1/2} = V_d \frac{0.693}{CL} \ \text{(text equation [3])}$$

$$= 80 \text{ L} \times \frac{0.693}{1.386 \text{ L/h}}$$

$$= 80 \text{ L} \times \frac{1}{2 \text{ L/h}}$$

$$= \textbf{40 hours}$$

The answer is **(D)**.

14. If the drug is cleared almost entirely by the kidney and creatinine clearance is reduced to one-third of normal, the total daily dose should also be reduced to one-third. The answer is **(B)**.

15. If the drug is given only once a day, 24 h/3 h (or eight half-lives) pass during which it declines in plasma concentration (Figure 3–3). Each half-life results in a decline by half of the preceding level, ie, a power of two (one half-life, to 50%; two half-lives, to 25%; etc). Since the dosing interval is eight times greater than the half-life of the drug, the peak concentration is roughly 2^8, or 256 times higher than the minimum (trough) concentration. If one assumes that the drug is still effective at its trough concentration, the "opening" of the therapeutic window would be at least 256. The answer is **(D)**.

4

Drug Metabolism

OBJECTIVES

You should be able to:

- List the major phase I and phase II metabolic reactions.
- Describe the mechanism of hepatic enzyme induction and list three drugs that are known to cause it.
- List three drugs that inhibit the metabolism of other drugs.
- List three drugs for which there are well-defined genetically determined differences in metabolism.
- Discuss the effects of smoking, liver disease, and kidney disease on drug elimination.
- Describe the pathways by which acetaminophen is metabolized (1) to harmless products if normal doses are taken and (2) to hepatotoxic products if an overdose is taken.

Learn the definitions that follow.

Table 4–1. Definitions.

Term	Definition
Phase I reactions	Reactions that convert the parent drug to more polar (water-soluble) or more reactive products by unmasking or inserting a polar functional group such as –OH, –SH, or –NH$_2$
Phase II reactions	Reactions that increase water solubility by conjugation of the drug molecule with a polar moiety such as glucuronate or sulfate
CYP isozymes	Cytochrome P450 enzyme species, eg, CYP2D6 and CYP3A4, that are responsible for much of drug metabolism. Many species of CYP enzymes have been recognized
Enzyme induction	Stimulation of drug-metabolizing capacity; usually manifested in the liver by increased synthesis of smooth endoplasmic reticulum (which contains a high concentration of phase I enzymes)

CONCEPTS

A. Need for Drug Metabolism: All higher organisms require mechanisms for ridding themselves of active foreign molecules that are absorbed from the environment as well as for excreting undesirable substances produced within the body. Biotransformation of drugs is one such mechanism. It is an important mechanism by which the body terminates the action of some drugs; in some cases, it serves to activate prodrugs. Most drugs are relatively lipid-soluble, which ensures good absorption. The same property would result in very slow removal from the body because the molecule would also be readily reabsorbed from the urine in the renal tubule. The body hastens excretion by transforming the drug to a less lipid-soluble, less readily reabsorbed form.

B. Types of Metabolic Reactions:
   1. **Phase I reactions:** Phase I reactions include oxidation (especially by the cytochrome P450 group of enzymes, also called mixed function oxidases), reduction, deamination, and hydrolysis. Examples are listed in Table 4–2.
   2. **Phase II reactions:** Phase II reactions are synthetic reactions that involve addition (conjugation) of subgroups to –OH, –NH$_2$, and –SH functions on the drug molecule. The subgroups that are added include glucuronate, acetate, glutathione, glycine, sulfate, and methyl groups. Most of these groups are relatively polar and make the product less lipid-soluble than the original drug molecule. Examples of phase II reactions are listed in Table 4–3.

C. Sites of Drug Metabolism: The most important organ for drug metabolism is the liver. The kidneys play an important role in the metabolism of some drugs. A few drugs (eg, esters) are metabolized in many tissues (liver, blood, intestinal wall, etc) because of the broad distribution of their enzymes.

30

Table 4–2. Examples of phase I drug-metabolizing reactions.

Reaction Type	Typical Drug Substrates
Oxidations, P450-dependent	
Hydroxylation	Barbiturates, amphetamines, phenylbutazone
N-Dealkylation	Morphine, caffeine, theophylline
O-Dealkylation	Codeine
N-Oxidation	Acetaminophen, nicotine, methaqualone
S-Oxidation	Thioridazine, cimetidine, chlorpromazine
Deamination	Amphetamine, diazepam
Oxidations, P450-independent	
Amine oxidation	Epinephrine
Dehydrogenation	Ethanol, chloral hydrate
Reductions	Chloramphenicol, clonazepam, dantrolene
Hydrolysis reactions	
Esters	Procaine, succinylcholine, aspirin, clofibrate
Amides	Procainamide, lidocaine, indomethacin

D. Determinants of Biotransformation Rate: The rate of biotransformation of a drug may vary markedly among different individuals. This variation is most often due to genetic or drug-induced differences. For a few drugs, age or disease-related differences in drug metabolism are significant. Gender is important for only a few drugs, eg, ethanol. (Women have lower first-pass metabolism of alcohol than do men.) Since the rate of biotransformation is often the primary determinant of clearance, variations in drug metabolism must be considered carefully when designing a dosage regimen. Smoking, a common cause of enzyme induction in the liver, may increase the metabolism of some drugs (eg, theophylline).

1. **Genetic factors:** Several drug-metabolizing systems have been shown to differ among families or populations in genetically determined ways.

   a. Hydrolysis of esters: Succinylcholine is an ester that is metabolized by plasma cholinesterase ("pseudocholinesterase" or butyrylcholinesterase). In most individuals, this process occurs very rapidly, and a single dose of the drug has a duration of action of about 5 minutes. Approximately one person in 2500 has an abnormal form of this enzyme that more slowly metabolizes succinylcholine and similar esters. In such individuals, the neuromuscular paralysis produced by a single dose of succinylcholine may last many hours.

   b. Acetylation of amines: Isoniazid and some other amines such as procainamide are inactivated by *N*-acetylation. Individuals deficient in acetylation capacity ("slow acetylators") may have prolonged or toxic responses to normal doses of these drugs. Slow acetylators constitute about 50% of white and African-American persons in the USA

Table 4–3. Examples of phase II drug-metabolizing reactions.[1]

Reaction Type	Typical Drug Substrates
Glucuronidation	Acetaminophen, morphine, diazepam, sulfathiazole, digoxin, digitoxin
Acetylation	Sulfonamides, isoniazid, clonazepam, mescaline, dapsone
Glutathione conjugation	Ethacrynic acid, reactive phase I metabolite of acetaminophen
Glycine conjugation	Salicylic acid, nicotinic acid (niacin), deoxycholic acid
Sulfate conjugation	Acetaminophen, methyldopa, estrone
Methylation	Epinephrine, norepinephrine, dopamine, histamine

[1]Adapted, with permission, from Katzung BG (editor): *Basic & Clinical Pharmacology,* 7th ed. Appleton & Lange, 1998.

Table 4–4. A partial list of CYP drug-metabolizing isozymes and the drugs that induce them in humans.

CYP Family Induced	Important Inducers	Important Drug Substrates
1A2	Benzo[a]pyrene (from tobacco smoke), rifampin, omeprazole	Acetaminophen, barbiturates, caffeine, clozapine, theophylline, tricyclic antidepressants (some), warfarin
2C9	Barbiturates (especially phenobarbital), rifampin	Barbiturates, chloramphenicol, doxorubicin, ibuprofen, phenytoin, chlorpromazine, steroids, tolbutamide, warfarin
2E1	Ethanol, isoniazid	Acetaminophen, ethanol (minor), halothane
3A4	Barbiturates, carbamazepine, corticosteroids, macrolides, phenytoin, rifampin	Antihistamines (nonsedating), carbamazepine, benzodiazepines (some), diltiazem, ketoconazole, quinidine, steroid hormones, tricyclics (some)

and a much smaller percentage of Asian and Inuit (Eskimo) populations. The slow acetylation trait is inherited as an autosomal recessive gene.

   c. **Oxidation:**   The rate of oxidation by certain P450 isozymes of debrisoquin, sparteine, phenformin, dextromethorphan, metoprolol, and some tricyclic antidepressants has been shown to be genetically determined.

2.   **Other drugs:**   Coadministration of certain agents may stimulate or inhibit the metabolism of many drugs. Mechanisms include the following:

   a. **Enzyme induction:**   As indicated above, induction usually results from increased synthesis of cytochrome P450-dependent drug-oxidizing enzymes in the liver. Many isozymes of the P450 family exist, and inducers selectively increase subgroups of isozymes. Common inducers of a few of these isozymes and some drugs whose metabolism is increased are indicated in Table 4–4. Several days are usually required to reach maximum induction; a similar amount of time is required to regress after withdrawal of the inducer.

   b. **Metabolism inhibitors:**   Common inhibitors and the drugs whose metabolism is diminished are listed in Table 4–5. **Suicide inhibitors** are drugs that are metabolized to products which irreversibly inhibit the metabolizing enzyme. Such agents include ethinyl estradiol, norethindrone, spironolactone, secobarbital, allobarbital, fluroxene, and propylthiouracil. Metabolism may also be decreased by pharmacodynamic factors such as a reduction in blood flow to the metabolizing organ (eg, propranolol reduces hepatic blood flow).

E.   **Toxic Metabolism:**   Drug metabolism is not synonymous with drug inactivation. Some drugs are converted to active products by metabolism. If these products are toxic, severe injury may result under some circumstances. An important example is acetaminophen—when it is taken in large overdose (Figure 4–1). Acetaminophen is conjugated to harmless glucuronide and sulfate

Table 4–5. A partial list of drugs that inhibit drug metabolism in humans.

Inhibitor	Drugs Whose Metabolism Is Inhibited
Allopurinol, isoniazid, chloramphenicol	Probenecid, tolbutamide, oral anticoagulants
Cimetidine	Benzodiazepines, warfarin, others
Dicumarol	Phenytoin
Disulfiram	Ethanol, phenytoin, warfarin
Erythromycin	Astemizole, terfenadine
Ethanol	Methanol, ethylene glycol
Ketoconazole, itraconazole	Cyclosporine, terfenadine, astemizole
Phenylbutazone	Phenytoin, tolbutamide
Secobarbital	Secobarbital

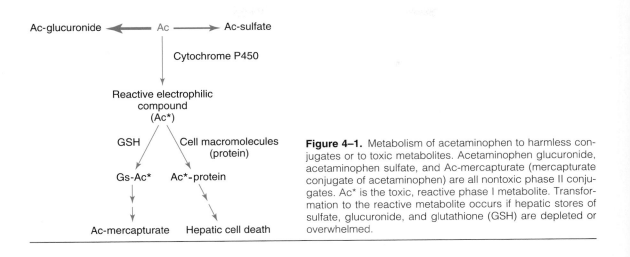

Figure 4–1. Metabolism of acetaminophen to harmless conjugates or to toxic metabolites. Acetaminophen glucuronide, acetaminophen sulfate, and Ac-mercapturate (mercapturate conjugate of acetaminophen) are all nontoxic phase II conjugates. Ac* is the toxic, reactive phase I metabolite. Transformation to the reactive metabolite occurs if hepatic stores of sulfate, glucuronide, and glutathione (GSH) are depleted or overwhelmed.

metabolites when it is taken in normal doses. If a large overdose is taken, however, the metabolic pathways are overwhelmed, and a P450-dependent system converts some of the drug to a reactive intermediate. The intermediate is conjugated with glutathione to a third harmless product if glutathione stores are adequate. If glutathione stores are exhausted, however, the reactive intermediate combines with essential hepatic cell proteins, resulting in cell death. Prompt administration of other sulfhydryl donors (eg, acetylcysteine) may be lifesaving after an overdose. In severe liver disease, stores of glucuronide, sulfate, and glutathione may be depleted, making the patient more susceptible to hepatic toxicity with near-normal doses of acetaminophen.

QUESTIONS

DIRECTIONS (Items 1–5): Each of the numbered items or incomplete statements in this section is followed by answers or by completions of the statement. Select the ONE lettered answer or completion that is BEST in each case.

Items 1–5: You have diagnosed asthma in a 19-year-old patient with recurrent attacks of bronchospasm with wheezing. Avoidance of allergens has been tried unsuccessfully. She is to receive therapy with several drugs.

1. You are concerned about drug interactions caused by changes in drug metabolism in your patient. Drug metabolism usually results in a product that is
   (A) More likely to distribute intracellularly
   (B) Less lipid-soluble than the original drug
   (C) More likely to be reabsorbed by kidney tubules
   (D) Less water-soluble than the original drug
   (E) More likely to produce adverse effects

2. If therapy with multiple drugs causes induction of drug metabolism in your asthma patient, it will
   (A) Result in increased smooth endoplasmic reticulum
   (B) Result in increased rough endoplasmic reticulum
   (C) Result in decreased enzymes in the soluble cytoplasmic fraction
   (D) Require 3–4 months to reach completion
   (E) Be irreversible

3. A factor that is likely to increase the duration of action of a drug that is partially metabolized in the liver is
   (A) Chronic administration of phenobarbital prior to and during therapy with the drug in question
   (B) Chronic therapy with cimetidine prior to and during therapy with the drug in question
   (C) Displacement from tissue binding sites by another drug

(D) Increased cardiac output
(E) Chronic administration of rifampin
4. Which of the following is NOT a phase I drug-metabolizing reaction?
(A) Acetylation
(B) Deamination
(C) Hydrolysis
(D) Oxidation
(E) Reduction
5. Reports of cardiac arrhythmias caused by unusually high blood levels of two antihistamines, terfenadine and astemizole, are best explained by
(A) Concomitant treatment with phenobarbital
(B) Use of these drugs by smokers
(C) Use of antihistamines by persons of Asian origin
(D) A genetic predisposition to metabolize succinylcholine slowly
(E) Concomitant treatment with ketoconazole, an antifungal agent

DIRECTIONS (Items 6–10): Each set of matching questions in this section consists of a list of four to twenty-six lettered options (some of which may be figures) followed by several numbered items. For each numbered item, select the ONE lettered option that is MOST closely associated with it. Each lettered option may be selected once, more than once, or not at all.
(A) Succinylcholine
(B) Quinidine
(C) Procainamide
(D) Rifampin
(E) Cimetidine
(F) Ethanol
(G) Ketoconazole
6. This drug is more slowly metabolized in Caucasians and African-Americans than in most Asians
7. This is a commonly used drug that may inhibit the hepatic microsomal P450 responsible for warfarin metabolism
8. An abnormal form of the enzyme that hydrolyzes this agent is found in the plasma of about one out of every 2500 humans
9. Pretreatment with this agent for 5–7 days might increase the toxicity of acetaminophen
10. This drug has higher first-pass metabolism in men than in women

ANSWERS

1. Biotransformation usually results in a product that is less lipid-soluble. The answer is **(B)**.
2. The smooth endoplasmic reticulum, which contains the mixed function oxidase drug-metabolizing enzymes, is selectively increased by "inducers." The answer is **(A)**.
3. Phenobarbital induces drug-metabolizing enzymes and thereby *reduces* their duration of action. Displacement of drug from tissue may transiently increase the intensity of the effect but will decrease the volume of distribution and thereby reduce the half-life. Cimetidine is recognized as an inhibitor of P450 and may also decrease hepatic blood flow under some circumstances. The answer is **(B)**.
4. Acetylation is a phase II reaction. The answer is **(A)**.
5. Treatment with phenobarbital and smoking are associated with increased drug metabolism and lower, not higher, blood levels. Persons of Asian genetic background have a high probability of metabolizing certain amides (isoniazid, procainamide) *more rapidly;* Asians do not appear to metabolize antihistamines differently from other ethnic groups. Ketoconazole, itraconazole, erythromycin, and a substance in grapefruit juice slow the metabolism of these "nonsedating" antihistamines. The answer is **(E)**.
6. Procainamide, like hydralazine and isoniazid, is metabolized by *N*-acetylation, an enzymatic process that is slower than average in about 20% of Asians and in about 50% of Caucasians and African-Americans. The answer is **(C)**.
7. Cimetidine is a very commonly used drug and has well-documented ability to inhibit the hepatic metabolism of many drugs. The answer is **(E)**.

8. Succinylcholine is normally hydrolyzed quite rapidly by plasma cholinesterase (pseudo-cholinesterase). This enzyme is abnormal in about 1/2500 of the human population, resulting in unusually long duration of action of succinylcholine in affected individuals. The answer is **(A)**.

9. Acetaminophen is normally eliminated by phase II conjugation reactions. The drug's toxicity is dependent on an oxidized reactive metabolite produced by phase I oxidizing P450 enzymes. Drugs that cause induction of P450 enzymes, such as rifampin, may increase the production of this toxic metabolite. The answer is **(D)**.

10. Ethanol is subject to metabolism in the stomach as well as in the liver. Men have greater gastric ethanol metabolism than women—independently of weight and other factors. The answer is **(F)**.

Drug Evaluation

5

OBJECTIVES

Learn the definitions that follow.

Table 5–1. Drug evaluation definitions.

Term	Definition
Single-blind study	A clinical trial in which the investigators, but not the subjects, know which subjects are receiving active drug and which are receiving placebo
Double-blind study	A clinical trial in which neither the subjects nor the investigators know which subjects are receiving placebo; the code is held by a third party
IND	Investigational New Drug Exemption; application for FDA approval to carry out new drug trials in humans; requires animal data
NDA	New Drug Application; application for FDA approval to market a new drug for ordinary clinical use
Placebo	A "dummy" medication made up to resemble the active investigational formulation as much as possible
Phases I, II, and III of clinical trials	Three parts of a clinical trial that must be carried out before submitting an NDA to the FDA
Positive control	A known standard therapy, to be used along with placebo, to fully evaluate the safety and efficacy of a new drug in relation to the others available
Mutagenic	Having an effect on the inheritable characteristics of a cell or organism—a mutation in the DNA; tested in microorganisms with the Ames test
Teratogenic	Having an effect on the prenatal development of an organism resulting in abnormal structure or function; not generally heritable
Carcinogenic	Having an effect of inducing malignant characteristics
Orphan drugs	Drugs developed for diseases in which the expected number of patients in the USA is less than 200,000; bestows certain advantages on companies that develop drugs for unusual diseases

CONCEPTS

A. **Safety & Efficacy:** Because society expects prescription drugs to be safe and effective, governments have regulated the development and marketing of new drugs. The **Food & Drug Administration (FDA)** is the regulatory body in the USA that proposes and administers these regulations. The FDA requires evidence of relative safety (derived from acute and subacute toxicity testing in animals) and probable therapeutic action (from the pharmacologic profile in animals) before human testing is permitted. Some information about the pharmacokinetics of a compound is also required before clinical evaluation is begun. Chronic toxicity test results are generally not required before human studies are started. The development of a new drug and its pathway through various levels of testing and regulation are illustrated in Figure 5–1. The cost of development of a new drug, including false starts and discarded molecules, is currently between $100 million and $500 million.

B. **Animal Testing:** The amount of animal testing required before human studies begin varies according to the proposed use and the urgency of the application. Thus, a drug proposed for occasional nonsystemic use requires less extensive testing than one destined for chronic systemic administration. Anticancer drugs and drugs proposed for use in AIDS, because of the urgency of the need for new agents, require less evidence of safety than do drugs used in less threatening diseases, and they are often investigated and approved on an accelerated schedule.

1. **Acute toxicity:** Acute toxicity studies are required for all drugs. These studies involve single administrations of the agent up to the lethal level in at least two species, eg, one rodent and one nonrodent.

2. **Subacute and chronic toxicity:** Subacute and chronic toxicity testing are required for most agents, especially those intended for chronic use. Tests are usually carried out for at least the amount of time proposed for human application, ie, 2–4 weeks (subacute) or 6–24 months (chronic), in at least two species.

C. **Types of Animal Tests:** Tests done with animals often include general screening tests for pharmacologic effects, hepatic and renal function monitoring, blood and urine tests, gross and histopathologic examination of tissues, and tests of reproductive effects and carcinogenicity.

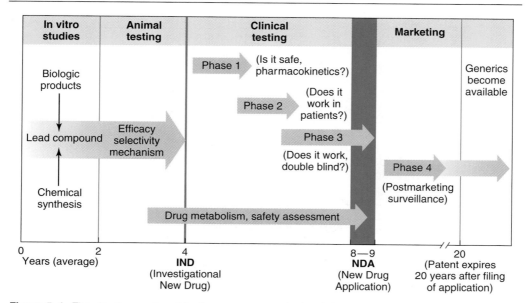

Figure 5–1. The development and testing process required to bring a new drug to market in the USA. Some requirements may be different for drugs used in life-threatening diseases. (Reproduced, with permission, from Katzung BG [editor]: *Basic and Clinical Pharmacology,* 7th ed. Appleton & Lange, 1998.)

1. **Pharmacologic profile:** The pharmacologic profile is a description of all the pharmacologic effects of a drug (eg, effects on blood pressure, gastrointestinal activity, respiration, renal function, endocrine function, the central nervous system).
2. **Reproductive toxicity:** Reproductive toxicity testing involves the study of the fertility effects of the candidate drug and its teratogenic and mutagenic effects. **Teratogenesis** can be defined as the induction of developmental defects in the fetus (by exposure of the fetus to a drug, radiation, etc). Teratogenesis is studied (1) by treating pregnant female animals of at least two species at selected times during early pregnancy when organogenesis is known to take place, and (2) later examining the fetuses or neonates for abnormalities. Examples of drugs known to have teratogenic effects include thalidomide, ethanol, glucocorticoids, valproic acid, isotretinoin, warfarin, lithium, and androgens. **Mutagenesis** is induction of changes in the genetic material of animals of any age and therefore induction of heritable abnormalities. The **Ames test,** the standard in vitro test for mutagenicity, uses a special strain of *Salmonella* bacteria that naturally depend on specific nutrients in the culture medium. Loss of this dependence during exposure to the test drug signals a mutation. The **dominant lethal test** is an in vivo mutagenicity test carried out in mice. Male animals are exposed to the test substance before mating. Abnormalities in the results of subsequent mating (loss of embryos, deformed fetuses, etc) signal a mutation in the male's germ cells. Many carcinogens (eg, aflatoxin, cancer chemotherapeutic drugs, and other agents that bind to DNA) have mutagenic effects.
3. **Carcinogenesis:** Carcinogenesis is the induction of malignant characteristics in cells. Because carcinogenicity is difficult and expensive to study, the Ames test is often used to screen chemicals, since there is a moderately high degree of correlation between mutagenicity in the Ames test and carcinogenicity in some animal tests. Agents with known carcinogenic effects include coal tar, aflatoxin, dimethylnitrosamine and other nitrosamines, urethan, vinyl chloride, and the polycyclic aromatic hydrocarbons in tobacco smoke, eg, benzo[*a*]pyrene.

D. **Clinical Trials:** Human testing in the USA requires the prior approval of an **Investigational New Drug (IND) Exemption** application, which has been submitted by the manufacturer to the FDA (see Figure 5–1). The major clinical testing process is informally divided into three phases before a **New Drug Application (NDA)** can be submitted. The NDA constitutes the request for approval of general marketing of the new agent for prescription use. A fourth phase of study follows NDA approval.
1. **Phase I:** A phase I trial consists of careful evaluation of the dose-response relationship in a small number of normal human volunteers (eg, 20–30). An exception is in phase I trials of cancer chemotherapeutic agents; these are carried out by administering the agents to patients with cancer. In phase I studies, the acute effects of the agent are studied over a broad range of dosages, starting with one that produces no detectable effect and progressing to one that produces a very minor toxic effect.
2. **Phase II:** A phase II trial involves evaluation of a drug in a moderate number of patients (eg, 100–300) with the target disease. A placebo or positive control drug is included in a single-blind or double-blind design. The goal is to determine whether the agent has the desired therapeutic effects at doses that are tolerated by sick patients.
3. **Phase III:** A phase III trial consists of a large design involving many patients (eg, 1000–5000 or more in many centers) and many clinicians who are using the drug in the manner proposed for its ultimate general use, eg, in outpatients. Such studies usually include placebo and positive controls in a double-blind crossover design. The goal is to explore further the spectrum of beneficial actions of the new drug, to compare it with older therapies, and to discover toxicities, if any, that occur so infrequently as to be undetectable in phase II studies.
4. **Phase IV:** Phase IV represents the postmarketing surveillance phase of evaluation after approval of the NDA, in which it is hoped that toxicities that occur very infrequently will be detected and reported early enough to prevent major therapeutic disasters. Unlike the first three phases, phase IV is not rigidly regulated by the FDA.

E. **Drug Legislation:** In the USA, many laws regulating drugs have been passed during this century. Refer to Table 5–2 for a partial list of this legislation.

Table 5–2. Selected legislation pertaining to drugs in the USA.*

Law	Purpose and Effect
Pure Food & Drug Act of 1906	Prohibited mislabeling and adulteration of drugs
Harrison Narcotics Act of 1914	Established regulations for the use of opium, opioids, and cocaine (marijuana added in 1937)
Food, Drug, & Cosmetic Act of 1938	Required that new drugs be safe as well as pure
Kefauver-Harris Amendment (1962)	Required proof of efficacy as well as safety for new drugs
Comprehensive Drug Abuse Prevention & Control Act (1970)	Outlined strict controls on the manufacture, distribution, and prescribing of habit-forming drugs; established programs for the treatment and prevention of addiction
Drug Price Competition & Patent Restoration Act of 1984	Abbreviated NDAs for generic drugs; required bioequivalence data; patent life extended by the amount of time drug was delayed by the review process; cannot exceed 5 years or extend to more than 14 years post-NDA

*Modified and reproduced, by permission, from Katzung BG (editor): *Basic & Clinical Pharmacology,* 7th ed, Appleton & Lange, 1998.

F. **Orphan Drugs:** An orphan drug is a drug for a rare disease (one affecting fewer than 200,000 people in the USA). The study of such agents has often been neglected because the sales of an effective agent for an uncommon ailment might not equal the costs of development. In the USA, current legislation provides regulatory and financial incentives encouraging the development of orphan drugs.

QUESTIONS

DIRECTIONS: Each of the numbered items or incomplete statements in this section is followed by answers or by completions of the statement. Select the ONE lettered answer or completion that is BEST in each case.

1. With regard to clinical trials of new drugs, all of the following are correct EXCEPT
   (A) Phase I involves the study of a small number of normal volunteers by highly trained clinical pharmacologists
   (B) Phase II involves the use of the new drug in a small number of patients (100–200) who have the disease to be treated
   (C) Phase III involves the determination of the drug's therapeutic index by the cautious induction of toxicity, conducted by highly trained clinical pharmacologists in a hospital setting
   (D) Phase IV involves the reporting by practitioners of unusual events, especially toxic reactions, after the drug is approved for general prescription use
   (E) Phase II does not require the use of a positive control (a known effective drug) or placebo, but these are often used in this phase

2. Animal testing of potential new therapeutic agents
   (A) Extends over a time period of at least 3 years in order to discover late toxicities
   (B) Requires the use of at least two primate species, eg, monkey and baboon
   (C) Requires the submission of histopathologic slides and specimens to the FDA for government evaluation
   (D) Has good predictability for drug allergy type reactions
   (E) May be abbreviated in the case of some very toxic agents used in cancer treatment

3. The "dominant lethal" test involves the treatment of a male adult animal with a chemical before mating; the pregnant female is later examined for fetal death and abnormalities. The dominant lethal test therefore is a test of
   (A) Teratogenicity
   (B) Mutagenicity
   (C) Carcinogenicity

   (D)   All of the above
   (E)   None of the above
4. An optimal phase III clinical trial of a new analgesic drug would include all of the following EXCEPT
   (A)   A negative control (placebo)
   (B)   A positive control (current standard therapy)
   (C)   Double-blind protocol (neither the patients nor immediate observers of the patients know which agent is active)
   (D)   A group of 1000–3000 subjects with a clinical condition requiring analgesia
   (E)   Prior approval of an NDA (New Drug Application) by the FDA
5. In the testing of new compounds (eg, antihypertensive drugs) for potential therapeutic use
   (A)   Animal tests cannot be used to predict the types of toxicities that may occur because there is no correlation with human toxicity
   (B)   Human studies in normal individuals will be done before the drug is used in diseased individuals
   (C)   Degree of risk must be assessed in at least three species of animals, including one primate species
   (D)   The animal therapeutic index must be known before trial of the agents in humans
6. The Ames test is a method for detecting
   (A)   Carcinogenesis in rodents
   (B)   Carcinogenesis in primates
   (C)   Teratogenesis in any mammalian species
   (D)   Teratogenesis in primates
   (E)   Mutagenesis in bacteria

ANSWERS

1. The induction of toxicity is not required in any phase of clinical testing, though some toxicity is usually seen. The answer is **(C)**.
2. Drugs proposed for short-term use may not require long-term chronic testing. For some drugs, no primates are used. The data from the tests, not the evidence itself, must be submitted to the FDA. Prediction of human drug allergy from animal testing is not very reliable. The answer is **(E)**.
3. The description of the test indicates that a chromosomal change (passed from father to fetus) is the toxicity detected. This is a mutation. The answer is **(B)**.
4. The first four items **(A–D)** are correct. An NDA cannot be acted upon until the first three phases of clinical trials have been completed. The answer is **(E)**.
5. Animal tests in a single species do not always predict human toxicities; but when these tests are carried out in several species, most acute toxicities that occur in humans will also appear in at least one animal species. According to current FDA rules, the "degree of risk" must be determined in at least two species. Use of primates is not always required. The therapeutic index is not required. Except for cancer chemotherapeutic and antiviral agents, phase I clinical trials are always carried out in normal subjects. The answer is **(B)**.
6. The Ames test is carried out in *Salmonella* and detects mutations in the bacterial DNA. Because mutagenic potential is associated with carcinogenic risk for many chemicals, the Ames test is often used to support a claim that a particular agent may be a carcinogen. However, the test itself detects only mutations. The answer is **(E)**.

6 Introduction to Autonomic Pharmacology

OBJECTIVES

You should be able to:

- Describe the steps in the synthesis, storage, release, and termination of action of the major autonomic transmitters.
- Name two cotransmitter substances.
- Describe the organ system effects of stimulation of the parasympathetic and sympathetic systems.
- Name examples of inhibitors of acetylcholine and norepinephrine synthesis, storage, and release. Predict the effects of these inhibitors on the function of the major organ systems.
- List the determinants of blood pressure and describe the baroreceptor reflex response to blood loss and to administration of (1) a vasodilator, (2) a vasoconstrictor, (3) a cardiac stimulant, and (4) a cardiac depressant.
- Name the major types of receptors found on autonomic effector tissues.
- Describe the differences between the effects of surgical sympathetic ganglionectomy (interruption of ganglionic transmission by surgical removal of the sympathetic ganglia) and those of pharmacologic ganglion block.
- Describe the actions of several toxins that affect nerve function: tetrodotoxin, saxitoxin, botulinum toxin, and latrotoxin.

Learn the definitions that follow.

Table 6–1. Autonomic definitions.

Term	Definition
Adrenergic	A term describing a nerve ending that releases norepinephrine as the primary transmitter; also, a synapse in which norepinephrine is the primary transmitter
Adrenoceptor	A receptor that binds, and is activated by, one of the catecholamine transmitters (norepinephrine, epinephrine, or dopamine) and related drugs
Autonomic effector cells or tissues	Cells or tissues that have adrenoceptors or cholinoceptors which, when activated, alter the function of those cells or tissues, eg, smooth muscle, heart, glands
Baroreceptor reflex	The neuronal homeostatic mechanism that the body uses in attempting to maintain constant blood pressure; the sensory limb originates in the baroreceptors of the carotid sinus
Cholinergic	Term for a nerve ending that releases acetylcholine as the primary transmitter; also, a synapse in which acetylcholine is the primary transmitter
Cholinoceptor	A receptor that binds, and is activated by, acetylcholine and related drugs
Dopaminergic	Term for a nerve ending that releases dopamine as the primary transmitter; also, a synapse in which dopamine is the primary transmitter
Homeostatic reflex	A neuronal compensatory mechanism for maintaining a body function at a predetermined level, eg, the baroreceptor reflex for blood pressure
Parasympathetic	Term for the part of the autonomic nervous system that originates in the cranial nerves and the sacral part of the spinal cord
Postsynaptic receptor	Receptor located on the distal side of the synapse, eg, on the effector cell; contrast with presynaptic receptors
Presynaptic receptor	Receptor located on the nerve ending in a synapse; modulates the release of transmitter
Sympathetic	Term for the part of the autonomic nervous system that originates in the thoracic and lumbar parts of the spinal cord

CONCEPTS

The autonomic nervous system (ANS) is the major involuntary, unconscious, automatic portion of the nervous system and differs in several ways from the somatic (voluntary) nervous system. The anatomy, neurotransmitter chemistry, receptor characteristics, and functional integration of the ANS are discussed below.

A. Anatomic Aspects of the ANS: The motor (efferent) portion of the ANS is the major pathway for information transmission from the central nervous system (CNS) to the involuntary effector tissues (smooth muscle, vascular endothelium, cardiac muscle, and exocrine glands; Figure 6–1). It has two major divisions: the sympathetic and the parasympathetic. The **enteric nervous system (ENS)** is a semiautonomous part of the ANS, with specific functions for the control of the gastrointestinal tract. The ENS consists of the myenteric plexus (plexus of Auerbach) and the submucosal plexus (plexus of Meissner) and includes inputs from the parasympathetic and sympathetic nervous systems.

There are many sensory (afferent) fibers in autonomic nerves. These are of considerable importance for the physiologic control of the involuntary organs but are directly influenced by only a few drugs.

1. Spinal roots of origin: The parasympathetic preganglionic motor fibers originate in cranial nerve nuclei III, VII, IX, and X and in sacral segments (usually S2–S4) of the spinal cord. The sympathetic preganglionic fibers originate in the thoracic (T1–T12) and lumbar (L1–L5) segments of the cord.

2. Location of ganglia: Most of the sympathetic ganglia are located in two paravertebral chains that lie along the spinal column. A few (the prevertebral ganglia) are located on the anterior aspect of the vertebral column. Most of the parasympathetic ganglia are located in the organs innervated.

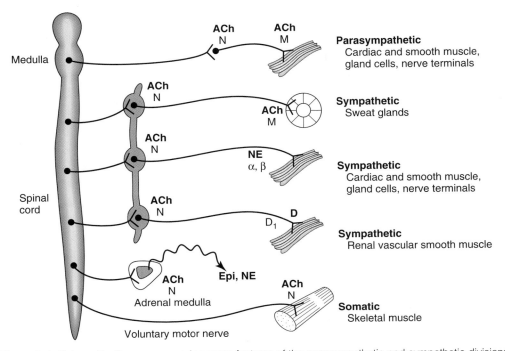

Figure 6–1. Schematic diagram comparing some features of the parasympathetic and sympathetic divisions of the autonomic nervous system with the somatic motor system. Parasympathetic ganglia are not shown as discrete structures because most of them are diffusely distributed in the walls of the organs innervated. ACh, acetylcholine; NE, norepinephrine; D, dopamine; N, nicotinic; M, muscarinic; α, β, alpha and beta adrenoceptors; D_1, dopamine$_1$ receptors. (Reproduced, with permission, from Katzung BG [editor]: *Basic & Clinical Pharmacology,* 7th ed. Appleton & Lange, 1998.)

3. **Length of pre- and postganglionic fibers:** Because of the locations of the ganglia noted above, the preganglionic sympathetic fibers are short and the postganglionic fibers are long. The opposite is true for the parasympathetic system: preganglionic fibers are long and postganglionic fibers are short.

4. **Uninnervated receptors:** Some receptors that respond to autonomic transmitters receive no innervation. These include muscarinic receptors on the endothelium of blood vessels, some presynaptic receptors, and in some species the adrenoceptors on apocrine sweat glands and α_2 and β adrenoceptors in some blood vessels.

B. **Neurotransmitter Aspects of the ANS:** The synthesis, storage, release, and termination of action of the neurotransmitters are very important in the action of autonomic drugs (Figure 6–2).

1. **Cholinergic transmission:** Acetylcholine (ACh) is the primary transmitter in all autonomic ganglia and at the parasympathetic postganglionic neuron-effector cell synapses.

   a. **Synthesis and storage:** ACh is synthesized from acetyl-CoA and choline by the enzyme choline acetyltransferase. The rate-limiting step is probably the transport of choline into the nerve terminal. This transport can be inhibited by **hemicholinium.** ACh is actively transported into vesicles for storage. This process can be inhibited by **vesamicol.**

   b. **Release of acetylcholine:** Release of transmitter stores from vesicles in the nerve ending requires the entry of **calcium** through calcium channels and the triggering of an interaction between several proteins associated with the vesicles and the nerve ending membrane (**synaptobrevin, synaptotagmin, SNAP,** and others). This interaction results in fusion of the vesicular and nerve ending membranes, opening of a pore to the

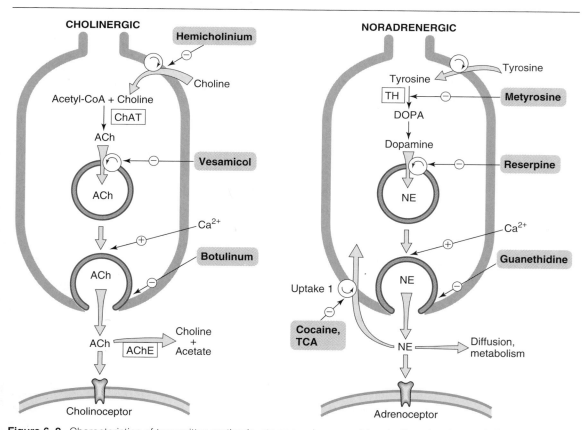

Figure 6–2. Characteristics of transmitter synthesis, storage, release, and termination of action at cholinergic and noradrenergic nerve terminals are shown from the top downward. Solid circles represent transporters; ACh, acetylcholine; AChE, acetylcholinesterase; ChAT, choline acetyltransferase; NE, norepinephrine; TH, tyrosine hydroxylase.

extracellular space, and release of the stored transmitter. **Botulinum toxin** enzymatically alters synaptobrevin to prevent the release process.

 c. **Termination of action of ACh:** The action of acetylcholine in the synapse is normally terminated by metabolism to acetate and choline by the enzyme **acetylcholinesterase.** The products are not excreted but are recycled in the body. Inhibition of acetylcholinesterase is an important therapeutic (and potentially toxic) effect of several drugs.

 d. **Drug effects on synthesis, storage, release, and termination of action of ACh:** Drugs that block the synthesis of ACh (eg, hemicholinium), its storage (eg, vesamicol), or its release (eg, botulinum toxin)* are not very useful in therapy because their effects are not sufficiently selective (ie, PANS and SANS ganglia as well as somatic neuromuscular junctions may all be blocked).

2. **Adrenergic transmission:** Norepinephrine is the primary transmitter at the sympathetic postganglionic neuron-effector cell synapses in most tissues. Important exceptions include sympathetic fibers to thermoregulatory (eccrine) sweat glands and probably vasodilator sympathetic fibers in skeletal muscle, which release ACh. Dopamine is an important vasodilator transmitter in renal blood vessels.

 a. **Synthesis and storage:** The synthesis of dopamine and norepinephrine is more complex than that of ACh (Figure 6–2). Tyrosine is hydroxylated by **tyrosine hydroxylase** (the rate-limiting step) to DOPA (dihydroxyphenylalanine), decarboxylated to dopamine, and (inside the vesicle) hydroxylated to norepinephrine. Tyrosine hydroxylase can be inhibited by **metyrosine.** Norepinephrine and dopamine are transported into vesicles and stored there. The vesicular transporter can be inhibited by **reserpine.**

 b. **Release and termination of action:** Dopamine and norepinephrine are released from their nerve endings by the same mechanism responsible for ACh release (see above). Termination of action, however, is quite different. Metabolism is not responsible for the termination of action of the catecholamine transmitters, norepinephrine and dopamine. Instead, **diffusion** and **reuptake** (especially uptake-1; Figure 6–2) reduce their concentration in the synaptic cleft and stop their action. However, these transmitters are also metabolized—by **monoamine oxidase (MAO)** and **catechol-O-methyltransferase (COMT)**—and the products of these enzymatic reactions are excreted. Determination of the 24-hour excretion of **metanephrine, normetanephrine, 3-methoxy-4-hydroxymandelic acid (VMA),** and other metabolites provides a measure of the total body production of catecholamines, a measure useful in diagnosing conditions such as pheochromocytoma. Blockade of MAO increases stores of neurotransmitter amines and has both therapeutic and toxicologic potential.

 c. **Drug effects on adrenergic transmission:** Drugs that block norepinephrine synthesis (eg, metyrosine) or catecholamine storage (eg, reserpine) or release (eg, guanethidine) are useful in several diseases (eg, hypertension) because they block sympathetic but not parasympathetic functions.

3. **Cotransmitters:** Many—perhaps all—autonomic nerves have transmitter vesicles that contain other transmitter molecules in addition to the primary agents (ACh or norepinephrine) described above. These cotransmitters may be localized in the same vesicles as the primary transmitter or in a separate population of vesicles. Substances recognized to date as cotransmitters include **ATP, enkephalins, vasoactive intestinal peptide (VIP), neuropeptide Y, substance P, neurotensin,** and **somatostatin,** as well as others. Their role in autonomic function appears to involve modulation of synaptic function. The same substances undoubtedly function as primary transmitters in other synapses.

C. **Receptor Characteristics:** The major receptor systems in the ANS include the following:

1. **Cholinoceptors:** Also referred to as cholinergic receptors, these molecules respond to acetylcholine and its analogs. Cholinoceptors are subdivided as follows (see Table 6–2):

 a. **Muscarinic receptors:** As their name suggests, these receptors respond to muscarine as well as acetylcholine. The effects of activation of these receptors resemble those of postganglionic parasympathetic nerve stimulation. Muscarinic receptors are located primarily in autonomic effector cells (including heart, vascular endothelium, smooth mus-

---

*Botulinum toxin can be used by local injection to achieve a medically useful selective action.

Table 6–2. Characteristics of the most important cholinoceptors in the peripheral nervous system.

Receptor	Location	Mechanism	Major Functions
M_1	Nerve endings	G_q-coupled	↑ IP_3, DAG cascade
M_2	Heart, some nerve endings	G_i-coupled	↓ cAMP, activates K^+ channels
M_3	Effector cells: smooth muscle, glands, endothelium	G_q-coupled	↑ IP_3, DAG cascade
N_N	ANS ganglia	Ion channel	Depolarizes, evokes action potential
N_M	Neuromuscular end plate	Ion channel	Depolarizes, evokes action potential

cle, presynaptic nerve terminals, and exocrine glands) and in the central nervous system. Evidence has been found for five subtypes, of which three are well-defined.

    b. Nicotinic receptors: These receptors respond to nicotine, another acetylcholine analog, but not to muscarine. The two major subtypes are located in ganglia, in skeletal muscle end plates, and in the central nervous system. The nicotinic receptors are the primary receptors for transmission at these sites.

2. Adrenoceptors: Also referred to as adrenergic receptors, adrenoceptors are divided into several subtypes (Table 6–3).

    a. Alpha receptors: Alpha receptors are located on vascular smooth muscle, presynaptic nerve terminals, blood platelets, fat cells (lipocytes), and neurons in the central nervous system. Alpha receptors are further divided into two major types: α_1 and α_2.

    b. Beta receptors: Beta receptors are located in most types of smooth muscle, cardiac muscle, some presynaptic nerve terminals, and lipocytes, as well as in the central nervous system. Beta receptors are divided into three major subtypes: β_1, β_2, and β_3.

3. Dopamine receptors: Dopamine receptors are a subclass of adrenoceptors but have rather different distribution and function. Dopamine receptors are especially important in the renal and splanchnic vessels and in the brain. Although at least four subtypes exist, the D_1 subtype appears to be the most important peripheral effector-cell dopamine receptor. D_2 receptors are found on presynaptic nerve terminals. D_1, D_2, and other types of dopamine receptors occur in the CNS.

D. Effects of Activating Autonomic Nerves: Each division of the ANS has specific effects on organ systems. These effects, summarized in Table 6–4, should be memorized.

    Dually innervated organs—such as the iris of the eye and the sinoatrial node of the heart—receive both sympathetic and parasympathetic innervation. The pupil has a natural, intrinsic diameter to which it returns if the influence of both divisions of the ANS is removed. Pharmacologic ganglionic blockade will therefore cause it to move to its intrinsic size. Similarly, the cardiac sinus rate has an intrinsic value in the absence of both ANS inputs. How will these vari-

Table 6–3. Characteristics of some important adrenoceptors in the ANS.

Receptor	Location	G Protein	Second Messenger	Major Functions
α_1	Effector tissues: smooth muscle, glands	G_q	↑ IP_3, DAG	↑ Ca^{2+}, causes contraction, secretion
α_2	Nerve endings, some smooth muscle	G_i	↓ cAMP	↓ Transmitter release, causes contraction
β_1	Cardiac muscle, juxtaglomerular apparatus	G_s	↑ cAMP	↑ Heart rate, ↑ force; ↑ renin release
β_2	Smooth muscle	G_s	↑ cAMP	Relax smooth muscle; ↑ glycogenolysis; ↑ heart rate, force of contraction
β_3	Adipose cells	G_s	↑ cAMP	↑ Lipolysis
D_1	Smooth muscle	G_s	↑ cAMP	Relax renal vascular smooth muscle

Table 6–4. Direct effects of autonomic nerve activity on some organ systems.*

Organ	Effect of			
	Sympathetic		Parasympathetic	
	Action[1]	Receptor[2]	Action	Receptor[2]
Eye				
Iris				
Radial muscle	Contracts	α_1	. . .	. . .
Circular muscle	. . .	. . .	Contracts	M_3
Ciliary muscle	[Relaxes]	β	Contracts	M_3
Heart				
Sinoatrial node	Accelerates	β_1, β_2	Decelerates	M_2
Ectopic pacemakers	Accelerates	β_1, β_2	. . .	. . .
Contractility	Increases	β_1, β_2	Decreases (atria)	M_2
Blood vessels				
Skin, splanchnic vessels	Contracts	α	. . .	. . .
Skeletal muscle vessels	Relaxes	β_2	. . .	. . .
	[Contracts]	α	. . .	. . .
	Relaxes	M^3	. . .	. . .
Endothelium			Releases EDRF	$M_3{}^4$
Bronchiolar smooth muscle	Relaxes	β_2	Contracts	M_3
Gastrointestinal tract				
Smooth muscle				
Walls	Relaxes	$\alpha_2{}^5, \beta_2$	Contracts	M_3
Sphincters	Contracts	α_1	Relaxes	M_3
Secretion	. . .		Increases	M_3
Myenteric plexus			Activates	M_1
Genitourinary smooth muscle				
Bladder wall	Relaxes	β_2	Contracts	M_3
Sphincter	Contracts	α_1	Relaxes	M_3
Uterus, pregnant	Relaxes	β_2	. . .	. . .
	Contracts	α	Contracts	M_3
Penis, seminal vesicles	Ejaculation	α	Erection	M
Skin				
Pilomotor smooth muscle	Contracts	α	. . .	. . .
Sweat glands			. . .	. . .
Thermoregulatory	Increases	M	. . .	. . .
Apocrine (stress)	Increases	α	. . .	. . .
Metabolic functions				
Liver	Gluconeogenesis	β_2, α	. . .	. . .
Liver	Glycogenolysis	β_2, α	. . .	. . .
Fat cells	Lipolysis	β_3	. . .	. . .
Kidney	Renin release	β_1	. . .	. . .
Autonomic nerve endings				
Sympathetic	. . .	. . .	Decreases NE release	M^6
Parasympathetic	Decreases ACh release	α	. . .	. . .

*Reproduced, with permission, from Katzung BG (editor): *Basic & Clinical Pharmacology*, 7th ed. Appleton & Lange, 1998.
[1]Less important actions are shown in brackets.
[2]Specific receptor type: α = alpha, β = beta, M = muscarinic.
[3]Vascular smooth muscle in skeletal muscle has sympathetic cholinergic dilator fibers.
[4]The endothelium of most blood vessels releases EDRF (endothelium-derived relaxing factor), which causes marked vasodilation, in response to muscarinic stimuli. However, unlike the receptors innervated by sympathetic cholinergic fibers in skeletal muscle blood vessels, these muscarinic receptors are not innervated and respond only to circulating muscarinic agonists.
[5]Probably through presynaptic inhibition of parasympathetic activity.
[6]Probably M_1, but M_2 may participate in some locations.

ables change (increase or decrease) if the ganglia are blocked? The answer is predictable if one knows which system is dominant. For example, both the pupil and, in young individuals, the sinoatrial node are dominated by the parasympathetic system. The resting pupillary diameter and the sinus rate are therefore under considerable PANS influence. Therefore, blockade of both systems, with removal of the dominant PANS and nondominant SANS effects, will result in mydriasis and tachycardia.

Table 6–5. Steps in autonomic transmission: Effects of drugs.*

Process	Drug Example	Site	Action
Action potential propagation	Local anesthetics, tetrodotoxin,[1] saxitoxin[2]	Nerve axons	Block sodium channels; block conduction
Transmitter synthesis	Hemicholinium	Cholinergic nerve terminals: membrane	Blocks uptake of choline and slows synthesis
	α-Methyltyrosine (metyrosine)	Adrenergic nerve terminals and adrenal medulla: cytoplasm	Blocks synthesis
Transmitter storage	Vesamicol	Cholinergic terminals: vesicles	Prevent storage, depletes transmitter
	Reserpine	Adrenergic terminals: vesicles	Prevents storage, depletes transmitter
Transmitter release	Many[3]	Nerve terminal membrane receptors	Modulate release
	ω-Conotoxin GVIA[4]	Nerve terminal calcium channels	Reduces transmitter release
	Botulinum toxin	Cholinergic vesicles	Prevents release
	Alpha-latrotoxin[5]	Cholinergic and adrenergic vesicles	Causes explosive release
	Tyramine, amphetamine	Adrenergic nerve terminals	Promote transmitter release
Transmitter uptake after release	Cocaine, tricyclic antidepressants	Adrenergic nerve terminals	Inhibit uptake; increase transmitter effect on postsynaptic receptors
	6-Hydroxydopamine	Adrenergic nerve terminals	Destroys the terminals
Receptor activation or blockade	Norepinephrine	Receptors at adrenergic junctions	Binds α receptors; causes activation
	Phentolamine	Receptors at adrenergic junctions	Binds α receptors; prevents activation
	Isoproterenol	Receptors at adrenergic junctions	Binds β receptors; causes activation
	Propranolol	Receptors at adrenergic junctions	Binds β receptors; prevents activation
	Nicotine	Receptors at nicotinic cholinergic junctions (autonomic ganglia, neuromuscular end plates)	Binds nicotinic receptors; opens ion channel in postsynaptic membrane
	Tubocurarine	Neuromuscular end plates	Prevents activation
	Bethanechol	Receptors, parasympathetic effector cells (smooth muscle, glands)	Binds and activates muscarinic receptors
	Atropine	Receptors, parasympathetic effector cells	Binds muscarinic receptors; prevents activation
Enzymatic inactivation of transmitter	Neostigmine	Cholinergic synapses (acetylcholinesterase)	Inhibits enzyme; prolongs and intensifies transmitter action
	Tranylcypromine	Adrenergic nerve terminals (monoamine oxidase)	Inhibits enzyme; increases stored transmitter pool

*Reproduced, with permission, from Katzung BG (editor): *Basic & Clinical Pharmacology,* 7th ed. Appleton & Lange, 1998.
[1]Toxin of puffer fish, California newt.
[2]Toxin of Gonyaulax (red tide organism).
[3]Norepinephrine, dopamine, acetylcholine, angiotensin II, various prostaglandins, etc.
[4]Toxin of marine snails of the genus *Conus.*
[5]Black widow spider venom.

E. Nonadrenergic, Noncholinergic Transmission: Some nerve fibers in autonomic effector tissues do not show the histochemical characteristics of either cholinergic or adrenergic fibers. Some of these are motor fibers that cause the release of ATP and possibly other purines related to it. Purine-evoked responses have been identified in the bronchi, gastrointestinal tract, and urinary tract. Other motor fibers are peptidergic, ie, they release peptides as the primary transmitters (see list above under Cotransmitters).

Other nonadrenergic, noncholinergic fibers have the anatomic characteristics of sensory fibers and contain peptides that are stored in and released from the fiber terminals. These fibers have been termed "sensory efferent" or "sensory local effector" fibers because when activated by a sensory input they are capable of releasing transmitter peptides from the sensory ending itself, from local axon branches, and from collaterals that terminate in the autonomic ganglia. These peptides are potent agonists in many autonomic effector tissues.

F. Sites of Autonomic Drug Action: Because of the number of steps in the transmission of autonomic commands from the CNS to the effectors, there are many sites at which autonomic drugs may act. These sites include the CNS centers, the ganglia, the postganglionic nerve terminals, the effector cell receptors, and the mechanisms responsible for termination of transmitter action. The most selective block is achieved by drugs acting at receptors that mediate very selective actions (see Table 6–5). In addition, many natural and synthetic toxins have significant effects on autonomic and somatic nerve function. Some of these toxins are listed in Table 6–5.

G. Integration of Autonomic Function: Functional integration is provided mainly through the mechanism of negative feedback. This process utilizes modulatory pre- and postsynaptic receptors at the local level and homeostatic reflexes at the system level.

    1. Local integration: Local feedback control has been found at the level of the nerve endings in all systems investigated. The best-documented of these is the negative feedback of norepinephrine upon its own release from the presynaptic adrenergic terminals. This effect is mediated by α_2 receptors located on the presynaptic nerve membrane (Figure 6–3).

        Presynaptic receptors that bind the primary transmitter substance and thereby regulate its release are called autoreceptors. Transmitter release is also modulated by other receptors (heteroreceptors); in the case of adrenergic nerve terminals, transmitter release is controlled by receptors for acetylcholine (M_1 receptors), histamine, serotonin, prostaglandins, peptides, and other substances. Presynaptic regulation by a variety of endogenous chemicals probably occurs in all nerve fibers.

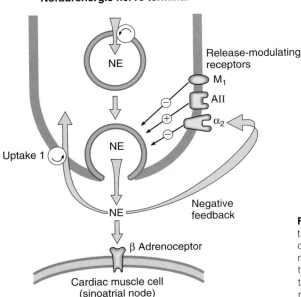

Noradrenergic nerve terminal

Figure 6–3. Local integration of ANS control via modulation of transmitter release. In the example shown, release of norepinephrine from a sympathetic nerve ending is modulated by norepinephrine itself, acting on presynaptic α_2 autoreceptors, and by acetylcholine and angiotensin II. Many other modulators (see text) influence the release process.

Postsynaptic receptors, including two types of muscarinic and at least one type of peptidergic receptor, have been found in ganglionic synapses where nicotinic transmission is primary. These receptors may facilitate or inhibit transmission by evoking slow excitatory or inhibitory postsynaptic potentials (EPSPs or IPSPs).

2. **System reflexes:** System reflexes include mechanisms that regulate blood pressure, especially the baroreceptor neural reflex and the renin-angiotensin-aldosterone hormonal response. (See Figure 6–4.) These homeostatic mechanisms have evolved to maintain mean arterial blood pressure at a level determined by the vasomotor center and renal sensors. Any deviation from this blood pressure "set point" causes a change in ANS activity and renin-angiotensin II-aldosterone levels. These changes are very important in determining the response to conditions or drugs that alter blood pressure. For example, a decrease in blood pressure caused by hemorrhage causes increases in SANS discharge and renin release. Peripheral vascular resistance, venous tone, heart rate, and cardiac force are increased by norepinephrine released from sympathetic nerves. Blood volume is replenished by retention of salt and water in the kidney under the influence of increased levels of aldosterone. These compensatory responses may be large enough to overcome some of the actions of drugs. For example, the treatment of hypertension with a vasodilator such as hydralazine will be unsuccessful if the compensatory tachycardia (via the baroreceptor reflex) and the salt and water retention (via the renin system response) are not prevented through the use of additional drugs. It is therefore essential that the student understand this homeostatic system.

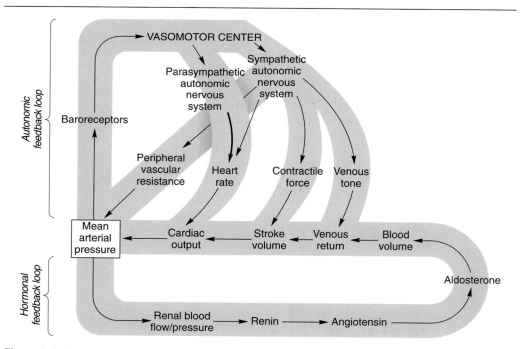

Figure 6–4. Autonomic and hormonal control of cardiovascular function. Note that two feedback loops are present, the autonomic nervous system loop and the hormonal loop. In addition, each major loop has several components. Thus, the sympathetic nervous system directly influences four major variables: peripheral vascular resistance, heart rate, force, and venous tone. The parasympathetic system directly influences heart rate. In addition, angiotensin II directly increases peripheral vascular resistance (not shown), and the sympathetic nervous system directly increases renin secretion (not shown). Because these control mechanisms have evolved to maintain normal blood pressure, the net feedback effect of each loop is negative; feedback tends to compensate for the change in arterial blood pressure that evoked the response. Thus, decreased blood pressure due to blood loss would be compensated by increased sympathetic outflow and renin release. Conversely, elevated pressure due to the administration of a vasoconstricting drug would cause reduced sympathetic outflow and renin release and increased parasympathetic (vagal) outflow.

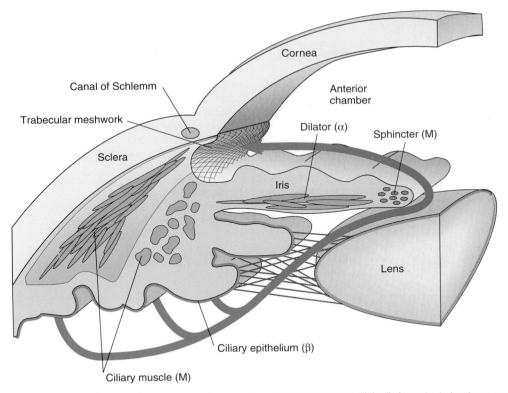

Figure 6–5. Some pharmacologic targets in the eye. The diagram illustrates clinically important structures and their receptors. The heavy arrow (color) illustrates the flow of aqueous humor from its secretion by the ciliary epithelium to its drainage through the canal of Schlemm. M, muscarinic; α, alpha receptor; β, beta receptor.

3. **Complex organ control—the eye:** The eye is composed of multiple tissues with various functions, most of them under autonomic control (Figure 6–5). The pupil, discussed above, is under reciprocal control by the SANS (via alpha receptors) and the PANS (via muscarinic receptors) acting on two different muscles in the iris. The ciliary muscle, which controls accommodation, is under primary control of muscarinic receptors innervated by the PANS, with insignificant contributions from the SANS. The ciliary *epithelium,* on the other hand, has important beta receptors that have a permissive effect on aqueous humor secretion. Each of these receptors is an important target of drugs that are discussed in the following chapters.

DRUG LIST

The following drugs or metabolites mentioned in this chapter are of special significance. It is important to know which ones occur in the normal ANS and what their functions are. For those not normally found in the ANS, it is important to know the effects of their administration.

Acetylcholine	3-Methoxy-4-hydroxymandelic acid (VMA)[1]
Amphetamine	Metyrosine (α-methyltyrosine)
Atropine	Neostigmine
Botulinum toxin[1]	Norepinephrine
Cocaine	Propranolol
DOPA	Reserpine
Dopamine	Saxitoxin[1]
Epinephrine	Tetrodotoxin[1]
Guanethidine	Tyramine
Metanephrine[1]	Vesamicol[1]

[1]Not discussed in succeeding chapters; should be learned with this chapter.

QUESTIONS

DIRECTIONS: Each of the numbered items or incomplete statements in this section is followed by answers or by completions of the statement. Select the ONE lettered answer or completion that is BEST in each case.

1. In the autonomic regulation of blood pressure
   (A) Cardiac output is maintained constant at the expense of other hemodynamic variables
   (B) Elevation of blood pressure results in elevated aldosterone secretion
   (C) Baroreceptor nerves decrease firing rate when arterial pressure increases
   (D) Stroke volume and mean arterial blood pressure are the primary direct determinants of cardiac output
   (E) A condition that reduces the sensitivity of the sensory baroreceptor nerve endings might cause an increase in sympathetic discharge

2. A child has swallowed the contents of two bottles of a nasal decongestant whose primary ingredient is a potent alpha adrenoceptor agonist drug. The signs of alpha activation that may occur in this patient include
   (A) Cardioacceleration (tachycardia)
   (B) Vasodepression (vasodilation)
   (C) Pupillary dilation (mydriasis)
   (D) Bronchodilation
   (E) All of the above

3. Ms Green has severe hypertension and is to receive minoxidil. Minoxidil is a powerful vasodilator that does not act on autonomic receptors. When used in severe hypertension, its effects would probably include
   (A) Tachycardia and increased cardiac contractility
   (B) Tachycardia and decreased cardiac output
   (C) Decreased mean arterial pressure and decreased cardiac contractility
   (D) No change in mean arterial pressure and decreased cardiac contractility
   (E) No change in mean arterial pressure and increased salt and water excretion by the kidney

4. Full activation of the sympathetic nervous system, as in maximal exercise, can produce all of the following responses EXCEPT
   (A) Mydriasis
   (B) Increased renal blood flow
   (C) Decreased intestinal motility
   (D) Bronchial relaxation
   (E) Increased heart rate (tachycardia)

Items 5–7: For the following three questions, use the accompanying diagram. Assume the diagram can represent either the sympathetic or the parasympathetic system.

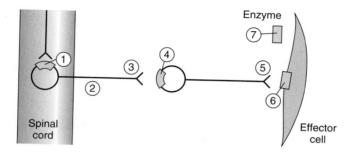

5. Which of the following drugs acts at site 3?
   (A) Botulinum toxin
   (B) Cocaine
   (C) Metyrosine
   (D) Reserpine
   (E) Tyramine

6. Acetylcholine does NOT interact at which one of the following sites in the diagram?
   (A) Site 2
   (B) Site 4
   (C) Site 5
   (D) Site 6
   (E) Site 7
7. Atropine is a useful antimuscarinic drug for dilating the pupil and paralyzing accommodation. These effects of atropine occur at which one of the following sites on the diagram?
   (A) Site 3
   (B) Site 4
   (C) Site 5
   (D) Site 6
   (E) Site 7
8. Mr Brown has recently had a successful cardiac transplant operation in which his badly damaged and failing heart was replaced by a healthy donor organ. Which of the following drugs would be expected to have the SMALLEST effect on his heart function as compared with the function of a normal heart?
   (A) Bethanechol
   (B) Isoproterenol
   (C) Norepinephrine
   (D) Propranolol
   (E) Tyramine
9. "Nicotinic" sites include all of the following EXCEPT
   (A) Parasympathetic ganglia
   (B) Sympathetic ganglia
   (C) Skeletal muscle
   (D) Excitatory receptors on Renshaw cells in the spinal cord
   (E) Bronchial smooth muscle
10. Several children at a summer camp are hospitalized with symptoms thought to be due to ingestion of food containing botulinum toxin. The anticholinergic effects of botulinum toxin
    (A) Are caused by acetylcholine receptor blockade
    (B) Occur in preganglionic nerve endings
    (C) Are permanent
    (D) Are treated with choline infusions
    (E) Are not seen at somatic motor nerve endings at skeletal muscle

DIRECTIONS (Items 11–15): Each set of matching questions in this section consists of a list of three to twenty-six lettered options (some of which may be figures) followed by several numbered items. For each numbered item, select the ONE lettered option that is MOST closely associated with it. Each lettered option may be selected once, more than once, or not at all.

(A) Acetylcholine	(F) Metyrosine	
(B) Amphetamine	(G) Norepinephrine	
(C) Botulinum toxin	(H) Reserpine	
(D) Dopamine	(I) Tetrodotoxin	
(E) Epinephrine	(J) Vesamicol	

11. Agent that is normally released from sympathetic nerve endings innervating thermoregulatory sweat glands
12. Drug that blocks propagation of action potentials in all nerves
13. Drug that inhibits the synthesis of catecholamines such as norepinephrine
14. Indirectly acting drug that releases norepinephrine and dopamine from their nerve endings
15. Drug that prevents the storage of acetylcholine in its vesicles

ANSWERS

1. Baroreceptors *increase* their firing rate with increased blood pressure. Therefore, a decrease in baroreceptor sensitivity would decrease input to the vasomotor center, which would be interpreted by the vasomotor center as a decrease in blood pressure. This would lead to an increase

in sympathetic outflow. The answer is **(E)**. (If you chose a different answer, review the components of the autonomic and hormonal feedback loops for the maintenance of blood pressure; Figure 6–4.)

2. Mydriasis can be caused by contraction of the radial fibers of the iris; these smooth muscle cells have alpha receptors. All the other responses are beta-mediated (Table 6–4). The answer is **(C)**.

3. Because of the baroreceptor reflex, a drug that directly decreases peripheral vascular resistance will cause a reflex increase in sympathetic outflow, a decrease in parasympathetic outflow, and an increase in renin release. As a result, heart rate and cardiac force will increase. (In addition, salt and water retention will occur.) The answer is **(A)**.

4. Sympathetic autonomic outflow causes constriction of the renal resistance vessels and a fall in renal blood flow. This is the typical response in severe exercise or hypotension. The answer is **(B)**.

5. Each of these agents has a different mechanism of action, yet all but one act on the sympathetic postganglionic nerve terminal (site 5). Site 3 is a cholinergic nerve ending. The answer is **(A)**.

6. Acetylcholine acts both at the nicotinic ganglionic receptor (site 4) and at muscarinic receptors on effector cells (site 6) and presynaptic nerve endings (site 5). ACh also interacts with acetylcholinesterase (site 7) but does not influence electrical transmission in axons (site 2). The answer is **(A)**.

7. In the simplified diagram, the muscarinic receptors blocked by atropine are located only at the smooth muscle effector cells and postganglionic nerve terminals. This type of receptor is also found in ganglia, but higher concentrations of atropine are required to block it. Blocking presynaptic muscarinic receptors would not produce mydriasis and cycloplegia. The answer is **(D)**.

8. Cardiac transplantation requires cutting all postsynaptic sympathetic and presynaptic parasympathetic nerves to the heart. As a result, sympathetic postganglionic nerve endings degenerate and stores of norepinephrine diminish markedly. A drug that acts by releasing stored norepinephrine (ie, an indirectly acting sympathomimetic such as tyramine) will have a greatly reduced effect on a transplanted heart. Directly acting drugs will be unaffected or may produce a greater effect due to receptor up-regulation. The answer is **(E)**.

9. Both types of ganglia and the neuromuscular junction have nicotinic cholinoceptors. Bronchial smooth muscle contains muscarinic cholinoceptors. The Renshaw cell was one of the first central neurons shown to respond to acetylcholine and nicotinic cholinomimetics (review the physiology of the spinal cord). The answer is **(E)**.

10. Botulinum toxin impairs all types of cholinergic transmission, including preganglionic nerve endings and somatic motor nerve endings. The toxin does so by preventing discharge of vesicular transmitter content from cholinergic nerve endings. Synthesis of the transmitter is not impaired, so infusion of choline is of no value. The effects of this toxin are very long-lasting (signs and symptoms may persist for several months), but they are not permanent. The answer is **(B)**.

11. Acetylcholine is the transmitter at sympathetic nerve endings innervating thermoregulatory sweat glands. Cholinergic transmission at sympathetic postganglionic nerve endings also occurs to a limited extent in the blood vessels of skeletal muscle. The answer is **(A)**.

12. Tetrodotoxin (and saxitoxin) block propagation of action potentials in all vertebrate nerve axons by blocking voltage-gated sodium channels. The answer is **(I)**.

13. Metyrosine reduces the synthesis of catecholamines such as norepinephrine by inhibiting the rate-limiting enzyme tyrosine hydroxylase (Figure 6–2). The answer is **(F)**.

14. Amphetamine causes the release of norepinephrine and dopamine from their nerve endings. Tyramine, a component of certain fermented foods (eg, cheeses, pickled fish, and some wines) has the same effect. The answer is **(B)**.

15. Vesamicol prevents the storage of acetylcholine in its vesicles by inhibiting the carrier molecule that normally transports acetylcholine into the vesicle (Figure 6–2). The answer is **(J)**.

Cholinoceptor-Activating & Cholinesterase-Inhibiting Drugs

7

OBJECTIVES

You should be able to:

- List the locations and types of acetylcholine receptors in the major organ systems (CNS, autonomic ganglia, eye, heart, vessels, bronchi, gut, genitourinary tract, skeletal muscle, exocrine glands).
- Describe the effects of acetylcholine on the major organs.
- Relate the different pharmacokinetic properties of the various choline esters and cholinomimetic alkaloids to their chemical properties.
- List the major clinical uses of cholinomimetic agonists.
- Describe the pharmacodynamic differences between direct- and indirect-acting cholinomimetic agents.
- List the major signs and symptoms of (1) acute nicotine toxicity and (2) organophosphate insecticide poisoning.

Learn the definitions that follow.

Table 7–1. Definitions.

Term	Definition
Choline ester	A cholinomimetic drug consisting of choline (an alcohol) esterified with an acidic substance, eg, acetic or carbamic acid
Cholinergic crisis	The clinical condition of excessive activation of cholinoceptors
Cholinomimetic alkaloid	A drug with weakly basic properties (usually of plant origin) whose effects resemble those of acetylcholine
Cyclospasm	Marked contraction of the ciliary muscle; maximum accommodation
Direct-acting cholinomimetic drug	One that binds and activates cholinoceptors; the effects mimic those of acetylcholine
Endothelium-derived relaxing factor, EDRF	A potent vasodilator substance, largely nitric oxide, that is released from vascular endothelial cells
Indirect-acting cholinomimetic drug	One that amplifies the effects of endogenous acetylcholine by inhibiting acetylcholinesterase
Muscarinic agonist	A cholinomimetic drug with primarily muscarine-like actions
Myasthenic crisis	In patients with myasthenia, an acute condition caused by inadequate cholinomimetic treatment
Nicotinic agonist	A cholinomimetic drug with primarily nicotine-like actions
Organophosphate	An ester of phosphoric acid and an organic alcohol that inhibits cholinesterase
Organophosphate aging	A process whereby the organophosphate, after binding to cholinesterase, is chemically modified and becomes more firmly bound to the enzyme
Parasympathomimetic drug	One whose effects resemble those of stimulating the parasympathetic nerves

CONCEPTS

Acetylcholine-like drugs (cholinomimetics) are subdivided in two ways: on the basis of their **mode of action** (ie, whether they act directly at the acetylcholine receptor or indirectly through inhibition of cholinesterase) and, for those that act directly, on the basis of their **spectrum of action** (ie, whether they act on muscarinic or nicotinic cholinoceptors; see Figure 7–1). Acetylcholine may be

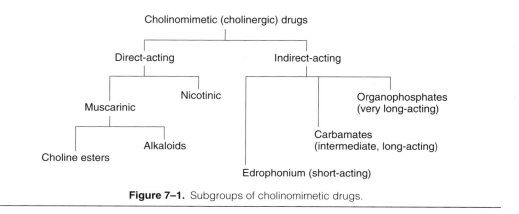

Figure 7–1. Subgroups of cholinomimetic drugs.

considered the prototype that acts directly at both muscarinic and nicotinic receptors. Neostigmine is a prototype for the indirect-acting cholinesterase inhibitors (see Appendix I: Key Words for Key Drugs).

DIRECT-ACTING CHOLINOMIMETIC AGONISTS

A group of choline esters (acetylcholine, methacholine, carbachol, and bethanechol) and a second group of naturally occurring alkaloids (muscarine, pilocarpine, nicotine, and lobeline) comprise this subclass. The members differ in their spectrum of action (amount of muscarinic versus nicotinic stimulation) and in their pharmacokinetic properties (Table 7–2). Both factors influence their clinical use.

A. Classification: Muscarinic agonists are parasympathomimetic, ie, they mimic the actions of parasympathetic nerve stimulation. Five subgroups of muscarinic receptors have been identified

Table 7–2. Cholinomimetics: Spectrum of action and pharmacokinetics.

Drug	Spectrum of Action[1]	Pharmacokinetic Features
Direct-acting		
Acetylcholine	B	Rapidly hydrolyzed by cholinesterase (ChE); duration of action 5–30 seconds
Bethanechol	M	Resistant to ChE, orally active, poor lipid solubility; duration of action 30 minutes to 2 hours
Carbachol	B	Like bethanechol
Pilocarpine	M	Not an ester, good lipid solubility; duration of action 30 minutes to 2 hours
Nicotine	N	Like pilocarpine; duration of action 1–6 hours
Indirect-acting		
Edrophonium	B	Alcohol, quarternary amine, poor lipid solubility, not orally active; 5–15 minutes duration of action
Neostigmine	B	Carbamate, quarternary amine, poor lipid solubility, orally active, duration of action 30 minutes to 2 hours
Physostigmine	B	Carbamate, tertiary amine, lipid soluble; duration of action 30 minutes to 2 hours
Pyridostigmine, ambenonium	B	Carbamates like neostigmine, but longer duration of action (4–8 hours)
Echothiophate	B	Organophosphate, moderate lipid solubility; duration of action 2–7 days
Parathion	B	Oranophosphate, high lipid solubility; duration of action 7–30 days

[1]M, muscarinic; N, nicotinic; B, both.

(Table 7–3), but selective agonists for these receptor subtypes are not available for clinical use. Nicotinic agonists are classified on the basis of whether ganglionic or neuromuscular stimulation predominates, though agonist selectivity is very limited. Relatively selective *antagonists* are available for the two nicotinic receptor types (Chapter 8).

B. Molecular Mechanisms of Action:

1. **Muscarinic mechanism:** Several molecular mechanisms of muscarinic action have been defined (Table 7–3). One involves G protein-coupling of muscarinic receptors (especially M_1 and M_3 receptors) to phospholipase C, a membrane-bound enzyme, leading to the release of the second messengers diacylglycerol (DAG) and inositol-1,4,5-trisphosphate (IP_3). DAG modulates the action of protein kinase C, an enzyme important in secretion, while IP_3 evokes the release of calcium from intracellular storage sites, which results in contraction. A second mechanism couples muscarinic receptors (especially M_2 receptors) to adenylyl cyclase through the inhibitory G_i coupling protein. A third mechanism couples the same receptors directly to potassium channels in the heart and elsewhere; muscarinic agonists facilitate opening of these channels.

2. **Nicotinic mechanism:** The mechanism of nicotinic action has been clearly defined as a direct coupling of the nicotinic receptor to the opening of ion channels selective for sodium and potassium (ACh channels) on ganglion cells (both sympathetic and parasympathetic) and the neuromuscular end plate. The ACh receptor is located on the channel protein. When the receptor is activated, the channel opens and depolarization of the cell (an excitatory postsynaptic potential, EPSP) results. If large enough, the EPSP evokes a propagated action potential in the surrounding membrane.

C. Tissue and Organ Effects: The tissue and organ system effects are summarized in Table 7–4. Note that vasodilation is not parasympathomimetic (ie, it is not evoked by parasympathetic nerve discharge, even though directly acting cholinomimetics cause vasodilation). This action results from the release of endothelium-derived relaxing factor (EDRF: nitric oxide and perhaps other substances) in the vessels, mediated by uninnervated muscarinic receptors on the endothelial cells. Note also that decreased blood pressure evokes the baroreceptor reflex, resulting in strong compensatory sympathetic discharge to the heart. As a result, injections of small to moderate amounts of direct-acting muscarinic cholinomimetics cause *tachycardia, not bradycardia*. Another effect seen with cholinomimetic drugs but not with parasympathetic nerve stimulation is thermoregulatory sweating; this is a *sympathetic cholinergic* effect (see Chapter 6).

The tissue and organ level effects of nicotinic ganglionic stimulation depend on the autonomic innervation of the organ involved. The blood vessels are dominated by sympathetic innervation; therefore, nicotinic receptor activation results in vasoconstriction mediated by sympathetic postganglionic nerve discharge. The gut is dominated by parasympathetic control; nicotinic drugs increase motility and secretion because of increased parasympathetic postganglionic neuron discharge. Nicotinic neuromuscular end plate activation by direct-acting drugs results in fasciculations and spasm of the muscles involved. Prolonged activation, which results in paralysis (see Chapter 27), is an important hazard of exposure to nicotine-containing and organophosphate insecticides.

Table 7–3. Identified or cloned cholinoceptors and their mechanisms.

Receptor Type	Other Names	G Protein	Postreceptor Mechanisms
M_1	M_{1a}	G_q	↑ IP_3, DAG cascade
M_2	M_{2a}, cardiac M_2	G_i	↓ cAMP production
M_3	M_{2b}, glandular M_2	G_q	↑ IP_3, DAG cascade
m_4[1]	...	G_i	↓ cAMP production
m_5[1]	...	G_q	↑ IP_3, DAG cascade
N_M	End plate receptor	None	Na^+/K^+ depolarizing current
N_N	Ganglion receptor	None	Na, K depolarizing current

[1]Cloned but functional receptors have not been identified conclusively.

Table 7–4. Effects of direct-acting cholinoceptor stimulants. Only the direct effects are indicated; compensatory responses to these direct actions may be important.

Organ	Response
Central nervous system	Complex stimulatory effects; eg, nicotine (elevation of mood), physostigmine (convulsions)
Eye	
Sphincter muscle of iris	Contraction (miosis)
Ciliary muscle	Contraction for near vision
Heart	
Sinoatrial node	Decrease in rate (negative chronotropy), but note important reflex response (see text)
Atria	Decrease in contractile strength (negative inotropy); decrease in refractory period
Atrioventricular node	Decrease in conduction velocity (negative dromotropy); increase in refractory period
Ventricles	Small decrease in contractile strength
Blood vessels	Dilation (via EDRF)
Bronchi	Contraction (bronchoconstriction)
Gastrointestinal tract	
Motility	Increase
Sphincters	Relaxation (via enteric nervous system)
Urinary bladder	
Detrusor	Contraction
Trigone and sphincter	Relaxation
Skeletal muscle	Activation of neuromuscular end plates; contraction of muscle
Glands	Increased secretion: thermoregulatory sweat, lacrimal, salivary, bronchial, gastric, intestinal glands

D. Clinical Use: We can predict the major clinical applications of the muscarinic agonists from a consideration of organs and diseases that benefit from an increase in cholinergic activity. They are summarized in Table 7–5. Direct-acting nicotinic agonists have no therapeutic applications except in producing skeletal muscle paralysis (succinylcholine; Chapter 27); indirect-acting agents are superior when increased nicotinic activation is needed (see below).

E. Toxicity: The signs and symptoms of overdosage are readily predicted from the general pharmacology of acetylcholine.

   1. Muscarinic toxicity: These include CNS stimulation (uncommon with direct-acting agonists), miosis, spasm of accommodation, bronchoconstriction, increased gastrointestinal and genitourinary smooth muscle activity, increased secretory activity (sweat glands, air-

Table 7–5. Clinical applications of some cholinomimetics.

Drug	Clinical Applications	Action
Direct-acting agonists		
Bethanechol	Postoperative and neurogenic ileus and urinary retention	Activates bowel and bladder smooth muscle
Carbachol, pilocarpine	Glaucoma	Activates pupillary sphincter and ciliary muscles of eye
Indirect-acting agonists		
Neostigmine	Postoperative and neurogenic ileus and urinary retention	Amplifies endogenous acetylcholine
Neostigmine, pyridostigmine, edrophonium	Myasthenia gravis, reversal of neuromuscular blockade	Amplifies endogenous acetylcholine; ↑ strength
Physostigmine, echothiophate	Glaucoma	Amplifies effects of ACh

way, gastrointestinal tract), vasodilation, and transient bradycardia if administered as an intravenous bolus—reflex tachycardia otherwise.

2. **Nicotinic toxicity:** These include CNS stimulation, ganglionic stimulation, and neuromuscular end plate depolarization leading to fasciculations and paralysis. Nicotine is still used in some insecticides.

INDIRECT-ACTING AGONISTS

A. **Classification and Prototypes:** The indirect-acting cholinomimetic drugs fall into two major chemical classes: carbamic acid esters (**carbamates;** neostigmine is a prototype) and phosphoric acid esters (**phosphates, organophosphates;** echothiophate is a prototype). A third class has only one member: **edrophonium** is an alcohol (not an ester) with a very short duration of action.

B. **Mechanism of Action:** Both carbamate and organophosphate inhibitors bind to cholinesterase and undergo prompt hydrolysis. The alcohol portion of the molecule is then released. The acidic portion (carbamate or phosphate) is released much more slowly, thus preventing the binding and hydrolysis of acetylcholine.

1. **Carbamates:** Carbamates are hydrolyzed, and the carbamate residue is released by cholinesterase over a period of 2–8 hours.
2. **Organophosphates:** Organophosphates are long-acting drugs; they form an extremely stable phosphate complex with the enzyme and are released over periods of days to weeks.

C. **Effects:** By inhibiting cholinesterase, the indirect-acting agonists "amplify" the action of endogenous acetylcholine; ie, these agents cause an increase in the concentration and half-life of acetylcholine in synapses where ACh is released physiologically. Therefore, the indirect agents have muscarinic or nicotinic effects depending on which organ system is under consideration. Cholinesterase inhibitors do not have therapeutic actions at sites where acetylcholine is not normally released.

D. **Clinical Use:** The major clinical applications of the indirect-acting cholinomimetics include both muscarinic and nicotinic effects. These effects are predictable based on a consideration of the organs and the diseases that benefit from an increase in cholinergic activity. The effects are summarized in Table 7–5. The carbamates, which include neostigmine, physostigmine, ambenonium, and pyridostigmine, are used more commonly in therapeutics than are organophosphates. Some carbamates (eg, carbaryl) are used in agriculture as insecticides. Three organophosphates used in medicine are echothiophate (an antiglaucoma drug), malathion (a scabicide), and metrifonate (an anthelmintic agent). A special use of edrophonium is in the diagnosis of myasthenia and in differentiating myasthenic from cholinergic crisis in patients with this disease. Because cholinergic crisis can result in muscle weakness like that of myasthenic crisis, distinguishing the two conditions may be difficult. Administration of a short-acting cholinomimetic such as edrophonium will improve myasthenic crisis but worsen cholinergic crisis.

E. **Toxicity:** In addition to their therapeutic uses, some indirect-acting agents have toxicologic importance because of potential accidental exposures to toxic amounts of pesticides. An example of intoxication is described in Case 1 (Appendix IV). The most toxic of these drugs (eg, parathion) are rapidly fatal if exposure is not immediately recognized and treated. Treatment is described in Chapter 8. After first binding to cholinesterase, most organophosphate inhibitors can be removed from the enzyme by the use of "regenerator" compounds such as pralidoxime (see Chapter 8). If the enzyme-inhibitor binding is allowed to persist, however, aging (a further chemical change) occurs and regenerator drugs can no longer remove the inhibitor. Because of their toxicity, organophosphates are used extensively in agriculture as insecticides and anthelmintic agents; examples include malathion and parathion. Some of these agents (eg, malathion, dichlorvos) are relatively safe in humans because they are metabolized rapidly to inactive products in mammals (and birds) but not in insects. Some are prodrugs (eg, malathion, parathion) and must be metabolized to the active product (malaoxon from malathion, paraoxon from parathion). The signs and symptoms of poisoning are the same as those described for the direct-acting agents with the following exceptions: vasodilation is a late and uncommon effect; bradycardia is more common than tachycardia; CNS stimulation is common with organophosphate and physostigmine overdosage and includes convulsions, followed by respiratory and cardiovascular depression. The spectrum of toxicity can be remembered with the aid of the mnemonic "DUMBELS," which stands for diarrhea, urination, miosis, bronchoconstriction, excitation (of skeletal muscle and CNS), lacrimation, and salivation and sweating.

DRUG LIST

The following drugs are important members of the group discussed in this chapter. Prototypes should be learned in detail; features of the major variants should be known well enough so that the variants can be distinguished from prototypes and from each other.

Subclass	Prototypes	Major Variants
Direct-acting drugs Muscarinic agonists	Acetylcholine	Muscarine, carbachol, bethanechol, pilocarpine
Nicotinic agonists	Acetylcholine	Nicotine, carbachol, succinylcholine
Indirect-acting drugs Alcohol	Edrophonium	
Carbamates	Neostigmine	Pyridostigmine, physostigmine, carbaryl
Organophosphates	Echothiophate	Parathion, DFP, malathion, dichlorvos

QUESTIONS

DIRECTIONS: Each of the numbered items or incomplete statements in this section is followed by answers or by completions of the statement. Select the ONE lettered answer or completion that is BEST in each case.

1. A patient requires mild cholinomimetic stimulation following surgery. Physostigmine and bethanechol in small doses have similar effects on all of the following EXCEPT
   (A) Neuromuscular junction (skeletal muscle)
   (B) Salivary glands
   (C) Ureteral tone
   (D) Sweat glands
   (E) Gastric secretion
2. Parathion has all of the following characteristics EXCEPT
   (A) It is less persistent in the environment than DDT
   (B) It is more toxic to humans than malathion
   (C) It is inactivated by conversion to paraoxon
   (D) It is very lipid-soluble and is well absorbed through skin and lungs
   (E) Its toxicity, if treated early, may be partly reversed by pralidoxime
3. Ms Smith has had myasthenia gravis for several years. She reports to the emergency department complaining of rapid onset of weakness of her hands, diplopia, and difficulty swallowing. She may be suffering from a change in response to her myasthenia therapy, ie, a cholinergic or a myasthenic crisis. The best drug for distinguishing between myasthenic crisis (insufficient therapy) and cholinergic crisis (excessive therapy) is
   (A) Atropine
   (B) Echothiophate
   (C) Edrophonium
   (D) Physostigmine
   (E) Pralidoxime
4. A crop duster pilot has been accidentally exposed to a high concentration of an agricultural organophosphate insecticide. The cause of death from such a poisoning would probably be

(A) Cardiac arrhythmia
(B) Congestive heart failure
(C) Gastrointestinal bleeding
(D) Hypertension
(E) Respiratory failure

5. Mr Brown has just been diagnosed with myasthenia gravis. You are considering different therapies for his disease. Pyridostigmine and neostigmine may cause all of the following EXCEPT
(A) Bronchoconstriction
(B) Constipation
(C) Reversible inhibition of acetylcholinesterase
(D) Some direct nicotinic effects at the neuromuscular end plate
(E) Spasm of accommodation

6. Parasympathetic nerve stimulation and a slow infusion of bethanechol will each increase
(A) Heart rate
(B) Bladder tone
(C) Both (A) and (B) are correct
(D) Neither (A) nor (B) is correct

7. In the human eye, echothiophate can cause all of the following EXCEPT
(A) Miosis
(B) Ciliary spasm
(C) Reversal of the cycloplegic action of atropine
(D) Decrease in the incidence of cataracts
(E) Reduction in intraocular pressure

8. In the comparison of bethanechol and pilocarpine, all of the following are correct EXCEPT
(A) Both are hydrolyzed by cholinesterase
(B) Both may cause tachycardia
(C) Both may increase sweating
(D) Both activate muscarinic receptors
(E) Both may increase gastrointestinal motility

9. A distraught parent calls the poison control center because her three-year-old has just ingested what may be some old insecticide in the garage. Typical symptoms of cholinesterase inhibitor toxicity include all of the following EXCEPT
(A) Nausea, vomiting, diarrhea
(B) Salivation, sweating
(C) Miosis
(D) Paralysis of skeletal muscles
(E) Paralysis of accommodation

10. Actions of cholinoceptor agonists include
(A) Cyclospasm and improved aqueous humor drainage in glaucoma
(B) Decreased gastrointestinal motility with resulting postoperative gastrointestinal stasis and ileus
(C) Improved neuromuscular transmission and accelerated recovery from neuromuscular blockade
(D) Improved neuromuscular transmission and prevention of cholinergic crisis in myasthenia
(E) Both (A) and (C) are correct

DIRECTIONS (Items 11–15): Each set of matching questions in this section consists of a list of three to twenty-six lettered options (some of which may be figures) followed by several numbered items. For each numbered item, select the ONE lettered option that is MOST closely associated with it. Each lettered option may be selected once, more than once, or not at all.
(A) Acetylcholine
(B) Bethanechol
(C) Echothiophate
(D) Malathion

  (E) Muscarine
  (F) Neostigmine
  (G) Nicotine
  (H) Parathion
  (I) Physostigmine
  (J) Pilocarpine

11. Direct-acting cholinomimetic that is lipid-soluble and is favored in the treatment of glaucoma

12. Indirect-acting cholinomimetic with a duration of many days; used in the treatment of glaucoma

13. Indirect-acting carbamate cholinomimetic; poor lipid solubility; duration of action about 2–4 hours

14. Direct-acting cholinomimetic used for its mood-elevating action and as an insecticide

15. Direct-acting cholinomimetic derived from mushrooms; mainly muscarinic spectrum of action

ANSWERS

1. Because physostigmine acts on the enzyme cholinesterase—which is present at all cholinergic synapses—this drug increases acetylcholine effects at the nicotinic junctions as well as muscarinic ones. Bethanechol, on the other hand, is a direct-acting agent that is selective for muscarinic junctions. The answer is **(A)**.

2. The "-thion" organophosphates (those containing the P=S) are activated, not inactivated, by conversion to "-oxon" (P=O) derivatives. They are less stable than halogenated hydrocarbon insecticides of the DDT type; therefore, they are less persistent in the environment. The answer is **(C)**.

3. Since short-acting drugs are usually preferable for diagnostic use, we choose the shortest-acting cholinesterase inhibitor, edrophonium. The answer is **(C)**.

4. Respiratory failure, from neuromuscular paralysis or central nervous system depression, is by far the most important cause of acute deaths in cholinesterase inhibitor toxicity. The answer is **(E)**.

5. Cholinesterase inhibition is typically associated with increased (never decreased) bowel activity. The answer is **(B)**.

6. Choice **(A)** is not correct because the vagus slows the heart. The answer is **(B)**.

7. The long-acting cholinesterase inhibitors are associated with an increased incidence of cataracts in patients who receive them for long periods for glaucoma. All the other effects are typical muscarinic actions. The answer is **(D)**.

8. Neither bethanechol nor pilocarpine is hydrolyzed by acetylcholinesterase. The answer is **(A)**.

9. Questions referring to cholinesterase inhibitor toxicity are very common. Skeletal muscle paralysis results from prolonged depolarization of neuromuscular end plates (depolarizing blockade). Cholinomimetics cause cyclospasm, the opposite of paralysis of accommodation (cycloplegia). The answer is **(E)**.

10. Cholinesterase inhibitors may either improve or impair neuromuscular transmission: cholinergic crisis is caused by too much acetylcholine at the end plate. Cholinomimetics never decrease gastrointestinal motility—they may in fact be used to reverse postoperative ileus. The answer is **(E)**.

11. Pilocarpine is the only direct-acting cholinomimetic in the list that is lipid-soluble and also favored in the treatment of glaucoma. Nicotine is also direct-acting and lipid-soluble, but it is of no value in glaucoma. The answer is **(J)**.

12. Echothiophate is an organophosphate acetylcholinesterase inhibitor with a duration of many days; it is used also in the treatment of glaucoma. The answer is **(C)**.

13. Neostigmine is the prototypical indirect-acting cholinomimetic; it is a quaternary (charged) substance with poor lipid solubility; its duration of action is about 2–4 hours. The answer is **(F)**.

14. Nicotine is a direct-acting cholinomimetic alkaloid with the properties noted. The answer is **(G)**.

15. Muscarine is derived from mushrooms, though the yield from its namesake fungus *Amanita muscaria* is relatively low. Larger amounts are found in other mushrooms, especially those of the *Inocybe* genus. The answer is **(E)**.

Cholinoceptor Blockers & Cholinesterase Regenerators

8

OBJECTIVES

You should be able to:

- Describe the effects of atropine on the major organ systems (CNS, eye, heart, vessels, bronchi, gut, genitourinary tract, exocrine glands, skeletal muscle).
- List the signs, symptoms, and treatment of atropine poisoning.
- List the major clinical indications and contraindications for the use of muscarinic antagonists.
- Describe the autonomic effects of the ganglion-blocking nicotinic antagonists.
- List one antimuscarinic agent promoted for each of the following special uses: mydriasis and cycloplegia; parkinsonism; peptic ulcer; asthma.

Learn the definitions that follow.

Table 8–1. Definitions.

Term	Definition
Atropine fever	Hyperthermia induced by antimuscarinic drugs; caused mainly by inhibition of sweating
Atropine flush	Marked cutaneous vasodilation of the arms and upper torso and head by antimuscarinic drugs; mechanism unknown
Cholinesterase regenerator	A chemical antagonist that binds the phosphorus of organophosphates and displaces acetylcholinesterase
Cycloplegia	Paralysis of accommodation
Depolarizing blockade	Flaccid skeletal muscle paralysis caused by persistent depolarization of the neuromuscular end plate
Miotic	A drug that constricts the pupil
Mydriatic	A drug that dilates the pupil
Nondepolarizing blockade	Flaccid skeletal muscle paralysis caused by blockade of the nicotinic end plate receptor
Organophosphate aging	A chemical change in the organophosphate molecule that occurs after binding of the organophosphate to cholinesterase for a period of time; aging renders the enzyme-inhibitor complex less susceptible to regeneration by pralidoxime
Parasympatholytic	A drug that blocks the muscarinic receptors of autonomic effector tissues and reduces the effects of parasympathetic nerve stimulation
Pharmacokinetic selectivity	Selectivity of effect that is achieved by local administration or special distribution of a drug, not by receptor selectivity

CONCEPTS

The cholinoceptor antagonists are readily grouped into subclasses on the basis of their spectrum of action (ie, whether they block muscarinic or nicotinic receptors; Figure 8–1). These drugs are pharmacologic antagonists. A special subgroup, the cholinesterase regenerators, are not receptor blockers but rather are chemical antagonists of organophosphate cholinesterase inhibitors.

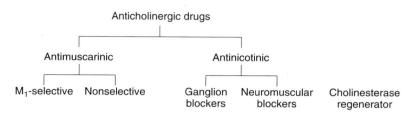

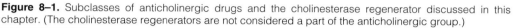

Figure 8–1. Subclasses of anticholinergic drugs and the cholinesterase regenerator discussed in this chapter. (The cholinesterase regenerators are not considered a part of the anticholinergic group.)

MUSCARINIC ANTAGONISTS

A. Classification & Pharmacokinetics:

1. **Classification of the muscarinic antagonists:** Muscarinic antagonists can be subdivided according to their selectivity for M_1 receptors or their lack of such selectivity. Although the division of muscarinic receptors into subgroups is well documented (Chapters 6, 7), only a few receptor-selective antagonists have reached clinical trials in the USA (eg, pirenzepine, telenzepine). All of the drugs in general use at present are nonselective. These blockers can be further subdivided on the basis of their primary clinical target organs (CNS, eye, bronchi, or gastrointestinal and genitourinary tracts). Drugs used for their effects on the CNS or the eyes must be sufficiently lipid-soluble to cross lipid barriers. A major determinant of this property is the presence or absence of a permanently charged (quaternary) amine group in the drug. This is because charged molecules are more polar and therefore less likely to penetrate a lipid barrier such as the blood-brain barrier or the cornea of the eye. Atropine is the prototypical nonselective muscarinic blocker.

2. **Pharmacokinetics of atropine:** Atropine is an alkaloid found in *Atropa belladonna* and many other plants. Because it is a tertiary amine, atropine is relatively lipid-soluble and readily crosses membrane barriers. The drug is well-distributed into the CNS and other organs and is eliminated partially by metabolism in the liver and partially by renal excretion. The elimination half-life is approximately 2 hours, and the duration of action of customary doses is 4–8 hours except in the eye, where effects last for 72 hours or longer.

3. **Pharmacokinetics of other muscarinic blockers:** In ophthalmology, topical activity (the ability to enter the eye after conjunctival administration) and duration of action are important in determining the usefulness of several antimuscarinic drugs (see Clinical Uses). Similar ability to cross lipid barriers is important for agents used in parkinsonism. In contrast, the drugs used for their antisecretory or antispastic actions in the gut and the bronchi are selected for minimal CNS activity; these drugs often incorporate quaternary amine groups to limit penetration through the blood-brain barrier.

B. Mechanism of Action: The muscarinic blocking agents act as competitive (surmountable) pharmacologic antagonists; their blocking effects can be overcome by increased concentrations of muscarinic agonists.

C. Effects: The peripheral actions of muscarinic blockers are mostly predictable effects derived from cholinoceptor blockade (Table 8–2). These include the ocular, gastrointestinal, genitourinary, and secretory effects. The CNS effects are less predictable. Those seen at therapeutic concentrations include sedation, amelioration of motion sickness, and, as noted above, reduction of some of the signs of parkinsonism. Cardiovascular effects at therapeutic doses include an initial slowing of heart rate caused by central or presynaptic vagal effects followed by the tachycardia and decreased atrioventricular conduction time that would be predicted from peripheral vagal blockade.

D. Clinical Uses: The muscarinic blockers have several therapeutic applications in the CNS, eye, bronchi, gut, and urinary bladder. These uses are summarized in Table 8–3.

1. **CNS:** Scopolamine is standard therapy for motion sickness; this drug is one of the most effective agents available. A transdermal patch formulation has been available. Benztropine, biperiden, and trihexyphenidyl are representative of several antimuscarinic agents used in

Table 8–2. Effects of muscarinic blocking drugs.

Organ	Effect	Mechanism
CNS	Sedation, antimotion sickness action, antiparkinson action, amnesia, delirium	Block of muscarinic receptors, unknown subtypes
Eye	Cycloplegia, mydriasis	Block of M_3 receptors
Bronchi	Bronchodilation, especially if constricted	Block of M_3 receptors
GI tract	Relaxation, slowed peristalsis	Block of M_1, M_3 receptors
GU tract	Relaxation of bladder wall, urinary retention	Block of M_3 receptors
Heart	Initial bradycardia, especially at low doses; then tachycardia	Initial bradycardia from increased vagal effect; tachycardia from block of M_2 receptors in the heart
Vessels	Block of muscarinic vasodilation; not manifest unless a muscarinic agonist is present	Block of M_3 receptors on endothelium of vessels
Exocrine glands	Marked reduction of salivation; moderate reduction of lacrimation, sweating; less reduction of gastric secretion	Block of M_1, M_3 receptors
Skeletal muscle	No effect	

parkinsonism. Although not as effective as levodopa (see Chapter 28), these agents may be useful as adjuncts or when patients become unresponsive to levodopa. Benztropine is sometimes used parenterally to treat acute dystonias caused by antipsychotic medications.

2. **Eye:** Antimuscarinic drugs are used to dilate the pupil and to paralyze accommodation. They include (in descending order of duration of action) atropine (> 72 hours), homatropine (24 hours), cyclopentolate (2–12 hours), and tropicamide (0.5–4 hours). These agents are all well-absorbed from the conjunctival sac into the eye.

3. **Bronchi:** Parenteral atropine has long been used to reduce airway secretions during surgery. Ipratropium is a quaternary antimuscarinic agent used by inhalation to reduce bronchoconstriction in asthma and chronic obstructive pulmonary disease (COPD). Although not as efficacious as beta agonists, ipratropium is less likely to cause cardiac arrhythmias in sensitive patients. It has very few antimuscarinic effects outside the lungs because it is poorly absorbed and rapidly metabolized.

4. **Gut:** Atropine, methscopolamine, and propantheline were used in acid-peptic disease to reduce acid secretion, but they are not as effective as H_2 blockers such as cimetidine, and they cause more adverse effects. Pirenzepine is an investigational M_1-selective muscarinic blocker that may be more useful in peptic ulcer. Muscarinic blockers can also be used to reduce cramping and hypermotility in transient diarrheas, but opioids such as diphenoxylate (Chapter 31) are more effective.

5. **Bladder:** Glycopyrrolate, oxybutynin, methscopolamine, or similar agents may be used to reduce urgency in mild cystitis and to reduce bladder spasms following urologic surgery. Glycopyrrolate and methscopolamine are quaternary molecules that may have fewer CNS effects.

Table 8–3. Some clinical applications of antimuscarinic drugs.

Organ	Drugs[1]	Application
CNS	Benztropine, trihexyphenidyl, biperiden	To treat the manifestations of Parkinson's disease
	Scopolamine	To prevent or reduce motion sickness
Eye	Atropine, homatropine, cyclopentolate, tropicamide	To produce mydriasis and cycloplegia
Bronchi	Ipratropium	To cause bronchodilation in asthma and COPD[2]
GI tract	Glycopyrrolate, dicyclomine, methscopolamine	To reduce transient hypermotility
GU tract	Oxybutynin, glycopyrrolate, dicyclomine	To treat transient cystitis, postoperative bladder spasms, or incontinence (rare)

[1]Only a few of many drugs are listed.
[2]COPD, chronic obstructive pulmonary disease.

E. **Toxicity:** A traditional mnemonic for atropine toxicity is "dry as a bone, red as a beet, mad as a hatter, blind as a bat." This description reflects both predictable antimuscarinic effects and some unpredictable actions.

1. **Predictable toxicities:** Antimuscarinic actions lead to several important and potentially dangerous effects. Blockade of thermoregulatory sweating may result in hyperthermia, or "atropine fever." This is the most dangerous effect of the antimuscarinic drugs and is potentially lethal in infants. In adults, the condition is described by "dry as a bone" because sweating, salivation, and lacrimation are all significantly reduced or stopped. In the elderly, important additional targets of toxicity include the eye (acute angle-closure glaucoma may occur) and the bladder (urinary retention is possible). Constipation and blurred vision are common adverse effects in all age groups.

2. **Other toxicities:** Toxicities not predictable from peripheral autonomic actions include the following.

   a. **CNS effects:** CNS toxicity includes sedation, amnesia, and delirium or hallucinations ("mad as a hatter"); convulsions may also develop. Central muscarinic receptors are probably involved.

   b. **Cardiovascular effects:** At toxic doses, intraventricular conduction may be blocked; this action is probably not mediated by muscarinic blockade and is difficult to treat. Dilation of the cutaneous vessels of the arms, head, neck, and trunk also occurs at these doses; the resulting "atropine flush" ("red as a beet") may be diagnostic of overdose with these drugs.

F. **Contraindications:** The antimuscarinic agents should be used cautiously in infants because of the danger of hyperthermia. The drugs are relatively contraindicated in persons with glaucoma, especially the closed-angle form, and in men with prostatic hyperplasia.

NICOTINIC ANTAGONISTS

A. **Classification:** Nicotinic receptor antagonists are divided into ganglion-blocking drugs and neuromuscular blocking drugs.

B. **Ganglion-Blocking Drugs:** Blockers of ganglionic nicotinic receptors are now of largely academic interest, though they were important historically for introducing the era of successful therapy of hypertension. Hexamethonium (C6, a prototype), mecamylamine, and several other ganglion blockers were extensively used for this disease. Unfortunately, the adverse effects of ganglion blockade are so severe (both sympathetic and parasympathetic divisions are blocked) that patients are unable to tolerate them for long periods (Table 8–4). Trimethaphan was the ganglion blocker most recently used in clinical practice, but it too has been withdrawn because of lack of use. Its action is like that of a competitive pharmacologic antagonist. It is poorly lipid-soluble, inactive orally, and has a short half-life. It was used intravenously to treat severe accelerated ("malignant") hypertension and to produce controlled hypotension. Because ganglion blockers interrupt sympathetic control of venous tone, they cause marked venous pooling; postural hypotension is a major manifestation of this effect. Toxicities of ganglion-blocking drugs include dry mouth, blurred vision, marked orthostatic hypotension, constipation, and severe sexual dysfunction that includes both impotence and inability to ejaculate (see Table 8–4).

Table 8–4. Effects of ganglion-blocking drugs.

Organ	Effects
Eye	Moderate mydriasis and cycloplegia
Bronchi	Little effect; asthmatics may note some bronchodilation
GI tract	Markedly reduced motility; constipation may be severe
GU tract	Reduced contractility of the bladder; impairment of erection and ejaculation
Heart	Slight tachycardia in young adults; reduction in force of contraction and cardiac output
Vessels	Reduction in arteriolar tone, marked reduction in venous tone; blood pressure decreases and orthostatic hypotension may be severe
Exocrine glands	Reductions in salivation, lacrimation, sweating, and gastric secretion
Skeletal muscle	No significant effect

C. **Neuromuscular Blocking Drugs:** Neuromuscular blocking drugs are important for producing complete skeletal muscle relaxation in surgery; new ones are frequently introduced. They are discussed in greater detail in Chapter 27.

   1. **Nondepolarizing group:** Tubocurarine is the prototype. It produces a competitive block at the end plate, causing flaccid paralysis that lasts 30–60 minutes (longer if large doses have been given). Pancuronium, atracurium, vecuronium, and several newer drugs are shorter-acting, nondepolarizing blockers. Gallamine is an older nondepolarizing drug that is used rarely in the USA.

   2. **Depolarizing group:** Although these drugs are nicotinic agonists, not antagonists, they cause a flaccid paralysis (see Chapter 27). Succinylcholine, the only member of this group used in the USA, produces fasciculations during induction of paralysis; patients may complain of muscle pain after its use. The drug is hydrolyzed by pseudocholinesterase (plasma cholinesterase) and has a half-life of a few minutes in persons with normal plasma cholinesterase. Approximately one in 2500 individuals produces a genetically determined form of abnormal cholinesterase that does not metabolize succinylcholine effectively. The drug's duration of action is greatly prolonged in such individuals.

   3. **Toxicity:** The toxicity of neuromuscular blockers is discussed in Chapter 27.

CHOLINESTERASE REGENERATORS

The cholinesterase regenerators are not receptor antagonists but belong to a class of *chemical* antagonists. These molecules contain an oxime group, which has an extremely high affinity for the phosphorus atom in organophosphate insecticides. Because the affinity of the oxime group for phosphorus exceeds that of the enzyme active site, these agents are able to bind the inhibitor and displace the enzyme (if aging has not occurred). The active enzyme is thus regenerated. **Pralidoxime,** the oxime currently available in the USA, is often used in the emergency department to treat patients exposed to insecticides such as parathion.

DRUG LIST

The following drugs are important members of the group discussed in this chapter. Prototypes should be learned in detail; features of the major variants should be known well enough so that the variants can be distinguished from prototypes and from each other; the other significant agents should be recognized as belonging to a specific subclass.

Subclass	Prototype	Major Variants	Other Significant Agents
Muscarinic blockers Nonselective	Atropine	Scopolamine, glycopyrrolate, ipratropium, cyclopentolate, benztropine	Homatropine, methscopolamine, tropicamide
M_1-selective	Pirenzepine		Telenzepine
Nicotinic blockers Ganglion blockers	Hexamethonium	Trimethaphan	
Neuromuscular blockers	Tubocurarine		Pancuronium, atracurium
Cholinesterase regenerator	Pralidoxime		

QUESTIONS

DIRECTIONS: Each of the numbered items or incomplete statements in this section is followed by answers or by completions of the statement. Select the ONE lettered answer or completion that is BEST in each case.

Items 1–2: A 3-year-old child has been admitted to the emergency room. Antimuscarinic drug overdose is suspected.

   1. Atropine overdose may cause all of the following EXCEPT
      (A) Blurred vision
      (B) Relaxation of gastrointestinal smooth muscle

    (C)   Decrease in gastric secretion
    (D)   Pupillary constriction
    (E)   Increase in cardiac rate

  2. In very young children, the most common cause of death due to belladonna alkaloids is
    (A)   Intraventricular heart block
    (B)   Dehydration
    (C)   Hypertension
    (D)   Hyperthermia
    (E)   Hallucinations

  3. Which of the following pairs of drugs and drug properties are properly matched?
    (A)   Atropine: Poorly absorbed after oral administration
    (B)   Cyclopentolate: Well-absorbed from conjunctival sac into the eye
    (C)   Scopolamine: Short duration of action when used as anti-motion sickness agent
    (D)   Ipratropium: Well-absorbed, long elimination half-life
    (E)   Benztropine: Quaternary, poor CNS penetration

  4. All of the following can be blocked by atropine pretreatment EXCEPT
    (A)   Vagal bradycardia (slowing of rate caused by vagal stimulation)
    (B)   Tachycardia induced by infusion of acetylcholine
    (C)   Sweating induced by injection of pilocarpine
    (D)   Increased blood pressure induced by nicotine poisoning
    (E)   Salivation induced by neostigmine

  5. In using topical antimuscarinic drugs in the eye
    (A)   Atropine is longer-acting than cyclopentolate and more efficacious than methscopolamine
    (B)   Reversal of excess antimuscarinic effect is more easily achieved with physostigmine than with neostigmine
    (C)   Both (A) and (B) are correct
    (D)   Neither (A) nor (B) is correct

Items 6 and 7: Two new synthetic drugs (X and Y) are to be studied for their cardiovascular effects. The drugs are given to three anesthetized animals while the blood pressure is recorded. The first animal has received no pretreatment (control), the second has received an effective dose of a long-acting ganglion blocker, and the third has received an effective dose of a long-acting muscarinic antagonist.

  6. Drug X caused a 50 mm Hg rise in mean blood pressure in the control animal, no blood pressure change in the ganglion-blocked animal, and a 75 mm Hg mean blood pressure rise in the atropine-pretreated animal. Drug X is probably a drug similar to
    (A)   Acetylcholine
    (B)   Atropine
    (C)   Epinephrine
    (D)   Hexamethonium
    (E)   Nicotine

  7. The net changes induced by drug Y are shown in the graph below. Drug Y is probably a drug similar to
    (A)   Acetylcholine
    (B)   Edrophonium
    (C)   Hexamethonium
    (D)   Nicotine
    (E)   Pralidoxime

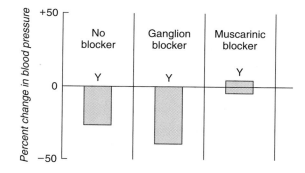

8. A 30-year-old man has been treated with several autonomic drugs over a period of weeks. He is now admitted to the emergency department showing signs of drug toxicity. Which of the following signs would distinguish between an overdose of a ganglion blocker versus a muscarinic blocker?
   (A) Mydriasis
   (B) Tachycardia
   (C) Postural hypotension
   (D) Blurred vision
   (E) Dry mouth, constipation

9. All of the following may cause cycloplegia (paralysis of accommodation) when used topically in the eye EXCEPT
   (A) Atropine
   (B) Cyclopentolate
   (C) Physostigmine
   (D) Scopolamine
   (E) Tropicamide

10. You have been asked to consult in the treatment of an 80-year-old patient. An antimuscarinic drug is being considered. Atropine therapy in the elderly may be hazardous because
    (A) Atropine can elevate intraocular pressure in patients with glaucoma
    (B) Atropine frequently causes ventricular tachycardia
    (C) Urinary retention may be precipitated by atropine in women
    (D) The elderly are particularly prone to develop dangerous hyperthermia when given atropine
    (E) Atropine often causes excessive vasodilation and hypotension in the elderly

11. When a dose-response study of atropine is carried out in young adults, which of the following effects may be observed?
    (A) Bradycardia
    (B) Tachycardia
    (C) Central nervous system stimulation, eg, hallucinations
    (D) Central nervous system depression, eg, sedation
    (E) All of the above

12. Accepted therapeutic indications for the use of antimuscarinic drugs include all of the following EXCEPT
    (A) Parkinson's disease
    (B) Hypertension
    (C) Traveler's diarrhea
    (D) Motion sickness
    (E) Postoperative bladder spasm

DIRECTIONS (Items 13–15): Each set of matching questions in this section consists of a list of three to twenty-six lettered options (some of which may be figures) followed by several numbered items. For each numbered item, select the ONE lettered option that is MOST closely associated with it. Each lettered option may be selected once, more than once, or not at all.
   (A) Atropine
   (B) Benztropine
   (C) Bethanechol
   (D) Botulinum
   (E) Cyclopentolate
   (F) Neostigmine
   (G) Pralidoxime
   (H) Scopolamine
   (I) Trimethaphan
   (J) Tubocurarine

13. This drug is used exclusively in ophthalmology for inducing cycloplegia and mydriasis
14. This drug causes vasodilation that can be blocked by atropine
15. This drug has a very high affinity for the phosphorus atom in parathion and is often used to treat insecticide toxicity

ANSWERS

1. Pupillary dilation, not constriction, is a characteristic atropine effect, as indicated by the origin of the name belladonna ("beautiful lady") from the ancient cosmetic use of extracts of the *Atropa belladonna* plant to dilate the pupils. The answer is **(D).**

2. Choices **(A), (D),** and **(E)** are possible effects of the atropine group. In small children, however, the most dangerous effect is hyperthermia. Deaths with body temperatures in excess of 42 °C have occurred after the use of atropine-containing eye drops in children. The answer is **(D).**

3. Atropine is very well absorbed. Scopolamine has a relatively long duration of action, especially when used as an anti-motion sickness transdermal patch. Ipratropium is quaternary and poorly absorbed from the airways. Benztropine is tertiary, lipid-soluble, and penetrates into the CNS well. Only **(B)** is correct.

4. Atropine blocks muscarinic receptors and inhibits parasympathomimetic effects. Nicotine can induce both parasympathomimetic and sympathomimetic effects by virtue of its ganglion-stimulating action. Hypertension reflects sympathetic discharge and therefore would not be blocked by atropine. The answer is **(D).**

5. Atropine is considerably longer-acting in the eye (about 72 hours) than cyclopentolate (about 2 hours) and is also more efficacious, especially in children. Physostigmine (a tertiary amine) penetrates the surface of the eye better than neostigmine (a quaternary amine; Chapter 7). The answer is **(C).**

6. Drug X causes an increase in blood pressure that is blocked by a ganglion blocker but not by a muscarinic blocker. The pressor response is actually increased by pretreatment with a muscarinic blocker, suggesting that compensatory vagal discharge might have blunted the full response. This description fits a ganglion stimulant like nicotine but not epinephrine, since epinephrine's pressor effects are produced at alpha receptors, not in the ganglia. The answer is **(E).**

7. Drug Y causes a decrease in blood pressure that is blocked by a muscarinic blocker but not by a ganglion blocker. Therefore, the depressor effect must be evoked at a site distal to the ganglia. In fact, the drop in blood pressure is actually greater in the presence of ganglion blockade, suggesting that compensatory sympathetic discharge might have blunted the full depressor action of drug Y in the untreated animal. The description fits a direct-acting muscarinic stimulant such as acetylcholine (given in high dosage). Indirect-acting cholinomimetics (cholinesterase inhibitors) would not produce this pattern because the vascular muscarinic receptors involved in the depressor response are not innervated and are therefore unresponsive to indirectly acting agents. The answer is **(A).**

8. Ganglion blockers and muscarinic blockers can both cause mydriasis, increase resting heart rate, blur vision, and cause dry mouth and constipation, because these are determined largely by parasympathetic tone. Postural hypotension, on the other hand, is a sign of sympathetic blockade, which would occur with ganglion blockers but not muscarinic blockers (Chapter 6). The answer is **(C).**

9. All antimuscarinic agents are, in theory, capable of causing cycloplegia. Physostigmine, on the other hand, is an indirect-acting cholinomimetic and has the opposite effect. The answer is **(C).**

10. The elderly have a much higher incidence of glaucoma than younger people (and may be unaware of the disease until late in its course). Antimuscarinic agents may increase intraocular pressure in individuals with glaucoma. Elderly men (not women) have a much higher probability of developing urinary retention—because they have a high incidence of prostatic hyperplasia. Cardiac and hyperthermic reactions to atropine are not common in the elderly. The answer is **(A).**

11. All of the effects listed may be observed. The answer is **(E).**

12. Hypertension is not responsive to antimuscarinic agents. The answer is **(B).**

13. Cyclopentolate is used in ophthalmology to produce mydriasis and cycloplegia. The answer is **(E).**

14. Bethanechol (Chapter 7) causes vasodilation by activating muscarinic receptors on the endothelium of blood vessels. This effect can be blocked by atropine. The answer is **(C).**

15. Pralidoxime has a very high affinity for the phosphorus atom in organophosphate insecticides. The answer is **(G).**

Sympathomimetics

9

OBJECTIVES

You should be able to:

- List tissues that contain significant numbers of alpha receptors of the α_1 or α_2 type.
- List tissues that contain significant numbers of β_1 or β_2 receptors.
- Describe the major organ system effects of a pure alpha agonist, a pure beta agonist, and a mixed alpha and beta agonist. Give examples of each type of drug.
- Describe a clinical situation in which the effects of an indirect sympathomimetic would differ from those of a direct agonist.
- List the major clinical applications of the adrenoceptor agonists.

Learn the definitions that follow.

Table 9–1. Definitions.

Term	Definition
Anorexiant	A drug that causes loss of appetite (anorexia)
Catecholamine	A dihydroxyphenylethylamine derivative, eg, norepinephrine, epinephrine
Decongestant	A drug that reduces nasal or oropharyngeal mucosal swelling, usually by constricting blood vessels in the submucosal tissue
Direct agonist, indirect agonist	A direct agonist binds and activates the receptor; an indirect one brings about receptor activation by binding to some other molecule, eg, a reuptake carrier, and causing an increase in the synaptic concentration of the normal transmitter
Mydriatic	A drug that causes dilation of the pupil; opposite of miotic
Phenylisopropyl-amine derivative	A drug like amphetamine, ephedrine. Unlike catecholamines, phenylisopropylamines usually have oral activity, a long half-life, some CNS activity, and an indirect mode of action
Selective α agonist, β agonist	Drugs that have relatively greater effects on alpha or beta adrenoceptors; none are *absolutely* selective
Sympathomimetic	A drug that mimics stimulation of the sympathetic autonomic nervous system
Reuptake inhibitor	An indirectly acting drug that increases the activity of transmitters in the synapse by inhibiting their reuptake into the presynaptic nerve ending; may act selectively on noradrenergic, serotonergic, or both types of nerve endings

CONCEPTS

A. Classification: The adrenoceptor agonists are subdivided in two ways: by mode of action and by spectrum of action (Figure 9–1).

    1. Mode of action: The adrenoceptor agonists may directly activate their receptors or may act indirectly to increase the concentration of catecholamine transmitter in the synapse. Amphetamine derivatives and tyramine cause the release of stored catecholamines; these sympathomimetics are therefore mainly indirect in their mode of action. Another form of indirect action is seen with cocaine and the tricyclic antidepressants; these drugs inhibit reuptake of catecholamines by nerve terminals and thus increase the synaptic activity of released transmitter.

        Blockade of metabolism (ie, block of catechol-*O*-methyltransferase [COMT] and monoamine oxidase [MAO]) has little direct effect on autonomic activity, but MAO inhibition increases the stores of catecholamines in storage vesicles and thus may potentiate the action of indirectly acting sympathomimetics.

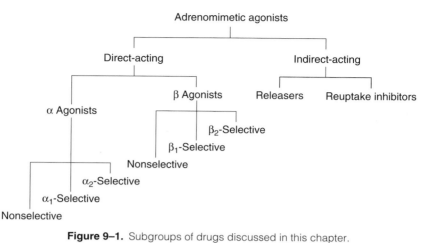

Figure 9–1. Subgroups of drugs discussed in this chapter.

2. **Spectrum of action:** The adrenoceptors are classified as alpha or beta receptors; both groups are further subdivided into two or more subgroups. The distribution of these receptors is set forth in Table 9–2. Epinephrine may be considered a single prototype with effects at all receptor types (α_1, α_2, β_1, β_2, and β_3). Alternatively, separate prototypes, phenylephrine (alpha) and isoproterenol (beta) may be defined. Dopamine receptors constitute a third class of adrenoceptors. The above-mentioned drugs have relatively little effect on dopamine receptors, but dopamine itself is a potent dopamine receptor agonist and when given as a drug can also activate beta (intermediate doses) and alpha receptors (large doses).

B. **Chemistry and Pharmacokinetics:** The endogenous adrenoceptor agonists (epinephrine, norepinephrine, and dopamine) are catecholamines and are rapidly metabolized by COMT and MAO. As a result, these adrenoceptor agonists are inactive when given by the oral route. After

Table 9–2. Types of adrenoceptors, some of the peripheral tissues in which they are found, and the major effects of their activation. Adrenoceptor distribution in the CNS is discussed in Chapter 21.

Type	Tissue	Actions
Alpha$_1$	Most vascular smooth muscle	Contracts ($\uparrow$ vascular resistance)
	Pupillary dilator muscle	Contracts (mydriasis)
	Pilomotor smooth muscle	Contracts (erects hair)
	Liver (in some species, eg, rat)	Stimulates glycogenolysis
Alpha$_2$	Adrenergic and cholinergic nerve terminals	Inhibits transmitter release
	Platelets	Stimulates aggregation
	Some vascular smooth muscle	Contracts
	Fat cells	Inhibits lipolysis
	Pancreatic B cells	Inhibits insulin release
Beta$_1$	Heart	Stimulates rate and force
	Juxtaglomerular cells	Stimulates renin release
Beta$_2$	Respiratory, uterine, and vascular smooth muscle	Relaxes
	Liver (human)	Stimulates glycogenolysis
	Pancreatic B cells	Stimulates insulin release
	Somatic motor nerve terminals (voluntary muscle)	Causes tremor
Beta$_3$ (β_1, β_2 may also contribute)	Fat cells	Stimulates lipolysis
Dopamine$_1$	Renal and other splanchnic blood vessels	Relaxes (reduces resistance)
Dopamine$_2$	Nerve terminals	Inhibits adenylyl cyclase

their release from nerve endings, they are again taken up into nerve endings and into perisynaptic cells; these agonists have a short duration of action. When given parenterally, they do not enter the CNS in significant amounts. Isoproterenol, a synthetic catecholamine, is similar to the endogenous transmitters but is not readily taken up into the nerve ending. Phenylisopropyl-amines (eg, amphetamine) are resistant to MAO; most of them are not catecholamines and are therefore also resistant to COMT. These agents are orally active; they enter the CNS, and their effects last much longer than do those of catecholamines. Tyramine, which is not a phenyliso-propylamine, is rapidly metabolized by MAO except in patients who are taking an MAO inhibitor drug.

C. Mechanisms of Action:
1. **Alpha$_1$ receptor effects:** Alpha$_1$ receptor effects are mediated primarily by the coupling protein G$_q$, which leads to activation of the phosphoinositide cascade and the release of ino-sitol-1,4,5-trisphosphate (IP$_3$) and diacylglycerol (DAG). Calcium is subsequently released in smooth muscle cells, and enzymes are activated. Direct gating of calcium channels may also play a role in increasing intracellular calcium concentration.
2. **Alpha$_2$ receptor effects:** Alpha$_2$ receptor activation results in inhibition of adenylyl cy-clase via the coupling protein G$_i$.
3. **Beta receptor effects:** Beta receptors (β_1, β_2, and β_3) stimulate adenylyl cyclase via the coupling protein G$_s$, which leads to an increase in cAMP concentration in the cell.
4. **Dopamine receptor effects:** Dopamine D$_1$ receptors activate adenylyl cyclase in neurons and vascular smooth muscle. Dopamine D$_2$ receptors are more important in the brain but probably also play a significant role as presynaptic receptors on peripheral nerves.

D. Organ System Effects:
1. **CNS:** Catecholamines do not enter the CNS effectively. Sympathomimetics that do enter the CNS (eg, amphetamines) have a spectrum of stimulant effects, beginning with mild alerting or reduction of fatigue and progressing to anorexia, euphoria, and insomnia. These effects probably represent the release of dopamine in certain dopaminergic tracts. Very high doses lead to marked anxiety or aggressiveness, paranoia, and sometimes convulsions.
2. **Eye:** The smooth muscle of the pupillary dilator responds to topical phenylephrine and similar alpha agonists with mydriasis. Accommodation is not significantly affected. Outflow of aqueous humor may be facilitated by alpha agonists, with a subsequent reduction of intraocular pressure.
3. **Bronchi:** The smooth muscle of the bronchi relaxes markedly in response to beta$_2$ agonists. These agents are the most efficacious and reliable drugs available for reversing bron-chospasm.
4. **Gastrointestinal tract:** The gastrointestinal tract is well endowed with both alpha and beta receptors, located on both smooth muscle and on neurons of the enteric nervous system. Activation of either alpha or beta receptors leads to relaxation of the smooth muscle. Alpha$_2$ agonists may decrease salt and water secretion in the intestine.
5. **Genitourinary tract:** The genitourinary tract contains alpha receptors in the bladder trigone and sphincter area; the receptors mediate contraction of the sphincter. Sympatho-mimetics are sometimes used to increase sphincter tone. Beta$_2$ agonists may cause significant uterine relaxation in pregnant women near term, but the doses required also cause significant tachycardia.
6. **Vascular system:**
   a. **Alpha$_1$ agonists:** Alpha$_1$ agonists (eg, phenylephrine) constrict skin and splanchnic blood vessels and increase peripheral vascular resistance and venous pressure. Because these drugs increase blood pressure, they often evoke a compensatory reflex bradycardia.
   b. **Alpha$_2$ agonists:** Alpha$_2$ agonists (eg, clonidine) cause vasoconstriction when administered intravenously or topically (eg, as a nasal spray), but when given orally they accumulate in the CNS and *reduce* sympathetic outflow and blood pressure, as described in Chapter 11.
   c. **Beta$_2$ agonists:** Beta$_2$ agonists (eg, terbutaline) cause significant reduction in arteriolar tone in the skeletal muscle vascular bed and can reduce peripheral vascular resistance and arterial blood pressure.
   d. **Dopamine:** Dopamine causes vasodilation in the splanchnic and renal vascular beds by activating D$_1$ receptors. This effect can be very useful in the treatment of renal fail-

ure associated with shock. At higher doses, dopamine activates beta receptors; at still higher doses, alpha receptors are activated.

7. **Heart:** The heart is well supplied with β_1 and β_2 receptors. The β_1 receptors predominate in some parts of the heart; both beta receptors, however, mediate increased rate of cardiac pacemakers (normal and abnormal), increased atrioventricular node conduction velocity, and increased cardiac force.

8. **Net cardiovascular actions:** Sympathomimetics with both alpha and beta$_1$ effects (eg, norepinephrine) may cause a reflex increase in vagal outflow because they increase blood pressure and evoke the baroreceptor reflex. This reflex bradycardia often dominates any direct beta effects on the heart rate, so that a slow infusion of norepinephrine typically causes increased blood pressure and *bradycardia* (see Figure 9–2). If the reflex is blocked (eg, by a ganglion blocker), norepinephrine may cause a direct beta$_1$-mediated tachycardia. A pure alpha agonist, eg, phenylephrine, will routinely slow heart rate via the baroreceptor reflex, while a pure beta agonist, eg, isoproterenol, almost always increases the heart rate.

The diastolic blood pressure is affected mainly by peripheral vascular resistance and the heart rate. The adrenoceptors with the greatest effects on vascular resistance are alpha and beta$_2$ receptors. The systolic pressure is the sum of the diastolic and the pulse pressures. The pulse pressure is determined mainly by the stroke volume (a function of force of cardiac contraction), which is influenced by beta$_1$ receptors.

9. **Metabolic and hormonal effects:** Beta$_1$ agonists increase renin secretion. Beta$_2$ agonists increase insulin secretion by the pancreas. They also increase glycogenolysis in the liver. The resulting hyperglycemia is countered by the increased insulin levels. Transport of glucose out of the liver is associated initially with hyperkalemia; transport into peripheral organs (especially skeletal muscle) is accompanied by movement of potassium into these cells, resulting in a later hypokalemia. All beta agonists appear to stimulate lipolysis.

E. **Clinical Uses:** See Table 9–3.

1. **Anaphylaxis:** Epinephrine is the drug of choice for the immediate treatment of anaphylactic shock. The catecholamine is sometimes supplemented with antihistamines and corticosteroids, but these agents are not as efficacious as epinephrine nor as rapid-acting.

2. **CNS:** The phenylisopropylamines such as amphetamine are widely used and abused for their CNS effects. Legitimate indications include narcolepsy, attention deficit disorder, and, with appropriate controls, weight reduction. The anorexiant effect is insufficient to maintain weight loss in patients who do not also receive intensive dietary and psychologic coun-

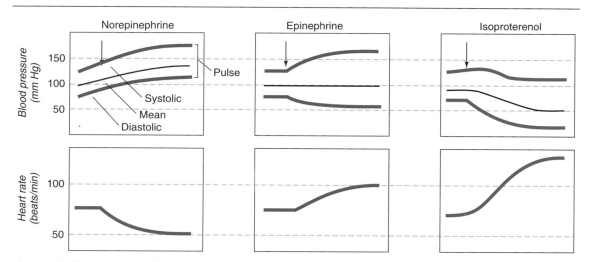

Figure 9–2. Typical effects of the principal catecholamines on blood pressure and heart rate. Note that the pulse pressure ("Pulse") is only slightly increased by norepinephrine but is markedly increased by epinephrine and isoproterenol. The reduction in heart rate caused by norepinephrine is the result of baroreceptor reflex activation of vagal outflow to the heart. The blood pressure effects of epinephrine are typically dose-dependent: small doses exhibit more beta effect (isoproterenol-like); large doses exhibit more alpha effect (norepinephrine-like).

Table 9–3. Pharmacokinetics and clinical applications of some sympathomimetics.

Drug	Oral Activity	Duration of Action	Clinical Applications
Catecholamines			
Epinephrine	No	Minutes	Anaphylaxis, glaucoma, asthma, and to cause vasoconstriction
Norepinephrine	No	Minutes	To cause vasoconstriction in hypotension
Isoproterenol	Poor	Minutes	Asthma, atrioventricular block (rare)
Dopamine	No	Minutes	Shock, heart failure
Dobutamine	No	Minutes	Shock, heart failure
Other sympathomimetics			
Amphetamine, phenmetrazine, others	Yes	Hours	Narcolepsy, obesity, attention deficit disorder
Ephedrine	Yes	Hours	Asthma (obsolete), urinary incontinence, and to cause vasoconstriction in hypotension
Phenylephrine	Poor	Hours	To cause mydriasis, vasoconstriction, decongestion
Albuterol, metaproterenol, terbutaline	Yes	Hours	Asthma, premature labor
Oxymetazoline, xylometazoline	Yes	Hours	To cause nasal decongestion (long action)
Cocaine	No	Minutes to hours	To cause vasoconstriction and local anesthesia

seling. The drugs are abused or misused for the purpose of deferring sleep and for their mood-elevating, euphoria-producing action.

3. **Eye:** The alpha agonists, especially phenylephrine, are often used topically to produce mydriasis and to reduce the conjunctival itching and congestion caused by irritation or allergy. These drugs do not cause cycloplegia. Epinephrine and a prodrug, dipivefrin, are sometimes used topically in the treatment of glaucoma. Phenylephrine has also been used for glaucoma, mainly outside the USA. Newer α_2 agonists introduced for use in glaucoma include apraclonidine and brimonidine.

4. **Bronchi:** The beta agonists, especially the β_2-selective agonists, are drugs of choice in the treatment of acute asthmatic bronchoconstriction.

5. **Cardiovascular applications:**
   a. **Conditions in which an increase in blood flow is desired:** In acute heart failure and some types of shock, an increase in cardiac output and blood flow to the tissues is needed. Beta$_1$ agonists may be useful in this situation because they increase cardiac contractility and reduce afterload (by decreasing the impedance to ventricular ejection through their partial beta$_2$ effect).
   b. **Conditions in which a decrease in blood flow or increase in blood pressure is desired:** Alpha$_1$ agonists are useful in situations in which vasoconstriction is appropriate. These include local hemostatic and decongestant applications as well as spinal shock, in which temporary maintenance of blood pressure may help maintain perfusion of the brain, heart, and kidneys. Shock due to septicemia or myocardial infarction, on the other hand, is usually made worse by vasoconstrictors, since the afterload is increased and tissue perfusion often declines. Alpha agonists are often mixed with local anesthetics to reduce the loss of anesthetic into the circulation from the area of injection. Chronic orthostatic hypotension due to inadequate sympathetic tone can be treated with a new α_1 agonist, midodrine.

6. **Genitourinary tract:** Beta$_2$ agonists (ritodrine, terbutaline) have been used in premature labor, but the cardiac stimulant effect may be hazardous to both mother and fetus.

   Long-acting sympathomimetics such as ephedrine are sometimes used to improve urinary continence in children with enuresis and in the elderly. This action is mediated by alpha receptors in the trigone of the bladder and, in men, the smooth muscle of the prostate.

F. Toxicity:

    1. Catecholamines: Because of their limited penetration into the brain, these drugs have little CNS toxicity when given systemically. In the periphery, their adverse effects are extensions of their pharmacologic alpha or beta actions: excessive vasoconstriction, cardiac arrhythmias, myocardial infarction, and pulmonary edema or hemorrhage.

    2. Other sympathomimetics: The phenylisopropylamines may produce mild to severe CNS toxicity, depending on dosage. In small doses, they induce nervousness, anorexia, and insomnia; in higher doses, they may cause anxiety, aggressiveness, or paranoid behavior. Convulsions may occur. Peripherally acting agents have toxicities that are predictable on the basis of the receptors they activate. Thus, α_1 agonists cause hypertension and β_1 agonists cause sinus tachycardia and serious arrhythmias. Beta$_2$ agonists cause skeletal muscle tremor. It is important to note that none of these drugs are perfectly selective; at high doses, β_1-selective agents have β_2 actions and vice versa. Cocaine is of special importance as a drug of abuse: its major toxicities include cardiac arrhythmias or infarction and convulsions. A fatal outcome is far more common with acute cocaine overdose than with any other sympathomimetic.

DRUG LIST

The following drugs are important members of the group discussed in this chapter. Prototypes should be learned in detail; features of the major variants should be known well enough so that the variants can be distinguished from prototypes and from each other; the other significant agents should be recognized as belonging to a specific subclass.

Subclass	Prototype	Major Variants	Other Significant Agents
General agonists Direct (α_1, α_2, β_1, β_2)	Epinephrine		
Indirect, releasers	Tyramine	Amphetamine	Ephedrine
Indirect, uptake inhibitors	Cocaine	Tricyclic antidepressants	
Selective agonists α_1, α_2, β_1	Norepinephrine		
$\alpha_1 > \alpha_2$	Phenylephrine		Methoxamine, metaraminol, midodrine
$\alpha_2 > \alpha_1$	Clonidine	Methylnorepinephrine[1]	Apraclonidine, brimonidine
$\beta_1 = \beta_2$	Isoproterenol		
$\beta_1 > \beta_2$	Dobutamine		
$\beta_2 > \beta_1$	Terbutaline		Albuterol, metaproterenol, ritodrine
Dopamine agonist	Dopamine	Bromocriptine[2]	

[1]Active metabolite of methyldopa.
[2]Ergot derivative with CNS dopamine agonist action, discussed in Chapter 28.

QUESTIONS

DIRECTIONS: Each of the numbered items or incomplete statements in this section is followed by answers or by completions of the statement. Select the ONE lettered answer or completion that is BEST in each case.

    1. Dilation of vessels in muscle, constriction of cutaneous vessels, and positive inotropic and chronotropic effects on the heart are all actions of

        (A) Metaproterenol

        (B) Norepinephrine

        (C) Acetylcholine

        (D) Epinephrine

        (E) Isoproterenol

2. A 7-year-old boy has a significant bed-wetting problem. A long-acting indirect sympatho-mimetic agent sometimes used by the oral route for this and other indications is
  (A) Epinephrine
  (B) Ephedrine
  (C) Dobutamine
  (D) Isoproterenol
  (E) Phenylephrine

3. When pupillary dilation—but not cycloplegia—is desired, a good choice is
  (A) Homatropine
  (B) Isoproterenol
  (C) Phenylephrine
  (D) Pilocarpine
  (E) Tropicamide

4. Which of the following drugs acts primarily on a receptor located on the membrane of the au-tonomic effector cell, ie, muscle or glandular tissue?
  (A) Clonidine
  (B) Cocaine
  (C) Norepinephrine
  (D) Tyramine
  (E) All of the above

5. When a moderate pressor dose of norepinephrine is given after pretreatment with a large dose of atropine, which of the following is most probable?
  (A) A decrease in heart rate caused by direct cardiac effect
  (B) A decrease in heart rate caused by indirect reflex effect
  (C) An increase in heart rate caused by direct cardiac action
  (D) An increase in heart rate caused by indirect reflex action
  (E) No change in heart rate

6. Which of the following may stimulate the central nervous system?
  (A) Sympathomimetic drugs
  (B) Antimuscarinic drugs
  (C) Both (A) and (B) are correct
  (D) Neither (A) nor (B) is correct

Items 7–8: Your patient is to receive a selective β_2 stimulant drug.

7. Beta$_2$-selective stimulants are often effective in
  (A) Raynaud's syndrome
  (B) Delayed or insufficiently strong labor
  (C) Ischemic ulcers of the skin
  (D) Asthma
  (E) Coronary insufficiency manifested by angina

8. In considering possible drug effects in this patient, you would note that beta$_2$ stimulants fre-quently cause
  (A) Skeletal muscle tremor
  (B) Direct stimulation of renin release
  (C) Vasodilation in the skin
  (D) Increased cGMP in mast cells
  (E) All of the above

9. Epinephrine increases the concentration of all of the following EXCEPT
  (A) Glucose in the blood
  (B) Free fatty acids in the blood
  (C) Lactate in the blood
  (D) cAMP in the heart
  (E) Triglycerides in the fat cells

10. Phenylephrine
  (A) Increases skin temperature
  (B) Causes miosis in the eye
  (C) Constricts small vessels in the nasal mucosa
  (D) Increases gastric secretion and motility
  (E) All of the above

11. A patient was given an IV infusion containing an intermediate dose of a sympathomimetic drug. The blood pressure changed as shown in the diagram. Which of the following drugs was given?
    (A) Albuterol
    (B) Epinephrine
    (C) Isoproterenol
    (D) Norepinephrine
    (E) Phenylephrine

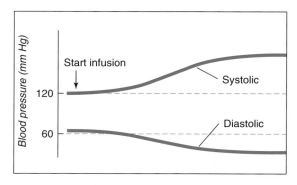

12. A new drug was given by subcutaneous injection to 20 normal subjects in a phase I clinical trial. The cardiovascular effects are summarized in the table below.

Variable	Control	Peak Drug Effect
Systolic BP (mm Hg)	116	144
Diastolic BP (mm Hg)	76	96
Cardiac output (L/min)	5.4	4.7
Heart rate (beats/min)	71.2	54.3

Which of the following drugs does the new experimental agent most resemble?
    (A) Bethanechol
    (B) Epinephrine
    (C) Isoproterenol
    (D) Neostigmine
    (E) Phenylephrine

DIRECTIONS (Items 13–15): Each set of matching questions in this section consists of a list of three to twenty-six lettered options (some of which may be figures) followed by several numbered items. For each numbered item, select the ONE lettered option that is MOST closely associated with it. Each lettered option may be selected once, more than once, or not at all.
    (A) Cocaine
    (B) Epinephrine
    (C) Isoproterenol
    (D) Norepinephrine
    (E) Phenylephrine
    (F) Terbutaline
    (G) Tyramine

13. This drug will decrease heart rate in the control situation but if given after a ganglion blocker will cause no change in heart rate
14. This β₂-selective drug is a drug of choice in acute asthmatic bronchoconstriction
15. This drug is the drug of choice in anaphylaxis

ANSWERS

1. The actions describe the effects of activating alpha, β_1, and β_2 receptors. Of the drugs listed, only epinephrine has all of these actions. The answer is **(D)**.

2. Phenylephrine and ephedrine are the only orally effective agents listed. Phenylephrine has a direct and relatively short action. The answer is **(B)**.

3. Antimuscarinics (homatropine, tropicamide) are mydriatic and cycloplegic; alpha sympathomimetic agonists are only mydriatic. Pilocarpine causes **miosis**. The answer is **(C)**.

4. The indirect-acting agents (cocaine and tyramine) act on stores of catecholamines in the nerve terminal; clonidine acts primarily on the α_2 receptor of the presynaptic nerve terminal. The answer is **(C)**.

5. Atropine will prevent the normal reflex bradycardia, since that requires integrity of the vagal pathway. The direct action of norepinephrine on the sinus node will be unmasked. The answer is **(C)**.

6. Phenylisopropylamines such as amphetamine are traditional stimulants with a spectrum of effects from mild alerting to paranoid schizophrenia and convulsions; antimuscarinic agents are capable of inducing hallucinations and convulsions. The answer is **(C)**.

7. The absence of β_2 receptors in the cutaneous vascular bed makes beta agonists useless in conditions involving reduced skin blood flow. Furthermore, ischemic ulcers are usually associated with structural occlusion of vessels that is not reversible with vasodilators. Beta agonists increase cardiac rate and force and increase myocardial oxygen demand; they are generally contraindicated in angina. Uterine and bronchiolar smooth muscle are relaxed by beta$_2$ agonists. The answer is **(D)**.

8. Tremor is a common β_2 effect. Blood vessels in the skin have almost exclusively alpha (vasoconstrictor) receptors. Stimulation of renin release is a β_1 effect. The answer is **(A)**.

9. Epinephrine increases free fatty acids by activating lipolysis of triglycerides in fat cells. The answer is **(E)**.

10. Choice **(A)** is incorrect; cutaneous vasoconstriction reduces skin temperature. Choice **(B)** is incorrect also; phenylephrine is a good mydriatic. Alpha agonists in ordinary dosage have little effect on the gut but may inhibit it. The answer is **(C)**.

11. The drug infusion caused a decrease in diastolic blood pressure and an increase in systolic pressure. Thus, there was a significant increase in pulse pressure. The decrease in diastolic pressure with no change in mean pressure suggests that the drug decreased vascular resistance in some beds while increasing it in others—ie, it must have significant alpha *and* beta agonist effects. The fact that it also markedly increased pulse pressure suggests that it strongly increased stroke volume, a beta-agonist effect. The drug with this balance of alpha and beta effects is epinephrine (Figure 9–2). The answer is **(B)**.

12. The investigational agent caused a marked increase in diastolic pressure but little increase in pulse pressure (from 40 to 48 mm Hg). These changes suggest a strong alpha effect on vessels but little beta-agonist action in the heart. The heart rate decreased markedly, reflecting a baroreceptor reflex compensatory response. Note that the stroke volume increased slightly (cardiac output divided by heart rate; from 75.8 mL to 86.6 mL). This is to be expected even in the absence of beta effects if venoconstriction causes an increase in venous return to the heart. The drug behaves most like a pure alpha agonist. The answer is **(E)**.

13. A pure alpha agonist will cause reflex bradycardia in a subject with intact reflexes but no change in heart rate if the reflexes are blocked. The answer is **(E)**.

14. The drugs of choice in asthmatic bronchoconstriction are the beta$_2$ agonists such as terbutaline, albuterol, and metaproterenol. The answer is **(F)**.

15. The drug of choice in anaphylaxis is epinephrine. The answer is **(B)**.

10

Adrenoceptor Blockers

OBJECTIVES

You should be able to:

- Describe the effects of epinephrine and norephinephrine in the presence and in the absence of phentolamine.
- Compare the effects of propranolol, metoprolol, and pindolol.
- Compare the pharmacokinetics of propranolol, atenolol, esmolol, and nadolol.
- Describe the clinical applications and toxicities of typical alpha- and beta-blockers.

Learn the definitions that follow.

Table 10–1. Definitions.

Term	Definition
Competitive blocker	A surmountable antagonist; one that can be overcome by increasing the dose of agonist
Covalently bound inhibitor	An antagonist that binds irreversibly to its receptor or other binding site
Epinephrine reversal	Conversion of the pressor response (typical of large doses of epinephrine) to a blood pressure-lowering effect; caused by alpha blockers
Intrinsic sympathomimetic activity (ISA)	Partial agonist action by adrenoceptor blockers; typical of several beta blockers, eg, pindolol, acebutolol
Irreversible blocker	A nonsurmountable inhibitor, usually because of covalent bond formation; eg, phenoxybenzamine
Membrane stabilizing activity (MSA)	Local anesthetic action; typical of several beta-blockers, eg, propranolol
Orthostatic hypotension	Hypotension that is most marked in the upright position; caused by venous pooling or inadequate blood volume; typical of alpha blockade
Partial agonist	A drug (eg, pindolol) that produces a smaller maximal effect than a full agonist and therefore can inhibit the effect of a full agonist
Pheochromocytoma	A tumor that resembles the adrenal medulla; consisting of cells that release varying amounts of norepinephrine, epinephrine, or both into the circulation
Presynaptic receptor	A receptor located on the presynaptic nerve terminal; the receptor modulates transmitter release from the terminal

CONCEPTS

Alpha- and beta-blocking agents are divided into primary subgroups on the basis of their receptor selectivity (Figure 10–1). Because they differ markedly in their effects and clinical applications, these drugs are considered separately in the following discussion.

ALPHA-BLOCKING DRUGS

A. Classification: Subdivisions of the alpha-blockers are based on selective affinity for α_1 versus α_2 receptors. Other features used to classify the alpha-blocking drugs are their reversibility and duration of action.

1. **Irreversible, long-acting: Phenoxybenzamine** is the prototypical long-acting, irreversible alpha-blocker. It is slightly α_1-selective.
2. **Reversible, shorter-acting: Phentolamine** (nonselective) and **tolazoline** (slightly α_2-selective) are competitive, reversible blocking agents.

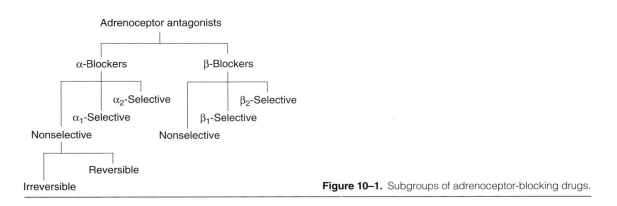

Figure 10–1. Subgroups of adrenoceptor-blocking drugs.

3. **Alpha₁-selective:** **Prazosin** is a selective, reversible pharmacologic α_1-blocker. Doxazosin and terazosin have similar properties. The advantage of α_1 selectivity is discussed below.

4. **Alpha₂-selective:** **Yohimbine** and **rauwolscine** are alpha₂-selective competitive pharmacologic antagonists. They are used primarily in research applications.

B. **Pharmacokinetics:** These drugs are all active when given by the oral as well as the parenteral route, though phentolamine and tolazoline are rarely given orally. Phenoxybenzamine has a short elimination half-life but a long duration of action—about 48 hours—because it binds covalently to its receptor. Phentolamine and tolazoline have durations of action of 2–4 hours when used orally and 20–40 minutes when given parenterally. Prazosin acts for 8–10 hours.

C. **Mechanism of Action:** Phenoxybenzamine binds covalently to the alpha receptor, thereby producing an irreversible (insurmountable) blockade. The other agents are competitive pharmacologic antagonists—ie, their effects can be surmounted by increased concentrations of agonist. This difference may be important in the treatment of pheochromocytoma, because a massive release of catecholamines from the tumor may overcome a reversible blockade.

D. **Effects:**
1. **Nonselective blockers:** These agents cause a predictable blockade of alpha-mediated responses to sympathetic nervous system discharge and exogenous sympathomimetics (ie, the alpha responses listed in Table 9–2). The most important effects of nonselective alpha-blockers are those on the cardiovascular system: a reduction in vascular tone with a reduction of both arterial and venous pressures. There are no significant direct cardiac effects. However, the nonselective alpha-blockers do cause baroreceptor reflex-mediated tachycardia as a result of the drop in mean arterial pressure (Figure 6–4). This tachycardia may be exaggerated because the alpha₂ receptors on adrenergic nerve terminals, which normally reduce the net release of norepinephrine, are also blocked (Figure 6–3).

   Epinephrine reversal is a predictable result of the use of this agonist in a patient who has received an alpha-blocker. The term refers to a reversal in the blood pressure effect of moderate to large doses of epinephrine, from a pressor response (mediated by alpha-receptors) to a depressor effect (mediated by β_2 receptors) (Figure 10–2). The effect is not observed with phenylephrine or norepinephrine because these drugs lack β_2 effects. Epinephrine reversal is occasionally seen as an unexpected (but predictable) effect of drugs for which alpha blockade is an adverse effect (eg, some phenothiazine tranquilizers, antihistamines).

2. **Selective alpha-blockers:** Because prazosin blocks vascular α_1 receptors much more effectively than the α_2-modulatory receptors associated with cardiac sympathetic nerve endings, this drug causes much less tachycardia than the nonselective alpha-blockers when reducing blood pressure.

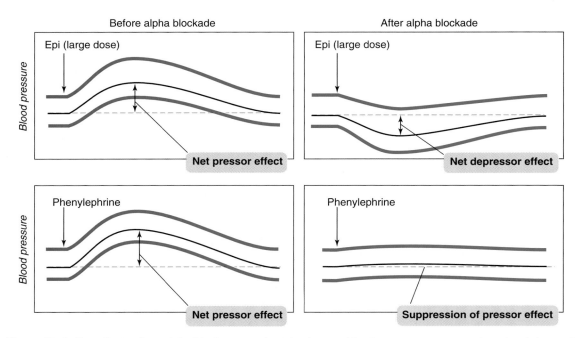

Figure 10–2. The effects of an alpha-blocker, eg, phentolamine, on blood pressure responses to epinephrine and phenylephrine. The epinephrine response exhibits reversal of the mean blood pressure change, from a net increase (the alpha response) to a net decrease (the beta$_2$ response). The response to phenylephrine is suppressed but not reversed, because phenylephrine is a "pure" alpha agonist without beta action.

E. **Clinical Uses:**
1. **Nonselective alpha-blockers:** Nonselective alpha-blockers have limited clinical applications. The best-documented application is in the presurgical management of pheochromocytoma. Such patients may have severe hypertension and reduced blood volume, which should be corrected before subjecting the patient to the stress of surgery. Phenoxybenzamine is usually used during this preparatory phase; phentolamine is sometimes used during surgery. Phenoxybenzamine also has serotonin receptor-blocking effects, which justify its occasional use in carcinoid tumor, and H$_1$ antihistamine effects, which lead to its use in mastocytosis.

   Accidental local infiltration of potent alpha agonists such as norepinephrine may lead to tissue ischemia and necrosis if not promptly reversed; infiltration of the ischemic area with phentolamine is sometimes used to prevent tissue damage. Overdose with drugs of abuse such as amphetamine, cocaine, or phenylpropanolamine may lead to severe hypertension because of their indirect sympathomimetic actions. This hypertension will usually respond well to alpha-blockers.

   Raynaud's phenomenon sometimes responds to phenoxybenzamine or phentolamine, but their efficacy is not well documented in this condition. Phentolamine or yohimbine is sometimes used by direct injection to cause penile erection in men with impotence.

2. **Selective alpha-blockers:** Prazosin and other α_1 blockers are used in hypertension (see Chapter 11). Selective α_1-blockers have also found increasing use in the management of urinary hesitancy and prevention of urinary retention in men with prostatic hyperplasia.

F. **Toxicity:** The most important toxicities of the alpha-blockers are simple extensions of their alpha-blocking effects. The main manifestations are orthostatic hypotension and, for the nonselective agents, reflex tachycardia. Phentolamine and tolazoline also have some non-alpha-mediated vasodilating effects. In patients with coronary disease, angina may be precipitated by the tachycardia. Oral administration of any of these drugs can cause nausea and vomiting. In some patients, α_1-selective blockers are associated with an exaggerated orthostatic hypotensive response to the first dose. Therefore, the first dose is usually small and taken just before going to bed.

BETA-BLOCKING DRUGS

A. **Classification, Subgroups, and Mechanisms:** All of the clinically used beta-blockers are competitive pharmacologic antagonists. Propranolol is the prototype. Drugs in this group are usually classified into subgroups on the basis of β_1 versus β_2 selectivity, partial agonist activity, local anesthetic action, and lipid solubility (Table 10–2).

1. **Receptor selectivity:** Beta$_1$ receptor selectivity (β_1 block > β_2 block), is a property of **metoprolol, atenolol, acebutolol,** and some other beta-blockers. This property may be an advantage when treating patients with asthma. **Butoxamine,** a β_2-selective drug, is used only in research.

    Labetalol is an unusual agent with combined alpha- and beta-blocking action. This drug has four diastereomers; the alpha-blocking activity resides in the SR enantiomer and the beta-blocking action in the RR enantiomer. The other two enantiomers (RS and SS) are virtually inactive. **Carvedilol,** a newer drug, has alpha- and beta-blocking actions in its two isomers.

2. **Partial agonist activity:** Partial agonist activity ("intrinsic sympathomimetic activity") may be an advantage in treating patients with asthma because, even at maximum dosage, these drugs (eg, **pindolol, acebutolol**) will—at least in theory—cause some bronchodilation. In contrast, the full antagonists such as propranolol may cause severe asthma in patients with airway disease.

3. **Local anesthetic activity:** Local anesthetic activity ("membrane-stabilizing activity") is a disadvantage when beta-blockers are used topically in the eye. Local anesthetic effects are absent from **timolol** and several newer beta-blockers.

4. **Pharmacokinetics:** The systemic agents have been developed for chronic oral use, but bioavailability and duration of action vary widely (Table 10–2). Esmolol is a short-acting ester beta-blocker that is used only parenterally. Nadolol is the longest-acting beta-blocker. Acebutolol and atenolol are less lipid-soluble than the older beta-blockers and probably enter the CNS to a lesser extent.

B. **Effects and Clinical Uses:** Most of the organ level effects of beta-blockers (Table 10–3) are predictable from blockade of the beta-receptor-mediated effects of sympathetic discharge. Effects of beta blockade not previously emphasized (and not recognized until beta-blockers became widely used) include reduction of aqueous humor formation in the eye and reduction of skeletal muscle tremor. The cardiovascular and ophthalmic applications are extremely important. The treatment of open-angle glaucoma involves the use of several groups of autonomic drugs; see Table 10–4. Treatment of congestive heart failure is a novel application of beta-

Table 10–2. Properties of several beta receptor-blocking drugs.*

Drug	Selectivity	Partial Agonist Activity	Local Anesthetic Action	Lipid Solubility	Elimination Half-Life	Approximate Bioavailability (%)
Acebutolol	β_1	Yes	Yes	Low	3–4 hours	50
Atenolol	β_1	No	No	Low	6–9 hours	40
Esmolol	β_1	No	No	Low	10 minutes	....
Carvedilol[1]	None	No	No	No data	7–10 hours	25–35
Labetalol[1]	None	Yes[2]	Yes	Moderate	5 hours	30
Metoprolol	β_1	No	Yes	Moderate	3–4 hours	50
Nadolol	None	No	No	Low	14–24 hours	33
Pindolol	None	Yes[2]	Yes	Moderate	3–4 hours	90
Propranolol	None	No	Yes	High	3.5–6 hours	30[3]
Timolol	None	No	No	Moderate	4–5 hours	50

*Modified and reproduced, with permission, from Katzung BG (editor): *Basic & Clinical Pharmacology,* 7th ed. Appleton & Lange, 1998.
[1]Also cause α_1 receptor blockade.
[2]Partial agonist effects at β_2 receptors.
[3]Bioavailability is dose-dependent.

Table 10–3. Clinical applications of beta-blockers.

Application	Drugs	Effect
Hypertension	Propranolol, metoprolol, timolol, others	Reduced cardiac output, reduced renin secretion
Angina pectoris	Propranolol, nadolol, others	Reduced cardiac rate and force
Arrhythmia prophylaxis after myocardial infarction	Propranolol, metoprolol, timolol	Reduced automaticity of all cardiac pacemakers
Supraventricular tachycardias	Propranolol, esmolol, acebutolol	Slowed AV conduction velocity
Hypertrophic cardiomyopathy	Propranolol	Slowed rate of cardiac contraction
Congestive heart failure	Carvedilol, labetalol, possibly others	Mechanism not understood
Migraine	Propranolol	Prophylactic; mechanism uncertain
Familial tremor, other types of tremor, "stage fright"	Propranolol	Reduced β_2 alteration of neuromuscular transmission; possible CNS effects
Thyroid storm, thyrotoxicosis	Propranolol	Reduced cardiac rate and arrhythmogenesis; other mechanisms may be involved
Glaucoma[1]	Timolol, others	Reduced secretion of aqueous humor

[1]See Table 10–4 for additional drugs used in glaucoma.

blockers, but studies suggest that several, including labetalol and carvedilol, may be beneficial when used in low dosage and titrated very carefully. It is not certain how much the alpha-blocking action of these agents contributes to their effect.

C. **Toxicity:** Cardiovascular adverse effects, which are extensions of the beta blockade induced by these agents, include bradycardia, atrioventricular blockade, and congestive heart failure. Patients with airway disease may suffer asthmatic attacks. Premonitory symptoms of hypoglycemia from insulin overdosage—eg, tachycardia, tremor, and anxiety—may be masked, and mobilization of glucose from the liver may be impaired. CNS adverse effects include sedation, fatigue, and sleep alterations. Atenolol, nadolol, and several other less lipid-soluble beta-blockers are claimed to have less marked CNS action because they do not enter the CNS as readily as other members of this group.

Table 10–4. Drugs used in glaucoma.*

Group, Drugs	Mechanism	Methods of Administration
Cholinomimetics Pilocarpine, carbachol, physostigmine, echothiophate	Ciliary muscle contraction, opening of trabecular meshwork; increased outflow	Topical drops or gel; plastic film slow-release insert
Alpha agonists, nonselective Epinephrine, dipivefrin	Increased outflow, probably via the uveoscleral veins	Topical drops
Alpha$_2$-selective agonists Apraclonidine, brimonidine	Decreased aqueous secretion	Topical drops
Beta-blockers Timolol, betaxolol, carteolol, levobunolol, metipranolol	Decreased aqueous secretion from the ciliary epithelium	Topical drops
Diuretics Acetazolamide, dorzolamide	Decreased secretion due to lack of HCO_3^- ion	Oral (acetazolamide) or topical (dorzolamide)
Ethacrynic acid (investigational)	Decreased secretion	Intraocular injection at long intervals, eg, annually

*Modified and reproduced, with permission, from Katzung BG (editor): *Basic & Clinical Pharmacology,* 7th ed. Appleton & Lange, 1998.

DRUG LIST

The following drugs are important members of the group discussed in this chapter. Prototypes should be learned in detail; the features of major variants should be known well enough so that the variants can be distinguished from prototypes and from each other; the other significant agents should be recognized as belonging to a specific subclass.

Subgroup	Prototype	Major Variants	Other Significant Agents
Alpha-blockers Nonselective	Phenoxybenzamine[1]	Phentolamine	
α_1-Selective	Prazosin		Terazosin, doxazosin
α_2-Selective	Yohimbine		Rauwolscine
Beta-blockers Nonselective	Propranolol	Timolol, nadolol	Carvedilol, labetalol
β_1-Selective	Metoprolol	Atenolol, esmolol	
β_2-Selective	Butoxamine		

[1]Compared to prazosin, phenoxybenzamine is only slightly α_1-selective.

QUESTIONS

DIRECTIONS: Each of the numbered items or incomplete statements in this section is followed by answers or by completions of the statement. Select the ONE lettered answer or completion that is BEST in each case.

1. Which of the following effects of epinephrine would be blocked by phentolamine but not by metoprolol?
   (A) Cardiac stimulation
   (B) Contraction of radial smooth muscle in the iris
   (C) Increase of cAMP in fat
   (D) Relaxation of bronchial smooth muscle
   (E) Relaxation of the uterus

2. Phentolamine and tolazoline
   (A) Are inactive by the oral route
   (B) Block both alpha and beta receptors
   (C) Cause hypertension
   (D) Cause tachycardia
   (E) Induce vasospasm in large doses

3. Propranolol is useful in all of the following EXCEPT
   (A) Angina
   (B) Familial tremor
   (C) Hypertension
   (D) Idiopathic hypertrophic subaortic cardiomyopathy
   (E) Partial atrioventricular nodal block

4. Adverse effects that limit the use of adrenoceptor blockers include
   (A) Bronchoconstriction from alpha-blocking agents
   (B) Congestive heart failure from beta-blockers
   (C) Impaired blood sugar response with alpha-blockers
   (D) Increased intraocular pressure with beta-blockers
   (E) Sleep disturbances from alpha-blocking drugs

Items 5–8: Four new synthetic drugs (designated W, X, Y, and Z) are to be studied for their cardiovascular effects. They are given to four anesthetized rats while the heart rates are recorded. The first animal has received no pretreatment ("control"); the second has received an effective dose of hexamethonium; the third has received an effective dose of atropine; and the fourth has received an effective dose of phenoxybenzamine. The net changes induced by the new drugs (not by the blocking drugs) are described in the following questions.

5. Drug W increased heart rate in the control animal, the atropine-pretreated animal, and the phenoxybenzamine-pretreated animal. However, Drug W had no effect on heart rate in the hexamethonium-pretreated animal. Drug W is probably
   (A) A drug similar to acetylcholine
   (B) A vasodilator that does not affect ANS receptors
   (C) A drug similar to norepinephrine
   (D) A drug similar to isoproterenol
   (E) A drug similar to edrophonium

6. Drug X had the effects shown in the table below.

In the Rat Receiving	Heart Rate Response to Drug X Was
No pretreatment	↓
Hexamethonium	↑
Atropine	↑
Phenoxybenzamine	↑

   Drug X is probably
   (A) A drug similar to acetylcholine
   (B) A vasodilator that does not affect ANS receptors
   (C) A drug similar to norepinephrine
   (D) A drug similar to isoproterenol
   (E) A drug similar to edrophonium

7. Drug Y had the effects shown in the table below.

In the Rat Receiving	Heart Rate Response to Drug Y Was
No pretreatment	↑
Hexamethonium	↑
Atropine	↑
Phenoxybenzamine	↑

   Drug Y is probably
   (A) A drug similar to acetylcholine
   (B) A vasodilator that does not affect ANS receptors
   (C) A drug similar to norepinephrine
   (D) A drug similar to isoproterenol
   (E) A drug similar to edrophonium

8. The results of the test of Drug Z are shown in the graph.

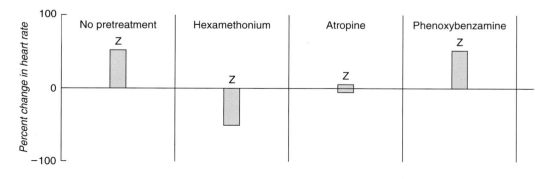

   Drug Z is probably
   (A) A drug similar to acetylcholine

    (B)   A vasodilator that does not affect ANS receptors
    (C)   A drug similar to norepinephrine
    (D)   A drug similar to isoproterenol
    (E)   A drug similar to edrophonium

9.   A traveler to your city visits you with a request for a renewal of his prescription for phenoxybenzamine. While preparing to telephone his physician, you recall that phenoxybenzamine is used in the treatment of all of the following EXCEPT
    (A)   Carcinoid
    (B)   Essential hypertension
    (C)   Mastocytosis
    (D)   Pheochromocytoma
    (E)   Raynaud's phenomenon

10.   When given to a patient, phentolamine blocks all of the following EXCEPT
    (A)   Vasoconstriction induced by norepinephrine
    (B)   Increased cardiac contractile force induced by norepinephrine
    (C)   Bradycardia induced by phenylephrine
    (D)   Pilomotor erection ("gooseflesh") induced by epinephrine
    (E)   Mydriasis induced by phenylephrine

11.   Pretreatment with propranolol will block which one of the following?
    (A)   Methacholine-induced tachycardia
    (B)   Nicotine-induced hypertension
    (C)   Norepinephrine-induced bradycardia
    (D)   Phenylephrine-induced mydriasis
    (E)   Pilocarpine-induced miosis

12.   Your 55-year-old patient with asthma and glaucoma is to receive a beta-blocking drug. Regarding beta-blocking drugs
    (A)   Esmolol's pharmacokinetics are compatible with chronic oral use
    (B)   Metoprolol blocks β_2 receptors selectively
    (C)   Nadolol lacks β_2-blocking action
    (D)   Pindolol is a beta antagonist with high membrane-stabilizing (local anesthetic) activity
    (E)   Timolol lacks the local anesthetic potency of propranolol

13.   Which of the following binds covalently to the site specified?
    (A)   Atenolol—beta receptor
    (B)   Carvedilol—cardiac beta receptors
    (C)   Labetalol—alpha and beta receptors
    (D)   Phenoxybenzamine—alpha receptor
    (E)   Pindolol—beta receptor

14.   A 60-year-old male patient presents with glaucoma. He also has mild prostatic hyperplasia. Your therapy might include
    (A)   Topical epinephrine
    (B)   Topical pilocarpine
    (C)   Topical timolol
    (D)   Oral acetazolamide
    (E)   Any of the above

15.   Your 38-year-old patient has symptoms highly suggestive of pheochromocytoma. Her urine VMA and metanephrine levels are highly elevated, but the normetanephrine level is below normal. She refuses treatment. A month later she enters a local hospital emergency room complaining of severe headache and chest pain. Imaging reveals a small subarachnoid hemorrhage, and ECG indicates a myocardial infarction. Her blood pressure is 230/150 mm Hg and her heart rate 150/min. She has been vomiting and is dehydrated. She is immediately given phentolamine intravenously, and an infusion of phenoxybenzamine is prepared. Ten minutes later, her blood pressure is 40/0 and she goes into shock. Vasoconstrictors are ineffective, and she dies after 6 hours. The cause of the exaggerated response to phentolamine in this patient is which one of the following?
    (A)   The patient's tumor secreted almost pure epinephrine with almost no norepinephrine
    (B)   The tumor had metastasized to the vasomotor center in the medulla
    (C)   The patient had abnormally low secretion of catecholamines from the tumor at the time of admission, so that the recommended dose of phentolamine constituted a major overdose
    (D)   The patient had a familial condition that limited autonomic nervous system control of the blood pressure

ANSWERS

1. Contraction of the pupillary dilator radial smooth muscle is mediated by alpha receptors. All the other effects are mediated by beta receptors. The answer is (**B**).

2. These alpha-blockers cause hypotension and significant reflex tachycardia. They have no beta-blocking action but do have histaminergic and cholinomimetic properties and never cause vasospasm. The answer is (**D**).

3. Atrioventricular block is an important **contraindication** to the use of beta-blockers. The answer is (**E**).

4. Congestive heart failure. Choices (**A**), (**C**), and (**E**) reverse the correct pairing of receptor subtype (alpha versus beta) with effect. Choice (**D**) reverses the direction of change of intraocular pressure. The answer is (**B**).

5. In developing a strategy for this type of question, consider first the actions of the known blocking drugs. Hexamethonium is very useful because it blocks reflexes as well as the direct action of nicotine. Atropine provides information regarding direct muscarinic effects of the unknown or reflex slowing of the heart mediated by the vagus. Phenoxybenzamine provides information only about alpha receptor-mediated processes. If the response produced in the nonpretreated animal is blocked or reversed by hexamethonium, it is probably a reflex response. In that case, consider all the receptors involved in mediating the reflex. Drug W causes tachycardia that is prevented by ganglion blockade and therefore is probably a compensatory reflex tachycardia. We do not have information about beta blockade, but a reflex tachycardia must be mediated by beta receptors in the heart. Two of the choices may cause a reflex tachycardia: the nonautonomic vasodilator and acetylcholine. However, the reflex tachycardia evoked by acetylcholine would be blocked by atropine (atropine would prevent the vasodilation that elicited the tachycardia). Thus, drug W must be a nonautonomic vasodilator. The answer is (**B**).

6. Drug X causes slowing of the heart rate, but this is converted into a tachycardia by hexamethonium and atropine—ie, the bradycardia is caused by reflex vagal discharge. Phenoxybenzamine also reverses the bradycardia to a tachycardia, suggesting that alpha receptors are needed to induce the reflex bradycardia and that X has direct beta agonist actions. The choices that evoke a vagal reflex bradycardia but can also cause a direct tachycardia are limited; the answer is (**C**).

7. Drug Y causes a tachycardia that is not significantly influenced by any of the blockers; therefore, drug Y must have a direct beta agonist effect on the heart. The answer is (**D**).

8. Drug Z causes tachycardia that is converted to bradycardia by hexamethonium and blocked completely by atropine. This indicates that the tachycardia is a reflex evoked by vasodilation. Drug Z causes bradycardia when the ganglia are blocked, indicating that it also has a direct muscarinic action on the heart. This is confirmed by the ability of atropine to block both the tachycardia and the bradycardia. The answer is (**A**).

9. Phenoxybenzamine is not useful in essential hypertension because it causes tachycardia and marked orthostatic hypotension. The drug is used in Raynaud's phenomenon, but efficacy in this application is controversial. The answer is (**B**).

10. Phenylephrine induces bradycardia through the baroreceptor reflex. Blockade of this drug's vasoconstrictor effect will prevent the bradycardia. Pilomotor erection is mediated by alpha receptors. The increase in cardiac force is mediated largely by beta receptors. The answer is (**B**).

11. The beta-blocker will not block the vagal slowing resulting from norepinephrine-induced hypertension. Nicotine-induced hypertension and phenylephrine-induced mydriasis are mediated by alpha receptors. Pilocarpine is a muscarinic agonist. The answer is (**A**).

12. Esmolol is a short-acting beta blocker for parenteral use only. Nadolol is a nonselective beta-blocker, and metoprolol is a β_1-selective blocker. Timolol is useful in glaucoma because it does not anesthetize the cornea. The answer is (**E**).

13. Phenoxybenzamine is the only autonomic receptor blocker in clinical use that binds covalently with its receptor. The answer is (**D**).

14. All of the drugs listed are used in glaucoma (see Table 10–4). Acetazolamide and dorzolamide are discussed in Chapter 15. The answer is (**E**).

15. Note that the original workup of the patient showed highly elevated metanephrine but lower than normal normetanephrine. This suggests that the tumor produced almost pure epinephrine and little or no norepinephrine (recall the metabolites of epinephrine and norepinephrine from Chapter 6). A patient with this type of tumor may have a dramatic *epinephrine reversal* response to any alpha-blocker, plunging the blood pressure to shock levels. This is especially true if the blood volume is low. Although most pheochromocytomas produce a mixture of norepinephrine and epinephrine, cases like the one described have been reported in the literature. The answer is (**A**).

Part III: Cardiovascular Drugs

Drugs Used in Hypertension

11

OBJECTIVES

You should be able to:

- List the four major groups of antihypertensive drugs and give examples of drugs in each group.
- Describe the compensatory responses to each of the four major types of antihypertensive drugs.
- List the major sites of action of sympathoplegic drugs and give examples of drugs that act at each site.
- List the major antihypertensive vasodilator drugs and describe their actions.
- List the major toxicities of the prototype antihypertensive agents.
- Explain why some combinations of antihypertensive drugs are rational and appropriate and others are not.

Learn the definitions that follow.

Table 11–1. Definitions.

Term	Definition
Baroreceptor reflex	Primary autonomic mechanism for blood pressure homeostasis; involves sensory input from carotid sinus to the vasomotor center and output via the parasympathetic and sympathetic motor nerves
Catecholamine reuptake pump	Nerve terminal transporter responsible for recycling catecholamine transmitters after release into the synapse
Catecholamine vesicle pump	Storage vesicle transporter that pumps amine from cytoplasm into vesicle
End organ damage	Vascular damage in heart, kidney, retina, or brain; usually caused by hypertension
Essential hypertension	Hypertension of unknown cause; also called "primary" hypertension
False transmitter	Substance stored in vesicles and released into synaptic cleft but lacking the effect of the true transmitter
Malignant hypertension	Accelerated hypertension causing rapid damage to vessels in end organs; a medical emergency
Orthostatic hypotension	Hypotension on assuming upright posture; postural hypotension
Postganglionic neuron blocker	Drug that blocks transmission by an action in the presynaptic postganglionic nerve terminal
Rebound hypertension	Elevated blood pressure resulting from loss of antihypertensive drug effect
Reflex tachycardia	Tachycardia resulting from lowering of blood pressure; mediated by the baroreceptor reflex
Stepped care	Progressive addition of drugs to a regimen, starting with one (usually a diuretic) and adding in stepwise fashion a sympatholytic, a vasodilator, and (sometimes) an ACE inhibitor
Sympatholytic, sympathoplegic	Drug that reduces effects of the sympathetic nervous system

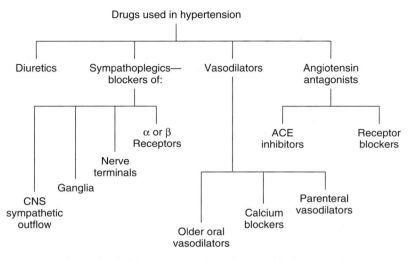

Figure 11–1. Subgroups of drugs discussed in this chapter.

CONCEPTS

Antihypertensive drugs are organized around a clinical indication—the need to treat a disease—rather than a receptor type. As a result, the drugs covered in this unit are much more heterogeneous than those in the preceding chapters on autonomic drugs. The antihypertensive drugs include diuretics, sympathoplegics, vasodilators, and angiotensin antagonists (Figure 11–1).

The strategies for treating high blood pressure are based on the determinants of arterial pressure (see Figure 6–4). These strategies include reduction of blood volume, sympathetic tone, vascular smooth muscle tone, and angiotensin effects. Because of the baroreceptor reflex, the compensatory homeostatic responses to these drugs may be significant (Table 11–2).

As indicated in Figure 11–2, the compensatory responses can be counteracted with β-blockers or reserpine (for tachycardia) and diuretics or ACE inhibitors (for salt and water retention).

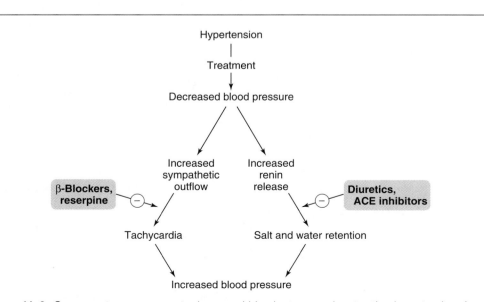

Figure 11–2. Compensatory responses to decreased blood pressure when treating hypertension. Arrows with minus signs indicate drugs used to minimize the compensatory responses.

DIURETICS

These drugs are covered in greater detail in Chapter 15 but are mentioned in this chapter because of their importance in hypertension. Diuretics lower blood pressure by reduction of blood volume and by a direct vascular effect that is not yet understood. The diuretics most important for treating hypertension are the **thiazides** (eg, hydrochlorothiazide). The **loop diuretics** (eg, furosemide) are used in severe and in malignant hypertension. Compensatory responses to blood pressure lowering by diuretics are minimal (Table 11–2). The maximum antihypertensive effect of thiazides is often achieved with doses less than those required for maximum diuretic effect.

SYMPATHOPLEGICS

Sympathoplegic drugs interfere with sympathetic nerve function in several ways. The result is a reduction of one or more of the following: venous tone, heart rate, contractile force of the heart, cardiac output, and total peripheral resistance. Compensatory responses and adverse effects are marked for some of these agents (Table 11–2). Sympathoplegics are subdivided by anatomic site of action (Figure 11–3).

Table 11–2. Compensatory responses to antihypertensive drugs and some of their adverse effects.

Class and Drug	Compensatory Responses	Adverse Effects of Drugs
Diuretics		
Hydrochlorothiazide	Minimal	Hypokalemia, slight hyperlipidemia, hyperuricemia, hyperglycemia, lassitude, weakness, impotence
Sympathoplegics		
Veratrum alkaloids	Salt and water retention	Vomiting, diarrhea
Clonidine	Salt and water retention	Dry mouth, severe rebound hypertension if drug is suddenly stopped
Methyldopa	Salt and water retention	Sedation, positive Coombs test, hemolytic anemia
Ganglion blockers	Salt and water retention	Orthostatic hypotension, constipation, blurred vision, sexual dysfunction
Reserpine (low dose)	Minimal	Diarrhea, nasal stuffiness, sedation, depression
Guanethidine	Salt and water retention	Orthostatic hypotension, retrograde ejaculation
α_1-Selective blockers	Salt and water retention, slight tachycardia	Orthostatic hypotension (limited to first few doses)
β-Blockers	Minimal	Sleep disturbances, sedation, impotence, cardiac disturbances, asthma
Vasodilators		
Hydralazine	Salt and water retention, marked tachycardia	Lupus-like syndrome (but lacking renal effects)
Minoxidil	Marked salt and water retention, very marked tachycardia	Hirsutism, pericardial effusion
Nifedipine	Minor salt and water retention	Constipation, cardiac disturbances, flushing
Nitroprusside	Salt and water retention	Cyanide toxicity (CN^- released)
Angiotensin antagonists		
ACE inhibitors (eg, captopril)	Minimal	Cough, renal damage in preexisting renal disease and in the fetus
Angiotensin II receptor blockers (eg, losartan)	Minimal	Renal damage in preexisting renal disease and in the fetus

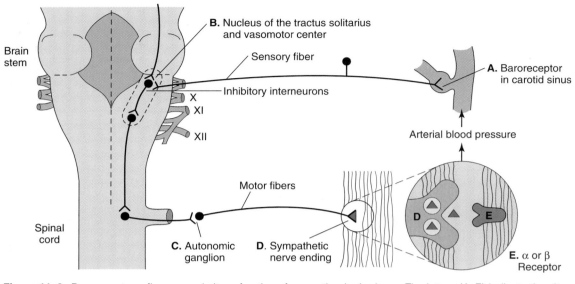

Figure 11–3. Baroreceptor reflex arc and sites of action of sympathoplegic drugs. The letters (A–E) indicate the sites of action of subgroups of sympathoplegics.

A. Baroreceptor-Active Agents: The veratrum alkaloids sensitize the carotid sinus baroreceptors. This leads to a reduction in sympathetic outflow and an increase in parasympathetic outflow. These drugs produce significant adverse gastrointestinal effects and are obsolete.

B. CNS-Active Agents: Alpha$_2$-selective agonists (eg, **clonidine, methyldopa**) cause a decrease in sympathetic outflow by a mechanism that involves activation of α_2 receptors in the CNS. These drugs readily enter the CNS when given orally. Methyldopa is a prodrug; it is converted to methylnorepinephrine in the brain. Clonidine and methyldopa both reduce blood pressure by reducing cardiac output or vascular resistance (or both) to some degree. The major compensatory response is salt retention. Sudden discontinuation of clonidine causes rebound hypertension, which may be quite severe. This rebound increase in blood pressure can be controlled by reinstitution of clonidine therapy or administration of alpha-blockers such as phentolamine. Methyldopa causes hematologic immunotoxicity, initially with agglutination of sheep red blood cells (positive Coombs test) and in some patients progressing to hemolytic anemia. Both drugs may cause sedation—methyldopa more so.

C. Ganglion-Blocking Drugs: Nicotinic blockers are very efficacious but because of their severe adverse effects (Table 11–2) are now considered obsolete. **Hexamethonium** and **trimethaphan** are extremely powerful blood pressure-lowering drugs. The major compensatory response is salt retention. Toxicities include parasympathetic blockade (blurred vision, constipation, urinary hesitancy, impotence) and sympathetic blockade (retrograde ejaculation, orthostatic hypotension).

D. Postganglionic Sympathetic Nerve Terminal Blockers: Drugs that deplete the adrenergic nerve terminal of its norepinephrine stores (eg, **reserpine**), block release of these stores, or both deplete and block release (eg, **guanethidine**) may be useful antihypertensive drugs. The major compensatory response is salt retention. In high doses, both reserpine and guanethidine produce a high incidence of adverse effects. Reserpine is still sometimes used in low doses as an adjunct to other agents. Guanethidine is now rarely used. Reserpine readily enters the CNS; guanethidine does not. Both have long durations of action (days to weeks). The most serious toxicity of reserpine is behavioral depression, which may require discontinuation of the drug. The major toxicities of guanethidine are orthostatic hypotension and sexual dysfunction. Guanethidine requires the catecholamine reuptake pump (uptake 1; see Figure 6–2) to reach its intracellular site of action. Therefore, drugs that inhibit this pump (eg, cocaine, tricyclic antidepressants) will interfere with the action of guanethidine.

MAO inhibitors are of interest in hypertension because they cause the formation of a false transmitter (octopamine) in sympathetic postganglionic neuron terminals and lower blood pressure. Octopamine is stored in the adrenergic vesicles along with norepinephrine. Normal nerve action potentials release this weak false transmitter with reduced amounts of norepinephrine, resulting in diminished vascular and cardiac responses. However, large doses of indirect-acting sympathomimetics (eg, the tyramine in a meal of fermented foods) may cause release of large amounts of stored norepinephrine and result in a hypertensive crisis. Because of this risk and the availability of better drugs, MAO inhibitors are no longer used in hypertension.

E. **Adrenoceptor Blockers:** An α_1-selective agent (eg, **prazosin**) or one of many beta-blockers (eg, **propranolol**) is often used. Alpha-blockers reduce vascular resistance. The nonselective alpha-blockers (phentolamine, phenoxybenzamine) are of no value in chronic hypertension because of excessive compensatory responses, especially tachycardia. Alpha$_1$-selective adrenoceptor blockers are relatively free of the severe adverse effects of the nonselective alpha-blockers and postganglionic nerve terminal sympathoplegic agents.

Beta-blockers initially reduce cardiac output, but after a few days their action may include a decrease in vascular resistance as a contributing effect. The latter effect may result from reduced angiotensin levels (beta-blockers reduce renin release from the kidney). The beta-blockers are among the most heavily used antihypertensive drugs. Beta-blocker therapy is associated with slightly elevated triglyceride and diminished high-density lipoprotein levels in the blood; other potential adverse effects are listed in Table 11–2.

VASODILATORS

Drugs that dilate blood vessels by acting directly on smooth muscle cells through nonautonomic mechanisms are useful in treating many hypertensive patients. Three major mechanisms are utilized by vasodilators: release of nitric oxide, opening of potassium channels (which leads to hyperpolarization), and blockade of calcium channels. Compensatory responses may be marked and include salt retention and tachycardia (Table 11–2).

A. **Hydralazine and Minoxidil:** These older vasodilators have more effect on arterioles than on veins. They are orally active and suitable for chronic therapy. The mechanism of hydralazine's action is uncertain but may involve release of nitric oxide. The toxicity of hydralazine includes compensatory responses (tachycardia, salt and water retention; see Table 11–2) and a risk of drug-induced lupus erythematosus that is reversible upon stopping the drug. However, lupus is uncommon at dosage levels below 200 mg/d.

Minoxidil is extremely efficacious and is thus reserved for severe hypertension. Minoxidil is a prodrug; its metabolite, minoxidil sulfate, is a potassium channel opener that hyperpolarizes and relaxes vascular smooth muscle. The toxicity of minoxidil consists of severe compensatory responses (Table 11–2, Figure 11–2), hirsutism, and pericardial abnormalities.

B. **Calcium Channel-Blocking Agents:** Calcium channel blockers (eg, **nifedipine, verapamil, diltiazem**) are effective vasodilators; because they are orally active, these drugs are suitable for chronic use in hypertension of any severity. Many analogs of nifedipine are also available. Because they produce fewer compensatory responses, the calcium channel blockers are usually preferred to hydralazine and minoxidil. Their mechanism of action and toxicities are discussed in Chapter 12.

C. **Nitroprusside and Diazoxide:** These parenteral vasodilators are used in hypertensive emergencies. Nitroprusside is a short-acting agent (duration of action is a few minutes) that must be infused continuously. The drug's mechanism of action is probably similar to that of the nitrates: the release of nitric oxide stimulates guanylyl cyclase and increases cGMP concentration in smooth muscle. The toxicity of nitroprusside includes excessive hypotension, tachycardia, and, if infusion is continued over several days, cumulation of cyanide or thiocyanate in the blood.

Diazoxide is given as intravenous boluses and has a duration of action of several hours. Diazoxide opens potassium channels, thus hyperpolarizing and relaxing smooth muscle cells. This drug also reduces insulin release and can be used to treat hypoglycemia caused by an insulin-producing tumor. The toxicity of diazoxide includes hypotension, hyperglycemia, and salt and water retention.

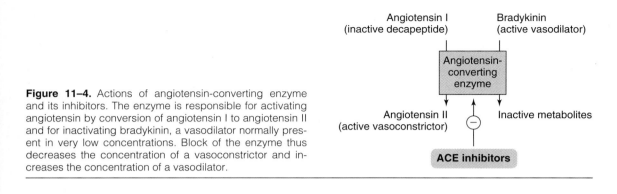

Figure 11–4. Actions of angiotensin-converting enzyme and its inhibitors. The enzyme is responsible for activating angiotensin by conversion of angiotensin I to angiotensin II and for inactivating bradykinin, a vasodilator normally present in very low concentrations. Block of the enzyme thus decreases the concentration of a vasoconstrictor and increases the concentration of a vasodilator.

ANGIOTENSIN ANTAGONISTS

The two primary groups of angiotensin antagonists are the **ACE inhibitors** and the **angiotensin II receptor blockers.** The more extensively used drugs are the ACE inhibitors (eg, **captopril**), which inhibit the enzyme variously known as angiotensin-converting enzyme, kininase II, and peptidyl dipeptidase. The result is a *reduction* in blood levels of angiotensin II and aldosterone and probably an *increase* in endogenous vasodilators of the kinin family (bradykinin; Figure 11–4). ACE inhibitors have a low incidence of serious adverse effects when given in normal doses and produce minimal compensatory responses (Table 11–2). The toxicities of ACE inhibitors include cough (up to 30% of patients), renal damage in occasional patients with preexisting renal disease (though they *protect* the diabetic kidney), and renal damage in the fetus. These drugs should not be used during pregnancy.

The second group of angiotensin antagonists, the receptor blockers, are represented by the orally active agents **losartan** and **valsartan** plus an older parenteral drug, **saralasin,** all of which competitively inhibit angiotensin II at its AT_1 receptor site (saralasin is a partial agonist used only in research). Losartan and valsartan appear to be as effective in lowering blood pressure as the ACE inhibitors and have the advantage of a much lower incidence of cough. However, they do cause fetal renal toxicity like that of the ACE inhibitors.

These drugs reduce aldosterone levels (angiotensin II is a major stimulant of aldosterone release) and cause potassium retention. Potassium accumulation may be marked, especially if the patient is consuming a high-potassium diet or taking other drugs that tend to conserve potassium, eg, "potassium-sparing" diuretics. Under these circumstances, potassium concentrations may reach toxic levels.

CLINICAL USES OF ANTIHYPERTENSIVE DRUGS

A. **Stepped Care:**   Therapy of hypertension requires attention to the problem of patient compliance, because the disease is symptomless until far advanced and the drugs are expensive and sometimes cause significant toxicities. This requirement gave rise to the concept of using multiple drugs to minimize individual drug toxicities. This approach is still used in patients with severe hypertension. Typically, drugs are added to a patient's regimen in stepwise fashion ("stepped care"); each additional agent is chosen from a different subgroup until adequate blood pressure control has been achieved. The usual steps include (1) lifestyle measures such as salt restriction and weight reduction, (2) diuretics, (3) sympathoplegics, (4) vasodilators, and (5) ACE inhibitors. The ability of drugs in steps 2 and 3 to control the compensatory responses induced by the others should be noted (eg, propranolol reduces the tachycardia induced by hydralazine).

B. **Monotherapy:**   It has been found in large clinical studies that many patients do well on a single drug (eg, an ACE inhibitor, calcium channel blocker, or alpha$_1$-blocker). This approach to the treatment of mild and moderate hypertension has become more popular than stepped care because of its simplicity, better patient compliance, and relatively low incidence of toxicity.

C. **Age and Ethnicity:**   Older patients of most races respond better to diuretics and beta-blockers than to ACE inhibitors. African-Americans of all ages respond better to diuretics and calcium channel blockers, less well to ACE inhibitors.

D. Malignant Hypertension: Malignant hypertension is an accelerated phase of severe hypertension associated with rapidly progressing damage to end organs and rising blood pressure. This condition may be signaled by deterioration of renal function, encephalopathy, and retinal hemorrhages, or by angina, stroke, or myocardial infarction. Management of malignant hypertension must be conducted on an emergency basis in the hospital. Powerful vasodilators (nitroprusside or diazoxide) are combined with diuretics (furosemide if necessary) and beta-blockers to lower the blood pressure promptly (within a few hours) to the 140–160/90–110 mm Hg range. Further reduction can then be pursued more slowly.

DRUG LIST

The following drugs are important members of the group discussed in this chapter. Prototypes should be learned in detail; features of the major variants should be known well enough so that the variants can be distinguished from prototypes and from each other; the other significant agents should be recognized as belonging to a specific subclass.

Subgroups	Prototypes	Major Variants	Other Significant Agents
Diuretics	Thiazides or loop diuretics, see Chapter 15		

Sympathoplegics
  Carotid sinus
    sensitizers
	Veratrum alkaloids
	  (obsolete)		

CNS action	Clonidine, methyldopa		
Ganglion blockers	Hexamethonium		Trimethaphan
Postganglionic neuron blockers	Reserpine, guanethidine		
Receptor blockers	Prazosin, propranolol	See Chapter 10	
Vasodilators	Hydralazine, nifedipine, nitroprusside	Minoxidil, verapamil, diazoxide	
Angiotensin antagonists ACE inhibitors	Captopril		Enalapril, lisinopril
Angiotensin II receptor blockers	Losartan		Valsartan, saralasin

QUESTIONS

DIRECTIONS: Each of the numbered items or incomplete statements in this section is followed by answers or by completions of the statement. Select the ONE lettered answer or completion that is BEST in each case.

1. A friend of yours has very severe hypertension and asks about a drug her doctor wishes to prescribe. Her physician has explained that this drug is associated with tachycardia and fluid retention (which may be marked) and increased hair growth. Which of the following is most likely to produce the effects your friend has described?
    (A) Captopril
    (B) Guanethidine
    (C) Minoxidil
    (D) Prazosin
    (E) Propranolol

2. A patient is admitted to the emergency department with severe bradycardia following a drug overdose. His family reports that he has been depressed about his hypertension. Each of the following can slow the heart rate EXCEPT
    (A) Clonidine
    (B) Guanethidine
    (C) Hydralazine
    (D) Propranolol
    (E) Reserpine

3. In comparing methyldopa and guanethidine, which of the following is correct?
    (A) Guanethidine—but not methyldopa—results in salt and water retention if used without a diuretic
    (B) Guanethidine is less efficacious than methyldopa in severe hypertension
    (C) Guanethidine causes fewer CNS adverse effects (such as sedation) than methyldopa
    (D) Methyldopa causes more orthostatic hypotension than guanethidine
    (E) Guanethidine causes more immunologic adverse effects (eg, hemolytic anemia) than methyldopa

4. Captopril and enalapril do all of the following EXCEPT
    (A) Increase renin concentration in the blood
    (B) Inhibit an enzyme
    (C) Competitively block angiotensin II at its receptor
    (D) Decrease angiotensin II concentration in the blood
    (E) Increase sodium and decrease potassium in the urine

5. A patient is admitted to the hematology service with moderately severe hemolytic anemia. After a thorough workup, the only positive finding is a history of several months' treatment with an antihypertensive drug. The most likely cause of the patient's blood disorder is
    (A) Atenolol
    (B) Captopril
    (C) Hydralazine
    (D) Methyldopa
    (E) Minoxidil

6. Postural hypotension is a recognized adverse effect of all of the following types of drugs EXCEPT
    (A) Venodilators
    (B) Ganglion blockers
    (C) Alpha-receptor blockers
    (D) Beta-receptor blockers
    (E) Powerful diuretics

7. A visitor from another city comes to your office complaining of incessant cough. He has diabetes and hypertension and has recently started taking a new antihypertensive medication. The most likely cause of his cough is
    (A) Enalapril
    (B) Losartan
    (C) Minoxidil
    (D) Propranolol
    (E) Verapamil

8. Important (though uncommon) adverse effects of vasodilators include all of the following EXCEPT
    (A) Lupus erythematosus with hydralazine
    (B) Reduced cardiac output or atrioventricular block with verapamil
    (C) Hypoglycemia with diazoxide
    (D) Pericardial abnormalities with minoxidil
    (E) Cyanide toxicity with nitroprusside

9. Comparison of prazosin with propranolol shows that
    (A) Both increase heart rate
    (B) Both increase central sympathetic outflow
    (C) Both decrease cardiac output
    (D) Both produce orthostatic hypotension
    (E) Both decrease renin secretion

10. Reserpine, an alkaloid derived from the root of *Rauwolfia serpentina*
    (A) Has been used in large doses to control hyperglycemia
    (B) Can cause psychiatric depression
    (C) Can decrease gastrointestinal secretion and motility
    (D) Often causes a reflex increase in heart rate when the drug lowers blood pressure
    (E) Is the safest of the sympathoplegic agents

DIRECTIONS (Items 11–16): The following section consists of a list of four to twenty-six lettered options followed by several numbered items. For each numbered item, select the ONE option that is MOST closely associated with it. Each answer may be selected once, more than once, or not at all.

(A) Captopril
(B) Cocaine
(C) Diazoxide
(D) Guanethidine
(E) Hydralazine
(F) Minoxidil
(G) Nifedipine
(H) Nitroprusside
(I) Prazosin
(J) Propranolol
(K) Reserpine
(L) Vesamicol

11. A drug used in severe hypertensive emergencies; very short acting; must be given by IV infusion
12. A vasodilator that causes hirsutism
13. A postganglionic nerve terminal blocker that has insignificant CNS effects
14. A calcium channel blocker useful in hypertension
15. A drug that may cause renal damage in the fetus if given during pregnancy
16. A drug that will interfere with the action of guanethidine

ANSWERS

1. Marked tachycardia and fluid retention are compensatory responses usually seen with strong vasodilators. The fact that the unknown drug also increases hair growth points strongly at minoxidil. The answer is (C).
2. Except for alpha-blockers, any sympathoplegic can, in sufficient dosage, cause bradycardia. Conversely, any vasodilator may induce tachycardia and, unless it is also sympathoplegic or a calcium channel blocker, will never slow heart rate. The answer is (C).
3. Guanethidine causes many peripheral adverse effects but is poorly distributed into the CNS, so it is relatively free of CNS effects. The answer is (C).
4. These converting enzyme inhibitors act on the enzyme, not on the angiotensin receptor. The plasma renin level may increase owing to the compensatory response to reduced angiotensin II. The answer is (C).
5. Methyldopa is the only antihypertensive drug associated with hemolytic anemia (usually preceded by a positive Coombs test). Hydralazine is also associated with autoimmune toxicity, but this takes the form of a lupus-like syndrome with butterfly facial rash, fever, joint and muscle pain, and antinuclear antibodies. The answer is (D).
6. Beta-blocking drugs do not cause orthostatic hypotension unless the patient is also suffering from severe heart failure, eg, following a myocardial infarction. The answer is (D).
7. Chronic cough is a common adverse effect of ACE inhibitors. It may sometimes be prevented by prior administration of aspirin. Angiotensin II receptor blockers such as losartan and valsartan cause a much lower incidence of cough but do cause renal damage in the fetus. The answer is (A).
8. Diazoxide is sometimes used to *treat* hypoglycemia because it can inhibit insulin release. It does not cause hypoglycemia. The answer is (C).
9. Prazosin—but not propranolol—may increase heart rate. Propranolol—but not prazosin—may decrease cardiac output. Propranolol does not cause orthostatic hypotension. Prazosin may increase renin output (a compensatory response), but beta-blockers inhibit its release by the kidney. By reducing blood pressure, both may increase central sympathetic outflow (a compensatory response). The answer is (B).
10. Reserpine is of no value in hyperglycemia. The drug does not induce reflex tachycardia because it reduces sympathetic neurotransmitter release in the heart as well as the vessels. This drug can cause dangerous psychiatric depression. The answer is (B).
11. Diazoxide, nitroprusside, and (rarely) nifedipine are the drugs in the list that are used in hypertensive emergencies. Diazoxide has a long duration of action and is given by intermittent injection, not by infusion. Nifedipine is almost always given orally. The answer is (H).
12. Minoxidil is the only drug in this list that regularly causes hirsutism. In fact, the drug is also marketed for the treatment of baldness. The answer is (F).
13. Reserpine and guanethidine are both sympathoplegics that act on the postganglionic sympathetic nerve terminal. Reserpine enters the CNS readily and causes important CNS toxicity.

Guanethidine, on the other hand, is too polar to cross the blood-brain barrier easily and is almost devoid of central toxicity. The answer is **(D)**.

14. Most of the calcium channel blockers are useful in hypertension; nifedipine is one of them. The answer is **(G)**.

15. All ACE inhibitors can cause renal damage in patients with preexisting renal disease and in the developing fetus. Captopril has been shown to have these effects. (The angiotensin II receptor antagonists appear to have similar renal toxicity.) The answer is **(A)**.

16. Cocaine can prevent the uptake of guanethidine into the nerve terminal because the drug blocks uptake 1, the catecholamine reuptake transporter in the nerve terminal membrane. The answer is **(B)**.

12 Vasodilators & the Treatment of Angina

OBJECTIVES

You should be able to:

- List the major determinants of cardiac oxygen consumption.
- List the strategies for relief of anginal pain.
- Contrast the therapeutic and adverse effects of nitrates, beta-blockers, and calcium channel blockers when used for angina.
- Explain why a combination of a nitrate with a beta-blocker or a calcium channel blocker may be extremely effective.
- Contrast the effects of medical therapy and surgical therapy of angina.

Learn the definitions that follow.

Table 12–1. Definitions.

Term	Definition
Angina of effort, classic angina, atherosclerotic angina	Angina (crushing, strangling, chest pain) that is precipitated by exertion, ie, increased O_2 demand that cannot be met because of irreversible atherosclerotic obstruction of coronary arteries
Vasospastic angina, variant angina, Prinzmetal's angina	Angina precipitated by reversible spasm of coronary vessels
Coronary vasodilator	Older, incorrect name for drugs useful in angina; drugs that relieve angina of effort do not act primarily through coronary vasodilation; some potent coronary vasodilators are ineffective in angina
Venodilator	Drug that selectively dilates veins, eg, nitroglycerin
"Monday disease"	Industrial disease caused by chronic exposure to vasodilating concentrations of organic nitrates in the workplace; characterized by headache, dizziness, and tachycardia on Mondays
Nitrate tolerance	Loss of effect of a nitrate venodilator when exposure is prolonged
Unstable angina	Rapidly progressing increase in frequency and severity of anginal attacks, especially pain at rest; probably heralds imminent myocardial infarction
Preload	Filling pressure of the heart; determines end-diastolic fiber length and tension
Afterload	Resistance to ejection of stroke volume; determined by arterial blood pressure and arterial stiffness
Intramyocardial fiber tension	Force exerted by myocardial fibers, especially ventricular fibers at any given time; a primary determinant of O_2 requirement
Double product	The product of heart rate and systolic blood pressure; an estimate of cardiac work
Myocardial revascularization	Mechanical intervention to improve O_2 delivery to the myocardium by angioplasty or bypass grafting

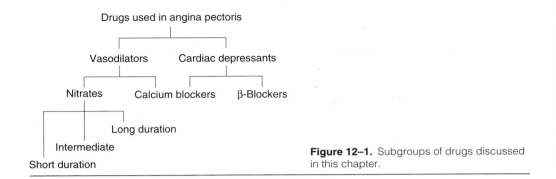

Figure 12–1. Subgroups of drugs discussed in this chapter.

CONCEPTS

PATHOPHYSIOLOGY OF ANGINA

A. Determinants of Cardiac Oxygen Requirement: The treatment of coronary insufficiency is based on physiologic factors that control the myocardial oxygen requirement. A major determinant is **myocardial fiber tension,** ie, the higher the tension, the greater the oxygen requirement (Figure 12–2).

Several variables contribute to fiber tension.

1. **Preload:**   Preload (diastolic filling pressure) is a function of blood volume and venous tone. Because venous tone is mainly controlled by sympathetic outflow, activities that increase sympathetic activity usually increase preload.

2. **Afterload:**   Afterload or arterial blood pressure is one of the systolic determinants of oxygen requirement. Arterial blood pressure depends on peripheral vascular resistance, which is determined by sympathetic outflow to the arteriolar vessels and other factors.

3. **Heart rate:**   Heart rate contributes to time-integrated fiber tension because at fast heart rates, fibers spend more time at systolic tension levels; at faster rates, diastole is abbreviated, and diastole constitutes the time available for coronary flow (coronary blood flow is low or nil during systole). Systolic blood pressure and heart rate may be multiplied to yield the **double product,** a measure of cardiac work and therefore oxygen requirement. In patients with atherosclerotic angina, effective drugs reduce the double product.

4. **Cardiac contractility:**   Force of cardiac contraction is another systolic factor controlled mainly by sympathetic outflow to the heart. Ejection time for ventricular contraction is inversely related to force of contraction but is also influenced by impedance to outflow. Increased ejection time increases oxygen requirement.

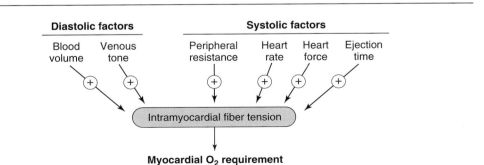

Figure 12–2. Determinants of MVO$_2$, the minute volume of oxygen required by the heart. Both diastolic and systolic factors contribute to the MVO$_2$; most of these factors are directly influenced by sympathetic discharge (venous tone, peripheral resistance, heart rate, and heart force).

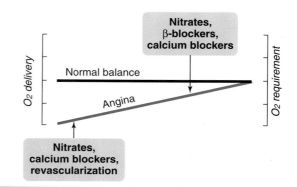

Figure 12–3. Strategies for the treatment of angina pectoris. Angina is characterized by reduced coronary oxygen delivery versus oxygen requirement. In some cases, this can be corrected by increasing oxygen delivery (box on left: revascularization or, in the case of reversible vasospasm, nitrates and calcium channel blockers). More often, drugs are used to reduce oxygen requirement (box on right: nitrates, β-blockers, and calcium channel blockers).

B. Types of Angina: There are three forms of angina pectoris.

   1. Atherosclerotic angina: Atherosclerotic angina is also known as angina of effort or classic angina. It is associated with atheromatous plaques that partially occlude one or more coronaries. When cardiac work increases (eg, in exercise), the obstruction of flow results in the accumulation of acidic metabolites and ischemic changes stimulate myocardial pain-mediating nerve endings. Atherosclerotic angina constitutes about 90% of angina cases and—depending on the rate of progression of the atheromas—may last for years with little change.

   2. Vasospastic angina: Vasospastic angina is also known as variant angina or Prinzmetal's angina. It involves reversible spasm of coronaries, usually at the site of an atherosclerotic plaque. Spasm may occur at any time, even during sleep. Vasospastic angina may deteriorate into unstable angina.

   3. Unstable angina: The third type of angina, unstable or crescendo angina, is caused by diminished coronary flow that results from a combination of atherosclerotic plaques, platelet aggregation at fractured plaques, and vasospasm. Unstable angina is thought to be the immediate precursor of a myocardial infarction and is treated as a medical emergency.

C. Therapeutic Strategies: The defect that causes anginal pain is coronary oxygen delivery inadequate for the myocardial oxygen requirement. This defect can be corrected in two ways: by **increasing oxygen delivery** or by **reducing oxygen requirement** (Figure 12–3). Pharmacologic therapies include the nitrates, the calcium channel blockers, and the beta-blockers. All three groups reduce oxygen requirement in atherosclerotic angina; nitrates and calcium channel blockers (but not beta-blockers) can also increase oxygen delivery by reducing vasospasm—but only in the vasospastic form. **Myocardial revascularization** corrects coronary obstruction either by bypass grafting or by angioplasty (enlargement of the lumen by means of a special catheter).

NITRATES

A. Classification and Pharmacokinetics: Nitroglycerin (the active ingredient in dynamite) is the most important of the nitrates and is available in forms that provide a range of durations of action from 10–20 minutes (sublingual) to 8–10 hours (transdermal) (Table 12–2). Because

Category	Example	Duration of Action
Very short	Inhaled amyl nitrite	3–5 minutes
Short	Sublingual nitroglycerin or isosorbide dinitrate	10–30 minutes (isosorbide dinitrate has a somewhat longer half-life than nitroglycerin)
Intermediate	Oral regular or sustained-release nitroglycerin or isosorbide dinitrate	4–8 hours (much of the effect is due to active metabolites)
Long	Transdermal nitroglycerin patch	8–10 hours (blood levels may persist for 24 hours, but tolerance limits the duration of action)

Table 12–2. Pharmacokinetically distinct forms of nitrate and nitrite drugs used in angina.

treatment of acute attacks and prevention of attacks are both important aspects of therapy, the pharmacokinetics of these different dosage forms are clinically significant.

Nitroglycerin (glyceryl trinitrate) is rapidly denitrated in the liver—first to the dinitrate (glyceryl dinitrate), which retains a significant vasodilating effect, and more slowly to the mononitrate, which is much less active. Because of the high enzyme activity in the liver, the first-pass effect for nitroglycerin is large—about 90%. The efficacy of oral (swallowed) nitroglycerin probably results from the high levels of glyceryl dinitrate in the blood. The effects of sublingual nitroglycerin are mainly the result of the unchanged drug.

Other nitrates are similar to nitroglycerin in their pharmacokinetics and pharmacodynamics. After nitroglycerin, isosorbide dinitrate is used most extensively; it is available in sublingual and oral forms. Isosorbide dinitrate is rapidly denitrated in the liver to isosorbide mononitrate, which like glyceryl dinitrate is active. Isosorbide mononitrate is available as a separate drug for oral use. Several other nitrates are available for oral use and, like the oral nitroglycerin preparation, have an intermediate duration of action (4–6 hours). Amyl nitrite is a volatile and rapidly acting vasodilator that was used for angina by inhalation but is now rarely prescribed.

B. Mechanism of Action: Denitration of the nitrates within smooth muscle cells releases nitric oxide (NO), which stimulates guanylyl cyclase, causes an increase of the second messenger cGMP, and leads to smooth muscle relaxation, probably by dephosphorylation of myosin light chain phosphate. Note that this mechanism is identical to that of nitroprusside (Chapter 11).

C. Organ System Effects:
   1. Cardiovascular: Smooth muscle relaxation leads to peripheral venodilation, which results in reduced cardiac size and cardiac output through reduced preload. Reduced afterload—from arteriolar dilation—may contribute to an increase in ejection and a further decrease in cardiac size. Some studies suggest that of the vascular beds, the veins are the most sensitive, arteries less so, and arterioles least sensitive. Venodilation leads to decreased diastolic heart size and fiber tension. Arteriolar dilation leads to reduced peripheral resistance and blood pressure. These changes contribute to an overall reduction in myocardial fiber tension, oxygen consumption, and the double product. Thus, the primary mechanism of therapeutic benefit in atherosclerotic angina is reduction of the oxygen requirement; an increase in coronary flow in ischemic areas is less likely. In vasospastic angina, on the other hand, a reversal of coronary spasm and increased flow can be demonstrated. A significant reflex tachycardia is predictable when nitroglycerin reduces the blood pressure.
   2. Other organs: Nitrates relax the smooth muscle of the bronchi, gastrointestinal tract, and genitourinary tract, but these effects are too small to be clinically useful. Intravenous nitroglycerin (sometimes used in unstable angina) reduces platelet aggregation. There are no significant effects on other tissues.

D. Clinical Uses: As previously noted, nitroglycerin is available in several formulations (Table 12–2). The standard form for treatment of acute anginal pain is the sublingual tablet, which has a duration of action of 10–20 minutes. Oral (swallowed) normal-release nitroglycerin has a duration of 4–6 hours. Sustained-release oral forms have a somewhat longer duration (Table 12–2). Transdermal formulations (ointment or patch) can maintain blood levels for up to 24 hours. Tolerance develops after about 8 hours, however, with markedly diminishing effectiveness thereafter. It is therefore recommended that nitroglycerin patches be removed after 10–12 hours to allow recovery of sensitivity to the drug.

E. Toxicity of Nitrates and Nitrites: The most common toxic effects of nitrates are the responses evoked by vasodilation. These include tachycardia (from the baroreceptor reflex), orthostatic hypotension (a direct extension of the venodilator effect), and throbbing headache from meningeal artery vasodilation. Nitrites are of greater toxicologic importance because they cause methemoglobinemia at high blood concentrations. This same effect has a potential antidotal action in cyanide poisoning (see below). The nitrates do not cause methemoglobinemia. In the past, the nitrates were responsible for several occupational diseases in munitions plants in which workplace contamination by these volatile chemicals was severe. The most common of these diseases was "Monday disease," or the alternating development of tolerance (during the work week) and loss of tolerance (over the weekend) for the vasodilating action, resulting in headache, tachycardia, and dizziness every Monday.

F. Nitrites in the Treatment of Cyanide Poisoning: Cyanide ion rapidly complexes with the iron in cytochrome oxidase, resulting in a block of oxidative metabolism and cell death. Fortunately, the iron in methemoglobin has a higher affinity for cyanide than does the iron in cytochrome oxidase. Nitrites convert the ferrous iron in hemoglobin to the ferric form, yielding methemoglobin. Therefore, cyanide poisoning can be treated by (1) immediate exposure to amyl nitrite, followed by (2) intravenous administration of sodium nitrite, which rapidly increases the methemoglobin level to the degree necessary to remove a significant amount of cyanide from cytochrome oxidase. This is followed by (3) intravenous sodium thiosulfate, which converts cyanmethemoglobin resulting from step 2 to thiocyanate and methemoglobin. Thiocyanate is much less toxic than cyanide and is excreted by the kidney. (It should be noted that excessive methemoglobinemia is fatal, since methemoglobin is a very poor oxygen carrier.)

CALCIUM CHANNEL-BLOCKING DRUGS

A. Classification and Pharmacokinetics: Several types of calcium channel blockers are approved for use in angina; these drugs are typified by **nifedipine,** a **dihydropyridine,** and several other dihydropyridines; **diltiazem;** and **verapamil.** Although calcium channel blockers differ markedly in structure, all are orally active and most have half-lives of 3–6 hours. Nimodipine is another member of the dihydropyridine family with similar properties, but it is approved only for the management of stroke associated with subarachnoid hemorrhage. Bepridil, a drug that is somewhat similar in structure to verapamil, has a longer duration of action but greater cardiovascular toxicity than the older calcium channel blockers.

B. Mechanism of Action: Almost all of these drugs block voltage-dependent "L-type" calcium channels, the calcium channels most important in cardiac and smooth muscle. By decreasing calcium influx during action potentials in a frequency- and voltage-dependent manner, these agents reduce intracellular calcium concentration and muscle contractility. **Mibefradil** is the newest of the calcium blockers to be approved for use in the USA. It is not a dihydropyridine and is said to block cardiac "T-type" calcium channels as well as "L-type" channels. None of the channel blockers interfere with calcium-dependent neurotransmitter or hormone release because these processes do not utilize "L-" or "T-type" channels.

C. Effects: Calcium channel blockers relax blood vessels, and, to a lesser extent, the uterus, bronchi, and gut. The rate and contractility of the heart are reduced by diltiazem and verapamil. Because they block calcium-dependent conduction in the AV node of the heart, verapamil and diltiazem may be used to treat AV nodal arrhythmias (Chapter 14). Nifedipine and other dihydropyridines evoke greater vasodilation, and the resulting sympathetic reflex prevents bradycardia and may actually increase the heart rate. All the calcium channel blockers reduce blood pressure and reduce the double product in patients with angina.

D. Clinical Use: Calcium channel blockers are effective as prophylactic therapy in both types of angina; nifedipine can also be used to abort an acute anginal attack. In atherosclerotic angina, these drugs are particularly valuable when combined with nitrates (Table 12–3). In addition to

Table 12–3. Effects of nitrates alone and with β-blockers or calcium channel blockers in angina pectoris.[1]

	Nitrates Alone	β-Blockers or Calcium Channel Blockers Alone	Combined Nitrate and β-Blockers or Calcium Channel Blockers
Heart rate	Reflex increase	**Decrease**	**Decrease**
Arterial pressure	Decrease	Decrease	**Decrease**
End-diastolic pressure	**Decrease**	Increase	**Decrease**
Contractility	Reflex increase	**Decrease**	No effect or **decrease**
Ejection time	Reflex decrease	Increase	No effect

[1]Undesirable effects (effects that increase myocardial oxygen requirement) are shown in italics; major therapeutic effects are shown in bold.

well-established uses in angina, hypertension, and supraventricular tachycardia, these agents are being tried in migraine, preterm labor, stroke, and Raynaud's phenomenon. As noted above, nimodipine is approved for use in hemorrhagic stroke.

E. **Toxicity:** The calcium channel blockers cause constipation, edema, nausea, flushing, and dizziness. More serious adverse effects include congestive heart failure, atrioventricular block-ade, and sinus node depression; these are more common with verapamil than with the dihy-dropyridines. Bepridil may induce **torsade de pointes** and other arrhythmias.

BETA-BLOCKING DRUGS

A. **Classification and Mechanism of Action:** These drugs are described in detail in Chapter 10. All beta-blockers are effective in the prophylaxis of atherosclerotic angina attacks.

B. **Effects:** Actions include both beneficial effects (decreased heart rate, cardiac force, blood pressure) and detrimental effects (increased heart size, longer ejection period) (Table 12–3). Like the nitrates and calcium channel blockers, the beta-blockers reduce the double product.

C. **Clinical Use:** Beta-blockers are used only for prophylactic therapy of angina; they are of no value in an acute attack. They are effective in preventing exercise-induced angina but are inef-fective against the vasospastic form. The combination of beta-blockers with nitrates is useful because the undesirable compensatory effects evoked by the nitrates (tachycardia and increased cardiac force) are prevented or reduced by beta blockade. (See Table 12–3.)

D. **Toxicity:** See Chapter 10.

NONPHARMACOLOGIC THERAPY

Myocardial revascularization by coronary artery bypass grafting (CABG) or percutaneous transluminal coronary angioplasty (PTCA) are important therapies in severe angina. These are the only methods capa-ble of consistently increasing coronary flow in atherosclerotic angina and increasing the double product.

DRUG LIST

The following drugs are important members of the group discussed in this chapter. Prototypes should be learned in detail; features of the major variants should be known well enough so that the variants can be distinguished from prototypes and from each other; the other significant agents should be recognized as belonging to a specific subclass.

Subclass	Prototype	Major Variants	Other Significant Agents
Nitrates	Nitroglycerin	Different dosage forms (sublin-gual, oral, transdermal)	Isosorbide dinitrate, amyl nitrite
Calcium channel blockers	Nifedipine Verapamil Diltiazem	Nimodipine	Bepridil, mibefradil
Beta-blockers	Propranolol	See Chapter 10	

QUESTIONS

DIRECTIONS: Each of the numbered items or incomplete statements in this section is followed by answers or by completions of the statement. Select the ONE lettered answer or completion that is BEST in each case.

Items 1–3: Mr Green, 60 years old, has severe chest pain when he attempts to carry parcels up-stairs to his apartment. The pain rapidly disappears when he rests. A decision is made to treat Mr Green with nitroglycerin.

1. Nitroglycerin, either directly or through reflexes, results in all of the following EXCEPT
   (A) Increased heart rate
   (B) Decreased cardiac force
   (C) Increased venous capacitance
   (D) Decreased intramyocardial fiber tension
   (E) Decreased afterload

2. In advising Mr Green about the adverse effects he may notice, you point out that nitroglycerin in moderate doses often produces certain symptoms. These toxicities result from all of the following EXCEPT
   (A) Meningeal vasodilation
   (B) Reflex tachycardia
   (C) Increased cardiac force
   (D) Methemoglobinemia
   (E) Sympathetic discharge

3. Two years later, Mr Green returns complaining that his nitroglycerin works well when he takes it for an acute attack, but he is having frequent attacks now and would like something to *prevent* them. Effective drugs for the prophylaxis of angina of effort include all of the following EXCEPT
   (A) Transdermal nitroglycerin
   (B) Amyl nitrite
   (C) Diltiazem
   (D) Nadolol
   (E) Oral isosorbide dinitrate

4. The antianginal effect of propranolol may be attributed to all of the following EXCEPT
   (A) Block of exercise-induced tachycardia
   (B) Reduced resting heart rate
   (C) Decreased cardiac force
   (D) Increased end-diastolic ventricular volume
   (E) Decreased systolic fiber tension

5. The major common determinant of myocardial oxygen consumption is
   (A) Blood volume
   (B) Cardiac output
   (C) Diastolic blood pressure
   (D) Heart rate
   (E) Myocardial fiber tension

6. A new patient presents with severe hypertension and angina. You are considering therapeutic options for her. In considering adverse effects, you note that an adverse effect that nitroglycerin, guanethidine, and ganglion blockers have in common is
   (A) Bradycardia
   (B) Impaired sexual function
   (C) Lupus erythematosus syndrome
   (D) Orthostatic hypotension
   (E) Throbbing headache

7. Epidemiologic surveys suggest that, in the past, workers exposed to high levels of organic nitrates in the workplace had
   (A) A high incidence of methemoglobinemia on the job
   (B) An increased incidence of angina at work as compared to at home
   (C) A high incidence of cyanide poisoning in the workplace
   (D) An increased incidence of headaches on Mondays as compared to other days
   (E) All of the above

8. A patient is admitted to the emergency department with marked tachycardia. She has been receiving therapy for hypertension and angina. A drug that often causes tachycardia when given in ordinary doses is
   (A) Isosorbide dinitrate
   (B) Verapamil
   (C) Guanethidine
   (D) Propranolol
   (E) Diltiazem

9. A patient being treated for another condition complains that whenever he takes that medication, his angina becomes worse. Drugs that may precipitate angina when used for other indications include all of the following EXCEPT
 (A) Hydralazine
 (B) Terbutaline
 (C) Isoproterenol
 (D) Reserpine
 (E) Amphetamine

10. When using nitrates in combination with other drugs for the treatment of angina,
 (A) The actions of beta-blockers and nitrates on end-diastolic cardiac size are additive
 (B) The actions of calcium channel blockers and nitrates on cardiac force are antagonistic
 (C) The actions of calcium channel blockers and nitrates on vascular tone are antagonistic
 (D) The actions of beta-blockers and nitrates on heart rate are additive
 (E) The actions of calcium channel blockers and beta-blockers on cardiac force are antagonistic

DIRECTIONS (Items 11–15): Each set of matching questions in this section consists of a list of three to twenty-six lettered options (some of which may be figures) followed by several numbered items. For each numbered item, select the ONE lettered option that is MOST closely associated with it. Each lettered option may be selected once, more than once, or not at all.

 (A) Amyl nitrite
 (B) Hydralazine
 (C) Isosorbide mononitrate
 (D) Nifedipine
 (E) Nimodipine
 (F) Nitroglycerin (sublingual)
 (G) Nitroglycerin (transdermal)
 (H) Propranolol
 (I) Terbutaline
 (J) Verapamil

11. A drug that is approved for the treatment of hemorrhagic stroke
12. A drug used by inhalation; very rapid onset but brief effect (2–5 minutes)
13. A drug capable of maintaining blood levels for 24 hours, but useful therapeutic effects last only about 10 hours
14. An antihypertensive vasodilator drug that lacks a direct effect on autonomic receptors but may provoke anginal attacks
15. An active metabolite of another drug and an active antianginal drug for oral administration in its own right

ANSWERS

1. Nitroglycerin increases cardiac force because the decrease in blood pressure evokes a compensatory increase in sympathetic discharge. The answer is **(B)**.

2. Methemoglobinemia never occurs from the doses of nitroglycerin (or other nitrates) used to treat angina. The *nitrites* (in large doses) cause methemoglobinemia. The answer is **(D)**.

3. The calcium channel blockers and the beta-blockers are generally effective in reducing the number of attacks of angina of effort and have durations of 4–8 hours. Oral and transdermal nitrates have similar or longer durations. Amyl nitrite has the shortest duration of action (3–5 minutes) of any drug used in angina and thus is of no value in prophylaxis. The answer is **(B)**.

4. Propranolol has all the effects listed, but the increase in end-diastolic volume is not advantageous—it tends to *increase* oxygen consumption. The answer is **(D)**.

5. The answer is **(E)**, fiber tension. The other variables contribute to this determinant.

6. These drugs all reduce venous return sufficiently to cause some degree of postural hypotension (not very prolonged in the case of nitroglycerin). Throbbing headache is a problem only with the nitrates, bradycardia only with guanethidine, sexual problems only with sympathoplegics (ganglion blockers and guanethidine), and lupus with none of them. The answer is **(D)**.

7. Nitrites, not nitrates, cause methemoglobinemia in adults. Headache, not angina, increased upon returning to work on Monday. Neither nitrates nor nitrites are related to causation of cyanide poisoning, but nitrites are used as one part of the antidote for cyanide intoxication. The answer is **(D)**.

8. Isosorbide dinitrate (like all the nitrates) causes reflex tachycardia, but all the other drugs listed here slow heart rate. The answer is **(A)**.

9. In general, drugs that induce hypertension or tachycardia—whether directly or by reflex—tend to precipitate angina in individuals with coronary obstruction, unless cardiac work is greatly reduced (as in the case of the nitrates). The answer is **(D)**.

10. The effects of beta-blockers (or calcium channel blockers) and nitrates on heart size are opposite. The answer is **(B)**.

11. Nimodipine, a dihydropyridine calcium channel blocker, is approved only for the treatment of hemorrhagic stroke. The answer is **(E)**.

12. Amyl nitrite, a very volatile liquid, is the only antianginal drug in this list that is usually used by the inhalation route. (Terbutaline is used by aerosol, but it has a longer duration of action and *causes* angina in susceptible patients.) The answer is **(A)**.

13. Transdermal formulations of nitroglycerin are capable of maintaining blood concentrations for up to 24 hours. Unfortunately, tolerance develops after about 10 hours of continued exposure, so the effect is limited to about 8–10 hours. The answer is **(G)**.

14. Hydralazine, a direct-acting vasodilator, often precipitates angina in susceptible individuals; the drug should never be used in patients with coronary disease unless heart rate is appropriately controlled. The answer is **(B)**.

15. The organic nitrates are denitrated in the liver after oral administration. Glyceryl dinitrate and isosorbide mononitrate are active metabolites. The latter agent is available as a separate drug. The answer is **(C)**.

13   Cardiac Glycosides & Congestive Heart Failure

OBJECTIVES

You should be able to:

- Describe the strategies and list the major drug groups used in the treatment of congestive heart failure.
- Describe the probable mechanism of action of digitalis.
- Describe the nature and mechanism of the toxic effects of digitalis on the heart.
- List some positive inotropic drugs that have been investigated as digitalis substitutes.
- Explain the beneficial effects of vasodilators and ACE inhibitors in congestive heart failure.

Learn the definitions that follow.

Table 13–1. Definitions.

Term	Definition
Bigeminy	An arrhythmia consisting of normal sinus beats coupled with ventricular extrasystoles, ie, "twinned beats"
Cardenolide	The basic chemical structure required for cardiac glycoside action, consisting of a steroid nucleus and a lactone ring at the 17 position
Congestive heart failure	A condition in which cardiac output is insufficient for the needs of the body. Low-output failure is the more common form and is more responsive to positive inotropic drugs than high-output failure
End-diastolic fiber length	The length of the ventricular fibers at the end of diastole; a determinant of the force of the following contraction
PDE inhibitor	Phosphodiesterase inhibitor; a drug that inhibits one or more enzymes that degrade cAMP (and other cyclic nucleotides). *Example:* high concentrations of theophylline
Premature ventricular beats	Abnormal beats arising from a cell below the AV node; often from a Purkinje fiber, sometimes from a ventricular fiber
Sodium pump (Na$^+$/K$^+$ ATPase)	A transport molecule in the membranes of all vertebrate cells; responsible for the maintenance of normal low intracellular sodium and high intracellular potassium concentrations
Sodium-calcium exchanger	A transport molecule in the membrane of many cells (eg, cardiac cells) that pumps one calcium atom against its concentration gradient (outward) in exchange for three sodium ions (moving down their concentration gradient)
Ventricular function curve	The curve that relates cardiac output, stroke volume, etc, to filling pressure or end-diastolic fiber length; also known as the Frank-Starling curve
Ventricular tachycardia	An arrhythmia consisting entirely or largely of beats originating below the AV node

CONCEPTS

PATHOPHYSIOLOGY OF CONGESTIVE HEART FAILURE & TREATMENT STRATEGIES

A. **Pathophysiology:** The fundamental physiologic defect in congestive heart failure is a decrease in cardiac contractility. The result of the defect is that cardiac output is inadequate for the needs of the body. This is best shown by the ventricular function curve (Frank-Starling curve; Figure 13–1). The homeostatic responses of the body to depressed cardiac output are mediated mainly by the sympathetic nervous system and the renin-angiotensin-aldosterone system. While these compensatory responses may temporarily improve cardiac output, they also increase the load on the heart; the increased load contributes to a further decline in cardiac function. The ventricular function curve reflects some of these deleterious compensatory responses and may also be used to demonstrate the response to drugs. As ventricular ejection decreases, the end-diastolic fiber length increases as shown by the shift from point A to point B in Figure 13–1. Operation at point B is intrinsically less efficient than operation at shorter fiber lengths because of the increase in myocardial oxygen requirement associated with increased fiber stretch (Figure 12–2).

Other compensatory responses include the following: (1) Tachycardia: an early manifestation of increased sympathetic tone. (2) Increased peripheral vascular resistance: another early response, also mediated by increased sympathetic tone. (3) Retention of salt and water by the kidney: an early compensatory response, mediated by the renin-angiotensin-aldosterone system and by increased sympathetic outflow. Increased blood volume results in edema and pulmonary congestion and contributes to the increased end-diastolic fiber length. (4) Cardiomegaly: enlargement of the heart is a slower compensatory response, mediated at least in part by sympathetic discharge. Angiotensin II also plays an important role.

B. **Therapeutic Strategies in Congestive Heart Failure:** Pharmacologic therapies for congestive heart failure include the removal of retained salt and water with diuretics; direct treatment of the depressed heart with positive inotropic drugs such as digitalis glycosides; reduction of preload or afterload with vasodilators; and reduction of afterload and retained salt and water by angiotensin-converting enzyme inhibitors. In addition, recent evidence suggests that ACE inhibitors also alter the structural changes (remodeling) that often follow myocardial infarction and lead to congestive failure. The use of diuretics is discussed in Chapter 15.

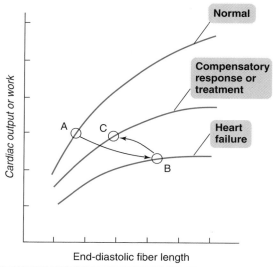

Figure 13–1. Ventricular function (Frank-Starling) curves. The abscissa can be any measure of preload—fiber length, filling pressure, pulmonary capillary wedge pressure, etc. The ordinate is a measure of useful external cardiac work—stroke volume, cardiac output, etc. In congestive heart failure, output is reduced at all fiber lengths and the heart expands because ejection fraction is decreased. As a result, the heart moves from point A to point B. Compensatory sympathetic discharge or effective treatment allows the heart to eject more blood, whereupon the heart moves to point C on the middle curve.

DIGITALIS GLYCOSIDES

A. Prototypes and Pharmacokinetics: All cardiac glycosides include a steroid nucleus and a lactone ring; most also have one or more sugar residues. The sugar residues constitute the glycoside portion of the molecule, and the steroid nucleus plus lactone ring comprise the "genin" portion. The cardiac glycosides are often called "digitalis" because several come from the digitalis (foxglove) plant. **Digoxin** is the prototype agent and the one most commonly used in the USA. A very similar molecule, digitoxin, now rarely used, also comes from the foxglove. Digitalis-like drugs come from many other plants, and a few come from animals. Ouabain, a shorter-acting glycoside, is derived from a tropical plant, though some evidence suggests that ouabain is synthesized in mammals as well. The pharmacokinetics of digoxin, digitoxin, and ouabain are summarized in Table 13–2.

B. Mechanism of Action: Inhibition of Na^+/K^+ ATPase of the cell membrane by digitalis is well documented and is considered to be the primary biochemical mechanism of action of digitalis (Figure 13–3). The translation of this effect into an increase in cardiac contractility involves the Na^+/Ca^{2+} exchange mechanism. Inhibition of Na^+/K^+ ATPase results in an increase in intracellular sodium. The increased sodium alters the driving force for sodium-calcium exchange so that less calcium is removed from the cell. The increased intracellular calcium is stored in the sarcoplasmic reticulum and upon release increases contractile force. Other mechanisms of action for digitalis have been proposed, but they are probably not as important as the ATPase effect. The consequences of Na^+/K^+ ATPase inhibition are seen in both the mechanical and the

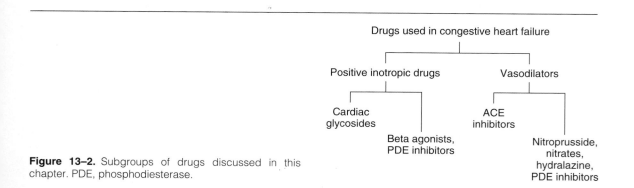

Figure 13–2. Subgroups of drugs discussed in this chapter. PDE, phosphodiesterase.

Table 13–2. Pharmacokinetic parameters of typical cardiac glycosides in adults. Digoxin is the cardiac glycoside most commonly used in the USA.

	Digoxin	Digitoxin	Ouabain
Oral bioavailability (%)	60–85	90–100	0
Half-life (hours)	36–40	168	20
Primary organ of elimination	Kidney	Liver	Kidney
Volume of distribution (L/kg)	6–8	0.6	18
Protein bound in plasma (%)	20–40	> 90	0

electrical function of the heart. Digitalis also modifies autonomic outflow, and this action has effects on the electrical properties of the heart.

C. Cardiac Effects:

1. **Mechanical effects:** The increase in contractility evoked by digitalis results in increased ventricular ejection, decreased end-systolic and end-diastolic size, increased cardiac output, and increased renal perfusion. These beneficial effects permit a decrease in the compensatory sympathetic and renal responses previously described. The decrease in sympathetic tone is especially beneficial: reduced heart rate, preload, and afterload permit the heart to function more efficiently (point C in Figure 13–1).

2. **Electrical effects:** Electrical effects include early cardiac parasympathomimetic responses and later arrhythmogenic responses. They are summarized in Table 13–3.

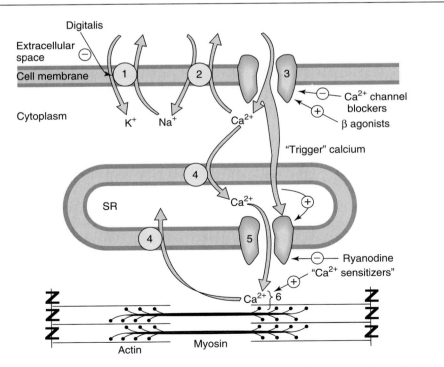

Figure 13–3. Schematic diagram of a cardiac sarcomere with the cellular components involved in excitation-contraction coupling. Factors involved in excitation-contraction coupling are numbered. 1, Na+/K+ ATPase; 2, Na+-Ca2+ exchanger; 3, voltage-gated calcium channel; 4, calcium pump in the wall of the sarcoplasmic reticulum (SR); 5, calcium release channel in the SR; 6, site of calcium interaction with troponin-tropomyosin system. (Reproduced, with permission, from Katzung BG [editor]: *Basic & Clinical Pharmacology,* 7th ed. Appleton & Lange, 1998.)

Table 13–3. Major actions of cardiac glycosides on cardiac electrical functions. (PANS, parasympathomimetic actions; direct, direct membrane actions.)

Variable	Tissue		
	Atrial Muscle	AV Node	Purkinje System, Ventricles
Effective refractory period	↓ (PANS)	↑ (PANS)	↓ (Direct)
Conduction velocity	↑ (PANS)	↓ (PANS)	Negligible
Automaticity	↑ (Direct)	↑ (Direct)	↑ (Direct)
Electrocardiogram Before arrhythmias	Negligible	↑ PR interval	↓ QT interval; T wave inversion; ST segment depression
Arrhythmias	Atrial tachycardia, fibrillation	AV nodal tachycardia; AV blockade	Premature ventricular contractions, ventricular tachycardia, ventricular fibrillation

    a. Early responses: Increased PR interval, caused by the decrease in atrioventricular conduction velocity, and flattening of the T wave are often seen. The effects on the atria and AV node are largely parasympathetic in origin and can be partially blocked by atropine. The increase in the atrioventricular nodal refractory period is particularly important when atrial flutter or fibrillation is present because the refractoriness of the AV node determines the ventricular rate in these arrhythmias. The effect of digitalis is to slow ventricular rate. Inversion of the T wave and ST depression may occur later.

    b. Toxic responses: Increased automaticity, caused by intracellular calcium overload, is the most important manifestation of toxicity. It results from delayed afterdepolarizations, which may evoke extrasystoles, tachycardia, or fibrillation in any part of the heart. In the ventricles, the extrasystoles are recognized as premature ventricular beats (PVBs). When PVBs are coupled to normal beats in a 1:1 fashion, the rhythm is called bigeminy (Figure 13–4).

D. Clinical Uses:

    1. Congestive heart failure: Digitalis is the traditional positive inotropic agent used in the treatment of congestive heart failure. However, other agents (diuretics, ACE inhibitors, vasodilators) may be equally effective and less toxic in some patients. Because the half-lives of both digoxin and digitoxin are long, the drugs accumulate significantly in the body, and dosing regimens must be carefully designed and monitored.

    2. Atrial fibrillation: In atrial flutter and fibrillation, it is desirable to reduce the conduction velocity or increase the refractory period of the atrioventricular node so that ventricular rate is decreased. The parasympathomimetic action of digitalis effectively accomplishes this therapeutic objective.

E. Interactions: Quinidine causes a well-documented reduction in digoxin clearance and often increases the serum digoxin level if digoxin dosage is not adjusted. Several other drugs (amiodarone, verapamil, others) have been shown to have the same effect, but the interactions with these drugs are not clinically significant. Digitalis effects are inhibited by extracellular potassium and magnesium and facilitated by extracellular calcium. Loop diuretics and thiazides, often used in treating heart failure, may significantly reduce serum potassium and thus precipitate

Figure 13–4. ECG record showing digitalis-induced bigeminy. The complexes marked NSR are normal sinus rhythm beats; an inverted T wave and depressed ST segment are present. The complexes marked PVB are premature ventricular beats.

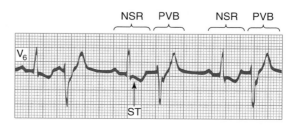

digitalis toxicity. Digitalis-induced vomiting may deplete serum magnesium and similarly facilitate toxicity. These ion interactions are important in treating digitalis toxicity (see below).

F. Digitalis Toxicity: The major signs of digitalis toxicity are arrhythmias, nausea, vomiting, and diarrhea. Rarely, confusion or hallucinations and visual aberrations may occur. The treatment of digitalis arrhythmias is important because this manifestation of digitalis toxicity is common and dangerous. Chronic intoxication is an extension of the therapeutic effect of the drug and is caused by excessive calcium accumulation in cardiac cells (calcium overload). This overload triggers abnormal automaticity and the arrhythmias noted in Table 13–3. Digitalis arrhythmia is more likely if serum potassium or magnesium is lower than normal or if serum calcium is higher than normal.

Severe acute intoxication is caused by suicidal or accidental extreme overdose and results in cardiac depression leading to cardiac arrest rather than tachycardia or fibrillation. A case of severe intoxication is described in Case 2 (Appendix IV).

Treatment of digitalis toxicity includes the following:

1. Correction of potassium or magnesium deficiency: Correction of potassium deficiency (caused, for example, by diuretics) is useful in chronic digitalis intoxication. Mild toxicity may often be managed by omitting one or two doses of digitalis and giving oral or parenteral K^+ supplements. Similarly, if hypomagnesemia is present, it should be treated by normalizing serum magnesium. Severe acute intoxication (as in suicidal overdoses) usually causes marked hyperkalemia and should not be treated with supplemental potassium.

2. Antiarrhythmic drugs: Antiarrhythmic drugs may be useful if increased automaticity is prominent and does not respond to normalization of serum potassium. Agents that do not severely impair cardiac contractility (eg, lidocaine) are favored. Severe acute digitalis overdose usually causes suppression of all pacemaker cells. Antiarrhythmic drugs would be dangerous in such patients.

3. Digoxin antibodies: Digoxin antibodies (FAB fragments, Digibind) are extremely effective and should always be used if other therapies appear to be failing. They are effective for both digoxin and digitoxin overdose and may save severely poisoned patients who would otherwise die.

OTHER DRUGS USED IN CONGESTIVE HEART FAILURE

The major agents used with or as alternatives to digitalis in heart failure include diuretics, ACE inhibitors, β_1-selective sympathomimetics, phosphodiesterase inhibitors, and vasodilators.

A. Diuretics: Diuretics are often used in congestive heart failure before digitalis and other drugs are considered. Furosemide is a very useful agent for immediate reduction of the pulmonary congestion and severe edema associated with acute congestive heart failure or severe chronic failure. Thiazides such as hydrochlorothiazide are often used in the management of mild chronic failure. The pharmacologic characteristics of the diuretics are discussed in Chapter 15.

B. Angiotensin-Converting Enzyme Inhibitors: These agents have been shown to be as effective as digitalis—or more so—in the management of chronic heart failure. Although they have no direct positive inotropic action, ACE inhibitors reduce aldosterone secretion, salt and water retention, and vascular resistance. They reduce symptoms and are the only drugs that have been shown to prolong life in patients with heart failure. Along with diuretics and digitalis, they are now considered among the first-line drugs for chronic heart failure.

C. Beta₁-Selective Adrenoceptor Agonists: Dobutamine and dopamine are useful in some cases of acute failure. However, they are not appropriate for chronic failure because of tolerance, lack of oral efficacy, and significant arrhythmogenic effects.

D. Phosphodiesterase Inhibitors: Amrinone and milrinone are the major representatives of this infrequently used group, though theophylline (in the form of its salt, aminophylline) was commonly used in the past. These drugs increase cAMP by inhibiting its breakdown by phosphodiesterase and cause an increase in cardiac intracellular calcium similar to that produced by beta-adrenoceptor agonists. Phosphodiesterase inhibitors also cause vasodilation, which may be responsible for a major part of their beneficial effect. At very high concentrations, these agents may also increase the sensitivity of the contractile protein system to calcium (site 6 in Figure 13–3).

E. Vasodilators: Vasodilator therapy with nitroprusside or nitroglycerin is often used for acute severe congestive failure. The use of these vasodilator drugs is based on the reduction in cardiac size and improved efficiency that can be realized with proper adjustment of venous return and reduction of resistance to ventricular ejection. Vasodilator therapy can be dramatically effective, especially in cases in which excessive afterload is a major factor in causing the failure (eg, continuing hypertension in an individual who has just had an infarct). Chronic congestive heart failure sometimes responds favorably to oral vasodilators such as hydralazine or isosorbide dinitrate.

DRUG LIST

The following drugs are important members of the group discussed in this chapter. Prototypes should be learned in detail; features of the major variants should be known well enough so that the variants can be distinguished from the prototypes and from each other; the other significant agents should be recognized as belonging to a specific subclass.

Subclass	Prototype	Major Variants	Other Significant Agents
Cardiac glycosides	Digoxin	Digitoxin	Ouabain
Positive inotropic digitalis substitutes	Dobutamine, amrinone		Milrinone, theophylline
ACE inhibitors	Captopril		Enalapril, lisinopril
Diuretics	Furosemide, hydrochlorothiazide		
Vasodilators	Nitroprusside	Nitroglycerin, hydralazine	Isosorbide dinitrate, theophylline

QUESTIONS

DIRECTIONS: Each of the numbered items or incomplete statements in this section is followed by answers or by completions of the statement. Select the ONE lettered answer or completion that is BEST in each case.

1. Drugs that have been found to be useful in one or more types of heart failure include all of the following EXCEPT
   (A) Na^+/K^+ ATPase inhibitors
   (B) Alpha adrenoceptor agonists
   (C) Beta adrenoceptor agonists
   (D) Thiazide diuretics
   (E) ACE inhibitors

2. The biochemical mechanism of action of digitalis is associated with
   (A) A shortening of the action potential duration
   (B) An increase in ATP synthesis
   (C) A modification of the actin molecule
   (D) An increase in systolic intracellular calcium levels
   (E) A block of sodium-calcium exchange

3. A patient who has been taking digoxin for several years for chronic heart failure is about to receive atropine for another condition. A common effect of digoxin (at therapeutic blood levels) that can be almost entirely blocked by atropine is
   (A) Tachycardia
   (B) Decreased appetite

(C) Increased atrial contractility
(D) Increased PR interval on the ECG
(E) Headaches

Items 4–6: A 65-year-old woman has been admitted to the coronary care unit with a myocardial infarction.

4. If this patient develops acute severe congestive failure, all of the following might be useful EXCEPT
   (A) Nitroprusside
   (B) Digoxin
   (C) Furosemide
   (D) Propranolol
   (E) Dobutamine

5. The patient might be given a cardiac glycoside. Important effects of digitalis on the heart include
   (A) Increased force of contraction
   (B) Decreased atrioventricular conduction velocity
   (C) Increased ectopic automaticity
   (D) Decreased ejection time
   (E) All of the above

6. Which of the following situations constitutes an added risk of drug toxicity in this patient?
   (A) Digoxin therapy in a patient with hypocalcemia
   (B) Digoxin therapy in a patient with hyperkalemia
   (C) Digoxin therapy in a patient with hypermagnesemia
   (D) Digoxin therapy in a patient taking captopril
   (E) Digoxin therapy in a patient taking quinidine

7. Which row in the following table correctly shows the major pharmacokinetic characteristics of the cardiac glycosides?

Row	Variable	Digoxin	Digitoxin	Ouabain
(A)	Oral bioavailability	75%	28%	98%
(B)	Half-life	168 hours	36 hours	20 hours
(C)	Volume of distribution	6.3 L/kg	0.6 L/kg	18 L/kg
(D)	Percent protein bound in plasma	50–60%	> 90%	40%
(E)	Organ of excretion	Kidney	Liver	Liver

8. Effects of digitalis on electrical functions of the heart include all of the following EXCEPT
   (A) Prolonged atrioventricular refractory period
   (B) Slowed sinoatrial nodal rate
   (C) Increased atrial rate in atrial flutter
   (D) Decreased ventricular rate in atrial fibrillation
   (E) Decreased ectopic automaticity

9. Drugs associated with clinically useful or physiologically important positive inotropic effects include all of the following EXCEPT
   (A) Amrinone
   (B) Captopril
   (C) Digoxin
   (D) Dobutamine
   (E) Norepinephrine

10. The effects of digoxin include all of the following EXCEPT
    (A) Increased cardiac intracellular potassium
    (B) Increased cardiac intracellular sodium
    (C) Increased cardiac intracellular calcium
    (D) Increased force of cardiac contraction
    (E) Reduced sympathetic outflow to the heart

DIRECTIONS (Items 11–15): Each set of matching questions in this section consists of a list of four to twenty-six lettered options (some of which may be figures) followed by several numbered items. For each numbered item, select the ONE lettered option that is MOST closely associated with it. Each lettered option may be selected once, more than once, or not at all.

    (A) Digibind antibodies
    (B) Digitoxin
    (C) Digoxin
    (D) Dobutamine
    (E) Enalapril
    (F) Furosemide
    (G) Lidocaine
    (H) Magnesium
    (I) Potassium
    (J) Quinidine

11.   Administration of this monovalent cation would tend to decrease or reverse a mild-to-moderate digitalis-induced arrhythmia

12.   Shown to prolong life in patients with chronic congestive failure but has no direct positive inotropic action

13.   A β_1-selective agent sometimes used in acute congestive failure

14.   Drug of choice in treating suicidal overdose of digoxin

15.   Antiarrhythmic drug that is used to suppress digoxin-induced arrhythmias in some patients

ANSWERS

1.   All the drugs listed are commonly used in heart failure except alpha agonists. Alpha agonist drugs *increase* vascular resistance and would *decrease* the stroke volume of the weakened heart even more. The answer is **(B)**.

2.   Digitalis does shorten the action potential in some parts of the heart and at some doses, but this action is another *result,* not the *mechanism,* of its biochemical action. Sodium-calcium exchange is not blocked, it is merely altered. The most accurate description of the mechanism of action of digitalis in this list is that it increases intracellular calcium. The answer is **(D)**.

3.   The parasympathomimetic effects of digitalis can be blocked by muscarinic blockers such as atropine. The only parasympathomimetic effect in the list provided is increased PR interval, representing slowing of AV conduction. The answer is **(D)**.

4.   Acute severe congestive failure often requires vasodilators to reduce intravascular pressures in the lungs and the periphery. Both nitroprusside and furosemide have such vasodilating actions in the context of acute failure. Positive inotropic agents such as digoxin and dobutamine are traditional agents for heart failure. Beta antagonists such as propranolol, on the other hand, are usually contraindicated in acute heart failure; they are used only if the failure is due to certain cardiomyopathies. The answer is **(D)**.

5.   The effects of digitalis include all the effects listed. The answer is **(E)**.

6.   Digitalis toxicity is facilitated by hypercalcemia, hypokalemia, or hypomagnesemia. It is also more likely if a patient begins taking quinidine after being stabilized on a dose of digitalis, because quinidine reduces the clearance of digoxin. The answer is **(E)**.

7.   Review the pharmacokinetics of the cardiac glycosides. The answer is **(C)**.

8.   The major cause of digitalis arrhythmias is *increased* automaticity. All the other effects listed are seen frequently. The answer is **(E)**.

9.   Although they are extremely useful in congestive heart failure, captopril and the other ACE inhibitors have no positive inotropic effect on the heart. The answer is **(B)**.

10.   Digoxin increases intracellular sodium and calcium and reduces sympathetic outflow to the heart (because the drug replaces the need for constant sympathetic stimulation of contractility). However, digoxin does not increase intracellular potassium; blockade of Na^+/K^+ ATPase increases intracellular sodium and calcium and very slightly reduces intracellular potassium. The answer is **(A)**.

11.   Potassium is the only monovalent cation in the list that is used for reversing mild to moderate digitalis toxicity. The answer is **(I)**.

12. The ACE inhibitors have been shown to prolong life in heart failure patients even though these drugs have no direct positive inotropic action on the heart. The answer is (**E**).
13. Dobutamine is a β_1-selective agonist often used in acute heart failure. The answer is (**D**).
14. The drug of choice in severe, massive digitalis overdose is digitalis antibody, Digibind. The answer is (**A**).
15. Although quinidine may have this beneficial effect, it is also much more likely than lidocaine to precipitate digitalis toxicity. The answer is (**G**).

Antiarrhythmic Drugs   **14**

OBJECTIVES

You should be able to:

- Describe the distinguishing features of the four major groups of antiarrhythmic drugs and adenosine.
- List two or three of the most important drugs in each of the four groups.
- List the major toxicities of those drugs.
- Describe the mechanism of selective depression by local anesthetic antiarrhythmic agents.
- Explain how hyperkalemia, hypokalemia, or an antiarrhythmic drug can cause an arrhythmia.

Learn the definitions that follow.

Table 14–1. Definitions.

Term	Definition
Abnormal automaticity	Pacemaker activity that originates anywhere other than in the sinoatrial node
Abnormal conduction	Conduction of an impulse that does not follow the path defined in Figure 14–1 or reenters tissue previously excited
Atrial fibrillation, ventricular fibrillation	Arrhythmias involving rapid reentry and chaotic movement of impulses through the tissue of the atria or ventricles; ventricular—but not atrial—fibrillation is fatal if not terminated within a few minutes
Groups I, II, III, and IV drugs	A method for classifying antiarrhythmic drugs, sometimes called the Vaughan Williams classification; based loosely on the channel or receptor affected
Reentrant arrhythmia	Arrhythmias of abnormal conduction; they involve the repetitive movement of an impulse through tissue previously excited by the same impulse
Effective refractory period	The period that must pass after the upstroke of a conducted impulse before a new action potential can be propagated in that cell or tissue
Selective depression	The ability of certain drugs to selectively depress areas of excitable membrane that are most susceptible, leaving other areas relatively unaffected
Supraventricular tachycardia	A reentrant arrhythmia that travels through the AV node; it may also include atrial and ventricular tissue as part of the reentrant circuit
Ventricular tachycardia	A very common arrhythmia, associated often with myocardial infarction; ventricular tachycardia may involve abnormal automaticity or abnormal conduction, usually impairs cardiac output, and may deteriorate into ventricular fibrillation; for these reasons, it requires prompt management
Action potential	The change in membrane voltage when the membrane is excited

CONCEPTS

Cardiac arrhythmias usually occur in the presence of preexisting heart disease. They are the most common cause of death in patients who have had a myocardial infarction. They are also the most serious manifestation of digitalis toxicity.

PATHOPHYSIOLOGY

A. What Is an Arrhythmia? Normal cardiac function is dependent on generation of an impulse in the normal pacemaker (the sinoatrial [SA] node), and its conduction through the atrial muscle, through the atrioventricular (AV) node, through the Purkinje conduction system, to the ventricular muscle (Figure 14–1). Normal pacemaking and conduction require normal action potentials (dependent on sodium, calcium, and potassium channel activity) under appropriate autonomic control. Arrhythmias are therefore defined by exclusion—ie, any rhythm that is not a normal sinus rhythm (NSR) is an arrhythmia.

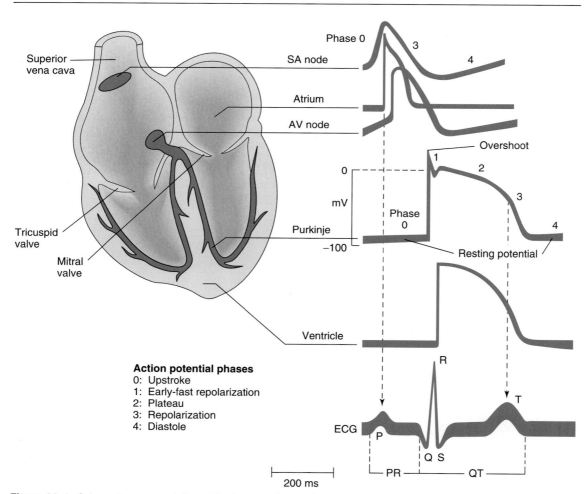

Figure 14–1. Schematic representation of the heart and normal cardiac electrical activity (intracellular recordings from areas indicated and ECG). The ECG is the body surface manifestation of the depolarization and repolarization waves of the heart. The P wave is generated by atrial depolarization, the QRS by ventricular muscle depolarization, and the T wave by ventricular repolarization. The PR interval is a measure of conduction time from atrium to ventricle, and the QRS duration indicates the time required for all of the ventricular cells to be activated (ie, the intraventricular conduction time). The QT interval reflects the duration of the ventricular action potential.

B. Arrhythmogenic Mechanisms: Abnormal automaticity and abnormal (reentry) conduction are the two major mechanisms for arrhythmias. A few of the clinically important arrhythmias are atrial flutter, atrial fibrillation (AF), atrioventricular nodal reentry (a common type of supraventricular tachycardia [SVT]), premature ventricular beats (PVBs), ventricular tachycardia (VT), and ventricular fibrillation (VF). Examples of electrocardiographic recordings of normal sinus rhythm and some of these common arrhythmias are shown in Figure 14–2.

C. Normal Electrical Activity in the Cardiac Cell: The cellular action potentials shown in Figure 14–1 are the result of ion fluxes through voltage-gated channels and carrier mechanisms. These processes are diagrammed in Figure 14–3. In most parts of the heart, sodium current (I_{Na}) dominates the upstroke of the action potential and is the most important determinant of conduction of

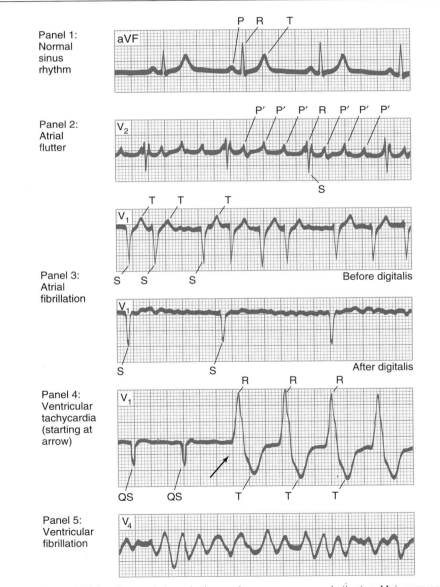

Figure 14–2. Typical ECGs of normal sinus rhythm and some common arrhythmias. Major waves (P, Q, R, S, and T) are labeled in each electrocardiographic record except in panel 5, in which electrical activity is completely disorganized and none of these deflections are recognizable. (Modified and reproduced, with permission, from Goldman MJ: *Principles of Clinical Electrocardiography,* 11th ed. Lange, 1982.)

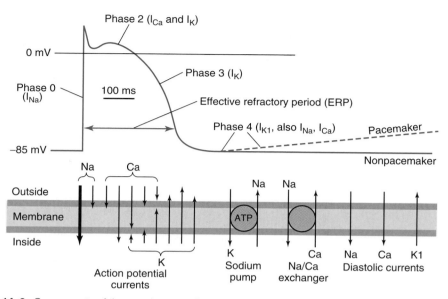

Figure 14–3. Components of the membrane action potential (AP) in a typical Purkinje or ventricular cardiac cell. The deflections of the AP, designated as phases 0 through 3, are generated by different ionic currents. The actions of the sodium pump and sodium-calcium exchanger are mainly involved in maintaining ionic steady state during repetitive activity. Note that small but significant currents occur during diastole (phase 4) in addition to the pump and exchanger activity. In nonpacemaker cells, the outward potassium current during phase 4 is sufficient to maintain a stable negative resting potential, as shown by the solid line at the right end of the tracing. In pacemaker cells, however, the potassium current is smaller and the depolarizing currents (sodium, calcium, or both) during phase 4 are large enough to gradually depolarize the cell during diastole (shown by the dashed line).

that action potential. In the AV node, calcium current (I_{Ca}) dominates the upstroke. The carrier processes (sodium pump and sodium-calcium exchanger) contribute little to the shape of the action potential (but they are critical for the maintenance of the ion gradients on which the sodium, calcium, and potassium currents depend). Antiarrhythmic drugs act on one or more of the three major currents (I_{Na}, I_{Ca}, I_K) or on the second-messenger systems that modulate these currents.

D. Drug Group Classification: The antiarrhythmic agents are often classified using a system loosely based on the channel or receptor involved (Figure 14–4). This system specifies four groups, usually denoted by Roman numerals I–IV:

    I. Sodium channel blockers
   II. Beta-adrenoceptor blockers
  III. Potassium channel blockers
  IV. Calcium channel blockers

A miscellaneous group includes adenosine, digitalis, potassium ion, and magnesium ion.

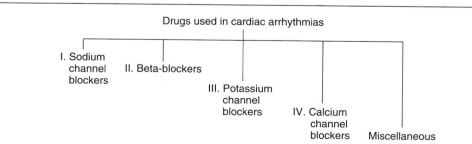

Figure 14–4. Subgroups of drugs discussed in this chapter.

GROUP I (LOCAL ANESTHETICS)

A. **Prototypes:** The group I drugs are further characterized on the basis of their effects on action potential duration. Group IA agents (prototype quinidine) prolong the action potential. Group IB drugs shorten the action potential in some cardiac tissues (prototype lidocaine). Group IC drugs have no effect on action potential duration (prototype flecainide).

B. **Mechanism of Action:** As local anesthetics, all group I drugs slow or block conduction (especially in depolarized cells) and slow or abolish abnormal pacemakers wherever these processes depend on sodium channels. Useful sodium channel-blocking drugs bind to their receptors much more readily when the channel is open or inactivated than when it is fully repolarized and recovered from its previous activity. Ion channels in arrhythmic tissue spend more time in the open or inactivated states than do channels in normal tissue. Therefore, these antiarrhythmic drugs block channels in abnormal tissue more effectively than channels in normal tissue. As a result, antiarrhythmic sodium channel blockers are state-dependent in their action, ie, selectively depressant on tissue that is frequently depolarizing (eg, during a fast tachycardia) or is relatively depolarized during rest (eg, by hypoxia). The effects of the major antiarrhythmic group I drugs are summarized in Table 14–2 and Figure 14–5.

1. **Drugs with group IA action:** Quinidine is the Group IA prototype. Other drugs with IA actions include amiodarone, procainamide, and disopyramide. They affect both atrial and ventricular arrhythmias. These drugs increase action potential (AP) duration and the effective refractory period (ERP). The increase in action potential duration generates an increase in QT interval (Table 14–2). Amiodarone has similar effects on sodium current and has the greatest AP-prolonging effect. It is often considered a group III drug even though it also blocks sodium channels, a group I action.

2. **Drugs with group IB actions:** Lidocaine is the prototype IB drug. Mexiletine and tocainide are other IB agents. Lidocaine affects ischemic or depolarized Purkinje and ventricular tissue and has little effect on atrial tissue; the drug reduces action potential duration, but because it slows recovery of sodium channels from inactivation, it does not shorten (or may even prolong) the effective refractory period. Mexiletine and tocainide have similar effects. Because these agents have little effect on normal cardiac cells, they have little effect on the ECG (Table 14–2).

Table 14–2. Properties of the prototype antiarrhythmic drugs.

Drug	Group	Half-Life	Route	PR Interval	QRS Duration	QT Interval
Adenosine	Misc	3 s	IV	↑	...	...
Amiodarone	IA, III	1–10 wks	Oral, parenteral	↑	↑↑	↑↑↑↑
Bretylium	III	4 h	IV	...	...	...[1]
Disopyramide	IA	6–8 h	Oral	↓ or ↑[2]	↑	↑
Esmolol	II	10 min	IV	↑↑	...	...
Flecainide	IC	20 h	Oral	↑ (slight)	↑↑	...
Ibutilide	III	6 h	Oral	↑	...	↑↑
Lidocaine	IB	1–2 h	IV	...	...[3]	...
Mexiletine, tocainide	IB	12 h	Oral	...	...[3]	...
Procainamide	IA	3–4 h	Oral, IV	↓ or ↑[2]	↑	↑↑
Propranolol	II	8 h	Oral, IV	↑↑	...	...
Quinidine	IA	6 h	Oral, IV	↓ or ↑[2]	↑	↑↑↑
Sotalol	III	7 h	Oral	↑	...	↑↑↑
Verapamil	IV	7 h	Oral, IV	↑↑	...	...

[1]Bretylium increases action potential duration in ischemic cells.
[2]PR may decrease through antimuscarinic action or increase through channel blocking action.
[3]Lidocaine, mexiletine, and tocainide slow conduction velocity in ischemic, depolarized ventricular cells but not in normal tissue.

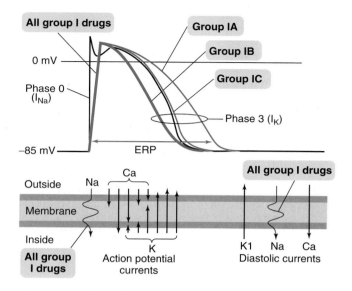

Figure 14–5. Schematic diagram of the effects of group I agents. Note that all group I drugs reduce both phase 0 and phase 4 sodium currents in susceptible cells (shown as wavy lines). Group IA drugs also reduce potassium current (I_K) and prolong the AP duration. This results in significant prolongation of the effective refractory period. Group IB and IC drugs have different (or no) effects on potassium current and thus shorten or have no effect on the action potential.

   3. **Drugs with group IC action:**   Flecainide is the prototype drug with group IC actions. Encainide (recently withdrawn), moricizine, and propafenone are also members of this group. These drugs have no effect on ventricular action potential duration or the QT interval. They are powerful depressants of sodium current, however, and can markedly slow conduction velocity in atrial and ventricular cells.

C. **Pharmacokinetics:**   See Table 14–2.

D. **Clinical Uses and Toxicities:**
   1. **Group IA drugs:**   Quinidine is used in all types of arrhythmias, especially chronic ones requiring outpatient treatment. Both atrial and ventricular arrhythmias may be responsive. Procainamide and disopyramide have similar uses.
      Quinidine causes cinchonism (headache, tinnitus), cardiac depression, gastrointestinal upset, and allergic reactions (eg, thrombocytopenic purpura). As noted in Chapter 13, quinidine reduces the clearance of digoxin and may increase the plasma concentration of the glycoside to dangerous levels. Procainamide causes a reversible syndrome similar to lupus erythematosus. Disopyramide has marked antimuscarinic effects and may precipitate congestive heart failure. All the group IA drugs may precipitate new arrhythmias. One arrhythmia, called **torsade de pointes,** is particularly associated with quinidine and other drugs that prolong action potential duration (except amiodarone).
      Hyperkalemia usually exacerbates the cardiac toxicity of group I drugs. Treatment of overdoses of these agents usually consists of giving sodium lactate (to reverse drug-induced arrhythmias) and pressor sympathomimetics (to reverse drug-induced hypotension).
   2. **Group IB drugs:**   Lidocaine is useful in acute ventricular arrhythmias, especially those involving ischemia, eg, following myocardial infarction. Atrial arrhythmias are not responsive unless caused by digitalis. Lidocaine is usually given intravenously, but IM administration is also possible. Mexiletine and tocainide have similar actions but can be given orally.
      Lidocaine, mexiletine, and tocainide cause typical local anesthetic toxicity (ie, CNS stimulation, including convulsions), cardiovascular depression (usually minor), and allergic reactions (usually rashes but may extend to anaphylaxis). Tocainide may cause agranulocy-

tosis. These drugs may also precipitate arrhythmias, but this is less common than with group IA drugs. Hyperkalemia increases cardiac toxicity.

3. **Group IC drugs:** Flecainide is effective in both atrial and ventricular arrhythmias but is approved only for refractory ventricular tachycardias that tend to progress to VF at unpredictable times, resulting in "sudden death"; and certain intractable supraventricular arrhythmias.

Flecainide and its congeners are more likely than other antiarrhythmic drugs to exacerbate or precipitate arrhythmias (proarrhythmic effect). For this reason, the group IC drugs are limited to last resort applications in refractory tachycardias. These drugs also cause local anesthetic-like CNS toxicity. Hyperkalemia increases the cardiac toxicity of these agents.

4. **Amiodarone, a special case:** Amiodarone is effective in most types of arrhythmias and may be considered the most efficacious antiarrhythmic drug. This may be because it has a broad spectrum: it blocks sodium, calcium, and potassium channels and beta adrenoceptors. Because of its toxicities, however, amiodarone must be reserved for use in arrhythmias that are resistant to other drugs.

Amiodarone causes thyroid dysfunction (hyper- or hypothyroidism), paresthesias, tremor, microcrystalline deposits in the cornea and skin, and pulmonary fibrosis. Amiodarone rarely causes new arrhythmias.

GROUP II (BETA-BLOCKERS)

A. **Prototypes, Mechanisms, and Effects:** Propranolol and esmolol are the prototype antiarrhythmic beta-blockers. Their mechanism in arrhythmias is primarily cardiac beta blockade and reduction in cAMP, which results in the reduction of both sodium and calcium currents and the suppression of abnormal pacemakers. The AV node is particularly sensitive to beta-blockers; the PR interval is frequently prolonged by group II drugs (Table 14–2). Under some conditions, these drugs may have some direct local anesthetic (membrane-stabilizing) effect in the heart, but this is probably rare at the concentrations achieved clinically.

B. **Clinical Uses and Toxicities:** Esmolol, a very short-acting beta-blocker for intravenous administration, is used almost exclusively in acute surgical arrhythmias. Propranolol, metoprolol, and timolol are commonly used as prophylactic drugs in patients who have had a myocardial infarction. These drugs provide a protective effect for 2 years or more after the infarct.

The toxicities of beta-blockers are the same in patients with arrhythmias as in patients with other conditions. However, patients with arrhythmias are often more prone to β-blocker-induced depression of cardiac output than are patients with normal hearts.

GROUP III (POTASSIUM CHANNEL BLOCKERS)

A. **Prototypes:** Sotalol and ibutilide are the prototypical group III drugs. Sotalol is a chiral compound, ie, it has two optical isomers. One isomer is an effective beta-blocker; the other provides part of the antiarrhythmic action. The clinical preparation contains both isomers. Ibutilide is a newer potassium channel-blocking drug. Amiodarone is often classified as a group III drug because it markedly prolongs AP duration as well as blocking sodium channels. Bretylium is an older drug that combines general sympathoplegic actions and a potassium channel-blocking effect in ischemic tissue.

B. **Mechanism and Effects:** The hallmark of group III drugs is prolongation of the action potential duration. This AP prolongation is caused by blockade of potassium channels that are responsible for the repolarization of the action potential (Figure 14–6). Sotalol, ibutilide, and amiodarone (and quinidine, see above) produce this effect on most cardiac cells; the action of these drugs is therefore apparent in the ECG. N-Acetylprocainamide (NAPA), a metabolite of procainamide, also significantly prolongs the action potential and the QT interval. Bretylium, on the other hand, produces AP prolongation mainly in ischemic cells, and causes little change in the ECG. AP prolongation results in an increase in effective refractory period and reduces the ability of the heart to respond to rapid tachycardias.

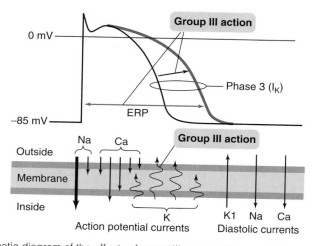

Figure 14–6. Schematic diagram of the effects of group III agents. All group III drugs prolong the AP duration in susceptible cardiac cells by reducing the outward phase 3 potassium current (I_K, wavy lines). The main effect is to prolong the effective refractory period. Note that the phase 4 diastolic potassium current (I_{K1}) is not affected by these drugs.

C. Clinical Uses and Toxicities: Bretylium is used only in the treatment of refractory post-myocardial infarction arrhythmias, eg, recurrent ventricular fibrillation. The drug is rarely used. It may precipitate new arrhythmias or marked hypotension. Sotalol is more generally useful and is available by the oral route (Table 14–2). Sotalol may precipitate torsade de pointes arrhythmia as well as signs of excessive beta blockade such as sinus bradycardia or asthma. Ibutilide is recommended for atrial flutter and fibrillation. Its most important toxicity is induction of torsade de pointes. The toxicities of amiodarone and other group IA drugs (which share the potassium channel-blocking action of group III agents) are discussed with the group IA drugs.

GROUP IV (CALCIUM CHANNEL BLOCKERS)

A. Prototype: Verapamil is the prototype. Diltiazem is also an effective antiarrhythmic drug although it is not approved for this purpose. Nifedipine and the other dihydropyridines are not useful as antiarrhythmics, probably because they decrease arterial pressure sufficiently to evoke a compensatory sympathetic discharge to the heart. The latter effect would facilitate rather than suppress arrhythmias.

B. Mechanism and Effects: Verapamil and diltiazem are effective in arrhythmias that must traverse calcium-dependent cardiac tissue (eg, the atrioventricular node). These agents cause a state- and use-dependent selective depression of calcium current in tissues that require the participation of L-type calcium channels (Figure 14–7). Conduction velocity is decreased and effective refractory period is increased by these drugs. The PR interval is consistently increased (Table 14–2).

C. Clinical Use and Toxicities: Calcium channel blockers were drugs of choice in atrioventricular nodal reentry (also known as nodal tachycardia and supraventricular tachycardia) until adenosine became available; they are highly effective in this type of arrhythmia. Their major use now is in the prevention of these nodal arrhythmias. These drugs are orally active; verapamil is also available for parenteral use (Table 14–2). The most important toxicity of verapamil as an antiarrhythmic relates to excessive pharmacologic effect, since cardiac contractility can be significantly depressed. See Chapter 12 for additional discussion of toxicity. Amiodarone has moderate calcium channel-blocking activity.

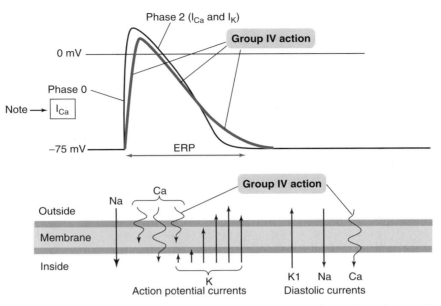

Figure 14–7. Schematic diagram of the effects of group IV drugs in a calcium-dependent cardiac cell in the AV node (note that the AP upstroke is due mainly to calcium current). Group IV drugs reduce inward calcium current during the action potential and during phase 4 (wavy lines). As a result, conduction velocity is slowed in the AV node and refractoriness is prolonged. Pacemaker depolarization during phase 4 is slowed as well if caused by the calcium current.

MISCELLANEOUS ANTIARRHYTHMIC DRUGS

A. Adenosine: Adenosine is a normal component of the body, but when it is given in high doses (6–12 mg) as an intravenous bolus, the drug markedly slows conduction in the atrioventricular node (Table 14–2), probably by hyperpolarizing this tissue and by reducing calcium current. Adenosine is extremely effective in abolishing AV nodal arrhythmias and, because of its very low toxicity, has become the drug of choice for this arrhythmia. Adenosine has an extremely short duration of action (about 15 seconds). Toxicity includes flushing and hypotension, but because of their short duration these effects do not limit the use of the drug.

B. Digitalis: The actions of digitalis were discussed in Chapter 13. The cardiac parasympathomimetic action of digoxin is sometimes exploited in the treatment of rapid atrial or AV nodal arrhythmias. In atrial flutter or fibrillation, digitalis slows AV conduction sufficiently to protect the ventricles from excessively high rates. In AV nodal reentrant arrhythmias, digitalis may exert enough depressant effect to abolish the arrhythmia. The latter application of digitalis has become less common since the development of calcium channel blockers and adenosine as antiarrhythmic drugs.

C. Potassium Ion: Potassium depresses ectopic pacemakers, including those caused by digitalis toxicity. Hypokalemia is associated with an increased incidence of arrhythmias, especially in patients receiving digitalis. Conversely, excessive potassium levels depress conduction and can cause reentry arrhythmias. Therefore, when treating arrhythmias, serum potassium should be measured and, if abnormal, normalized.

D. Magnesium Ion: Magnesium has not been as well studied as potassium but appears to have similar depressant effects on digitalis-induced arrhythmias. Magnesium also appears to be effective in some cases of torsade de pointes arrhythmia.

DRUG LIST: See Table 14–2.

QUESTIONS

DIRECTIONS: Each of the numbered items or incomplete statements in this section is followed by answers or by completions of the statement. Select the ONE lettered answer or completion that is BEST in each case.

Items 1–3: An elderly patient with rheumatoid arthritis and chronic heart disease is being considered for treatment with quinidine. She is already receiving digoxin, hydrochlorothiazide, and potassium supplements for her cardiac condition.

1. In making your decision to treat with quinidine, all of the following statements would be important EXCEPT
   (A) Quinidine may worsen or precipitate arrhythmias
   (B) Quinidine is not effective for atrial arrhythmias
   (C) Quinidine prolongs the effective refractory period in atrial and ventricular cells
   (D) Quinidine may induce thrombocytopenia
   (E) Quinidine may induce nausea, headache, and tinnitus

2. In deciding on a treatment regimen with quinidine for this patient, which of the following statements is MOST correct?
   (A) Quinidine is not active by the oral route
   (B) Quinidine has a duration of action of 20–30 hours
   (C) The serum potassium level should be as high as possible to reduce the likelihood of quinidine toxicity
   (D) Digoxin blood levels should be obtained before and after starting quinidine
   (E) Because of its beta-blocking effect, quinidine cannot be used if the patient has asthma

3. If this patient should manifest severe quinidine toxicity, rational therapy would entail the immediate administration of
   (A) A calcium chelator such as EDTA
   (B) Digitalis
   (C) KCl
   (D) Nitroprusside
   (E) Sodium lactate

4. When used as an antiarrhythmic drug, lidocaine typically
   (A) Reduces abnormal automaticity
   (B) Reduces resting potential
   (C) Increases action potential duration
   (D) Increases PR interval
   (E) Increases contractility

5. All of the following can be used for chronic oral therapy of arrhythmias EXCEPT
   (A) Amiodarone
   (B) Disopyramide
   (C) Esmolol
   (D) Procainamide
   (E) Verapamil

6. A 16-year-old girl is found to have paroxysmal attacks of rapid heart rate. The antiarrhythmic of choice in most cases of *acute* supraventricular tachycardia (nodal tachycardia) is
   (A) Adenosine
   (B) Amiodarone
   (C) Flecainide
   (D) Propranolol
   (E) Quinidine

7. A patient is admitted to the emergency department for evaluation of an abnormal ECG. Overdose of an antiarrhythmic drug is considered. Antiarrhythmic substances and their electrocardiographic effects include all of the following EXCEPT
   (A) Quinidine: increased QRS and QT intervals
   (B) Flecainide: increased PR, QRS, and QT intervals
   (C) Verapamil: increased PR interval

     (D) Lidocaine: no consistent electrocardiographic effect
     (E) Metoprolol: increased PR interval

8. Drugs that consistently reduce potassium (I_K) current and thereby prolong the action potential duration include all of the following EXCEPT
     (A) Amiodarone
     (B) Ibutilide
     (C) Lidocaine
     (D) Quinidine
     (E) Sotalol

9. Recognized adverse effects of quinidine include all of the following EXCEPT
     (A) Cinchonism
     (B) Constipation
     (C) Thrombocytopenic purpura
     (D) Reduction of digoxin clearance with possible digoxin toxicity
     (E) Precipitation of torsade de pointes arrhythmia

10. A drug that consistently hyperpolarizes the AV node and prevents conduction of impulses is
     (A) Adenosine
     (B) Digoxin
     (C) Lidocaine
     (D) Quinidine
     (E) Verapamil

DIRECTIONS (Items 11–20): Each set of matching questions in this section consists of a list of three to twenty-six lettered options (some of which may be figures) followed by several numbered items. For each numbered item, select the ONE lettered option that is MOST closely associated with it. Each lettered option may be selected once, more than once, or not at all.

     (A) Adenosine
     (B) Amiodarone
     (C) Disopyramide
     (D) Esmolol
     (E) Flecainide
     (F) Lidocaine
     (G) Mexiletine
     (H) Procainamide
     (I) Quinidine
     (J) Verapamil

11. Orally active drug that blocks sodium channels and decreases action potential duration

12. Slows conduction through the atrioventricular node; primary action is directly on calcium channels

13. Longest half-life of all antiarrhythmic drugs

14. Blocks sodium channels and prolongs action potential duration; duration of action is 6–8 hours

15. Very useful in supraventricular tachycardia; duration of action is 10–15 seconds

16. Causes thyroid abnormalities; may induce either hypo- or hyperthyroidism

17. Orally active drug that may cause purpuric rash

18. Derived from the bark of the cinchona tree; may cause tinnitus and diarrhea

19. Causes reversible lupus erythematosus

20. Sodium channel blocker with little effect on AP duration; high incidence of arrhythmia induction

ANSWERS

1. Quinidine is effective for both atrial and ventricular arrhythmias. All of the other statements are true. The answer is **(B)**.

2. Quinidine is active by the oral route and has a duration of action of 6–8 hours. Hyperkalemia facilitates quinidine toxicity. Quinidine does have a well-documented interaction with digoxin: the clearance of the latter is reduced. Quinidine has little or no beta-blocking action. The answer is **(D)**.

3. The most effective therapy for quinidine toxicity appears to be concentrated sodium lactate. This drug may (a) increase sodium current by increasing the ionic gradient and (b) reduce drug-receptor binding by alkalinizing the tissue. The answer is **(E)**.

4. Lidocaine reduces automaticity in the ventricles; the drug does not alter resting potential nor increase AP duration and does not increase contractility. The answer is **(A)**.

5. Esmolol is an ester that is rapidly metabolized even when given intravenously; it is inactive by the oral route. Therefore, esmolol would not be suitable for chronic therapy. The answer is **(C)**.

6. Calcium channel blockers are effective in supraventricular tachycardias. However, adenosine is just as effective in most acute supraventricular tachycardias and is less toxic because of its extremely short duration of action. The answer is **(A)**.

7. All the associations listed are correct except flecainide. This group IC drug has little effect on QT interval. The answer is **(B)**.

8. All of the group IA and group III agents reduce potassium current during phase 3 and prolong the action potential. Lidocaine, the prototype IB drug, actually shortens the duration under some circumstances. The answer is **(C)**.

9. Quinidine has a wide spectrum of adverse effects but causes increased, not decreased, gastrointestinal motility and often results in diarrhea. The answer is **(B)**.

10. The only antiarrhythmic agent that consistently alters the resting potential of the AV node is adenosine. It apparently activates potassium channels in the AV node, thus forcing the membrane potential closer to the Nernst potassium potential; adenosine therefore significantly hyperpolarizes this tissue, preventing the conduction of action potentials. The answer is **(A)**.

11. Group IB drugs such as lidocaine and mexiletine typically block sodium channels and decrease the action potential duration. Mexiletine, but not lidocaine, is orally active. The answer is **(G)**.

12. Verapamil is the calcium channel blocker in this list. (Adenosine and beta-blockers also slow AV conduction but do not act primarily on calcium channels.) The answer is **(J)**.

13. Amiodarone has the longest half-life of all the antiarrhythmics (Table 14–2). The answer is **(B)**.

14. Quinidine, procainamide, and amiodarone all block sodium channels and prolong the action potential. The duration of amiodarone action, however, is very long; that of procainamide is shorter than 6–8 hours (Table 14–2). The answer is **(I)**.

15. The only drug in the list with a half-life of seconds is adenosine. The answer is **(A)**.

16. Amiodarone is the only antiarrhythmic drug that is associated with thyroid toxicity. The answer is **(B)**.

17. Quinidine may cause thrombocytopenia; this can lead to punctate hemorrhages under the skin (purpura). The answer is **(I)**.

18. Quinidine is derived, along with quinine, from cinchona bark. The answer is **(I)**.

19. Procainamide frequently results in a positive antinuclear antibody (ANA) test after prolonged therapy; this may progress to typical signs of drug-induced lupus (joint, skin, and systemic but not renal changes). The answer is **(H)**.

20. The IC antiarrhythmic drugs have little effect on AP duration; they have been associated with a high incidence of drug-induced arrhythmias. The answer is **(E)**.

15

Diuretic Agents

OBJECTIVES

You should be able to:

- List five major types of diuretics and relate them to their sites of action.
- Describe two drugs that reduce potassium loss during sodium diuresis.
- Describe a therapy that will reduce calcium excretion in patients who have recurrent urinary stones.

- Describe a treatment for severe hypercalcemia in a patient with advanced carcinoma.
- Describe a method for reducing urine volume in nephrogenic diabetes insipidus.
- List the major applications and the toxicities of thiazides, loop diuretics, and potassium-sparing diuretics.

Learn the definitions that follow.

Table 15–1. Definitions.

Term	Definition
Bicarbonate diuretic	A diuretic that selectively increases sodium bicarbonate excretion. *Example:* a carbonic anhydrase inhibitor
Diluting segment	A segment of the nephron that removes solute without water; the thick ascending limb and the distal convoluted tubule are active salt-absorbing segments that are not permeant to water
Hyperchloremic metabolic acidosis	A shift in body electrolyte and pH balance involving elevated chloride, diminished bicarbonate concentration, and a decrease in pH in the blood. Typical result of bicarbonate diuresis
Hypokalemic metabolic alkalosis	A shift in body electrolyte balance and pH involving a decrease in serum potassium and an increase in blood pH. Typical result of loop and thiazide diuretics
Nephrogenic diabetes insipidus	Loss of urine-concentrating ability in the kidney caused by lack of responsiveness to antidiuretic hormone (ADH is present)
Pituitary diabetes insipidus	Loss of urine-concentrating ability in the kidney caused by lack of antidiuretic hormone (ADH is absent)
Potassium-sparing diuretic	A diuretic that reduces the exchange of potassium for sodium in the collecting tubule; a drug that increases sodium and reduces potassium excretion. *Example:* aldosterone antagonists
Uricosuric diuretic	A diuretic that increases uric acid excretion, usually by inhibiting uric acid reabsorption in the proximal tubule. *Example:* ethacrynic acid

CONCEPTS

RENAL TRANSPORT & DIURETIC DRUG GROUPS

A. **Renal Transport Mechanisms:** Each segment (proximal convoluted tubule, PCT; thick ascending limb of the loop of Henle, TAL; distal convoluted tubule, DCT; and cortical collecting tubule, CCT) has a different mechanism for reabsorbing sodium and other ions. The subgroups of the diuretics are based upon these sites in the nephron (Figure 15–1). The effects of the diuretic agents are predictable from a knowledge of the function of the segment of the nephron in which they act (Figure 15–2).

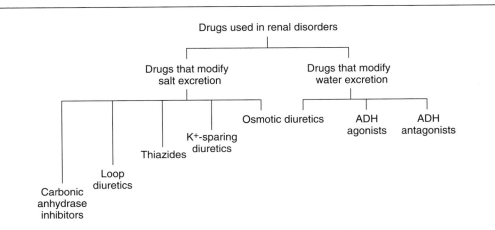

Figure 15–1. Subgroups of drugs discussed in this chapter.

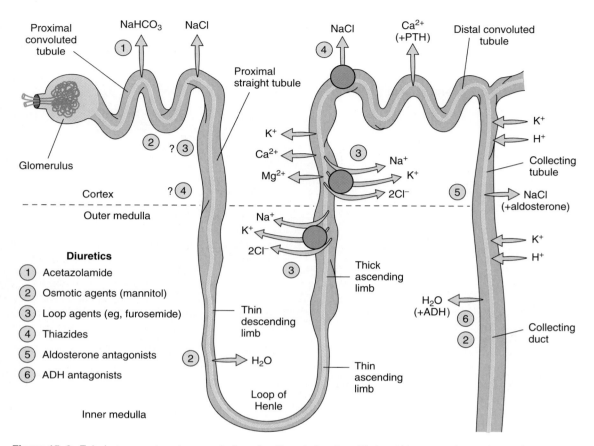

Figure 15–2. Tubule transport systems and sites of action of diuretics. Circles with arrows denote known ion cotransporters that are targets of the diuretics indicated by the numerals. Question marks denote preliminary or incompletely documented suggestions for the location of certain drug effects. (Reproduced, with permission, from Katzung BG [editor]: *Basic & Clinical Pharmacology,* 7th ed. Appleton & Lange, 1998.)

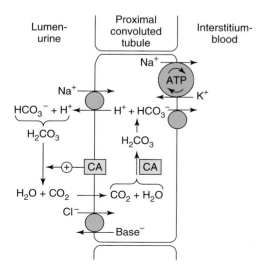

Figure 15–3. Mechanisms of sodium bicarbonate reabsorption in the proximal tubule cell. CA, carbonic anhydrase. (Reproduced, with permission, from Katzung BG [editor]: *Basic & Clinical Pharmacology,* 7th ed. Appleton & Lange, 1998.)

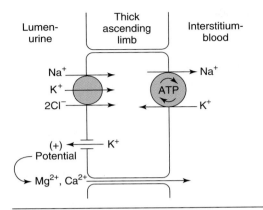

Figure 15–4. Mechanisms of sodium, potassium, and chloride reabsorption in the thick ascending limb of the loop of Henle. Note that pumping of potassium into the cell from both the lumen and the interstitium would result in unphysiologically high intracellular K^+ concentration. This is avoided by movement of K^+ down its concentration gradient back into the lumen, carrying with it excess positive charge. This positive charge drives the reabsorption of calcium and magnesium. (Reproduced, with permission, from Katzung BG [editor]: *Basic & Clinical Pharmacology,* 7th ed. Appleton & Lange, 1998.)

1. **Proximal convoluted tubule (PCT):** This segment carries out isosmotic reabsorption of amino acids, glucose, and cations. This is also the major site for bicarbonate reabsorption. The mechanism for bicarbonate reabsorption is shown in Figure 15–3. Although bicarbonate itself is not reabsorbed through the luminal membrane, conversion of bicarbonate to carbon dioxide permits rapid reabsorption; sodium is reabsorbed in exchange for hydrogen ions. Bicarbonate can then be regenerated within the tubular cell and reabsorbed back into the blood. Carbonic anhydrase, the enzyme required for this bicarbonate reabsorption process, is the target of carbonic anhydrase inhibitor diuretic drugs. The proximal tubule is responsible for 40–50% of the total reabsorption of sodium. Active secretion and reabsorption of weak acids and bases also occurs in the PCT. Most weak acid transport occurs in the S_2 segment; weak bases are transported in the S_1 and S_2 segments. Uric acid transport is especially important and is targeted by some of the drugs used in treating gout (Chapter 36).

2. **Thick portion of the ascending limb of the loop of Henle (TAL):** This segment pumps sodium, potassium, and chloride out of the lumen into the interstitium of the kidney. As shown in Figure 15–4, it is also a major site of calcium and magnesium reabsorption. Reabsorption of sodium, potassium, and chloride are all carried out by a single carrier, which is the target of the loop diuretics. This cotransporter provides the concentration gradient for the countercurrent-concentrating mechanism in the kidney and is responsible for the reabsorption of 30–40% of the sodium filtered at the glomerulus. Because potassium is pumped into the cell from both the luminal and basal sides, an escape route must be provided; this occurs into the lumen via a potassium channel. Since the potassium diffusing back is not accompanied by an anion, a net positive charge is set up in the lumen. This positive potential drives the reabsorption of calcium and magnesium.

3. **Distal convoluted tubule (DCT):** This segment actively pumps sodium and chloride out of the lumen of the nephron via the carrier shown in Figure 15–5. This cotransporter is the

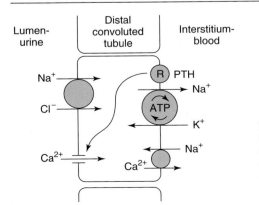

Figure 15–5. Mechanism of sodium and chloride reabsorption in the distal convoluted tubule. A separate reabsorptive mechanism, modulated by parathyroid hormone, is present for movement of calcium into the cell from the urine. This calcium must be transported via the sodium-calcium exchanger back into the blood. (Reproduced, with permission, from Katzung BG [editor]: *Basic & Clinical Pharmacology,* 7th ed. Appleton & Lange, 1998.)

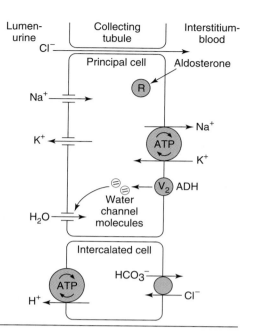

Figure 15–6. Mechanisms of sodium, potassium, and hydrogen ion movement and water reabsorption in the collecting tubule cells. Synthesis of Na^+/K^+ ATPase and sodium and potassium channels is under the control of aldosterone, which combines with an intracellular receptor, *R*, before entering the nucleus. ADH acts on its receptor, V_2, to facilitate the insertion of water channels from storage vesicles into the luminal membrane. (Reproduced, with permission, from Katzung BG [editor]: *Basic & Clinical Pharmacology*, 7th ed. Appleton & Lange, 1998.)

target of the thiazide diuretics. The distal convoluted tubule is responsible for approximately 10% of sodium reabsorption. Calcium is also reabsorbed in this segment under the control of parathyroid hormone (PTH). Removal of the reabsorbed calcium back into the blood requires the sodium-calcium exchange process, discussed in Chapter 13.

4. **Cortical collecting tubule (CCT):** The final segment of the nephron is the last tubular site of sodium reabsorption and is controlled by aldosterone (Figure 15–6). The aldosterone receptor and the sodium channels are sites of potassium-sparing diuretic action. This segment is responsible for reabsorbing 2–4% of the total filtered sodium. Reabsorption occurs via sodium channels and is accompanied by an equivalent loss of potassium or hydrogen ions. The CCT is thus the primary site of acidification of the urine. Reabsorption of water occurs here and in the medullary collecting tubule under the control of antidiuretic hormone (ADH).

B. **Diuretic Drug Groups:** Because the mechanisms of reabsorption of salt and water differ in each of the four segments discussed above, the diuretics acting in these segments each have differing mechanisms of action. Most diuretics act from the luminal side of the membrane and must be present in the urine. They are filtered at the glomerulus, and some are also secreted by the weak acid secretory carrier in the proximal tubule. An exception is the aldosterone receptor antagonist spironolactone, which enters from the basolateral side and binds to the cytoplasmic aldosterone receptor.

CARBONIC ANHYDRASE INHIBITORS

A. **Prototypes and Mechanism of Action:** Acetazolamide is the prototype agent. These diuretics are sulfonamide derivatives. The mechanism of action is inhibition of carbonic anhydrase in the brush border and intracellular carbonic anhydrase in the PCT cells (Figure 15–3). Inhibition of carbonic anhydrase by acetazolamide occurs in other tissues of the body as well as in the kidney.

B. **Effects:** The major renal effect is a bicarbonate diuresis (ie, sodium bicarbonate is excreted); body bicarbonate is depleted, and a metabolic acidosis results. As increased sodium is presented to the cortical collecting tubule, some of the excess sodium is reabsorbed and potassium is secreted, resulting in significant potassium "wasting" (Table 15–2). As a result of bicarbonate

Table 15–2. Electrolyte changes produced by diuretic drugs.

Drug Group	Urine[1]			Body	
	NaCl	NaHCO$_3$	K$^+$	Cl^{-2}	pH
Carbonic anhydrase inhibitors	↑	↑↑↑	↑	↑	Acidosis
Loop diuretics	↑↑↑↑	↓	↑	↓	Alkalosis
Thiazides	↑↑	↑, ↓	↑	↓	Alkalosis
Potassium-sparing diuretics	↑	↓	↓	↓, ↑	Acidosis

[1]Arrows indicate change in *amount* of salt or ion excreted.
[2]Arrows indicate change in *concentration* of chloride ion in blood.

depletion, sodium bicarbonate excretion slows—even with continued diuretic administration—and the diuresis is self-limiting within 2–3 days. The inhibitory effect of acetazolamide occurs throughout the body; secretion of bicarbonate into aqueous humor by the ciliary epithelium in the eye and into the cerebrospinal fluid by the choroid plexus is reduced. In the eye, a useful reduction in intraocular pressure can be achieved. This effect is not self-limiting. In the CNS, acidosis of the cerebrospinal fluid results in hyperventilation, which can protect against high altitude sickness.

C. Clinical Uses: The major application of carbonic anhydrase inhibitors is in the treatment of glaucoma. Acetazolamide must be used orally, but a topical analog is now available (dorzolamide). Carbonic anhydrase inhibitors are also used to prevent development of acute mountain (high-altitude) sickness. These agents are used for their diuretic effect only if edema is accompanied by significant metabolic alkalosis.

D. Toxicity: Drowsiness and paresthesias are commonly reported. Cross-allergenicity occurs between these and all other sulfonamide derivatives. Alkalinization of the urine by these drugs may cause precipitation of calcium salts and formation of renal stones. Renal potassium wasting may be marked. Patients with hepatic impairment may develop hepatic encephalopathy because of increased ammonia reabsorption.

LOOP DIURETICS

A. Prototypes and Mechanism of Action: Furosemide is the prototypical loop agent. Furosemide, bumetanide, and torsemide are sulfonamide derivatives. Ethacrynic acid is a phenoxyacetic acid derivative; it is not a sulfonamide but acts by the same mechanism. Loop diuretics inhibit the cotransport of sodium, potassium, and chloride (Figure 15–4). The loop diuretics are relatively short-acting (diuresis usually occurs over the 4 hours following a dose).

B. Effects: The loop of Henle is responsible for a large proportion of total renal sodium chloride reabsorption; therefore, a full dose of a loop diuretic produces massive sodium chloride diuresis. If tissue perfusion is adequate, edema fluid is rapidly excreted and blood volume may be significantly reduced. The diluting ability of the nephron is reduced because the loop of Henle is the site of significant dilution of urine. Inhibition of the transporter also results in loss of the lumen-positive potential, which reduces reabsorption of divalent cations as well. As a result, calcium excretion is significantly increased. Ethacrynic acid is a moderately effective uricosuric drug. The presentation of large amounts of sodium to the cortical collecting tubule may result in significant potassium wasting and excretion of protons; hypokalemic alkalosis may result (Table 15–2). The loop diuretics also have useful pulmonary vasodilating effects; the mechanism is not understood.

C. Clinical Use: The major application of loop diuretics is in the treatment of edematous states (eg, congestive heart failure and ascites). They are particularly valuable in acute pulmonary edema, in which the pulmonary vasodilating action plays a useful role. They are sometimes used in hypertension if response to thiazides is inadequate; but the short duration of action of loop diuretics is a disadvantage in this condition. A less common but important application is in the treatment of severe hypercalcemia (eg, that induced by malignancy). This life-threatening condition can often be managed with large doses of furosemide coupled with parenteral volume and electrolyte (sodium and potassium chloride) supplementation. It should be noted that diuresis *without* volume replacement will result in hemoconcentration; serum calcium concentration will then not diminish and may even increase further.

D. Toxicity: Loop diuretics usually induce hypokalemic metabolic alkalosis. Because large amounts of sodium are presented to the collecting tubules, wasting of potassium (which is excreted by the kidney, thus conserving sodium) may be severe. Because they are so efficacious, the loop diuretics can cause hypovolemia and cardiovascular complications. Ototoxicity is an important toxic effect of the loop agents. The sulfonamides in this group may cause typical sulfonamide allergy.

THIAZIDE DIURETICS

A. Prototypes and Mechanism of Action: Hydrochlorothiazide, the prototypical agent, is a sulfonamide derivative. A few sulfonamide derivatives that lack the typical thiazide ring in their structure nevertheless have effects identical to those of thiazides and are therefore considered thiazide-like. Indapamide is one of these thiazide-like agents and has a significant vasodilating effect. Thiazides are active by the oral route and have a duration of action of 6–12 hours, considerably longer than that of the loop diuretics. The major action of thiazides is to inhibit sodium chloride transport in the early segment of the distal convoluted tubule (Figure 15–5).

B. Effects: In full doses, thiazides produce moderate but sustained sodium and chloride diuresis. Hypokalemic metabolic alkalosis may occur. Reduction in the transport of sodium into the tubular cell reduces intracellular sodium and promotes sodium-calcium exchange. As a result, reabsorption of calcium from the urine is increased and urine calcium content is decreased—the *opposite* of the effect of loop diuretics.

Thiazides reduce the blood pressure (Chapter 11). Initially, the reduction reflects the reduction of blood volume, but with continued use these agents appear to reduce vascular resistance as well. The vascular effect is modest but significant and is maximal at doses lower than the maximal diuretic dosage. Compared with older thiazides and thiazide-like agents, indapamide may have a greater ratio of vasodilating effect relative to its sodium diuretic effect.

When a thiazide is used with a loop diuretic, a synergistic effect occurs with marked diuresis.

C. Clinical Use: The major application of thiazides is in hypertension, for which their long duration and moderate intensity of action are particularly useful. Chronic therapy of edematous conditions such as congestive heart failure is another common application. Chronic renal calcium stone formation can be reduced with thiazides because of their ability to reduce urine calcium concentration.

D. Toxicity: Massive sodium diuresis with hyponatremia is an uncommon but dangerous early effect of thiazides. Chronic therapy is often associated with potassium wasting, since an increased sodium load is presented to the collecting tubules. Diabetic patients may have significant hyperglycemia. Serum uric acid and lipid levels are also increased in some individuals. Thiazides are sulfonamides and share sulfonamide allergenicity.

POTASSIUM-SPARING DIURETICS

A. Prototypes and Mechanism of Action: Spironolactone, a steroid derivative, is a pharmacologic antagonist of aldosterone in the collecting tubules. By combining with the intracellular aldosterone receptor, spironolactone reduces expression of the genes controlling synthesis of sodium ion channels and Na+/K+ ATPase. Amiloride and triamterene act by blocking the sodium channels in the same portion of the nephron (Figure 15–6). Spironolactone has a slow onset and offset of action (24–72 hours). Amiloride and triamterene have durations of action of 12–24 hours.

B. **Effects:** All three drugs in this class cause an increase in sodium clearance and a decrease in potassium and hydrogen ion excretion and therefore qualify as "potassium-sparing" diuretics. These drugs may cause hyperkalemic metabolic acidosis.

C. **Clinical Use:** Aldosteronism (eg, the elevated serum aldosterone levels that occur in cirrhosis) is an important indication for spironolactone. Potassium wasting caused by chronic therapy with loop or thiazide diuretics, if not controlled by dietary potassium supplements, will usually respond to these drugs. The most common use is in the form of products that combine a thiazide with a potassium-sparing agent in a single pill.

D. **Toxicity:** The most important toxic effect is hyperkalemia. These drugs should never be given with potassium supplements. Other aldosterone antagonists (such as ACE inhibitors), if used at all, should be used with great caution. Spironolactone may cause endocrine abnormalities, including gynecomastia and antiandrogenic effects.

OSMOTIC DIURETICS

A. **Prototypes and Mechanism of Action:** Mannitol, the prototypical osmotic diuretic, is given intravenously. Other drugs often classified with mannitol (but rarely used) include glycerin, isosorbide, and urea. Because it is filtered at the glomerulus but poorly reabsorbed from the tubule, mannitol "holds" water in the lumen by virtue of its osmotic effect. The major location for this action is the proximal convoluted tubule, where the bulk of isosmotic reabsorption normally takes place. Reabsorption of water is also reduced in the descending limb of the loop of Henle and the collecting tubule.

B. **Effects:** The volume of urine is increased. Most filtered solutes will be excreted in larger amounts unless they are actively reabsorbed. Sodium excretion is usually increased because the rate of urine flow through the tubule is greatly accelerated and sodium transporters cannot handle the volume rapidly enough. Mannitol can also reduce brain volume and intracranial pressure by osmotically extracting water from the tissue into the blood. A similar effect occurs in the eye.

C. **Clinical Use:** These drugs are used to maintain high urine flow (eg, when renal blood flow is reduced and in conditions of solute overload from severe hemolysis or rhabdomyolysis). Mannitol and several other osmotic agents are useful in reducing intraocular pressure in acute glaucoma and intracranial pressure in neurologic conditions.

D. **Toxicity:** Removal of water from the intracellular compartment may cause hyponatremia and pulmonary edema. As the water is excreted, hypernatremia may follow. Headache, nausea, and vomiting are common.

ANTIDIURETIC HORMONE AGONISTS & ANTAGONISTS

A. **Prototypes and Mechanism of Action:** Antidiuretic hormone (ADH) and desmopressin are prototypical antidiuretic hormone agonists. They are peptides and must be given parenterally. Demeclocycline and lithium ion are ADH antagonists that can be used orally.

   ADH facilitates water reabsorption from the collecting tubule by activation of adenylyl cyclase. The increased cAMP causes the insertion of additional water channels into the luminal membrane in this part of the tubule (Figure 15–6). Demeclocycline and lithium inhibit the action of ADH at some point distal to the generation of cAMP and presumably interfere with the insertion of water channels into the membrane.

B. **Effects and Clinical Uses:** ADH and desmopressin reduce urine volume and increase its concentration. ADH and desmopressin are useful in pituitary diabetes insipidus. They are of no value in the nephrogenic form of the disease, but salt restriction, thiazides, and loop diuretics may be used.

ADH antagonists oppose the actions of ADH and other naturally occurring peptides that act on the same V_2 receptor. Such peptides are produced by certain tumors (eg, small cell carcinoma of the lung) and can cause significant water retention and dangerous hyponatremia. This syndrome of inappropriate ADH secretion (SIADH) can be treated with demeclocycline.

C. Toxicity: In the presence of ADH and desmopressin, a large water load may cause dangerous hyponatremia. Large doses of either peptide may cause hypertension in some individuals.

In children under 8 years of age, demeclocycline (like other tetracyclines) causes bone and teeth abnormalities. Lithium causes nephrogenic diabetes insipidus as a toxic effect; the drug is never used to treat SIADH because of its other toxicities.

DRUG LIST

The following drugs are important members of the group discussed in this chapter. Prototypes should be learned in detail; the features of major variants should be known well enough so that the variants can be distinguished from prototypes and from each other; the other significant agents should be recognized as belonging to a specific subclass.

Subclass	Prototype	Major Variants	Other Significant Drugs
Carbonic anhydrase inhibitors	Acetazolamide	Dorzolamide	
Loop diuretics	Furosemide	Ethacrynic acid	
Thiazides and thiazide-like drugs	Hydrochlorothiazide	Indapamide	Metolazone
Potassium-sparing diuretics	Spironolactone, amiloride		Triamterene
Osmotic diuretics	Mannitol		
ADH agonists	Vasopressin	Desmopressin	
ADH antagonists	Demeclocycline	Lithium	

QUESTIONS

DIRECTIONS: Each of the numbered items or incomplete statements in this section is followed by answers or by completions of the statement. Select the ONE lettered answer or completion that is BEST in each case.

1. A 70-year-old man is admitted with a history of heart failure and acute left ventricular myocardial infarction. He has severe pulmonary edema. Which of the following drugs has a rapid diuretic effect plus smooth muscle effects that prove useful in the treatment of acute pulmonary edema?
   (A) Furosemide
   (B) Hydrochlorothiazide
   (C) Spironolactone
   (D) Triamterene
   (E) Acetazolamide

2. A 50-year-old man has a history of frequent episodes of renal colic with high-calcium renal stones. The most useful agent in the treatment of recurrent calcium stones is
   (A) Mannitol
   (B) Furosemide
   (C) Spironolactone
   (D) Hydrochlorothiazide
   (E) Acetazolamide

3. When used chronically to treat hypertension, thiazide diuretics have all of the following properties or effects EXCEPT

    (A)   Reduction of blood volume or vascular resistance or both
    (B)   Maximal effects on blood pressure at dosages below the maximal diuretic dosage
    (C)   Elevation of plasma uric acid and triglyceride levels
    (D)   Reduction of the urinary excretion of calcium
    (E)   Ototoxicity

4. Which of the following drugs is correctly associated with its site of action and maximal diuretic efficacy?
    (A)   Thiazides—distal convoluted tubule—10% of filtered Na^+
    (B)   Spironolactone—distal convoluted tubule—10%
    (C)   Furosemide—thick ascending limb—15%
    (D)   Metolazone—collecting tubule—2%
    (E)   All of the above

5. A patient with long-standing diabetic renal disease and hyperkalemia and recent-onset congestive heart failure requires a diuretic. Which of the following agents would be LEAST harmful in a patient with severe hyperkalemia?
    (A)   Amiloride
    (B)   Captopril
    (C)   Hydrochlorothiazide
    (D)   Spironolactone
    (E)   Triamterene

6. Which of the following would be MOST useful in a patient with cerebral edema?
    (A)   Acetazolamide
    (B)   Amiloride
    (C)   Ethacrynic acid
    (D)   Furosemide
    (E)   Mannitol

7. Which of the following is NOT a complication of therapy with thiazide diuretics?
    (A)   Hypercalciuria
    (B)   Hyponatremia
    (C)   Hypokalemia
    (D)   Hyperuricemia
    (E)   Metabolic alkalosis

8. Which of the following therapies would be MOST useful in the management of severe hypercalcemia?
    (A)   Amiloride plus saline infusion
    (B)   Furosemide plus saline infusion
    (C)   Hydrochlorothiazide plus saline infusion
    (D)   Mannitol plus saline infusion
    (E)   Spironolactone plus saline infusion

9. A 70-year-old woman is admitted to the emergency room because of a "fainting spell" at home. She appears to have suffered no trauma from her fall, but her blood pressure is 110/60 when lying down and 60/40 when she sits up. Neurologic examination and an ECG are within normal limits when she is lying down. Questioning reveals that she has been on "water pills" for a heart condition. All of the following statements about this case are reasonable EXCEPT
    (A)   The fainting spell could have resulted from postural hypotension caused by an inadvertent overdose with furosemide
    (B)   The fainting spell could have resulted from a transient arrhythmia caused by furosemide-induced hypokalemia
    (C)   The fainting spell could be unrelated to her diuretic therapy
    (D)   The fainting spell could have resulted from furosemide-induced hyperuricemia
    (E)   Management should include careful evaluation of her blood volume

10. A patient complains of paresthesias and occasional nausea associated with one of her drugs. She is found to have hyperchloremic metabolic acidosis. She is probably taking
    (A)   Acetazolamide for glaucoma
    (B)   Amiloride for edema associated with aldosteronism
    (C)   Furosemide for severe hypertension and congestive failure
    (D)   Hydrochlorothiazide for hypertension
    (E)   Mannitol for cerebral edema

DIRECTIONS (Items 11–16):   Each set of matching questions in this section consists of a list of three to twenty-six lettered options (some of which may be figures) followed by several numbered items. For each numbered item, select the ONE lettered option that is MOST closely associated with it. Each lettered option may be selected once, more than once, or not at all.

    (A) Acetazolamide
    (B) Amiloride
    (C) Demeclocycline
    (D) Desmopressin
    (E) Ethacrynic acid
    (F) Furosemide
    (G) Metolazone
    (H) Mannitol
    (I) Spironolactone
    (J) Triamterene

11.   Causes a self-limiting diuresis and a hyperchloremic metabolic acidosis
12.   Is not a thiazide but has its major effect in the distal convoluted tubule
13.   Increases the formation of dilute urine in water-loaded subjects; used to treat SIADH
14.   Useful in glaucoma and high-altitude sickness
15.   Acts in the thick ascending limb of the loop of Henle; no cross-allergenicity with thiazides
16.   Can reduce the binding of aldosterone to its receptor

ANSWERS

1.   Furosemide has a rapid onset of action, is very efficacious, and appears to have significant direct smooth muscle-relaxing effects, especially in the pulmonary vessels. The answer is **(A)**.

2.   The thiazides are useful in the prevention of calcium stones because these drugs inhibit the renal excretion of calcium. In contrast, the loop agents facilitate calcium excretion. The answer is **(D)**.

3.   Thiazides do not cause ototoxicity; loop diuretics do. The answer is **(E)**.

4.   Spironolactone acts in the collecting tubule, not the distal convoluted tubule. This drug is not capable of causing a 10% sodium diuresis. Furosemide, a loop diuretic, can produce a 30–40% increase in sodium excretion. Metolazone, a thiazide-like drug, acts in the distal convoluted tubule, not in the collecting tubule. The answer is **(A)**.

5.   Hyperkalemia should not be treated with drugs that interfere with aldosterone production (eg, captopril) or collecting tubule potassium excretion (eg, amiloride, spironolactone, triamterene). These agents are all capable of increasing serum potassium. Hydrochlorothiazide would not reduce serum potassium rapidly, but neither would it increase it. The answer is **(C)**.

6.   An osmotic agent is needed to remove water from the cells of the edematous brain and reduce intracranial pressure. The answer is **(E)**.

7.   Thiazides produce all of the effects listed except hypercalciuria. They *reduce* urine calcium and for this reason are useful in chronic stone formers. The answer is **(A)**.

8.   Diuretic therapy of hypercalcemia requires reduction of calcium reabsorption in the thick ascending limb. However, a loop diuretic alone would reduce blood volume around the remaining calcium so that serum calcium would not decrease appropriately. Therefore, saline infusion should accompany the loop diuretic. The answer is **(B)**.

9.   The clinical vignette and the choice of answers suggest that the patient is taking a diuretic. Complications of diuretics that could result in syncope (fainting) include both postural hypotension (which this patient exhibits) due to excessive reduction of blood volume and arrhythmias due to excessive potassium loss. On the other hand, we have not ruled out other possible causes; the syncope may be unrelated to her diuretic therapy. Management would certainly include evaluation of her hemodynamic status, especially the level of hydration and blood volume, and her neurologic status. Both loop and thiazide diuretics may cause hyperuricemia. However, diuretic-induced hyperuricemia is not a cause of syncope but may cause acute gout in patients with gout as a preexisting condition. The answer is **(D)**.

10.   Paresthesias and gastrointestinal distress are common adverse effects of acetazolamide, especially when it is taken chronically, as in glaucoma. The observation that the patient has metabolic acidosis confirms the use of acetazolamide. The answer is **(A)**.

11. The carbonic anhydrase inhibitors, as suggested in question 10, cause metabolic acidosis; the diuresis is self-limiting because of bicarbonate depletion associated with this acidosis. The answer is (**A**).

12. Metolazone, though not a thiazide, is a sulfonamide that is often used as a thiazide substitute. The action and toxicities of metolazone (including sulfonamide allergy) are indistinguishable from those of the thiazides. The answer is (**G**).

13. Inability to form dilute urine in the fully hydrated condition is characteristic of SIADH. Antagonists of ADH are needed to treat this condition. The answer is (**C**).

14. Carbonic anhydrase inhibitors are useful in glaucoma and altitude sickness. The answer is (**A**).

15. A loop agent that does not demonstrate cross-allergenicity with thiazides is not a sulfonamide derivative. The answer is (**E**).

16. Spironolactone is a pharmacologic antagonist of aldosterone—ie, it binds to the same receptor as the salt-retaining hormone. The answer is (**I**).

Part IV: Drugs With Important Actions on Smooth Muscle

16 Histamine, Serotonin, & the Ergot Alkaloids

OBJECTIVES

You should be able to:

- List the major organ system effects of histamine and serotonin.
- List two or three different antihistamines of the H_1 and H_2 types.
- List two antiserotonin drugs and their major applications; describe the action of and indication for sumatriptan.
- List the major organ system effects of the ergot alkaloids.
- Describe the major clinical applications of the ergot drugs.

Learn the definitions that follow.

Table 16–1. Definitions.

Term	Definition
Acid-peptic disease	Disease of upper digestive tract caused by acid and pepsin; includes erosions and ulcers
Autacoids	Endogeneous substances with complex physiologic and pathophysiologic functions; commonly taken to include histamine, serotonin, prostaglandins, and vasoactive peptides
Carcinoid	A neoplasm of the bronchi or gastrointestinal tract that may secrete serotonin and a variety of peptides
Ergotism ("St. Anthony's Fire")	Disease caused by excess ergot alkaloids; classically an epidemic caused by consumption of grain (in bread, etc) contaminated by the ergot fungus
Gastrinoma	A tumor that produces large amounts of gastrin; associated with hypersecretion of gastric acid and pepsin, leading to ulceration
IgE-mediated immediate reaction	An allergic response caused by interaction of an antigen with IgE antibodies on mast cells; results in the release of histamine and other mediators of allergy
Oxytocic drug	One that causes contraction of the uterus
Prolactinoma	A tumor of the anterior pituitary that produces large amounts of prolactin and leads to amenorrhea or galactorrhea
Zollinger-Ellison syndrome	Syndrome of hypersecretion of gastric acid and pepsin, often caused by gastrinoma; it is associated with severe acid-peptic ulceration and diarrhea

CONCEPTS

Autacoids are endogenous molecules with powerful effects but poorly defined physiologic roles. Histamine and serotonin (5-hydroxytryptamine, 5-HT) are two of the most important autacoids.

Both are synthesized in the body from amino acid precursors and then eliminated by pathways very similar to those used for catecholamine synthesis and metabolism. The ergot alkaloids are a heterogeneous group of drugs that interact with serotonin receptors, dopamine receptors, and adrenoceptors. They are included in this chapter because of their effects on serotonin receptors and on smooth muscle.

HISTAMINE

Histamine is formed from the amino acid histidine and is stored in high concentrations in mast cells. Histamine is metabolized by amine oxidase enzymes. Excess production of histamine in the body can be detected by measurement of imidazoleacetic acid, its major metabolite, in the urine. Because it is released from mast cells in response to IgE-mediated (immediate) allergic reactions, this autacoid plays an important pathophysiologic role in seasonal rhinitis (hay fever), urticaria, and angioneurotic edema. Histamine also plays an important physiologic role in the control of acid secretion in the stomach.

    A. Receptors and Effects: Two receptors for histamine, H_1 and H_2, mediate most of the well-defined peripheral actions; a third (H_3) has been identified (Table 16–2).

        1. H_1 receptor: This receptor is important in smooth muscle effects, especially those caused by IgE-mediated responses. IP_3 and DAG are released. Typical responses include bronchoconstriction and vasodilation, the latter by release of endothelium-derived relaxing factor (EDRF). Capillary endothelium, in addition to releasing EDRF, also contracts, opening gaps in the permeability barrier and resulting in the formation of local edema. These effects are manifest in allergic reactions and in mastocytosis, a rare neoplasm of mast cells.

        2. H_2 receptor: This receptor mediates gastric acid secretion by parietal cells in the stomach. It also has a cardiac stimulant effect. A third action is to reduce histamine release from mast cells—a negative feedback effect. These actions are mediated by activation of adenylyl cyclase, which increases intracellular cAMP.

        3. H_3 receptor: This receptor appears to be involved mainly in presynaptic modulation of histaminergic neurotransmission in the central nervous system. In the periphery, it appears to be a presynaptic heteroreceptor with modulatory effects on the release of other transmitters.

    B. Clinical Use: Histamine has no therapeutic applications, but drugs that block histamine's effects are very important in clinical medicine.

HISTAMINE H_1 ANTAGONISTS

    A. Classification and Prototypes: A wide variety of antihistaminic H_1 blockers are available from several different chemical families. Diphenhydramine and chlorpheniramine may be considered prototypes. Because they have been developed for use in chronic conditions, H_1 blockers are all active by the oral route. Most are metabolized extensively in the liver. Half-lives of

Table 16–2. Histamine and serotonin receptor subtypes.[1]

Receptor Subtype	Distribution	Postreceptor Mechanisms	Prototype Antagonist
H_1	Smooth muscle	G_q; ↑ IP_3, DAG	Diphenhydramine
H_2	Stomach, heart, mast cells	G_s; ↑ cAMP	Cimetidine
H_3	Nerve endings, CNS	G protein-coupled	Impromidine[2]
$5\text{-}HT_{1d}$	Brain	G_i; ↓ cAMP	. . .
$5\text{-}HT_2$	Smooth muscle, platelets	G_q; ↑ IP_3, DAG	Ketanserin
$5\text{-}HT_3$	Area postrema (CNS), sensory and enteric nerves	Gated cation channel	Ondansetron

[1]Many other serotonin receptors are recognized in the CNS. They are discussed in Chapter 21.
[2]Research use only.

the older H_1 blockers vary from 4 hours to 12 hours. Several newer agents ("second-generation" antihistamines, eg, terfenadine, fexofenadine, astemizole, loratadine) have half-lives of 12–24 hours and decreased CNS penetration.

B. Mechanism and Effects: H_1 blockers are competitive pharmacologic antagonists at the H_1 receptor; these drugs have no effect on histamine release from storage sites. Because their structure closely resembles that of muscarinic blockers and alpha-adrenoceptor blockers, many of these agents are also pharmacologic antagonists at these autonomic receptors. A few also block serotonin receptors. However, they have negligible effects at H_2 receptors.

H_1-blocking drugs have sedative and anti-motion sickness effects in the CNS. In the periphery, they competitively inhibit the effects of histamine (especially if given before histamine release occurs). In addition, they may block muscarinic, alpha adrenoceptor-mediated, and some serotonin-mediated effects. Many H_1 blockers are potent local anesthetics.

C. Clinical Use: H_1 blockers have major applications in allergies of the immediate type (ie, those caused by antigens acting on IgE antibody-sensitized mast cells). These conditions include hay fever and urticaria. The drugs have a broad spectrum of adverse effects that limit their usefulness but can sometimes be used to good effect (eg, the sedative effect is used in over-the-counter sleep aids). Many H_1-blocking compounds are available.

D. Toxicity and Interactions: Sedation is common, especially with diphenhydramine and promethazine. It is much less common with newer agents that do not enter the CNS readily (eg, terfenadine, astemizole). Antimuscarinic effects such as dry mouth and blurred vision occur with some drugs in some patients. Alpha-blocking actions may cause orthostatic hypotension.

Interactions occur between older antihistamines and other drugs with sedative effects, eg, benzodiazepines and alcohol. Drugs that inhibit hepatic metabolism may result in dangerously high levels of nonsedating antihistaminic drugs that are taken concurrently. For example, ketoconazole inhibits metabolism of astemizole and terfenadine. In the presence of this antifungal drug, the plasma concentration of either antihistamine may increase and precipitate lethal arrhythmias.

Cardiac arrhythmias are effects of excessive concentrations of terfenadine and astemizole. However, terfenadine is the prodrug of the active antihistaminic molecule fexofenadine. Fexofenadine is not subject to the interaction described above and has become available as a prescription drug.

HISTAMINE H_2 ANTAGONISTS

A. Classification and Prototypes: (Figure 16–1.) Four H_2 blockers are available; cimetidine is the prototype. These drugs do not resemble H_1 blockers structurally. They are orally active, with half-lives of 1–3 hours. Because they are relatively nontoxic, they can be given in large doses, so that the duration of action of a single dose may be 12–24 hours.

B. Mechanism and Effects: These drugs produce a surmountable pharmacologic blockade of histamine H_2 receptors. They are relatively selective and have no significant blocking actions at H_1 or autonomic receptors.

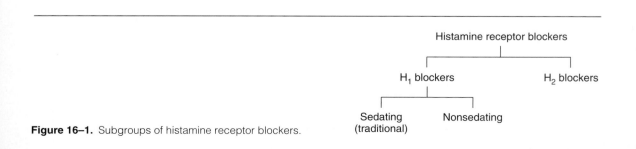

Figure 16–1. Subgroups of histamine receptor blockers.

The only therapeutic effect of clinical importance is the reduction of gastric acid secretion, but this is a very useful action. Blockade of cardiovascular H_2 receptor-mediated effects can be demonstrated but has no clinical significance.

C. Clinical Use: In acid-peptic disease, especially duodenal ulcer, these drugs reduce symptoms, accelerate healing, and prevent recurrences. Acute ulcer is usually treated with two or more doses per day, while recurrence of the ulcer can often be prevented with a single bedtime dose. H_2 blockers are also effective in accelerating healing and preventing recurrences of gastric peptic ulcers. In Zollinger-Ellison syndrome, these drugs are very helpful (though large doses are required and they are not as effective as omeprazole) in controlling symptoms (acid hypersecretion, severe recurrent peptic ulceration, gastrointestinal bleeding, and diarrhea). Similarly, the H_2 blockers have been used in gastroesophageal reflux disease (GERD), but they are not as effective as omeprazole in this condition.

D. Toxicity: Cimetidine is a potent inhibitor of hepatic drug-metabolizing enzymes and may reduce hepatic blood flow. Cimetidine also has significant antiandrogen effects in many patients. Ranitidine has a weaker inhibitory effect on hepatic drug metabolism; neither it nor the newer H_2 blockers appear to have endocrine effects.

SEROTONIN (5-HYDROXYTRYPTAMINE, 5-HT) & RELATED AGONISTS

Serotonin is produced from tryptophan and stored in the enterochromaffin cells of the gut and in the CNS. Excess production in the body can be detected by measuring its major metabolite, 5-hydroxyindoleacetic acid (5-HIAA), in the urine. Serotonin appears to play a physiologic role as a neurotransmitter in both the CNS and the enteric nervous system and perhaps as a local hormone that modulates gastrointestinal activity. Serotonin is also stored (but synthesized to only a minimal extent) in platelets. Only one drug is in use for its serotonin agonist effects; several are in use or under investigation as serotonin antagonists (Figure 16–2). Fourteen 5-HT receptors have been discovered.

A. Receptors and Effects:
1. **5-HT$_1$ receptors:** 5-HT$_1$ receptors are most important in the brain and mediate synaptic inhibition via increased potassium conductance (Table 16–2). Peripheral 5-HT$_1$ receptors mediate both excitatory and inhibitory effects in various smooth muscle tissues.
2. **5-HT$_2$ receptors:** 5-HT$_2$ receptors are important in both brain and peripheral tissues. These receptors mediate synaptic excitation in the CNS and smooth muscle contraction (gut, bronchi, uterus, vessels) or dilation (vessels). The mechanism involves (in different tissues) decreased potassium conductance, decreased cAMP, and increased IP$_3$. In carcinoid tumor, this receptor probably mediates some of the flushing, diarrhea, and bronchoconstriction characteristic of the disease.
3. **5-HT$_3$ receptors:** 5-HT$_3$ receptors are found in the CNS, especially in the chemoreceptive area and vomiting center, and in peripheral sensory and enteric nerves. These receptors mediate excitation via a 5-HT-gated cation channel (ie, the mechanism of serotonin at the 5-HT$_3$ receptor resembles that of ACh at nicotinic cholinergic cation channels). Antagonists acting at this receptor have proved to be useful antiemetic drugs.

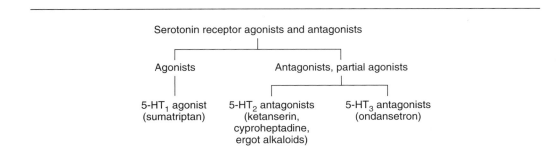

Figure 16–2. Subgroups of drugs acting at serotonin receptors and nerve endings.

B. Clinical Use: Serotonin has no clinical applications.

C. Other Serotonin Agonists:
1. **Sumatriptan, a receptor agonist:**   Sumatriptan, a substituted indole compound, is a 5-HT_{1d} agonist. It is effective in the treatment of acute migraine and cluster headache attacks—an observation that supports the association of serotonin abnormalities with these headache syndromes. It is available for oral, nasal, or parenteral administration. Ergot alkaloids, discussed below, are partial agonists at 5-HT receptors.
2. **Serotonin reuptake inhibitors:**   A number of important antidepressant drugs act at serotonergic synapses by inhibiting the reuptake carrier for 5-HT. These drugs are discussed in Chapter 29. **Dexfenfluramine,** a reuptake inhibitor with other effects, was used exclusively for its appetite-reducing effect. While effective as an anorexiant, it is toxic: cardiac disease in patients and neurologic damage in animals were reported. In the past, dexfenfluramine was sometimes combined with phentermine, an amphetamine-like anorexiant. Dexfenfluramine has been withdrawn.

SEROTONIN ANTAGONISTS

A. Classification and Prototypes: **Ketanserin** is a 5-HT_2 and alpha-adrenoceptor blocker. **Phenoxybenzamine** (an alpha-adrenoceptor blocker) and **cyproheptadine** (an H_1 blocker) are also good 5-HT_2 blockers. **Ondansetron** is a 5-HT_3 blocker. The **ergot alkaloids** are partial agonists at 5-HT (and other) receptors (see below).

B. Mechanisms and Effects: Ketanserin and cyproheptadine are competitive pharmacologic antagonists. Phenoxybenzamine is an irreversible blocker.
    Ketanserin, cyproheptadine, and phenoxybenzamine are weakly selective agents. In addition to inhibition of serotonin effects, they also have alpha-blocking effects (ketanserin, phenoxybenzamine) or H_1 blocking effects (cyproheptadine). Ondansetron, which is more selective for 5-HT_3 receptors, has a very significant central antiemetic action.

C. Clinical Uses: Ketanserin is under investigation as an antihypertension drug. Ketanserin, cyproheptadine, and phenoxybenzamine may be of value (separately or in combination) in the treatment of carcinoid tumor, a neoplasm that secretes large amounts of serotonin (and peptides) and causes diarrhea, bronchoconstriction, and flushing. Ondansetron is extremely useful in the control of postoperative vomiting and vomiting associated with cancer chemotherapy.

D. Toxicity: Adverse effects of ketanserin are those of alpha blockade and H_1 blockade. The toxicities of ondansetron include diarrhea and headache.

ERGOT ALKALOIDS

These complex molecules are produced by a fungus found in wet or spoiled grain. They are responsible for the epidemics of "St. Anthony's Fire" (ergotism) described during the Middle Ages. There are at least 20 naturally occurring members of the family, but only a few of these and a handful of semisynthetic derivatives are used as therapeutic agents. The ergot alkaloids are partial agonists at alpha adrenoceptors and 5-HT receptors. The balance of agonist-versus-antagonist effect varies from compound to compound. Some are also agonists at the dopamine receptor.

A. Classification and Prototypes: The ergot alkaloids may be subdivided into three major groups on the basis of the organ or tissue in which they have their primary effects (Figure 16–3). This division is not absolute, since most of the alkaloids have some effects on several tissues.
    The brain is a target organ for several natural ergot alkaloids that cause the hallucinations and chemical psychoses associated with epidemics of ergotism. The most important derivatives acting in the CNS, however, are the semisynthetic drugs **LSD** and **bromocriptine.** The uterus is very sensitive to ergot alkaloids as term pregnancy nears but less so at other times. **Ergonovine** is a prototypical oxytocic ergot alkaloid. Blood vessels are sensitive to ergonovine and other ergot drugs of which **ergotamine** is the prototype.

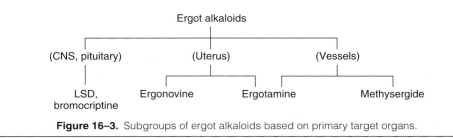

Figure 16–3. Subgroups of ergot alkaloids based on primary target organs.

B. Effects: The receptor effects of the ergot alkaloids are summarized in Table 16–3 and include the following:

1. **Vessels:** Ergot alkaloids can produce marked and prolonged alpha receptor-mediated vasoconstriction. An overdose can cause ischemia and gangrene of the limbs.

2. **Uterus:** A powerful contraction occurs in this tissue near term. This is sufficient to cause abortion or miscarriage. Earlier in pregnancy (and in the nonpregnant uterus), much higher doses of ergot alkaloids are needed to produce this effect. After delivery of the placenta, ergonovine or ergotamine can produce a useful contraction of the uterus that reduces blood loss.

3. **Brain:** Hallucinations may be prominent with the naturally occurring ergots and with LSD but are less common with therapeutic ergots. Although LSD is a potent 5-HT_2 blocker in peripheral tissues, its CNS effects may be due to actions at dopamine receptors. In the pituitary, some ergot alkaloids are potent dopamine-like inhibitors of prolactin secretion. Bromocriptine and pergolide are among the most potent of the semisynthetic derivatives at these dopamine D_2 receptors and at similar receptors in the basal ganglia.

C. Clinical Uses:

1. **Migraine:** Ergotamine is a mainstay of treatment of acute attacks. Methysergide and ergonovine are used prophylactically.

2. **Obstetric bleeding:** Ergonovine and ergotamine are effective agents for the reduction of postpartum bleeding.

3. **Hyperprolactinemia and parkinsonism:** Bromocriptine and pergolide are used to reduce prolactin secretion (dopamine is the physiologic prolactin release inhibitor). Bromocriptine also appears to reduce the size of pituitary tumors of the prolactin-secreting cells. This drug is useful also in the treatment of Parkinson's disease (Chapter 27).

4. **Other uses:** Methysergide has been used in carcinoid tumor.

D. Toxicity: The toxic effects of ergot alkaloids are quite important both from a public health standpoint (epidemics of ergotism from spoiled grain) and because of the toxicity of overdose or abuse by individuals.

1. **Vascular effects:** Severe prolonged vasoconstriction can result in ischemia and gangrene. The only consistently effective antagonist is nitroprusside. When used for long periods,

Table 16–3. Effects of ergot alkaloids at several receptors.*

Ergot Alkaloid	Alpha Adrenoceptor[1]	Dopamine Receptor (D_2)[1]	Serotonin Receptor (5-HT_2)[1]	Uterine Smooth Muscle Stimulation[1]
Bromocriptine	–	+++	–	0
Ergonovine	+	+	– (PA)	+++
Ergotamine	– – (PA)	0	+ (PA)	+++
Lysergic acid diethylamide (LSD)	0	+++	– –	++
Methysergide	0/+	+/0	– – – (PA)	+/0

*Reproduced, with permission, from Katzung BG (editor): *Basic & Clinical Pharmacology,* 7th ed. Appleton & Lange, 1998.
[1]Agonist effects are indicated by +, antagonist by –, no effect by 0. Relative affinity for the receptor is indicated by the number of + or – signs. PA means partial agonist.

methysergide produces an unusual hyperplasia of connective tissue. This fibroplasia may be retroperitoneal, retropleural, or subendocardial and can cause hydronephrosis or cardiac valvular and conduction system malfunction. Similar lesions are found in some patients with carcinoid, suggesting that this action is probably mediated by agonist effects at serotonin receptors.

2. **Gastrointestinal effects:** Most ergot alkaloids cause gastrointestinal upset (nausea, vomiting, diarrhea) in many individuals.

3. **Uterine effects:** Marked uterine contractions may be produced. The uterus becomes progressively more sensitive to ergot alkaloids during pregnancy. Although abortion due to use of ergot for migraine is rare, most obstetricians recommend avoidance or very conservative use of these drugs as pregnancy progresses.

4. **CNS effects:** Hallucinations resembling psychosis are common with LSD but less common with the other ergot alkaloids. Methysergide has occasionally been used as an LSD substitute by users of "recreational drugs."

DRUG LIST

The following drugs are important members of the group discussed in this chapter. Prototypes should be learned in detail; features of the major variants should be known well enough so that they can be distinguished from prototypes and from each other; the other significant agents should be recognized as belonging to a specific subclass.

Subclass	Prototype	Major Variants	Other Significant Agents
Histamine agonists	Histamine		
H₁ blockers	Diphenhydramine Fexofenadine		Chlorpheniramine, cyproheptadine, promethazine, astemizole, terfenadine
H₂ blockers	Cimetidine		Ranitidine, famotidine, nizatidine
5-HT agonists	Serotonin, sumatriptan	Dexfenfluramine	
5-HT antagonists	Ketanserin, ondansetron		Cyproheptadine, ergot alkaloids[1]
Ergot alkaloids	Bromocriptine Ergonovine Ergotamine	LSD, methysergide	Pergolide

[1]Partial agonists.

QUESTIONS

DIRECTIONS: Each of the numbered items or incomplete statements in this section is followed by answers or by completions of the sentence. Select the ONE lettered answer or completion that is BEST in each case.

Items 1–2: Your patient has been diagnosed with a rare metastatic carcinoid tumor. This neoplasm is releasing serotonin, bradykinin, and several unknown peptides.

1. The effects of serotonin in this patient may include all of the following EXCEPT
   (A) Episodes of bronchospasm
   (B) Diarrhea
   (C) Hypersecretion of gastric acid
   (D) Instability of blood pressure
   (E) Retroperitoneal fibroplasia

2. In recommending treatment for your carcinoid patient, you will consider all of the following EXCEPT
   (A) Cyproheptadine
   (B) Ketanserin
   (C) Methysergide
   (D) Phenoxybenzamine
   (E) Sumatriptan

3. Drugs that can reverse one or more smooth muscle effects of circulating histamine in humans include all of the following EXCEPT
   (A) Chlorpheniramine
   (B) Cyproheptadine
   (C) Epinephrine
   (D) Ketanserin
   (E) Phenylephrine

4. Many antihistamines (H_1 blockers) have additional effects; these are likely to include all of the following EXCEPT
   (A) Antimuscarinic reduction in bladder tone
   (B) Local anesthetic effects if the drug is injected
   (C) Anti-motion sickness effect
   (D) Increase in total peripheral resistance
   (E) Sedation

5. All of the following are H_2-blocking drugs EXCEPT
   (A) Cimetidine
   (B) Famotidine
   (C) Nizatidine
   (D) Ranitidine
   (E) Terfenadine

6. Toxicities of H_1 antihistamines include all of the following EXCEPT
   (A) Blurred vision
   (B) Diarrhea
   (C) Orthostatic hypotension
   (D) Sleepiness

7. All of the following statements about possible pharmacologic causes of sixteenth and seventeenth century accounts of witchcraft are reasonable EXCEPT
   (A) Ingestion of bread made with flour from spoiled grain could cause painful burning sensations in the limbs, leading naive individuals to suspect supernatural evil forces
   (B) Similar ingestion could cause "epidemics" of abortions, with similar interpretations
   (C) Similar ingestion by elderly women might cause them to have hallucinations and exhibit behaviors interpretable by others as "casting spells"
   (D) The major substance now known to occur in spoiled grain is methysergide, a substance similar to PCP

8. A patient undergoing cancer chemotherapy is vomiting frequently. A drug that might help in this situation is
   (A) Bromocriptine
   (B) Cimetidine
   (C) Ketanserin
   (D) Ondansetron
   (E) Terfenadine

9. Characteristics of H_2 histamine blockers include all of the following EXCEPT
   (A) All have short half-lives of 2–4 hours
   (B) All available H_2 blockers have approximately equal efficacy but widely varying potency
   (C) Cimetidine is associated with more drug interactions than other H_2 blockers because of inhibition of hepatic P450 systems
   (D) Cimetidine is associated with antiandrogenic effects in some patients
   (E) H_2 blockers must be given four or five times a day for therapeutic effect

10. Correct applications of drugs include all of the following clinical indications EXCEPT
    (A) Astemizole: for hay fever
    (B) Ergonovine: for postpartum bleeding
    (C) Methysergide: for recurrent migraine headache
    (D) Ondansetron: for acute migraine headache
    (E) Ranitidine: for prophylaxis of duodenal ulcer

DIRECTIONS (Items 11–16): Each set of matching questions in this section consists of a list of three to twenty-six lettered options (some of which may be figures) followed by several numbered items. For each numbered item, select the ONE lettered option that is MOST closely associated with it. Each lettered option may be selected once, more than once, or not at all.

(A) Bromocriptine
(B) Cimetidine
(C) Ergotamine
(D) Ketanserin
(E) LSD
(F) Methysergide
(G) Nitroprusside
(H) Ondansetron
(I) Phenoxybenzamine
(J) Sumatriptan

11. Useful in the treatment of hyperprolactinemia
12. Effective in the treatment of peptic ulcer disease
13. Serotonin agonist useful for aborting an acute migraine headache; not derived from a fungus
14. Used in management of severe ergot-induced vasospasm
15. Causes inhibition of hepatic metabolism of many drugs; some antiandrogenic effects
16. Useful irreversible antagonist for treatment of some carcinoid tumors

ANSWERS

1. The effects of serotonin include all of those listed except gastric acid hypersecretion; serotonin actually decreases acid secretion. The answer is **(C)**.
2. All of the drugs listed have significant blocking effects on 5-HT receptors except sumatriptan, which is an agonist at 5-HT_{1d} receptors. The answer is **(E)**.
3. Each of the drugs listed is a pharmacologic antagonist (chlorpheniramine, cyproheptadine) or physiologic antagonist (epinephrine, phenylephrine) of histamine except ketanserin, a pharmacologic antagonist of 5-HT at 5-HT_2 receptors. The answer is **(D)**.
4. H_1 blockers do not activate receptors that mediate vasoconstriction; some of these drugs actually block alpha adrenoceptors, causing significant vasodilation. The answer is **(D)**.
5. Terfenadine is a nonsedating H_1 blocker. The answer is **(E)**.
6. None of the H_1 blockers cause diarrhea as a prominent adverse effect, and many have antimuscarinic actions that result in constipation (see also question 4). The answer is **(B)**.
7. Historians have noted that many of the behaviors described for accused "witches" and their purported victims during the Salem witch trials period of American history resemble signs of ergotism. Ergotism is caused by a mixture of naturally occurring ergot alkaloids—not methysergide, a semisynthetic ergot derivative. Methysergide is not similar to PCP (phencyclidine). The answer is **(D)**.
8. Ondansetron has significant antiemetic effects. The answer is **(D)**.
9. H_2 blockers have short half-lives but can be given in very large doses that provide adequate blood levels for 12–24 hours. The answer is **(E)**.
10. Ondansetron has no value in migraine headache; the drug is used only as an antiemetic during chemotherapy and for postoperative vomiting. The answer is **(D)**.
11. Bromocriptine is an effective dopamine agonist in the CNS with the advantage of oral activity. The drug inhibits prolactin secretion by activating pituitary dopamine receptors. The answer is **(A)**.
12. An H_2 blocker is appropriate for peptic ulcer; cimetidine is such a drug. The answer is **(B)**.
13. Sumatriptan, an agonist at 5-HT_{1d} receptors, is indicated for treatment of acute migraine. Ergotamine is also effective for acute migraine, but it is produced by the fungus *Claviceps purpurea*. The answer is **(J)**.
14. A very powerful vasodilator is necessary to reverse ergot-induced vasospasm; nitroprusside is such a drug. The answer is **(G)**.
15. Cimetidine is well known for causing drug interactions because of its ability to inhibit hepatic P450 isozymes. The drug also has weak antiandrogenic effects. The answer is **(B)**.
16. Phenoxybenzamine is the only irreversible blocker in this list. The drug has significant affinity for histamine and 5-HT_2 receptors as well as for alpha receptors and has been found useful in some patients with carcinoid tumors, presumably because of this agent's ability to block 5-HT_2 receptors. The answer is **(I)**.

Vasoactive Peptides

17

OBJECTIVES

You should be able to:

- Name an antagonist of angiotensin at its receptor and at least two drugs that reduce the formation of angiotensin II.
- Outline the major effects of bradykinin and atrial natriuretic peptide.
- Describe the functions of converting enzyme (peptidyl dipeptidase, kininase II).
- Describe the effects of vasoactive intestinal peptide, substance P, and neuropeptide Y.

CONCEPTS

A. Classification and Prototypes: Vasoactive peptides comprise a large class of endogenous substances that function as neurotransmitters as well as local and systemic hormones. The better known peptides include angiotensin, bradykinin, atrial natriuretic peptide, vasoactive intestinal peptide, substance P, calcitonin gene-related peptide, vasopressin, glucagon, and several opioid peptides. Vasopressin is discussed in Chapters 15 and 36, the opioid peptides in Chapter 30, and glucagon in Chapter 40. The peptides discussed in this chapter and their effects are summarized in Table 17–1.

B. Mechanisms: These agents probably all act on cell surface receptors. As indicated in Table 17–1, most act via G protein-coupled receptors and cause the production of second messengers; a few may open ion channels.

ANGIOTENSIN & ITS ANTAGONISTS

A. Source and Disposition: **Angiotensin I** is produced from angiotensinogen by renin, an enzyme released from the juxtaglomerular apparatus of the kidney. An inactive decapeptide, angiotensin I is converted into **angiotensin II (AII),** an octapeptide, by **angiotensin-converting**

Table 17–1. Some vasoactive peptides and their properties.

Peptide	Properties
Angiotensin II (AII)	↑ IP_3, DAG. Constricts arterioles, increases aldosterone secretion
Atrial natriuretic peptide (ANP)	↑ cGMP. Dilates vessels, inhibits aldosterone secretion and effects, increases glomerular filtration
Bradykinin	↑ IP_3, DAG; ↑ cAMP, ↑ NO. Dilates arterioles, increases capillary permeability, stimulates sensory pain endings
Calcitonin gene-related peptide (CGRP)	Causes hypotension and tachycardia by unknown mechanisms
Endothelins	↑ IP_3, DAG. Synthesized in vascular endothelium. Constrict most vessels and contract other smooth muscle
Neuropeptide Y (NPY)	Causes vasoconstriction and stimulates the heart. Effects mediated in part by IP_3
Substance P	Dilates arterioles, contracts veins, intestinal, and bronchial smooth muscle, causes diuresis; and is a transmitter in sensory pain neurons
Vasoactive intestinal peptide (VIP)	Dilates vessels, relaxes bronchi and intestinal smooth muscle

enzyme (ACE), also known as peptidyl dipeptidase or kininase II (Figure 11–3). Angiotensin II, the active form of the peptide, is rapidly degraded by peptidases (angiotensinases).

B. Effects: Angiotensin II is a potent arteriolar vasoconstrictor and stimulant of aldosterone release. AII directly increases peripheral vascular resistance and, through aldosterone, causes renal sodium retention. AII also facilitates the release of norepinephrine from adrenergic nerve endings via presynaptic heteroreceptor action.

C. Clinical Role: Angiotensin II was used by intra-arterial infusion in the past to control bleeding in sites difficult to access. The peptide is no longer used for this indication. Its major clinical significance is as a pathophysiologic mediator in some cases of hypertension (high-renin hypertension) and in congestive heart failure. Therefore, AII antagonists are of considerable clinical interest.

D. Antagonists: As noted in Chapter 11, two types of antagonists are available. **Angiotensin II receptor-blockers (eg, losartan, valsartan)** are orally active nonpeptide inhibitors at the angiotensin II AT_1 receptor. **Saralasin,** a peptide partial agonist at this receptor, is not used clinically. **Angiotensin-converting enzyme inhibitors** (eg, captopril, enalapril) are important agents for the treatment of hypertension and heart failure. Blocking the effects of angiotensin by either of these drug types is often accompanied by a compensatory increase in renin and angiotensin I.

BRADYKININ

A. Source and Disposition: Bradykinin is one of several vasodilator kinins produced from kininogen by a family of enzymes, the kallikreins. Bradykinin is rapidly degraded by various peptidases, including angiotensin-converting enzyme.

B. Effects: Bradykinin is one of the most potent vasodilators known. The peptide is thought to be involved in inflammation and causes edema and pain when released or injected into tissue. Bradykinin can be found in saliva and may play a role in stimulating its secretion.

C. Clinical Role: Although it has no therapeutic application, bradykinin may play a role in the antihypertensive action of angiotensin-converting enzyme inhibitors, as previously noted (Chapter 11; Figure 11–4). There are no clinically important bradykinin antagonists.

ATRIAL NATRIURETIC PEPTIDE

A. Source and Disposition: Atrial natriuretic peptide (ANP; also known as atrial natriuretic factor, ANF) is synthesized and stored in the cardiac atria of mammals. Atrial natriuretic peptide is released from the atria in response to distention of the chambers.

B. Effects: Atrial natriuretic peptide activates guanylyl cyclase in many tissues. It is a vasodilator as well as a natriuretic (sodium excretion-enhancing) agent. Its renal action includes increased glomerular filtration, decreased proximal tubular sodium reabsorption, and inhibitory effects on renin secretion. The peptide also inhibits the actions of angiotensin II and aldosterone. Although it lacks positive inotropic action, atrial natriuretic peptide may play an important compensatory role in congestive heart failure by limiting sodium retention.

C. Clinical Role: Atrial natriuretic peptide has been studied for possible use in the treatment of congestive heart failure, as has a similar peptide from brain (BNF). There are no clinically important products that act as agonists or antagonists at atrial natriuretic peptide receptors.

ENDOTHELINS

Endothelins are peptide vasoconstrictors formed in and released by endothelial cells in blood vessels. Endothelins are believed to function as paracrine hormones in the vasculature. Three different endothelin peptides (ET-1, ET-2, and ET-3) with minor variations in amino acid sequence have been identified in humans. Two receptors have been identified, both of which are G protein-coupled.

Endothelins are much more potent than norepinephrine as vasoconstrictors and have a relatively long-lasting effect. The peptides also stimulate the heart, increase atrial natriuretic peptide release, and activate smooth muscle proliferation. The peptides may be involved in some forms of hypertension and other cardiovascular disorders. Antagonists have recently become available for research use.

VASOACTIVE INTESTINAL PEPTIDE, SUBSTANCE P, CALCITONIN GENE-RELATED PEPTIDE, & NEUROPEPTIDE Y

Vasoactive intestinal peptide (VIP) is an extremely potent vasodilator but probably is physiologically more important as a neurotransmitter. It is found in the central and peripheral nervous systems and in the gastrointestinal tract. No clinical application has been found for this peptide.

Substance P is another neurotransmitter peptide with potent vasodilator action on arterioles. However, substance P is a potent *stimulant* of veins and of intestinal and airway smooth muscle. The peptide may also function as a local hormone in the gastrointestinal tract. Highest concentrations of substance P are found in those parts of the nervous system that contain neurons subserving pain. At the present time, there are no clinical applications for substance P or its antagonists. However, **capsaicin,** the "hot" component of chili peppers, releases substance P from its stores in nerve endings and depletes the peptide. Capsaicin has been approved for topical use on arthritic joints.

Calcitonin gene-related peptide (CGRP) is found (along with calcitonin) in high concentrations in the thyroid and is also present in most smooth muscle tissues. The presence of CGRP in smooth muscle suggests a function as a cotransmitter in autonomic nerve endings. CGRP is the most potent hypotensive agent discovered to date and causes reflex tachycardia. There is no clinical application for this peptide at present.

Unlike the three peptides described above, neuropeptide Y (NPY) is a potent *vasoconstrictor* that stimulates the heart. NPY is found in both the CNS and the peripheral nerves. In the periphery, NPY is most commonly localized as a cotransmitter in adrenergic nerve endings. Several receptor subtypes have been identified.

DRUG LIST: See Table 17–1.

QUESTIONS

DIRECTIONS: Each of the numbered items or incomplete statements in this section is followed by answers or by completions of the statement. Select the ONE lettered answer or completion that is BEST in each case.

1. Regarding peptides,
    (A) Angiotensin I (a decapeptide) is the most potent of the series that includes angiotensinogen and angiotensin II (an octapeptide)
    (B) Bradykinin is a potent vasodilator with pain-inducing and edema-inducing effects
    (C) Atrial natriuretic peptide increases cardiac contractility in congestive heart failure
    (D) Because they cannot cross the blood-brain barrier, peptides are not found in the brain
    (E) Bradykinin is inactivated by the enzyme kallikrein
2. Which of the following——if given intravenously—will cause increased gastrointestinal motility and diarrhea?
    (A) Angiotensin II
    (B) Bethanechol
    (C) Bradykinin
    (D) Renin
    (E) All of the above
3. A peptide that causes increased capillary permeability and edema is
    (A) Angiotensin II
    (B) Bradykinin
    (C) Captopril
    (D) Histamine
    (E) Losartan

4. Agents that produce arteriolar vasoconstriction include all of the following EXCEPT
   (A) Angiotensin II
   (B) Epinephrine
   (C) Methysergide
   (D) Serotonin
   (E) Substance P

5. A vasodilator that can be inactivated by proteolytic enzymes is
   (A) Angiotensin I
   (B) Isoproterenol
   (C) Histamine
   (D) Neuropeptide Y
   (E) Vasoactive intestinal peptide

DIRECTIONS (Items 6–14): Each set of matching questions in this section consists of a list of three to twenty-six lettered options (some of which may be figures) followed by several numbered items. For each numbered item, select the ONE lettered option that is MOST closely associated with it. Each lettered option may be selected once, more than once, or not at all.
   (A) Angiotensin I
   (B) Angiotensin II
   (C) Atrial natriuretic peptide
   (D) Bradykinin
   (E) Calcitonin gene-related peptide
   (F) Endothelin
   (G) Neuropeptide Y
   (H) Renin
   (I) Substance P
   (J) Vasoactive intestinal peptide

6. Released in traumatized tissue; causes pain and edema; metabolized by angiotensin-converting enzyme

7. Decapeptide precursor of a vasoconstrictor substance

8. Arterial vasodilator found in peripheral and central nervous system nerves; causes contraction of veins and airway smooth muscle; found in afferent pain fibers

9. Octapeptide vasoconstrictor that increases in the blood of hypertensive patients treated with large doses of diuretics

10. Vasodilator that increases in the blood or tissues of patients treated with captopril

11. Most potent vasodilator discovered to date; found in high concentration in the thyroid

12. Peptide cotransmitter in many autonomic nerve endings; directly relaxes vascular, airway, and gastrointestinal smooth muscle

13. Peptide cotransmitter found in autonomic nerve endings; a vasoconstrictor

14. A potent vasoconstrictor peptide synthesized in the endothelium of blood vessels

ANSWERS

1. Angiotensin I is an inactive precursor. Atrial natriuretic peptide has no effect on cardiac contractility. Peptides are found in high concentrations in parts of the brain because they are synthesized there. The answer is **(B).**

2. The peptides listed here are not associated with marked increases in gastrointestinal motility. Bethanechol, a muscarinic cholinoceptor stimulant, is an effective stimulant of the gut. The answer is **(B).**

3. Histamine and bradykinin both cause marked increase in permeability that is often associated with edema, but histamine is not a peptide. The answer is **(B).**

4. Substance P is a potent arterial *vasodilator.* The answer is **(E).**

5. A peptide—but not an amine—would be altered by proteolytic enzymes. Vasoactive intestinal peptide is the only peptide in the list that is a vasodilator. The answer is **(E).**

6. Bradykinin is a mediator of tissue damage, pain, and edema. The answer is **(D).**

7. Angiotensin I is a decapeptide. The answer is **(A).**

8. Substance P is an arteriolar vasodilator that is also a pain-mediating neurotransmitter. The answer is **(I).**

9.   Angiotensin II, an octapeptide, increases when blood volume decreases because the compensatory cardiovascular response causes an increase in renin secretion. The answer is (**B**).
10. Bradykinin increases because converting enzyme, the enzyme inhibited by captopril, normally degrades kinins in addition to synthesizing angiotensin II (see Figure 11–4). The answer is (**D**).
11. The most potent vasodilator discovered to date is calcitonin gene-related peptide. The answer is (**E**).
12. Vasoactive intestinal peptide is a general smooth muscle relaxant that is also an important cotransmitter in ANS nerves. The answer is (**J**).
13. Neuropeptide Y is found in many sympathetic postganglionic nerve endings as a cotransmitter. Unlike vasoactive intestinal peptide (another autonomic cotransmitter), neuropeptide Y is a vasoconstrictor. The answer is (**G**).
14. Endothelins are synthesized in vascular endothelium and are powerful vasoconstrictors. The answer is (**F**).

Prostaglandins & Other Eicosanoids   18

OBJECTIVES

You should be able to:

- List the major effects of PGE_2, $PGF_{2\alpha}$, LTB_4, LTC_4, and LTD_4.
- List important sites of synthesis and the effects of thromboxane and prostacyclin in the vascular system.
- List the targets (receptors or enzymes) for currently available therapeutic antagonists of leukotrienes and prostaglandins.
- Explain the differing effects of aspirin on prostaglandin synthesis and on leukotriene synthesis.

Learn the definitions that follow.

Table 18–1. Definitions.

Term	Definition
Abortifacient	A drug used to cause an abortion. *Example:* prostaglandin $F_{2\alpha}$
Cyclooxygenase	Enzyme that converts arachidonic acid to PGG and PGH, the precursors of the prostaglandins
Dysmenorrhea	Painful uterine cramping activated by prostaglandins released during menstruation
Endoperoxide	General term for prostaglandin precursors, eg, PGG, PGH
Great vessel transposition	Congenital anomaly in which the pulmonary artery exits from the left ventricle and the aorta from the right ventricle. Incompatible with life unless a large patent ductus or ventricular septal defect is present
Lipoxygenase	Enzyme that converts arachidonic acid to leukotriene precursors (HPETEs)
NSAID	Nonsteroidal anti-inflammatory drug, eg, aspirin, ibuprofen. Inhibitor of cyclooxygenase.
Patent ductus arteriosus	Persistence after birth of the fetal connection between the pulmonary artery and the aorta
Phospholipase A_2	Enzyme in the cell membrane that generates arachidonic acid from membrane lipid constituents
Slow-reacting substance of anaphylaxis (SRS-A)	Material originally identified by bioassay from tissues of animals undergoing anaphylactic shock; now recognized as a mixture of leukotrienes, especially LTB_4, LTC_4, and LTD_4

CONCEPTS

The eicosanoids are an important group of endogenous fatty acid derivatives that are produced from arachidonic acid. Arachidonic acid is derived from cell membrane lipids.

EICOSANOID AGONISTS

A. Classification: The principal eicosanoid subgroups are the prostaglandins, prostacyclins, thromboxanes, and leukotrienes. Prostacyclin and thromboxane are often considered members of the prostaglandins since they are also cyclized derivatives. The leukotrienes retain the straight-chain configuration of arachidonic acid. There are several series for most of the principal subgroups; these series are based on different substituents (indicated by A, B, C, etc) and different numbers of double bonds (indicated by subscript 2, 3, 4, etc) in the molecule.

B. Synthesis: (See Figure 18–1.) Active eicosanoids are synthesized in response to various stimuli, eg, physical injury, immune reactions. These stimuli activate phospholipases in the cell membrane, and arachidonic acid is produced from membrane lipid. Arachidonic acid can be metabolized to straight-chain products by **lipoxygenase,** finally producing leukotrienes. Alternatively, cyclization by the enzyme **cyclooxygenase** may occur, resulting in the production of prostacyclin, prostaglandins, or thromboxane. Cyclooxygenase (COX) exists in at least two forms. **COX I** is found in many tissues; the prostaglandins produced in these tissues by COX I appear to be important for a variety of normal physiologic processes. In contrast, **COX II** is found primarily in inflammatory cells; the products of its actions play a major role in tissue injury, eg, inflammation. Thromboxane is preferentially synthesized in platelets, whereas prostacyclin is synthesized in the endothelial cells of vessels. Naturally occurring eicosanoids have very short half-lives (seconds to minutes) and are inactive when given by the oral route.

C. Mechanism of Action: Most eicosanoid effects appear to be brought about by activation of cell surface receptors that are coupled by G proteins to adenylyl cyclase (producing cAMP) or the phosphatidylinositol cascade (producing IP_3 and DAG second messengers).

D. Effects: A vast array of effects are produced on smooth muscle, platelets, the CNS, and other tissues. Some of the most important effects are summarized in Table 18–2. Eicosanoids most di-

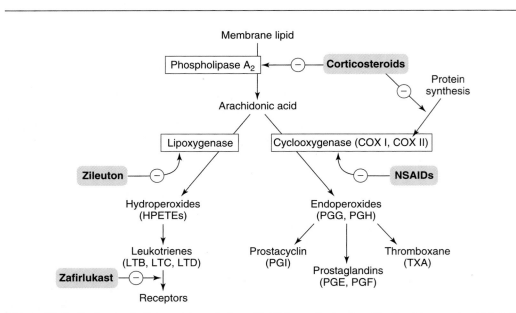

Figure 18–1. Synthesis of eicosanoids and sites of inhibitory effects of corticosteroids, nonsteroidal anti-inflammatory drugs (NSAIDs), and leukotriene antagonist drugs.

Table 18–2. Effects of some important eicosanoids. (? = unknown effect.)

Effect	PGE_2	PGF_{2a}	PGI_2	TXA_2	LTB_4	LTC_4	LTD_4
Vascular tone	↑	↑ or ↓	↓↓	↑↑↑	?	↑ or ↓	↑ or ↓
Bronchial tone	↓↓	↑	↓	↑↑↑	?	↑↑↑↑	↑↑↑↑
Uterine tone	↑↑	↑↑↑	↓		?	?	?
Platelet aggregation	↑ or ↓	?	↓↓↓	↑↑↑	?	?	?
Leukocyte chemotaxis	?	?	?	?	↑↑↑↑	?	?

rectly involved in pathologic processes include $PGF_{2\alpha}$, thromboxane (TXA_2), and the leukotrienes LTC_4 and LTD_4. LTC_4 and LTD_4 comprise **"slow-reacting substance of anaphylaxis" (SRS-A),** the important mediator of bronchoconstriction. Leukotriene LTB_4 is a chemotactic factor important in inflammation. PGE_2 and prostacyclin may play important roles as naturally occurring vasodilators. PGE_1 and its derivatives have significant protective effects on the gastric mucosa and relax smooth muscle. The gastric mechanism may involve increased secretion of bicarbonate and mucous, decreased acid secretion, or both. PGE_2 and $PGF_{2\alpha}$ are released in large amounts from the endometrium during menstruation and may play a physiologic role in labor. Dysmenorrhea is associated with uterine contractions induced by prostaglandins, especially $PGF_{2\alpha}$. Platelet clotting is strongly activated by thromboxane. Therapeutic effects of prostaglandins are described below.

E. Clinical Uses:
1. **Obstetrics:** PGE_2 and $PGF_{2\alpha}$ produce a strong contraction of the uterus. They are useful as abortifacients in the second trimester of pregnancy. Although effective in inducing labor at term, they produce more adverse effects (nausea, vomiting, diarrhea) than do other oxytocics used for this application. In Europe, the PGE_1 analog **misoprostol** has been used with mifepristone (RU 486) as an extremely effective and safe abortifacient combination.
2. **Pediatrics:** PGE_1 is given as an infusion to maintain patency of the ductus arteriosus in infants with transposition of the great vessels until surgical correction can be undertaken.
3. **Dialysis:** Prostacyclin (PGI_2) is occasionally used to prevent platelet aggregation in dialysis machines.
4. **Peptic ulcer associated with NSAID use:** Misoprostol is approved in the USA for the prevention of peptic ulcers in patients who must take high doses of nonsteroidal anti-inflammatory drugs for arthritis and have a history of ulcer associated with this use.
5. **Urology:** PGE_1 (as **alprostadil**) is used in the treatment of impotence. Preparations are available for injection into the penis as well as for insertion into the urethra.

EICOSANOID ANTAGONISTS

Phospholipase A_2 and cyclooxygenase can be inhibited by drugs; these inhibitors are mainstays in the treatment of inflammation (Figure 18–1; Chapter 35). **Zileuton** is a selective inhibitor of lipoxygenase; some cyclooxygenase inhibitors exert a mild inhibitory effect on leukotriene synthesis. Inhibitors of the receptors for the prostaglandins and the leukotrienes are being actively sought; **zafirlukast,** an inhibitor at the LTD_4 receptor, is currently available.

A. Corticosteroids: As indicated in Figure 18–1, corticosteroids inhibit the production of arachidonic acid by phospholipases in the membrane. This effect is mediated by intracellular steroid receptors that, when activated by an appropriate steroid, increase expression of specific proteins capable of inhibiting phospholipase. Steroids also inhibit the synthesis of COX II. These actions are thought to be the major mechanisms of the important anti-inflammatory action of corticosteroids.

B. NSAIDs: Aspirin and other nonsteroidal (ie, noncorticosteroid) anti-inflammatory drugs inhibit cyclooxygenase and the production of the thromboxane, prostaglandin, and prostacyclin branch of the synthetic path (Figure 18–1). Unfortunately, none of the currently available NSAIDs selectively inhibit COX II, the isoform of the enzyme thought to be responsible for the production of inflammatory prostaglandins. In fact, most inhibit COX I more effectively than COX II.

Inhibition of cyclooxygenase by aspirin, unlike that of other NSAIDs, is irreversible. It is thought that some cases of aspirin allergy result from diversion of arachidonic acid to the leukotriene pathway when the cyclooxygenase-catalyzed prostaglandin pathway is blocked. The antiplatelet action of aspirin results from the fact that inhibition of thromboxane synthesis is essentially permanent in platelets; they lack the machinery for new protein synthesis. In contrast, inhibition of prostacyclin synthesis in the vascular endothelium is temporary because these cells can synthesize new enzyme. Inhibition of prostaglandin synthesis also results in important anti-inflammatory effects. Inhibition of synthesis of fever-inducing prostaglandins in the brain produces the antipyretic action of NSAIDs. Closure of a patent ductus arteriosus in an otherwise normal infant can be accelerated with a potent NSAID such as indomethacin.

C. Leukotriene Antagonists: As noted above, an inhibitor of lipoxygenase (zileuton) and an LTD_4 (and LTE_4) receptor antagonist (zafirlukast) have become available for clinical use. At present, these agents are approved only for use in asthma.

DRUG LIST

The following drugs are important members of the group discussed in this chapter. Prototypes should be learned in detail; features of the major variants should be known well enough so that the variants can be distinguished from prototypes and from each other; the other significant agents should be recognized as belonging to a specific subclass.

Subclass	Prototype	Major Variants	Other Significant Agents
Prostaglandins	PGE_2, $PGF_{2\alpha}$	PGE_1	
Prostacyclin	PGI_2		
Thromboxane	TXA_2		
Leukotrienes	LTC_4	LTB_4	LTD_4
Leukotriene inhibitors	Zafirlukast, zileuton		
Phospholipase inhibitors	Prednisone, hydrocortisone	(See Chapter 38)	
Cyclooxygenase inhibitors	Aspirin	Ibuprofen, etc (see Chapter 35)	

QUESTIONS

DIRECTIONS: Each of the numbered items or incomplete statements in this section is followed by answers or by completions of the statement. Select the ONE lettered answer or completion that is BEST in each case.

1. Your patient calls the office complaining that your last prescription has caused severe diarrhea. Which of the following is frequently associated with increased gastrointestinal motility and diarrhea?
   (A) Corticosteroids
   (B) Leukotriene LTB_4
   (C) Prostaglandin E_1
   (D) Timolol
   (E) Zileuton

2. Which of the following drugs inhibits cyclooxygenase irreversibly?
   (A) Aspirin
   (B) Histamine
   (C) Hydrocortisone
   (D) Ibuprofen
   (E) Zileuton

3. Agents that often cause vasoconstriction include all of the following EXCEPT
   (A) Angiotensin II
   (B) Methysergide
   (C) $PGF_{2\alpha}$

      (D) Prostacyclin
      (E) Thromboxane

4. A uterine stimulant derived from membrane lipid is
      (A) Angiotensin II
      (B) Histamine
      (C) Prostacyclin (PGI$_2$)
      (D) Prostaglandin E$_2$
      (E) Serotonin

5. Inflammation is a complex tissue reaction that includes the release of cytokines, leukotrienes, prostaglandins, and peptides. Inflammatory prostaglandins are produced from arachidonic acid by
      (A) Cyclooxygenase I
      (B) Cyclooxygenase II
      (C) Glutathione-S-transferase
      (D) Lipoxygenase
      (E) Phospholipase A$_2$

6. Recognized clinical indications for eicosanoids or their inhibitors include all of the following EXCEPT
      (A) Abortion
      (B) Hypertension
      (C) Patent ductus arteriosus
      (D) Primary dysmenorrhea
      (E) Transposition of the great arteries

7. All of the following have direct or indirect bronchoconstrictor action EXCEPT
      (A) Leukotriene LTD$_4$
      (B) Prostaglandin E$_2$
      (C) Prostaglandin F$_{2\alpha}$
      (D) Slow-reacting substance of anaphylaxis (SRS-A)
      (E) Thromboxane A$_2$

DIRECTIONS (Items 8–15): Each set of matching questions in this section consists of a list of three to twenty-six lettered options (some of which may be figures) followed by several numbered items. For each numbered item, select the ONE lettered option that is MOST closely associated with it. Each lettered option may be selected once, more than once, or not at all.

      (A) Aspirin
      (B) Alprostadil
      (C) Ibuprofen
      (D) LTC$_4$
      (E) Misoprostol
      (F) Prednisone
      (G) Prostacyclin
      (H) Zafirlukast
      (I) Zileuton

8. Reversible inhibitor of platelet cyclooxygenase
9. Component of SRS-A (slow-reacting substance of anaphylaxis)
10. Reduces the activity of phospholipase A$_2$
11. Increased levels may be responsible, in part, for some cases of aspirin hypersensitivity
12. Extremely potent vasodilator produced in vascular endothelium
13. Leukotriene receptor blocker
14. Used in the treatment of impotence
15. Lipoxygenase inhibitor

ANSWERS

1. Beta-blockers (eg, timolol), corticosteroids, and zileuton do not cause diarrhea. LTB$_4$ is a chemotactic factor. The answer is **(C)**.
2. Hydrocortisone and other corticosteroids inhibit phospholipase, and histamine has no recognized effect on the enzymes involved in eicosanoid synthesis. Ibuprofen inhibits cyclooxygenase reversibly, while zileuton inhibits lipoxygenase. The answer is **(A)**, aspirin.
3. Prostacyclin PGI$_2$ is a very potent vasodilator. The answer is **(D)**.

4. While serotonin and, in some species, histamine may cause uterine stimulation, these substances are not derived from membrane lipid. Prostacyclin relaxes the uterus (Table 18–2). The answer is **(D)**.

5. Phospholipase A_2 converts membrane phospholipid to arachidonic acid. Cyclooxygenases convert arachidonic acid to prostaglandins. COX II is the enzyme believed to be responsible for this reaction in inflammatory cells. The answer is **(B)**.

6. None of the vasodilator eicosanoids have a long enough duration of action or sufficient bioavailability to be useful in hypertension. The answer is **(B)**.

7. PGE_2 is a very potent bronchodilator. Unfortunately, it is an irritant and causes coughing when inhaled. The answer is **(B)**.

8. NSAIDs other than aspirin are reversible inhibitors of cyclooxygenase. The answer is **(C)**.

9. Leukotrienes C and D are major components of SRS-A. The answer is **(D)**.

10. Corticosteroids cause inhibition of phospholipase A_2, the enzyme that produces arachidonic acid. The answer is **(F)**.

11. It is thought that the leukotrienes may be produced in increased amounts when cyclooxygenase is blocked; in patients with aspirin hypersensitivity, this might precipitate the bronchoconstriction often observed in this condition. The answer is **(D)**.

12. Prostacyclin is a potent vasodilator that is synthesized in vascular endothelium. The answer is **(G)**.

13. Zafirlukast is a blocker of LTD_4 receptors. The answer is **(H)**.

14. Alprostadil is used by injection into the corpus cavernosa or by absorption from the urethra in impotence. The answer is **(B)**.

15. Zileuton is an inhibitor of lipoxygenase. The answer is **(I)**.

19

Nitric Oxide: Donors & Inhibitors

Objectives

You should be able to:

- Name the enzyme responsible for the synthesis of nitric oxide in tissues.
- List the major beneficial and toxic effects of endogenous nitric oxide.
- List two drugs that cause release of endogenous nitric oxide.
- List two drugs that spontaneously or enzymatically break down in the body to release nitric oxide.

Learn the definitions that follow.

Table 19–1. Definitions.

Term	Definition
Endothelium-derived relaxing factor (EDRF)	A mixture of nitric oxide and other vasodilator substances synthesized in vascular endothelium
Nitric oxide donor	A molecule from which nitric oxide can be released, eg, arginine, nitroprusside, nitroglycerin
cNOS, iNOS, eNOS	Naturally occurring isoforms of nitric oxide synthase: constitutive, inducible, and endothelial isoforms, respectively

CONCEPTS

Nitric oxide (NO) is a common product of the metabolism of arginine in many tissues. It is thought to be an important paracrine vasodilator and may also play a role in cell death and neurotransmission. Nitric oxide is also released from several important vasodilator drug molecules.

A. **Endogenous Nitric Oxide:** Endogenous nitric oxide is synthesized by a family of enzymes collectively called **nitric oxide synthase (NOS).** These intracellular enzymes are activated by calcium influx or by cytokines. Arginine, the primary substrate, is converted by nitric oxide synthase to citrulline and nitric oxide. Three forms of nitric oxide synthase are known: isoform I (cNOS, a *constitutive* form found in epithelial and neuronal cells); isoform II (iNOS, an *inducible* form found in macrophages and smooth muscle cells); and isoform III (eNOS, a constitutive form found in *endothelial* cells). Nitric oxide synthase can be inhibited by arginine analogs such as N^G-monomethyl-L-arginine (L-NMMA). Nitric oxide is not stored in cells. Drugs that cause its release do so by stimulating its synthesis by nitric oxide synthase. Such drugs include **acetylcholine,** other **muscarinic agonists,** and **histamine.**

B. **Exogenous Nitric Oxide Donors:** Nitric oxide is released from several important drugs, including **nitroprusside** (Chapter 11), **nitrates** (Chapter 12), and **nitrites** (Chapter 12). Release from nitroprusside occurs spontaneously in the blood in the presence of oxygen, whereas release from nitrates and nitrites is intracellular and requires the presence of thiol compounds such as cysteine. Tolerance may develop to nitrates and nitrites if endogenous thiol compounds are depleted.

C. **Effects of Nitric Oxide:**
   1. **Smooth muscle:** Nitric oxide is a powerful vasodilator in all vascular beds and a potent relaxant in most other smooth muscle tissues. The mechanism of this effect involves activation of guanylyl cyclase and the synthesis of cGMP. cGMP in turn facilitates the dephosphorylation and inactivation of myosin light chains, which results in relaxation of the muscle cells. Nitric oxide may play a physiologic role in erectile tissue function, in which smooth muscle relaxation is required to bring about the influx of blood that causes erection.
   2. **Cell adhesion:** Nitric oxide has effects on cell adhesion that result in reduced platelet aggregation and reduced neutrophil adhesion to vascular endothelium. The latter effect is probably due to reduced expression of adhesion molecules by endothelial cells.
   3. **Inflammation:** Nitric oxide appears to *facilitate* inflammation, both directly and through the stimulation of prostaglandin synthesis by cyclooxygenase II.

D. **Clinical Applications of Nitric Oxide Inhibitors and Donors:** While *inhibitors* of nitric oxide synthesis are of great research interest, none are currently in clinical use. Nitric oxide can be *inactivated* by heme, but application of this approach is in preclinical research.

   In contrast, drugs that *release* endogenous nitric oxide and *donors* of the molecule were in use long before nitric oxide was discovered and continue to be very important in clinical medicine. The cardiovascular applications of nitroprusside (Chapter 11) and the nitrates and nitrites (Chapter 12) have been discussed. Uses in the treatment of preeclampsia and of pulmonary hypertension and acute respiratory distress syndrome are currently under clinical investigation. Early results from the pulmonary disease studies appear promising.

   Preclinical studies suggest that nitric oxide donor drugs or dietary supplementation with arginine may assist in slowing atherosclerosis, especially in grafted organs. In contrast, *acute rejection* of grafts may involve up-regulation of nitric oxide synthase enzymes, and inhibition of these enzymes may prolong graft survival.

QUESTIONS

DIRECTIONS: Each of the numbered items or incomplete statements in this section is followed by answers or by completions of the statement. Select the ONE lettered answer or completion that is BEST in each case.

1. Molecules from which nitric oxide can be released in vivo include all of the following EXCEPT
   (A) Amyl nitrite
   (B) Arginine
   (C) Histamine
   (D) Isosorbide dinitrate
   (E) Nitroprusside

2. A molecule that stimulates nitric oxide synthase, especially the eNOS isoform, is
   (A) Acetylcholine
   (B) Citrulline
   (C) Epinephrine
   (D) Nitroglycerin
   (E) Nitroprusside

3. The inducible isoform of nitric oxide synthase (iNOS, isoform II) is found primarily in
   (A) Cartilage
   (B) Eosinophils
   (C) Macrophages
   (D) Platelets
   (E) Vascular endothelial cells

4. The primary endogenous substrate for nitric oxide synthase is
   (A) Acetylcholine
   (B) Angiotensinogen
   (C) Arginine
   (D) Citrulline
   (E) Heme

5. Which of the following is a recognized effect of nitric oxide?
   (A) Arrhythmia
   (B) Bronchoconstriction
   (C) Constipation
   (D) Inhibition of graft rejection
   (E) Pulmonary vasodilation

ANSWERS

1. Nitroprusside and organic nitrites (eg, amyl nitrite) and nitrates (eg, isosorbide dinitrate, nitroglycerin) contain NO groups that can be released as nitric oxide. Arginine is the normal source of endogenous nitric oxide. Histamine stimulates the production of nitric oxide from arginine. The answer is **(C)**.

2. Acetylcholine is the only molecule in this list that stimulates the endogenous production of nitric oxide by nitric oxide synthase. The answer is **(A)**.

3. The inducible form of nitric oxide synthase is associated with inflammation, and the enzyme is found in macrophages. The answer is **(C)**.

4. Arginine is the substrate and citrulline (along with nitric oxide) the product of nitric oxide synthase. The answer is **(C)**.

5. Nitric oxide does not cause arrhythmias or constipation. It causes bronchodilation and may hasten graft rejection. Nitric oxide does cause pulmonary vasodilation. The answer is **(E)**.

Bronchodilators & Other Drugs Used in Asthma

20

OBJECTIVES

You should be able to:

- Describe the strategies of drug treatment of asthma.
- List the major classes of drugs used in asthma.
- Describe the mechanisms of action of these drug groups.
- List the major adverse effects of the most important anti-asthma drugs.

Learn the definitions that follow.

Table 20–1. Definitions.

Term	Definition
Bronchial hyperreactivity	Pathologic increase in the bronchoconstrictor response to antigens and irritants; caused by bronchial inflammation
IgE-mediated disease	Disease caused by excessive or misdirected immune response mediated by IgE antibodies. *Example:* asthma
Mast cell degranulation	Exocytosis of granules from mast cells with release of mediators of inflammation and bronchoconstriction
Phosphodiesterase, PDE	Enzyme that degrades cAMP (active) to AMP (inactive)
Tachyphylaxis	Rapid loss of responsiveness to a stimulus, eg, a drug

CONCEPTS

A. Pathophysiology of Asthma: Asthma is a disease characterized by airway inflammation and episodic, reversible bronchospasm. The immediate cause of the bronchial smooth muscle contraction is the release of several mediators from sensitized mast cells and other cells involved in immunologic responses (Figure 20–1). These mediators include the leukotrienes LTC_4 and LTD_4. In addition, chemoattractant mediators such as LTB_4 attract inflammatory cells to the airways. Chronic inflammation leads to marked bronchial hyperreactivity to various inhaled substances, including antigens, histamine, muscarinic agonists, and irritants such as SO_2 and cold air. This reactivity is partially mediated by vagal reflexes.

B. Subgroups of Anti-asthmatic Drugs: Drugs useful in asthma include bronchodilators (smooth muscle relaxants) and anti-inflammatory drugs (Figure 20–2). Leukotriene antagonists have been introduced recently.

Bronchodilators include sympathomimetics, especially β_2-selective agonists, muscarinic antagonists, methylxanthines, and, presumably, leukotriene receptor blockers.

The most important anti-inflammatory drugs in the treatment of asthma are the corticosteroids and drugs such as cromolyn and nedocromil that inhibit release of mediators from mast cells and other inflammatory cells. The lipoxygenase inhibitor zileuton probably also exerts an anti-inflammatory effect in asthma.

BETA-ADRENOCEPTOR AGONISTS

A. Prototypes and Pharmacokinetics: The most important sympathomimetics used to reverse asthmatic bronchoconstriction are the β_2-selective agonists, though epinephrine and isopro-

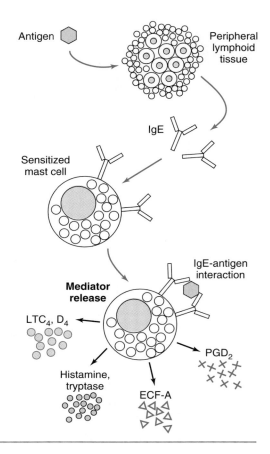

Figure 20–1. Immunologic model for the pathogenesis of asthma. Exposure to antigen causes synthesis of IgE, which binds to and sensitizes mast cells and other inflammatory cells. When such sensitized cells are challenged with antigen, a variety of mediators are released that can account for most of the signs of the early bronchoconstrictor response in asthma. (Modified and reproduced, with permission, from Gold WW: Cholinergic pharmacology in asthma. In: *Asthma Physiology, Immunopharmacology, and Treatment.* Austen KF, Lichtenstein LM [editors]. Academic Press, 1974.)

terenol are still used occasionally. Of the selective agents, **terbutaline, albuterol,** and **metaproterenol** are most important in the USA. **Salmeterol** is a newer, long-acting β_2 agonist that is available in the USA. Formoterol is a similar drug available outside the USA. Beta agonists are given almost exclusively by inhalation, usually from pressurized aerosol canisters but occasionally by nebulizer. The inhalation route decreases the systemic dose (and adverse effects) while delivering a locally effective dose to airway smooth muscle. The older drugs have durations of action of 6 hours or less; salmeterol acts for 12 hours or more.

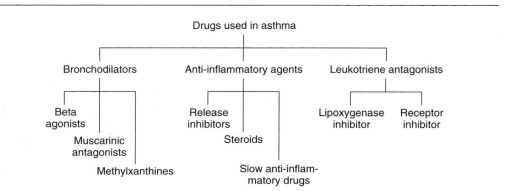

Figure 20–2. Subgroups of drugs discussed in this chapter. Leukotriene antagonists are shown as a separate category because it is not yet clear whether their benefits are primarily as bronchodilators or as anti-inflammatory agents.

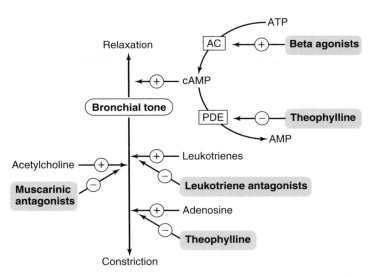

Figure 20–3. Possible mechanisms of beta agonists, muscarinic antagonists, theophylline, and leukotriene antagonists in altering bronchial tone in asthma. AC, adenylyl cyclase; PDE, phosphodiesterase.

B. Mechanism and Effects: Beta receptor activation, linked by G_s, results in stimulation of adenylyl cyclase and increased cAMP in smooth muscle cells (Figure 20–3). The increase in cAMP results in a powerful bronchodilator response.

C. Clinical Use: Sympathomimetics are used very extensively in asthma. In almost all patients, the beta agonists are the most effective bronchodilators available. Shorter-acting sympathomimetics (albuterol, metoprolol, terbutaline) should be used only for acute episodes of bronchospasm (not for prophylaxis), whereas the long-acting agents (salmeterol, formoterol) should be used for prophylaxis, not for acute episodes.

D. Toxicity: Skeletal muscle tremor is a common adverse β_2 effect. Beta$_2$ selectivity is relative. At high clinical dosage, these agents have significant β_1 effects. Even when they are given by inhalation, some cardiac effect (tachycardia) is common. Other adverse effects are rare. When the agents are used excessively, arrhythmias may occur. Loss of responsiveness (tolerance, tachyphylaxis) is an unwanted effect of excessive use of the short-acting sympathomimetics.

METHYLXANTHINES

A. Prototypes and Pharmacokinetics: The methylxanthines are purine derivatives. Three major methylxanthines are found in plants and provide the stimulant effects of three common beverages: **caffeine** (in coffee), **theophylline** (tea), and **theobromine** (cocoa). Theophylline is the only methylxanthine important in the treatment of asthma. The drug is orally active and available as various salts and as the base and is provided in rapid-release and slow-release forms. Theophylline is eliminated by P450 drug-metabolizing enzymes in the liver. Clearance varies with age (highest in young adolescents), smoking status (higher in smokers), and concurrent use of other drugs that inhibit or induce hepatic enzymes.

B. Mechanism of Action: The methylxanthines inhibit phosphodiesterase (PDE), the enzyme that degrades cAMP to AMP (Figure 20–3), and thus increase cAMP. This anti-PDE effect, however, requires high concentrations of the drug. Methylxanthines also block adenosine receptors in the CNS and elsewhere, but a relationship between this action and the bronchodilating effect has not been clearly established. It is possible that bronchodilation is caused by a third action as yet unrecognized.

C. **Effects:** In asthma, bronchodilation is the most important therapeutic action. Increased strength of contraction of the diaphragm has been demonstrated in some patients. Other effects of therapeutic doses include CNS stimulation, cardiac stimulation, vasodilation, a slight increase in blood pressure (probably caused by the release of norepinephrine from adrenergic nerves), and increased gastrointestinal motility.

D. **Clinical Use:** The major clinical indication for the use of any methylxanthine is asthma; theophylline is the most important methylxanthine in clinical use. Another methylxanthine derivative, **pentoxifylline,** is promoted as a remedy for intermittent claudication; this effect is said to result from decreased viscosity of the blood. Of course, the nonmedical use of the methylxanthines in coffee, tea, and cocoa is far greater, in total quantities consumed, than the medical uses of the drugs.

E. **Toxicity:** The common adverse effects include gastrointestinal distress, tremor, and insomnia. Severe nausea and vomiting, hypotension, cardiac arrhythmias, and convulsions may result from overdosage. Very large overdoses (eg, in suicide attempts) are potentially lethal because of the arrhythmias and convulsions. Beta-blockers and anticonvulsants are useful antidotes for severe theophylline toxicity.

MUSCARINIC ANTAGONISTS

A. **Prototypes and Pharmacokinetics:** Atropine and other naturally occurring belladonna alkaloids were used for many years in the treatment of asthma with only modest success. A quaternary antimuscarinic agent designed for aerosol use, **ipratropium,** has achieved much greater success. This drug is delivered to the airways by pressurized aerosol. When absorbed, ipratropium is rapidly metabolized and has little systemic action.

B. **Mechanism of Action:** When given as an aerosol, ipratropium competitively blocks muscarinic receptors in the airways and effectively prevents bronchoconstriction mediated by vagal discharge. Given systemically (not an approved use), the drug is indistinguishable from other short-acting muscarinic blockers. It has no effect on the inflammatory aspects of asthma.

C. **Effects:** Ipratropium reverses bronchoconstriction in some asthma patients (especially children) and in many patients with chronic obstructive pulmonary disease (COPD).

D. **Clinical Use:** Asthma. Muscarinic blockers are useful in one-third to two-thirds of asthmatic patients; β_2 agonists are effective in almost all. For acute bronchospasm, therefore, the beta agonists are usually preferred. However, in chronic obstructive pulmonary disease (which is often associated with acute episodes of bronchospasm), the antimuscarinic agents may be more effective and less toxic than beta agonists.

E. **Toxicity:** Because ipratropium is delivered directly to the airway and is minimally absorbed, systemic effects are small. When it is given in excessive dosage, minor atropine-like toxic effects may occur (Chapter 8). In contrast to the β_2 agonists, ipratropium does not cause tremor or arrhythmias.

CROMOLYN & NEDOCROMIL

A. **Prototypes and Pharmacokinetics:** Cromolyn (disodium cromoglycate) and nedocromil are unusual chemicals: they are extremely insoluble, so that even massive doses given orally or by aerosol result in negligible systemic blood levels. They are given by aerosol for asthma. Cromolyn is the older compound and is the prototype of this group.

B. **Mechanism of Action:** The mechanism of action of these drugs is poorly understood but appears to involve a decrease in the release of mediators (such as the leukotrienes and histamine) from mast cells. The drugs have no bronchodilator action but can prevent bronchoconstriction caused by a challenge with antigen to which the patient is allergic. Cromolyn and nedocromil are capable of preventing both early and late responses to challenge (Figure 20–4).

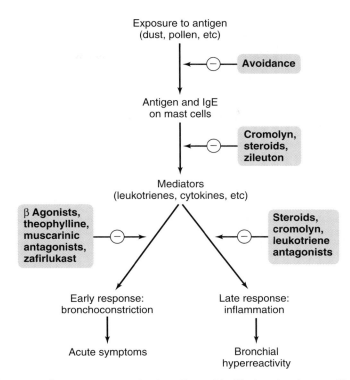

Figure 20–4. Summary of treatment strategies in asthma. (Modified and redrawn, with permission, from Cockcroft DW: The bronchial late response in the pathogenesis of asthma and its modulation by therapy. Ann Allergy 1985;55:857.)

C. **Effects:** Because they are not absorbed from the airway, cromolyn and nedocromil have only local effects. When administered orally, cromolyn has some efficacy in preventing food allergy. Similar actions have been demonstrated after local application in the conjunctiva and the nasopharyngeal tract.

D. **Clinical Uses:** Asthma (especially in children) is by far the most important use for cromolyn and nedocromil. Nasal inhaler and eyedrop formulations of cromolyn are available for hay fever, and an oral formulation is used for food allergy.

E. **Toxicity:** These drugs may cause cough and irritation of the airway when given by aerosol. Rare instances of drug allergy have been reported.

CORTICOSTEROIDS

A. **Prototypes and Pharmacokinetics:** All of the corticosteroids, eg, cortisol and prednisone, are potentially beneficial in severe asthma (see Chapter 39). However, because of their toxicity, systemic (oral or intravenous) corticosteroids are used only as a last resort. In contrast, local aerosol administration of surface-active corticosteroids (eg, **beclomethasone, budesonide, triamcinolone**) is relatively safe; inhaled corticosteroids are commonly used as first-line therapy for individuals with moderate to severe asthma.

B. **Mechanism of Action:** Corticosteroids reduce the synthesis of arachidonic acid by phospholipase A$_2$ and inhibit the expression of COX II, the inducible form of cyclooxygenase (see Chapter 18, Figure 18–1). It has also been suggested that corticosteroids increase the responsiveness of beta adrenoceptors in the airway.

C. Effects: See Chapter 39 for details. Glucocorticoids bind to intracellular receptors and activate glucocorticoid response elements (GREs) in the nucleus, resulting in synthesis of substances that prevent the full expression of inflammation and allergy. Reduced activity of phospholipase A_2 is thought to be particularly important in asthma because the leukotrienes that result from eicosanoid synthesis are extremely potent bronchoconstrictors and may also participate in the late inflammatory response (Figure 20–4).

D. Clinical Use: Inhaled glucocorticoids are now considered appropriate (even for children) in most cases of moderate asthma that are not fully responsive to beta agonists by aerosol. It is believed that such early use may prevent the severe, progressive inflammatory changes characteristic of long-standing asthma. This is a shift from earlier beliefs that steroids should be used only in severe, refractory asthma. In such cases of severe asthma, patients are usually hospitalized and stabilized on daily systemic prednisone and then switched to inhaled or alternate-day oral therapy before discharge. (See Chapter 39 for other uses.)

E. Toxicity: Local aerosol administration can occasionally result in a very small degree of adrenal suppression, but this is rarely significant. More commonly, changes in oropharyngeal flora result in candidiasis. If oral therapy is required, adrenal suppression can be reduced by using alternate-day therapy—ie, by giving the drug in slightly higher dosage every other day rather than in smaller doses every day. The major systemic toxicities of the glucocorticoids described in Chapter 39 are much more likely if systemic treatment is required for more than 2 weeks, as in severe refractory asthma.

LEUKOTRIENE ANTAGONISTS

Recognition of the importance of leukotrienes in the pathophysiology of asthma has led to the introduction of two newer drugs that interfere with the synthesis or the action of these arachidonic acid derivatives (see also Chapter 18). Although their value has been documented, these agents are not as effective as corticosteroids in severe asthma.

A. Zileuton: Zileuton is an orally active drug that selectively inhibits the enzyme 5-lipoxygenase, a key enzyme in the conversion of arachidonic acid to leukotrienes. The drug is effective against both exercise- and antigen-induced bronchospasm. It is also effective against "aspirin allergy," the bronchospasm that results from ingestion of aspirin by individuals who apparently divert all eicosanoid production to leukotrienes when the cyclooxygenase pathway is blocked.

B. Zafirlukast: Zafirlukast is an antagonist at the LTD_4 leukotriene receptor. The LTE_4 receptor is also blocked. Like zileuton, the drug is orally active and has been shown to be effective against exercise-, antigen-, and aspirin-induced bronchospastic attacks.

DRUG LIST

The following drugs are important members of the group discussed in this chapter. Prototypes should be learned in detail; features of the major variants should be known well enough so that the variants can be distinguished from prototypes and from each other; the other significant agents should be recognized as belonging to a specific subclass.

Subclass	Prototype	Major Variants	Other Significant Agents
Beta agonists	Terbutaline	Salmeterol	Metaproterenol, albuterol, formoterol
Methylxanthines	Theophylline	Aminophylline (a theophylline salt)	Caffeine, theobromine
Muscarinic antagonist	Ipratropium		
Release inhibitors	Cromolyn		Nedocromil
Glucocorticoids	Beclomethasone	Prednisone	
Leukotriene antagonists	Zileuton, zafirlukast		

QUESTIONS

DIRECTIONS: Each of the numbered items or incomplete statements in this section is followed by answers or by completions of the statement. Select the ONE lettered answer or completion that is BEST in each case.

1. One effect that theophylline, nitroglycerin, isoproterenol, and histamine have in common is
    (A) Direct stimulation of cardiac contractile force
    (B) Tachycardia
    (C) Increased gastric acid secretion
    (D) Postural hypotension
    (E) Throbbing headache

2. A 23-year-old woman is using a terbutaline inhaler for frequent acute episodes of asthma and describes symptoms that she attributes to the terbutaline. Which of the following is NOT a recognized action of terbutaline?
    (A) Diuretic effect
    (B) Positive inotropic effect
    (C) Skeletal muscle tremor
    (D) Smooth muscle relaxation
    (E) Tachycardia

3. A 10-year-old child has severe asthma and was hospitalized five times between the ages of 7 and 9. He is now receiving outpatient medications that have greatly reduced the frequency of severe attacks. Of the following, the most likely to cause adverse effects when used over long periods for severe asthma is
    (A) Daily administration of albuterol by aerosol
    (B) Daily administration of beclomethasone by aerosol
    (C) Daily administration of cromolyn by inhaler
    (D) Daily administration of prednisone by mouth
    (E) Daily administration of theophylline in its long-acting oral formulation

4. Cromolyn has as its major action
    (A) Block of calcium channels in lymphocytes
    (B) Block of mediator release from mast cells
    (C) Block of phosphodiesterase in mast cells and basophils
    (D) Smooth muscle relaxation in the bronchi
    (E) Stimulation of cortisol release by the adrenals

Items 5–6: A 16-year-old patient is in the emergency room. She has a heart rate of 135/min, a respiratory rate of 40/min, and an estimated 1-second forced expiratory volume less than 10% of normal. Wheezing and rales are audible without a stethoscope.

5. Drugs that can dilate bronchi during an acute asthmatic attack include all of the following EXCEPT
    (A) Epinephrine
    (B) Terbutaline
    (C) Nedocromil
    (D) Theophylline
    (E) Ipratropium

6. After successful treatment of the acute attack, the patient was referred to the outpatient clinic for follow-up treatment of her asthma. Successful strategies currently in use for asthma include all of the following EXCEPT
    (A) Avoidance of antigen exposure
    (B) Blockade of histamine receptors
    (C) Blockade of leukotriene receptors
    (D) Inhibition of phospholipase A_2
    (E) Inhibition of release of mediators from mast cells and leukocytes

DIRECTIONS (Items 7–15): Each set of matching questions in this section consists of a list of three to twenty-six lettered options (some of which may be figures) followed by several numbered items. For each numbered item, select the ONE lettered option that is MOST closely associated with it. Each lettered option may be selected once, more than once, or not at all.

    (A)   Aminophylline
    (B)   Cromolyn
    (C)   Epinephrine
    (D)   Ipratropium
    (E)   Metaproterenol
    (F)   Metoprolol
    (G)   Prednisone
    (H)   Salmeterol
    (I)   Zafirlukast
    (J)   Zileuton

7. Bronchodilator; useful in chronic obstructive pulmonary disease; of the listed bronchodilators, it is the one least likely to cause cardiac arrhythmia

8. Nonselective but very potent and efficacious bronchodilator; not active by the oral route

9. Prophylactic agent that appears to stabilize mast cells

10. Direct bronchodilator most often used in asthma by the oral route

11. Parenteral form is life-saving in severe status asthmaticus; inhibits phospholipase A_2

12. Overdose toxicity includes insomnia, arrhythmias, convulsions

13. A newer β_2-selective agonist with a long duration of action; used for prophylaxis

14. A drug that inhibits 5-lipoxygenase and reduces leukotriene synthesis

15. Inhibitor of LTD_4 receptors

ANSWERS

1. Theophylline does not cause headache. Nitroglycerin does not increase gastric acid secretion. Isoproterenol does not cause either. Histamine may cause all of the effects listed. The answer is **(B)**.

2. Terbutaline is a "selective" β_2-receptor agonist, but in moderate to high doses it induces β_1 cardiac effects as well as β_2-mediated smooth and skeletal muscle effects. The answer is **(A)**.

3. If oral corticosteroids must be used, alternate-day therapy is preferred because it interferes less with normal growth in children. The answer is **(D)**.

4. The answer is **(B)**, inhibition of mediator release from mast cells. The mechanism for this effect is not known.

5. Neither nedocromil nor cromolyn is capable of reversing bronchospasm; the action is prophylactic. The answer is **(C)**.

6. Histamine does not appear to play a significant role in asthma, and antihistaminic drugs, even in high doses, are of little or no value. The answer is **(B)**.

7. Ipratropium is the bronchodilator that is most likely to be useful in COPD without causing arrhythmias. The answer is **(D)**.

8. Epinephrine is still one of the most potent and efficacious agents available for asthma. However, because it is nonselective, β_2-selective agents are preferred. The answer is **(C)**.

9. Cromolyn is useful only for prophylaxis. The drug stabilizes mast cells, ie, prevents mediator release. The answer is **(B)**.

10. Aminophylline, a salt of theophylline, is a bronchodilator that is active by the oral and IV route. The answer is **(A)**.

11. Parenteral corticosteroids such as prednisone are life-saving in status asthmaticus. They probably act by reducing production of leukotrienes (see Chapter 18). The answer is **(G)**.

12. Aminophylline is a salt of theophylline. Like the base theophylline, aminophylline can cause severe and potentially lethal overdose toxicity. The answer is **(A)**.

13. Salmeterol is a newer, long-acting β_2-selective sympathomimetic agent that is approved for prophylactic use in asthma. The answer is **(H)**.

14. Zileuton is a selective inhibitor of 5-lipoxygenase. The answer is **(J)**.

15. Zafirlukast inhibits LTD_4 at its receptors. The answer is **(I)**.

Part V: Drugs That Act in the Central Nervous System

Introduction to CNS Pharmacology **21**

OBJECTIVES

You should be able to:

- List the criteria for accepting a chemical as a neurotransmitter.
- Describe the mechanisms by which drugs cause presynaptic and postsynaptic modulation of synaptic transmission.
- List the major excitatory central neurotransmitters.
- List the major inhibitory central neurotransmitters.
- Identify the major receptor subtypes of CNS neurotransmitters.

Learn the definitions that follow.

Table 21–1. Definitions.

Term	Definition
Voltage-sensitive ion channels	Transmembrane ion channels that are regulated by changes in membrane potential; also called electrically-gated or voltage-gated channels
Receptor-operated ion channels	Transmembrane ion channels that are regulated by interactions between neurotransmitters and their receptors; also called chemically gated channels
EPSP	Excitatory postsynaptic potential; a depolarizing potential change
IPSP	Inhibitory postsynaptic potential; a hyperpolarizing potential change
Synaptic mimicry	Ability of an administered drug to mimic the actions of the natural synaptic transmitter; a criterion for identification of a putative neurotransmitter

CONCEPTS

A. **Targets of CNS Drug Action:**   Most drugs that act on the CNS appear to do so by changing ion flow through transmembrane channels.

1. **Types of ion channels:**   Transmembrane ion channels can be divided into voltage-sensitive (electrically gated) and transmitter-sensitive (chemically gated or receptor-operated) groups. Voltage-sensitive channels are concentrated on the axons of nerve cells and include the sodium channels responsible for action potential propagation. Cell bodies and dendrites also have voltage-sensitive ion channels for potassium and calcium. Some voltage-gated channels (eg, calcium channels) are partly regulated by chemical transmitters. Chemically sensitive ion channels are found on cell bodies and on both pre- and postsynaptic sides of synapses.

2. **Types of receptor-channel coupling:**   In the case of chemically-sensitive ion channels, activation (or inhibition) is initiated by the interaction between chemical transmitters and their receptors. Coupling may be (1) through a receptor that acts directly on the channel protein, (2) through a receptor that is coupled to the ion channel through a G protein, or (3) through a receptor coupled to a G protein that modulates the formation of second messen-

gers—including cAMP, inositol trisphosphate (IP$_3$), and diacylglycerol (DAG)—which secondarily modulate a channel.

3. **Role of the ion current carried by the channel:** Excitatory postsynaptic potentials (EPSPs) are usually generated by the opening of sodium or calcium channels. In some synapses, similar depolarizing potentials result from the *closing* of potassium channels. Inhibitory postsynaptic potentials (IPSPs) are generated by the opening of potassium or chloride channels.

B. **Sites and Mechanisms of Drug Action:** A small number of neuropharmacologic agents exert their effects through direct interactions with molecular components of ion channels on axons. Examples include certain anticonvulsants (eg, carbamazepine, phenytoin), local anesthetics, and some drugs used in general anesthesia. However, the effects of most therapeutically important CNS drugs are exerted mainly at synapses. Possible mechanisms are indicated in Figure 21–1. Thus, drugs may act presynaptically to alter the synthesis, storage, release, reuptake, or metabolism of transmitter chemicals. Other drugs can activate or block both pre- and postsynaptic receptors for specific transmitters or interfere with the actions of second messengers. The selectivity of CNS drug action is largely based on the fact that different groups of neurons utilize different neurotransmitters and that they are segregated into networks that subserve different CNS functions. A few neurotoxic substances damage or kill nerve cells. For example, 1-methyl-4-phenyl-1,2,3,6-tetrahydropyridine (MPTP) is cytotoxic to neurons of the nigrostriatal dopaminergic pathway.

C. **Role of CNS Organization:** The CNS contains two types of neuronal systems: hierarchical and diffuse.

1. **Hierarchical systems:** Hierarchical systems are clearly delimited in their anatomic distribution and generally contain large myelinated rapidly conducting fibers. They control major sensory and motor functions. The major excitatory transmitters in these systems are aspartate and glutamate. These systems also include numerous small inhibitory interneurons, which utilize gamma-aminobutyric acid (GABA) or glycine as transmitters. Drugs that affect hierarchical systems often have profound effects on the overall excitability of the CNS.

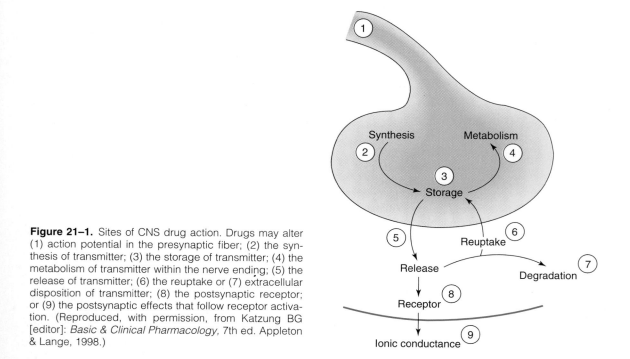

Figure 21–1. Sites of CNS drug action. Drugs may alter (1) action potential in the presynaptic fiber; (2) the synthesis of transmitter; (3) the storage of transmitter; (4) the metabolism of transmitter within the nerve ending; (5) the release of transmitter; (6) the reuptake or (7) extracellular disposition of transmitter; (8) the postsynaptic receptor; or (9) the postsynaptic effects that follow receptor activation. (Reproduced, with permission, from Katzung BG [editor]: *Basic & Clinical Pharmacology,* 7th ed. Appleton & Lange, 1998.)

2. **Diffuse systems:** Diffuse systems are broadly distributed, with single cells frequently sending processes to many different areas. The axons are fine and branch repeatedly to form synapses with many cells. Axons commonly have periodic enlargements (varicosities) that contain vesicles so that transmitter is released at many sites along the path of the axon. The transmitters in diffuse systems are often amines (norepinephrine, dopamine, serotonin) or peptides. Drugs that affect these systems will often have marked effects on such functions as attention, appetite, and emotional states.

D. **Transmitters at Central Synapses:**
   1. **Criteria for transmitter status:** To be accepted as a neurotransmitter, a candidate chemical must be present in higher concentration in the synaptic area than in other areas (ie, must be localized in appropriate areas), must be released by electrical or chemical stimulation, and must produce the same sort of postsynaptic response that is seen with physiologic activation of the synapse (ie, must exhibit synaptic mimicry). Table 21–2 lists the most important chemicals currently accepted as neurotransmitters in the CNS.
   2. **Acetylcholine:** Approximately 5% of brain neurons have receptors for ACh. Most CNS responses to ACh are mediated by a large family of G protein-coupled muscarinic M_1 receptors that lead to slow excitation when activated. Of the nicotinic receptors present in the CNS (they are less common than muscarinic receptors), the ones best characterized are those on the Renshaw cells activated by motor axon collaterals in the spinal cord. Drugs affecting the activity of cholinergic systems in the brain include the acetylcholinesterase inhibitors used in Alzheimer's disease and the muscarinic blocking agents used in parkinsonism.
   3. **Dopamine:** Dopamine exerts inhibitory actions at synapses in diffuse neuronal systems. The D_2 receptor is the main dopamine subtype in basal ganglia neurons, and it is widely distributed at the supraspinal level. In addition to the two receptors listed in Table 21–2, three other dopamine receptor subtypes have been identified (D_3, D_4, and D_5). Drugs affecting the activity of dopaminergic pathways include antipsychotics, CNS stimulants, and antiparkinsonism drugs.
   4. **Norepinephrine:** Noradrenergic neuron cell bodies are mainly located in the locus ceruleus and the lateral tegmental area of the pons. These neurons fan out broadly to provide most regions of the CNS with diffuse noradrenergic input. Excitatory effects are produced by activation of $alpha_1$ and $beta_1$ receptors. Inhibitory effects are caused by activation of $alpha_2$ and $beta_2$ receptors. CNS stimulants, monoamine oxidase inhibitors, and tricyclic antidepressants affect the activity of noradrenergic pathways.
   5. **Serotonin:** Most serotonergic pathways originate from cell bodies in the raphe or midline regions of the pons and upper brain stem; these pathways innervate most regions of the CNS. Serotonin is inhibitory at many CNS sites but can cause excitation of some neurons depending on the receptor subtype activated. Both excitatory and inhibitory actions can occur on the same neuron if appropriate receptors are present. Most of the agents used in the treatment of major depressive disorders affect serotonergic pathways (tricyclic antidepressants, selective serotonin reuptake inhibitors).
   6. **Excitatory amino acids:** Most neurons in the brain are excited by **glutamic acid** and **aspartic acid**. Receptors that directly gate cation-selective channels are called **ionotropic**. Subtypes include the NMDA (*N*-methyl-D-aspartate) receptor, which is blocked by phencyclidine (PCP) and ketamine. Glutamate receptors that modulate G protein-coupled second messenger systems are called **metabotropic**.
   7. **Inhibitory amino acids:** GABA is the primary neurotransmitter mediating IPSPs in neurons in the brain; it is also important in the spinal cord. Fast IPSPs are blocked by $GABA_A$ receptor antagonists and slow IPSPs are blocked by $GABA_B$ receptor antagonists. Drugs that influence GABAergic systems include sedatives, hypnotics, and some anticonvulsants. **Glycine** receptors, which are more numerous in the cord than in the brain, are blocked by strychnine, a spinal convulsant.
   8. **Peptide transmitters:** Many peptides have been identified in the CNS, and some meet most or all of the criteria for acceptance as neurotransmitters. The best-defined are the opioid peptides (beta-endorphin, met- and leu-enkephalin, and dynorphin), which are distributed at all levels of the neuraxis. Some of the important therapeutic actions of opioid analgesics (eg, morphine) are mediated by receptors for these endogenous peptides. Sub-

Table 21–2. Neurotransmitter pharmacology in the central nervous system.*

Transmitter	Anatomic Distribution	Receptor Subtypes	Receptor Mechanisms
Acetylcholine	Cell bodies at all levels, short and long axons	Muscarinic, M_1; blocked by pirenzepine and atropine	Excitatory; $\downarrow K^+$ conductance; $\uparrow IP_3$ and DAG
		Muscarinic, M_2; blocked by atropine	Inhibitory; $\uparrow K^+$ conductance; $\downarrow$ cAMP
	Motoneuron-Renshaw cell synapse	Nicotinic, N	Excitatory; $\uparrow$ cation conductance
Dopamine	Cell bodies at all levels, short, medium, and long axons	D_1; blocked by phenothiazines	Inhibitory; $\uparrow$ cAMP
		D_2; blocked by phenothiazines and haloperidol	Inhibitory (presynaptic); $\downarrow Ca^{2+}$ conductance
			Inhibitory (postsynaptic); $\uparrow K^+$ conductance; $\downarrow$ cAMP
Norepinephrine	Cell bodies in pons and brain stem project to all levels	Alpha$_1$; blocked by prazosin	Excitatory; $\downarrow K^+$ conductance; $\uparrow IP_3$ and DAG
		Alpha$_2$; activated by clonidine	Inhibitory (presynaptic); $\downarrow Ca^{2+}$ conductance
			Inhibitory (postsynaptic); $\uparrow K^+$ conductance; $\downarrow$ cAMP
		Beta$_1$; blocked by propranolol	Excitatory; $\downarrow K^+$ conductance; $\uparrow$ cAMP
		Beta$_2$; blocked by propranolol	Inhibitory; ? increase in electrogenic sodium pump; $\uparrow$ cAMP
Serotonin (5-hydroxy-tryptamine)	Cell bodies in midbrain and pons project to all levels	5-HT$_{1A}$; buspirone is a partial agonist	Inhibitory; $\uparrow K^+$ conductance
		5-HT$_{2A}$; blocked by clozapine, risperidone, and olanzapine	Excitatory; $\downarrow K^+$ conductance; $\uparrow IP_3$ and DAG
		5-HT$_3$; blocked by ondansetron	Excitatory; $\uparrow$ cation conductance
		5-HT$_4$	Excitatory; $\downarrow K^+$ conductance; $\downarrow$ cAMP
GABA	Supraspinal interneurons; spinal interneurons involved in presynaptic inhibition	GABA$_A$; facilitated by benzodiazepines and zolpidem	Inhibitory; $\uparrow Cl^-$ conductance
		GABA$_B$; activated by baclofen	Inhibitory (presynaptic); $\downarrow Ca^{2+}$ conductance
			Inhibitory (postsynaptic); $\uparrow K^+$ conductance
Glutamate, aspartate	Relay neurons at all levels	Three subtypes; NMDA subtype blocked by phencyclidine	Excitatory; $\uparrow Ca^{2+}$ or cation conductance; $\downarrow K^+$ conductance
Glycine	Interneurons in spinal cord and brain stem	Single subtype; blocked by strychnine	Inhibitory; $\uparrow Cl^-$ conductance
Opioid peptides	Cell bodies at all levels	Three subtypes: mu, delta, kappa	Inhibitory (presynaptic); $\downarrow Ca^{2+}$ conductance; $\downarrow$ cAMP
			Inhibitory (postsynaptic); $\uparrow K^+$ conductance; $\downarrow$ cAMP

*Adapted, with permission, from Katzung BG (editor): *Basic & Clinical Pharmacology,* 7th ed. Appleton & Lange, 1998.

stance P is localized in type C neurons involved in nociceptive sensory pathways in the spinal cord. Peptide transmitters differ from nonpeptide transmitters in two ways: (1) the peptides are synthesized in the cell body and transported to the nerve ending via axonal transport, and (2) no reuptake or specific enzyme mechanisms have been identified for terminating their actions.

QUESTIONS

DIRECTIONS: Each of the numbered items or incomplete statements in this section is followed by answers or by completions of the statement. Select the ONE lettered answer or completion that is BEST in each case.

1. Which one of the following chemicals does NOT satisfy the criteria for a neurotransmitter role in the CNS?
   (A) Aspartic acid
   (B) Dopamine
   (C) Glycine
   (D) Nitric oxide
   (E) Substance P

2. Many therapeutically useful drugs act via brain dopaminergic systems. The mechanisms by which they exert their actions include all of the following EXCEPT
   (A) Inhibition of dopamine reuptake
   (B) Increase in dopamine synthesis
   (C) Activation of dopamine receptors
   (D) Inhibition of dopamine metabolism
   (E) Blockade of dopamine receptors

3. Neurotransmitters may
   (A) Increase chloride conductance to cause inhibition
   (B) Increase potassium conductance to cause excitation
   (C) Increase sodium conductance to cause inhibition
   (D) Increase calcium conductance to cause inhibition
   (E) Exert all of the above actions

4. Which one of the following chemicals does NOT change membrane excitability by decreasing K^+ conductance?
   (A) Acetylcholine
   (B) Dopamine
   (C) Glutamic acid
   (D) Norepinephrine
   (E) Serotonin

5. Which one of the following receptors shares the same potassium channel as the $5\text{-}HT_{1A}$ receptor?
   (A) Delta opioid receptor
   (B) Dopamine D_2 receptor
   (C) $GABA_B$ receptor
   (D) Muscarinic M_1 receptor
   (E) Substance P receptor

6. Which one of the following chemicals is most likely to function as a neurotransmitter in hierarchical systems?
   (A) Dopamine
   (B) Glutamate
   (C) Met-enkephalin
   (D) Norepinephrine
   (E) Serotonin

7. Which one of the following statements about beta-endorphin is most accurate?
   (A) It is exclusively located in the spinal cord
   (B) Enzymes for its synthesis are located in nerve endings
   (C) It selectively activates delta opioid receptors
   (D) Its postsynaptic effects are terminated by active reuptake
   (E) Its actions are mainly inhibitory

DIRECTIONS (Items 8–12): Each set of matching questions in this section consists of a list of three to twenty-six lettered options (some of which may be figures) followed by several numbered items. For each numbered item, select the ONE lettered option that is MOST closely associated with it. Each lettered option may be selected once, more than once, or not at all.

    (A)   Acetylcholine
    (B)   Beta-endorphin
    (C)   cAMP
    (D)   Dopamine
    (E)   GABA
    (F)   Glutamine
    (G)   Glycine
    (H)   *N*-Methyl-D-aspartate
    (I)   Norepinephrine
    (J)   Reserpine
    (K)   Serotonin
    (L)   Strychnine
    (M)   Substance P

8. This agent blocks receptors in the spinal cord that are coupled to chloride ion channels

9. This amine is found in diffuse neuronal systems in the CNS, particularly in the raphe nuclei; it appears to play a major role in the expression of mood, since most antidepressant drugs are thought to increase its functional activity

10. Receptors activated by this chemical are antagonized by phencyclidine

11. This agent may cause extrapyramidal dysfunction by depleting transmitter at nigrostriatal dopaminergic nerve endings

12. This neurotransmitter is found in high concentrations in cell bodies in the locus ceruleus; at some sites, release of transmitter is autoregulated via presynaptic inhibition

ANSWERS

1. Nitric oxide synthase, the enzyme that generates nitric oxide, is found in some neurons in the CNS. However, a role for nitric oxide in synaptic transmission in the CNS has not been clearly established. Substance P is a neurotransmitter released from unmyelinated sensory neurons in the spinal cord involved in nociception. The answer is **(D)**.

2. Levodopa increases dopamine synthesis; bromocriptine activates dopamine receptors; selegiline inhibits dopamine metabolism; and haloperidol blocks dopamine receptors. Although cocaine's mood-elevating action may be due to inhibition of dopamine reuptake, drugs that have been shown to act through inhibition of brain dopamine transporters have not yet found a *therapeutic* niche. However, such drugs could have important therapeutic applications in Parkinson's disease and in the treatment of hyperprolactinemia. The answer is **(A)**.

3. Activation of chloride or potassium ion channels often generates inhibitory postsynaptic potentials (IPSPs) and inhibits nerve membranes. Activation of sodium and *inhibition* of potassium ion channels generate excitatory postsynaptic potentials (EPSPs). The answer is **(A)**.

4. A decrease in K^+ conductance is associated with neuronal excitation. All of the neurotransmitters listed are able to cause excitation by this mechanism at certain neurons in the CNS except dopamine. The answer is **(B)**.

5. Though not mentioned in the text, $GABA_B$ receptors and 5-HT_{1A} receptors share the same potassium ion channel, with a G protein involved in the coupling mechanism. The spasmolytic drug baclofen is an activator of $GABA_B$ receptors in the spinal cord. The anxiolytic drug buspirone may act as a partial agonist at brain 5-HT_{1A} receptors. The answer is **(C)**.

6. Catecholamines (dopamine, norepinephrine), opioid peptides, and serotonin act as neurotransmitters in nonspecific or diffuse neuronal systems. Glutamate is the primary excitatory transmitter in hierarchical neuronal systems. The answer is **(B)**.

7. The opioid peptides are widely distributed in the CNS at all levels of the neuraxis and are synthesized in the cell bodies. They activate several receptor subtypes and cause inhibition. No mechanism has been described for termination of the synaptic actions of endogenous peptides. The answer is **(E)**.

8. The $GABA_A$ and glycine receptors present on neurons in the spinal cord are both coupled to chloride ion channels. However, only the glycine receptor is inhibited by strychnine. The answer is **(L)**.

9. Several amine transmitters may be involved in the control of mood states, especially norepinephrine and serotonin. Many of the cell bodies of serotonergic neurons are found in the raphe nuclei. Most of the drugs used for the treatment of major depressive disorders increase serotonergic activity in the CNS. The answer is **(K)**.

10. Phencyclidine (and ketamine) are glutamate antagonists at a subtype of glutamate (not glutamine) receptor that is responsive to NMDA (*N*-methyl-D-aspartate). The answer is (**H**).

11. In addition to depleting vesicular stores of norepinephrine in sympathetic nerve endings, reserpine depletes brain dopamine and causes parkinsonian adverse effects. Reserpine also decreases vesicular stores of norepinephrine and serotonin, which can result in depression of mood. The answer is (**J**).

12. Cell bodies of many noradrenergic neurons are located in the locus ceruleus. Agents that activate presynaptic alpha$_2$ receptors on such neurons decrease their activity. The regulatory action of norepinephrine is thought to involve these presynaptic alpha$_2$ receptors. The answer is (**I**).

Sedative-Hypnotic Drugs

22

OBJECTIVES

You should be able to:

- Identify the major chemical classes of sedative-hypnotics.
- Describe the pharmacodynamics of benzodiazepines and barbiturates, including their mechanisms of action.
- Compare the pharmacokinetics of commonly used benzodiazepines and barbiturates and discuss how differences among them affect clinical use.
- Describe the clinical uses and the adverse effects of sedative-hypnotics.
- Identify the distinctive properties of buspirone and zolpidem.

Learn the definitions that follow.

Table 22–1. Definitions.

Term	Definition
Sedation	Reduction of anxiety
Anxiolytic	A drug that reduces anxiety, a sedative
Hypnosis	Induction of sleep
REM sleep	Phase of sleep associated with rapid eye movements; most dreaming takes place during REM sleep
Tolerance	Reduction in drug effect requiring an increase in dosage to maintain the same response
Physical dependence	The state of response to a drug in which removal of the drug evokes unpleasant symptoms, usually the opposite of the drug's effects
Psychologic dependence	The state of response to a drug in which the drug taker feels compelled to use the drug and suffers anxiety when separated from the drug
Anesthesia, general	Loss of consciousness associated with absence of response to pain
Coma	Extremely deep anesthesia or depression of brain activity; precursor to respiratory and circulatory failure

CONCEPTS

A. Classification and Pharmacokinetics:
    1. Subgroups: The sedative-hypnotics belong to a chemically heterogeneous class of drugs (Figure 22–1) almost all of which produce dose-dependent CNS depressant effects. The

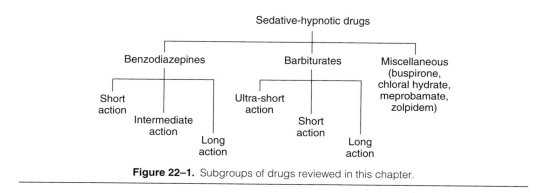

Figure 22–1. Subgroups of drugs reviewed in this chapter.

most important subgroup is the **benzodiazepines,** but representatives of other subgroups, including **barbiturates,** and miscellaneous agents (**carbamates, alcohols,** and **cyclic ethers**) are still in use. Newer drugs with distinctive characteristics include **buspirone** and **zolpidem.**

2. **Absorption and distribution:** Most of these drugs are lipid-soluble and are absorbed well from the gastrointestinal tract with good distribution to the brain. Drugs with the highest lipid solubility (eg, **thiopental**) enter the CNS rapidly and can be used as induction agents in anesthesia. The CNS effects of thiopental are terminated by rapid **redistribution** of the drug from brain to other tissues.

3. **Metabolism and excretion:** Sedative-hypnotics are metabolized prior to elimination from the body, mainly by hepatic enzymes. Metabolic rates and pathways vary among different drugs. Many benzodiazepines are converted initially to **active metabolites** with long half-lives. After several days of therapy with some drugs (eg, diazepam, flurazepam), accumulation of active metabolites can lead to excessive sedation. Lorazepam and oxazepam do not form active metabolites. With the exception of phenobarbital, a part of which is excreted unchanged in the urine, the barbiturates are extensively metabolized via oxidation at the C5 position. Chloral hydrate is oxidized to trichloroethanol, an active metabolite. The duration of CNS actions of sedative-hypnotic drugs ranges from a few hours (eg, chloral hydrate, pentobarbital, triazolam) to more than 30 hours (eg, chlordiazepoxide, clorazepate, diazepam, phenobarbital).

B. **Mechanism of Action:** No single mechanism of action for sedative-hypnotics has been identified, and the different chemical subgroups may have different actions. Certain drugs (eg, benzodiazepines) facilitate neuronal membrane inhibition by actions at specific receptors.

1. **Benzodiazepines:** Receptors for benzodiazepines (BZ receptors) are present in many brain regions, including the thalamus, limbic structures, and the cerebral cortex. The BZ receptors form part of a $GABA_A$ receptor-chloride ion channel macromolecular complex. Binding of benzodiazepines to these receptors appears to facilitate the inhibitory actions of GABA, which are exerted through increased chloride ion conductance (Figure 22–2). Benzodiazepines increase the *frequency* of GABA-mediated chloride ion channel opening. **Flumazenil** reverses the central nervous system effects of benzodiazepines and is classified as an **antagonist** at BZ receptors. Certain beta-carbolines have high affinity for BZ receptors and can elicit anxiogenic and convulsant effects. These drugs are classified as **inverse agonists.**

2. **Barbiturates:** Barbiturates depress neuronal activity in the midbrain reticular formation, facilitating and prolonging the inhibitory effects of GABA and glycine. They do not bind to BZ or GABA receptors but appear to interact with other sites on the chloride ion channel. Barbiturates increase the *duration* of GABA-mediated chloride ion channel opening. They may also block the excitatory transmitter, glutamic acid—and, at high concentration, sodium channels.

3. **Other drugs:** The newer anxiolytic drug **buspirone** interacts with the 5-HT_{1A} subclass of brain serotonin receptors as a partial agonist, but the precise mechanism of its anxiolytic effect is unknown. The hypnotic drug **zolpidem,** though not a benzodiazepine, appears to exert its CNS effects via interaction with certain benzodiazepine receptors, classified as BZ_1 or omega$_1$ subtypes. The effects of zolpidem are antagonized by flumazenil.

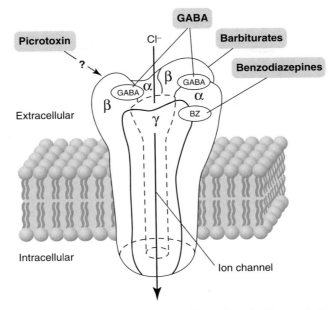

Figure 22–2. Mechanism of action of benzodiazepines. (Reproduced, with permission, from Zorumski CF, Isenberg KE: Insights into the structure and function of GABA-benzodiazepine receptors: Ion channels and psychiatry. Am J Psychiatry 1991;148:162.)

C. Pharmacodynamics: The CNS effects of most sedative-hypnotics depend on the dose, as shown in Figure 22–3. These effects range from sedation and relief of anxiety (anxiolysis), through hypnosis (facilitation of sleep), to anesthesia and coma. Depressant effects are additive when two or more drugs are given together. The steepness of the dose-response curve varies among drug groups; those with flatter curves, such as benzodiazepines, are safer for clinical use. Buspirone is a selective anxiolytic, with minimal depressant effects on the CNS.

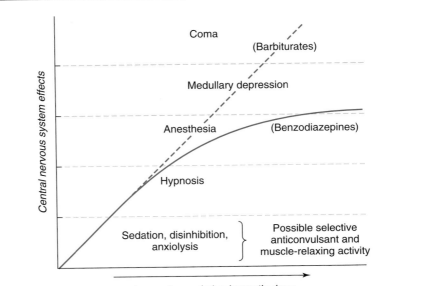

Figure 22–3. Relationships between doses of benzodiazepines and barbiturates and their CNS effects.

1. **Sedation:**   Sedative actions, with relief of anxiety, occur with all drugs in this class. Anxiolysis is usually accompanied by some impairment of psychomotor functions, and behavioral disinhibition may also occur. In animals, most sedative-hypnotics release punishment-suppressed behavior.
2. **Hypnosis:**   Sedative-hypnotics promote sleep onset and increase the duration of the sleep state. Rapid eye movement (REM) sleep duration is usually decreased at high doses; a rebound increase in REM sleep may occur upon withdrawal from chronic drug use.
3. **Anesthesia:**   At high doses, loss of consciousness may occur, with amnesia and suppression of reflexes. Anesthesia can be produced by most barbiturates (eg, thiopental) and certain benzodiazepines (eg, midazolam).
4. **Anticonvulsant actions:**   Suppression of seizure activity occurs with high doses of most of the barbiturates and some of the benzodiazepines, but this is usually at the cost of marked sedation. Selective anticonvulsant action (ie, suppression of convulsions at doses that do not cause severe sedation) occurs with only a few of these drugs (eg, phenobarbital, clonazepam). High doses of intravenous diazepam, lorazepam, or phenobarbital are used in status epilepticus. In this condition, heavy sedation is desirable.
5. **Muscle relaxation:**   Relaxation of skeletal muscle occurs with high doses of most sedative-hypnotics. Diazepam is effective at sedative dose levels for specific spasticity states, including cerebral palsy. Meprobamate also has some selectivity as a muscle relaxant.
6. **Medullary depression:**   High doses can cause depression of medullary neurons, leading to respiratory arrest, hypotension, and cardiovascular collapse. These effects are the cause of death in suicidal overdose.
7. **Tolerance and dependence:**   Tolerance—a decrease in responsiveness—occurs when sedative-hypnotics are used continuously or in high dosage. Cross-tolerance may occur among different chemical subgroups. Psychologic dependence occurs frequently with most sedative-hypnotics and involves the compulsive use of these drugs to reduce anxiety. Physical dependence constitutes an altered state that leads to an abstinence syndrome (withdrawal state) when the drug is discontinued. Withdrawal signs, which may include anxiety, tremors, hyperreflexia, and seizures, occur more commonly with shorter-acting drugs such as pentobarbital and secobarbital. Buspirone is not schedule-controlled because dependence is unlikely to occur with this drug. The dependence liability of zolpidem may be less than that of the benzodiazepines.

D. **Clinical Use:**   Most of these uses can be predicted from the pharmacodynamic effects outlined above.
   1. **Anxiety states:**   Benzodiazepines with intermediate or long durations of action are favored in the drug treatment of most anxiety states. Alprazolam and clonazepam have greater efficacy than other benzodiazepines in panic and phobic disorders. The anxiolytic effects of buspirone occur without sedation or cognitive impairment but take a week or more to develop. Buspirone is commonly used for generalized anxiety disorders in patients with a history of substance abuse.
   2. **Sleep disorders:**   Benzodiazepines, including estazolam, flurazepam, and triazolam, are widely used in primary insomnia and for the management of certain other sleep disorders. Zolpidem appears to cause less daytime cognitive impairment than most benzodiazepines and has minimal effects on sleep patterns.
   3. **Other uses:**   Thiopental is commonly used for the induction of anesthesia, and certain benzodiazepines (eg, diazepam, midazolam) are used as components of anesthesia protocols. Special uses include the management of seizure disorders (eg, clonazepam, phenobarbital) and muscle spasticity (diazepam). Longer-acting drugs (eg, chlordiazepoxide, diazepam) are used in the management of withdrawal states in persons physically dependent on ethanol and other sedative-hypnotics.

E. **Toxicity:**
   1. **Psychomotor dysfunction:**   This includes cognitive impairment, decreased psychomotor skills, and unwanted daytime sedation. These adverse effects are more common with benzodiazepines that have active metabolites with long half-lives (eg, diazepam, flurazepam). The dosage of a sedative-hypnotic should be reduced in elderly patients to avoid excessive daytime sedation, which has been shown to increase the risk of falls and fractures. Short-acting hypnotics, especially triazolam, may cause daytime anxiety and amnesia. Anterograde amnesia may also occur with other benzodiazepines when used at high dosage.

2. **Additive CNS depression:** This occurs when sedative-hypnotics are used with other drugs in the class as well as with alcoholic beverages, antihistamines, antipsychotic drugs, opioid analgesics, and tricyclic antidepressants. This is the most common type of drug interaction involving sedative-hypnotics. Additive CNS depression with buspirone is uncommon.

3. **Overdosage:** Overdosage causes severe respiratory and cardiovascular depression; these potentially lethal effects are more likely to occur with alcohols, barbiturates, and carbamates than with benzodiazepines. Management of intoxication requires maintenance of a patent airway and ventilatory support. Flumazenil may reverse CNS depressant effects of benzodiazepines and zolpidem but has no beneficial actions in overdosage with other sedative-hypnotics.

4. **Other adverse effects:** Barbiturates and carbamates (but not benzodiazepines, buspirone, or zolpidem) induce the formation of the liver microsomal enzymes that metabolize drugs. This enzyme induction may lead to multiple drug interactions. Barbiturates may also precipitate acute porphyria in susceptible patients. Chloral hydrate may displace coumarins from plasma protein binding sites and increase anticoagulant effects.

DRUG LIST

The following drugs are important members of the group discussed in this chapter. Prototypes should be learned in detail; features of the major variants should be known well enough so that the variants can be distinguished from prototypes and from each other; the other significant agents should be recognized as belonging to a specific subclass.

Subclass	Prototype	Major Variants	Other Significant Agents
Benzodiazepines	Chlordiazepoxide, diazepam, temazepam	Alprazolam, clonazepam	Flurazepam, lorazepam, nitrazepam, oxazepam, triazolam
Barbiturates	Phenobarbital, pentobarbital, thiopental		Secobarbital, methohexital
Carbamates	Meprobamate		
Alcohols	Ethanol	Chloral hydrate	
Others	Buspirone, zolpidem		

QUESTIONS

DIRECTIONS: Each of the numbered items or incomplete statements in this section is followed by answers or by completions of the statement. Select the ONE lettered answer or completion that is BEST in each case.

1. Which one of the following is LEAST likely to be caused by treatment with moderate to large doses of diazepam?
   (A) Decreased performance on tests of psychomotor function
   (B) Anterograde amnesia with continued use
   (C) Hyperreflexia and seizures with abrupt discontinuance after chronic use
   (D) Increased synthesis of porphyrins
   (E) Additive depression of the central nervous system with alcohol

2. A 56-year-old man, very overweight, complains of not sleeping well and feeling tired during the day. He tells his physician that his wife is the cause of the problem because she wakes him up several times during the night due to his loud snores. This appears to be a breathing-related sleep disorder, so you will probably write a prescription for
   (A) Clorazepate
   (B) Flurazepam
   (C) Secobarbital
   (D) Triazolam
   (E) None of the above

3. Which one of the following statements concerning the barbiturates is FALSE?
   (A) Symptoms of the abstinence syndrome are more severe during withdrawal from secobarbital than from phenobarbital
   (B) Compared with benzodiazepines, the barbiturates exhibit a steeper dose-response relationship
   (C) Barbiturates may decrease the half-lives of drugs metabolized by the liver
   (D) An increase in urinary pH will accelerate the elimination of phenobarbital
   (E) Respiratory depression caused by barbiturate overdosage can be reversed by flumazenil

4. Concerning the clinical uses of benzodiazepines, which one of the following statements is FALSE?
   (A) Alprazolam has selective anxiolytic effects in patients who suffer from agoraphobia
   (B) Clonazepam is approved for use in the management of obsessive-compulsive disorders
   (C) Diazepam is used for muscle spasticity in patients with cerebral palsy
   (D) Intravenous diazepam is useful in status epilepticus
   (E) Symptoms of the alcohol withdrawal state may be alleviated by treatment with chlordiazepoxide

Items 5–6: The wife of a 24-year-old computer programmer considers him to be of a "nervous disposition." He is easily startled, worries about inconsequential matters, and sometimes complains of stomach cramps. At night he grinds his teeth in his sleep. There is no current history of drug abuse.

5. Assuming that the symptoms experienced by this young man are not related to a medical condition, the most appropriate drug treatment would be the judicious use of
   (A) Buspirone
   (B) Midazolam
   (C) Phenobarbital
   (D) Triazolam
   (E) Zolpidem

6. Regarding the characteristic properties of the drug prescribed for this young man, the physician should inform the patient to anticipate
   (A) Additive CNS depression with alcoholic beverages
   (B) A significant effect on memory
   (C) That the drug will take a week or so to begin working
   (D) A need to gradually increase drug dosage because of tolerance
   (E) That if he stops taking the drug abruptly he will experience withdrawal signs

7. Which one of the following statements best describes the mechanism of action of benzodiazepines?
   (A) Benzodiazepines activate $GABA_B$ receptors in the spinal cord
   (B) Their inhibition of GABA transaminase leads to increased levels of GABA
   (C) Benzodiazepines block glutamate receptors in hierarchical neuronal pathways in the brain
   (D) They increase the frequency of opening of chloride ion channels that are coupled to $GABA_A$ receptors
   (E) They are direct-acting GABA receptor agonists in the CNS

Items 8–9: An 82-year-old woman, otherwise healthy for her age, has difficulty sleeping. Triazolam is prescribed for her at half the conventional adult dose.

8. Which one of the following statements about the use of triazolam in this elderly patient is FALSE?
   (A) The drug may cause ambulatory difficulties in the elderly patient
   (B) She may experience rebound insomnia when she stops taking the drug
   (C) Additive CNS depressant effects are likely if she takes over-the-counter cold medications
   (D) Hypertension is a common adverse effect of flurazepam in patients over 75 years of age
   (E) She may experience amnesia, especially if she also drinks alcoholic beverages

9. The most likely explanation for the increased sensitivity of elderly patients to a single dose of triazolam and other sedative-hypnotic drugs is
   (A) Changes in brain function that accompany the aging process
   (B) Decreased renal function
   (C) Increased cerebral blood flow

    (D) Decreased hepatic metabolism of lipid-soluble drugs
    (E) Changes in plasma protein binding

10. A 28-year-old woman has sporadic attacks of intense anxiety with marked physical symptoms including hyperventilation, tachycardia, and sweating. If she is diagnosed as suffering from a panic disorder, the most appropriate drug to use is
    (A) Chloral hydrate
    (B) Clonazepam
    (C) Flurazepam
    (D) Meprobamate
    (E) Propranolol

DIRECTIONS (Items 11–15): Each set of matching questions in this section consists of a list of three to twenty-six lettered options (some of which may be figures) followed by several numbered items. For each numbered item, select the ONE lettered option that is MOST closely associated with it. Each lettered option may be selected once, more than once, or not at all.

    (A) Alprazolam
    (B) Buspirone
    (C) Chloral hydrate
    (D) Clonazepam
    (E) Clorazepate
    (F) Diazepam
    (G) Flumazenil
    (H) Flurazepam
    (I) Meprobamate
    (J) Phenobarbital
    (K) Thiopental
    (L) Triazolam
    (M) Zolpidem

11. This prodrug is biotransformed to an active metabolite; it may increase anticoagulant effects by displacement of warfarin from plasma protein binding sites

12. This drug has been used in the management of alcohol withdrawal states and in maintenance treatment of patients with tonic-clonic or partial seizure states; chronic use may lead to an increase in the rates of metabolism of warfarin, phenytoin, and digitalis compounds

13. Used as a sleeping pill, this drug has caused a high incidence of unwanted daytime sedation in elderly patients; it has a long duration of action owing to the formation of several active metabolites with half-lives greater than 24 hours

14. Of the antianxiety drugs listed, this agent is least likely to alleviate withdrawal symptoms in a patient who has abruptly discontinued use of high doses of a barbiturate

15. This hypnotic drug binds to a subclass of benzodiazepine receptors; it has no anticonvulsant actions and minimal effects on sleep architecture

ANSWERS

1. In contrast to the barbiturates and carbamates, chronic therapy with benzodiazepines does not lead to increased activity of liver drug-metabolizing enzymes or of enzymes involved in porphyrin synthesis. However, the benzodiazepines are CNS depressants that exert additive effects with ethanol. With chronic use, tolerance and both psychologic and physical dependence occur. The answer is **(D)**.

2. Benzodiazepines and barbiturates are contraindicated in breathing-related sleep disorders because they will further compromise ventilation. In obstructive sleep apnea syndrome (pickwickian syndrome), obesity is a major risk factor. The best prescription you can give this patient is to lose weight. The answer is **(E)**.

3. Flumazenil is an antagonist at BZ receptors and is used in emergency and operating rooms to reverse CNS depressant effects of benzodiazepines. Flumazenil does not reverse the CNS depressant actions of alcohols, barbiturates, or carbamates. Note that, since it is a weak acid ($pK_a = 7$), phenobarbital will exist mainly in the ionized (nonprotonated) form in the urine at alkaline pH and will not be reabsorbed in the renal tubule. The answer is **(E)**.

4. None of the benzodiazepines have shown significant therapeutic benefit in the management of obsessive-compulsive disorders. Drugs effective for this condition increase the activity of serotonergic systems in the brain. The answer is (**B**).

5. The symptoms described suggest that this patient is suffering from a generalized anxiety disorder. Buspirone or longer-acting benzodiazepines are considered to be the drugs of choice for the management of such disorders. Midazolam and triazolam are short-acting benzodiazepines used in anesthesia protocols and for sleep disorders, respectively. The answer is (**A**).

6. Buspirone is a selective anxiolytic with pharmacologic characteristics quite different from those of most other drugs used in anxiety states. Buspirone has minimal effects on cognition or memory; it is not additive with ethanol in terms of CNS depression; tolerance is minimal; and it has no dependence liability. However, buspirone is not effective in *acute* anxiety because it has a slow onset of therapeutic action. The answer is (**C**).

7. Benzodiazepines are thought to exert most of their CNS effects by increasing the inhibitory effects of GABA. Benzodiazepines interact with specific receptors (BZ receptors) that are components of the $GABA_A$ receptor-chloride ion channel macromolecular complex and increase the frequency of chloride ion channel opening. Benzodiazepines are not GABA receptor agonists because they do not interact directly with this component of the complex. The answer is (**D**).

8. In elderly patients taking benzodiazepines, hypotension is far more likely than elevation of blood pressure. All of the other statements are accurate. The answer is (**D**).

9. Decreased blood flow to vital organs, including the liver and kidney, occurs during the aging process. These changes may contribute to cumulative effects of sedative-hypnotic drugs. However, this does not explain the enhanced sensitivity of the elderly patient to a *single* dose of a central depressant, which appears to be due to changes in brain function that accompany aging. The answer is (**A**).

10. Alprazolam (not listed) and clonazepam are the most effective of the benzodiazepines for the treatment of panic disorders. Propranolol has sometimes been used to attenuate excessive sympathomimetic activity in persons who suffer from performance anxiety ("stage fright"). The answer is (**B**).

11. Chloral hydrate is a prodrug and is metabolized to trichloroethanol, the active moiety. It displaces certain drugs from plasma protein binding sites and may cause bleeding when administered to patients given warfarin. The chronic use of chloral hydrate has been associated with an increased incidence of neoplastic disease. Clorazepate is also a prodrug that is hydrolyzed to form nordiazepam, the active metabolite. The benzodiazepines do not displace other drugs from plasma protein binding sites. The answer is (**C**).

12. Chronic administration of phenobarbital increases the activity of hepatic drug-metabolizing enzymes, including cytochrome P450 isozymes. This often increases the rate of metabolism of drugs administered concomitantly, with decreases in the intensity and duration of their effects. The answer is (**J**).

13. The formation of long-acting metabolites can lead to cumulative CNS depressant effects when flurazepam is used daily in the treatment of sleep disorders. The incidence of unwanted sedative actions is highest in the elderly patient. For such patients, it seems preferable to use a benzodiazepine such as lorazepam that does not form active metabolites. The answer is (**H**).

14. Buspirone is a novel anxiolytic drug that appears to interact with a subclass of brain serotonin receptors. Buspirone does not exhibit cross-tolerance with conventional sedative-hypnotics and does not reduce the severity of withdrawal symptoms in patients who have become physically dependent on such drugs. The answer is (**B**).

15. Though not a benzodiazepine, zolpidem acts on BZ_1 receptors in the CNS. Its effects can be reversed by flumazenil. Used as a hypnotic, zolpidem has minor effects on sleep patterns. Its dependence liability is lower than that of the benzodiazepines. The answer is (**M**).

Alcohols

23

OBJECTIVES

You should be able to:

- Describe the pharmacodynamics and pharmacokinetics of acute ethanol ingestion.
- List the toxic effects of chronic ethanol ingestion.
- Describe the treatment of ethanol overdosage.
- Outline the pharmacotherapy of (a) the alcohol withdrawal syndrome and (b) alcoholism.
- Describe the toxicity and treatment of acute poisoning with (a) methanol and (b) ethylene glycol.

Learn the definitions that follow.

Table 23–1. Definitions.

Term	Definition
Alcoholism	Compulsive use of ethanol
Psychologic and physical dependence	States wherein deprivation of the drug results in severe anxiety (psychologic dependence) and physical symptoms (physical dependence)
Tolerance, cross-tolerance	State of adaptation to a drug that results in reduced effects at a given dosage; cross-tolerance is tolerance to a second drug which develops as a result of exposure to a first drug
Acute ethanol intoxication	The signs and symptoms of acute ingestion of a large quantity of ethanol (see text)
Alcohol withdrawal syndrome	The syndrome engendered by alcohol deprivation in an individual who has become physically dependent
Fetal alcohol syndrome	The syndrome of teratogenic effects of alcohol consumed by a pregnant woman (see text)
Wernicke-Korsakoff syndrome	Destruction of brain neurons that results from acute thiamin deficiency; most commonly occurs in alcoholics (see text)

CONCEPTS

Ethanol, a sedative-hypnotic drug, is the most important alcohol of pharmacologic interest. It has few medical applications, but its abuse as a recreational drug is responsible for major medical and socio-economic problems. Other alcohols of toxicologic importance are methanol and ethylene glycol.

ETHANOL

A. **Pharmacokinetics:** After ingestion, ethanol is rapidly and almost completely absorbed (some is metabolized in the gut); the drug is then distributed to all body tissues, and its volume of distribution is equivalent to that of total body water (0.5–0.7 L/kg). Two enzyme systems metabolize ethanol to acetaldehyde.
1. **Alcohol dehydrogenase:** This cytosolic, NAD-dependent enzyme, found mainly in the liver and gut, accounts for the metabolism of low to moderate doses of ethanol. Because of the limited supply of the coenzyme NAD, the reaction has zero-order kinetics that result in a fixed capacity for ethanol metabolism of 7–10 g/h. With chronic ethanol use, the requirement of NAD for its metabolism may lead to a deficiency of the coenzyme for its normal metabolic functions. Gastrointestinal metabolism of ethanol is lower in women than in men.
2. **Microsomal ethanol-oxidizing system (MEOS):** At blood levels below 100 mg/dL, this liver microsomal mixed-function oxidase system contributes little to ethanol metabolism.

However, the MEOS increases in activity with chronic exposure to ethanol or inducing agents such as barbiturates, and this increase may be partially responsible for the development of tolerance.

Acetaldehyde formed from the oxidation of ethanol is rapidly metabolized to acetate by aldehyde dehydrogenase, a mitochondrial enzyme found in the liver and many other tissues. Aldehyde dehydrogenase is inhibited by **disulfiram** and by other drugs, including **metronidazole, oral hypoglycemics,** and certain **cephalosporins.**

B. Acute Effects:
1. **CNS:** The major acute effects of ethanol on the CNS include sedation, loss of inhibition, impaired judgment, slurred speech, and ataxia. Impairment of driving ability is thought to occur at ethanol blood levels between 50 and 80 mg/dL. Blood levels of 120–160 mg/dL are usually associated with gross drunkenness. Levels greater than 300 mg/dL lead to loss of consciousness, anesthesia, and coma, with possibly fatal respiratory and cardiovascular depression. Levels higher than 500 mg/dL are usually lethal. Chronic alcoholics function almost normally at much higher blood levels than occasional drinkers. Additive CNS depression occurs with concomitant administration of sedative-hypnotics, phenothiazines, and tricyclic antidepressants.

    The molecular mechanisms underlying the complex CNS effects of ethanol are not fully understood. Specific receptors for ethanol have not been identified, but ethanol appears to facilitate the action of GABA at $GABA_A$ receptors and inhibits the ability of glutamate to activate NMDA (*N*-methyl-D-aspartate) receptors.
2. **Other organ systems:** Ethanol, even at relatively low blood concentrations, significantly depresses the heart. Vascular smooth muscle is relaxed, which leads to vasodilation, sometimes with marked hypothermia. Ethanol relaxes uterine smooth muscle. The drug also enhances the hypoglycemic effects of sulfonylureas and the antiplatelet actions of aspirin.

C. Chronic Effects:
1. **Tolerance and dependence:** Tolerance occurs mainly as a result of CNS adaptation but may be partly caused by an increased rate of ethanol metabolism. There is cross-tolerance to other sedative-hypnotic drugs. Both psychologic and physical dependence are marked, the latter demonstrated by an abstinence syndrome that occurs if a heavy user abruptly discontinues ethanol intake.
2. **Liver:** Gluconeogenesis is reduced and hypoglycemia and fat accumulation may occur as a result of NAD depletion; nutritional deficiencies may contribute to this process. Progressive loss of liver function occurs, with hepatitis and cirrhosis. Hepatic dysfunction is often more severe in women than in men, perhaps because higher concentrations of alcohol reach the liver in women. Ethanol may induce an increase in the activity of hepatic microsomal drug-metabolizing enzymes. One form of cytochrome P450 that is inducible by ethanol converts acetaminophen to a hepatotoxic metabolite.
3. **Gastrointestinal system:** Irritation, inflammation, bleeding, and scarring of the gut wall occur after chronic heavy use of ethanol and may cause absorption defects and exacerbate nutritional deficiencies.
4. **CNS:** Peripheral neuropathies are the most common neurologic abnormalities in chronic alcoholics. More rarely, thiamin deficiency—along with ethanol use—leads to the **Wernicke-Korsakoff** syndrome, which is characterized by ataxia, confusion, and paralysis of the extraocular muscles. Prompt treatment with parenteral thiamine is essential to prevent permanent brain damage.
5. **Endocrine system:** Gynecomastia, testicular atrophy, and salt retention occur, partly because of altered steroid metabolism in the cirrhotic liver.
6. **Cardiovascular system:** Excessive ethanol use is associated with an increased incidence of hypertension, anemia, and myocardial infarction. However, the ingestion of modest quantities of ethanol (10–15 g daily) may *protect* against coronary heart disease.
7. **Fetal alcohol syndrome:** Ethanol use in pregnancy is associated with teratogenic effects that include mental retardation, growth deficiencies, microcephaly, and a characteristic underdevelopment of the mid face region.
8. **Neoplasia:** Ethanol is not a primary carcinogen, but its chronic use is associated with an increased incidence of neoplastic diseases, including breast carcinoma.

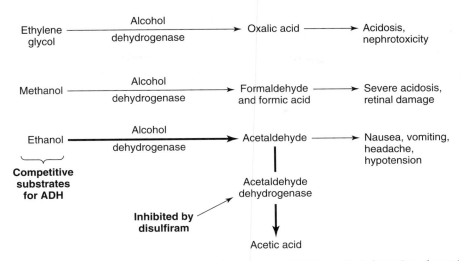

Figure 23–1. Oxidation of alcohols by alcohol dehydrogenase (ADH) results in formation of metabolites that cause serious toxicities. Ethanol, a preferred substrate for ADH, is used in methanol or ethylene glycol poisoning to slow the rate of formation of the toxic metabolites of these alcohols. Acetaldehyde formed from ethanol is oxidized rapidly by aldehyde dehydrogenase except in the presence of disulfiram.

D. Treatment of Acute and Chronic Alcoholism:

1. **Excessive CNS depression:** Intoxication due to acute ingestion of ethanol is managed by maintenance of vital signs and prevention of aspiration after vomiting. Intravenous dextrose is standard. Thiamine administration and correction of electrolyte imbalance may also be required.

2. **Alcohol withdrawal syndrome:** In the chronic user of ethanol, discontinuance can lead to a withdrawal syndrome characterized by insomnia, tremor, anxiety, and, in severe cases, delirium tremens (DTs) and life-threatening seizures. Peripheral effects include nausea, vomiting, diarrhea, and arrhythmias. The abstinence syndrome is usually managed by administration of a long-acting sedative-hypnotic (eg, chlordiazepoxide, diazepam) with gradual dose tapering. The intensity of the withdrawal syndrome may also be reduced by clonidine or propranolol.

3. **Treatment of alcoholism:** Alcoholism is a complex sociomedical problem, and the disease is characterized by a high relapse rate. The aldehyde dehydrogenase inhibitor disulfiram is used adjunctively in some treatment programs. If ethanol is consumed by a patient who has taken disulfiram, acetaldehyde accumulation leads to nausea, headache, flushing, and hypotension (Figure 23–1). Several CNS neurotransmitter systems appear to be targets for drugs that may reduce the craving for alcohol. The opioid antagonist naltrexone has proved to be useful in this context, presumably through its ability to decrease the effects of endogenous opioid peptides in the brain. The selective serotonin reuptake inhibitors (eg, fluoxetine), which can increase serotonergic activity in the CNS, may also be helpful in some patients.

OTHER ALCOHOLS

A. **Methanol:** Methanol is sometimes ingested by alcoholics when they are unable to obtain ethanol. Intoxication from methanol alone may include visual dysfunction, gastrointestinal distress, shortness of breath, loss of consciousness, and coma. Methanol is metabolized to formaldehyde, which can cause severe acidosis, retinal damage, and blindness. The formation of this toxic metabolite is retarded by prompt intravenous administration of ethanol, which acts as a preferred substrate for alcohol dehydrogenase and competitively inhibits the oxidation of methanol (Figure 23–1).

B. **Ethylene Glycol:** Industrial exposure to ethylene glycol (by inhalation or skin absorption) or self-administration (eg, by drinking antifreeze products) leads to severe acidosis and renal damage from the metabolism of ethylene glycol to oxalic acid. Prompt treatment with ethanol may slow or prevent formation of this toxic metabolite via competition for oxidation by alcohol dehydrogenase. Alcohol dehydrogenase is also inhibited by **fomepizole,** an orphan drug used as an antidote in methanol and ethylene glycol toxicity.

QUESTIONS

DIRECTIONS: Each of the numbered items or incomplete statements in this section is followed by answers or by completions of the statement. Select the ONE lettered answer or completion that is BEST in each case.

1. Which one of the following effects is LEAST likely to occur after acute ingestion of ethanol?
   (A) Additive CNS depression with over-the-counter antihistaminic drugs
   (B) Hypertension
   (C) Inhibition of liver microsomal drug-metabolizing enzymes
   (D) Myocardial depression
   (E) Relaxation of uterine smooth muscle

2. A 42-year-old man with a history of alcoholism is brought to the emergency room in a confused and delirious state. He has truncal ataxia and ophthalmoplegia. The most appropriate immediate course of action is to administer
   (A) Chlordiazepoxide
   (B) Disulfiram
   (C) Folic acid
   (D) Lorazepam
   (E) Thiamine

3. Which one of the following statements about the biodisposition of ethanol is FALSE?
   (A) Ethanol is absorbed at all levels of the gastrointestinal tract
   (B) Acetaldehyde is the initial product of ethanol metabolism
   (C) After an intravenous dose, plasma levels of ethanol are higher in women than in men
   (D) The elimination of ethanol follows zero-order kinetics
   (E) Aldehyde dehydrogenase exhibits genetic variability

4. A freshman student (weight 70 kg) attends a college party where he rapidly consumes a quantity of an alcoholic beverage that results in a blood level of 5 mg/mL. Assuming that this young man has not had an opportunity to develop tolerance to ethanol, his present condition is best characterized as
   (A) Alert and competent to drive a car
   (B) Slightly inebriated
   (C) Sedated with increased reaction times
   (D) Able to walk, but not in a straight line
   (E) Comatose and near death

5. The regular consumption of a glass or two of wine each day with meals may decrease the risk of
   (A) Cancer
   (B) Coronary heart disease
   (C) Gastritis
   (D) Psychologic dependence
   (E) Viral hepatitis

Items 6–7: A homeless middle-aged male patient presents in the emergency room in a state of intoxication. You note that he is behaviorally disinhibited and rowdy. He tells you that he has recently consumed about a pint of a red-colored liquid that his friends were using to "get high." He complains that his vision is blurred and that it is "like being in a snowstorm." His breath smells a bit like formaldehyde.

6. The most likely cause of this patient's intoxicated state is the ingestion of
   (A) Ethanol
   (B) Ethylene glycol

(C) Isopropanol
(D) Hexane
(E) Methanol

7. Your management of this patient is LEAST likely to include
   (A) Airway and respiratory support if needed
   (B) Administration of activated charcoal
   (C) Administration of bicarbonate to counteract metabolic acidosis
   (D) Administration of ethanol before laboratory diagnosis is confirmed
   (E) Initiation of dialysis procedures

DIRECTIONS (Items 8–12): Each set of matching questions in this section consists of a list of three to twenty-six lettered options (some of which may be figures) followed by several numbered items. For each numbered item, select the ONE lettered option that is MOST closely associated with it. Each lettered option may be selected once, more than once, or not at all.

   (A) Adenylyl cyclase
   (B) Alcohol dehydrogenase
   (C) Aldehyde dehydrogenase
   (D) Cytochrome P450
   (E) GABA transaminase
   (F) Microsomal ethanol-oxidizing system (MEOS)
   (G) Monoamine oxidase
   (H) NADH dehydrogenase
   (I) Pyruvate dehydrogenase

8. A cytosolic zinc-containing enzyme that is primarily responsible for the oxidation of low to moderate doses of ethanol

9. The clinical use of disulfiram depends on its ability to inhibit this enzyme

10. This enzyme utilizes NADPH as a coenzyme; its activity may be increased with chronic ingestion of ethanol

11. Heavy use of ethanol increases the activity of this enzyme, resulting in the formation of a toxic metabolite of acetaminophen

12. The activity of this enzyme is specifically decreased in the Wernicke-Korsakoff syndrome

ANSWERS

1. The emphasis in this question is on the word *acute*. An acute dose of ethanol relaxes both vascular and uterine smooth muscle. Vasodilation occurs and at high doses may lead to hypothermia. Blood pressure is not raised acutely, though chronic use of alcohol is a risk factor for hypertension. The effect of ethanol on the uterus is to prolong labor. Note that most nonprescription antihistaminic drugs act as sedatives and will cause additive CNS depression if ethanol is consumed. The answer is **(B)**.

2. This patient has the symptoms of Wernicke's encephalopathy, including delirium, gait disturbances, and paralysis of the external eye muscles. The condition results from thiamin deficiency but is rarely seen in the absence of alcoholism. The answer is **(E)**.

3. There are no differences between men and women in plasma levels of ethanol following its intravenous administration. The higher plasma levels of ethanol in women after its *oral* ingestion may be due to the fact that they have lower activity of gastric alcohol dehydrogenase than men. A characteristic feature of ethanol biodisposition is that its elimination via metabolism follows zero-order kinetics. Certain persons of Asian descent are deficient in aldehyde dehydrogenase and may experience a disulfiram-like reaction at low doses of ethanol. The answer is **(C)**.

4. The blood level of ethanol achieved in this person is equivalent to 500 mg/dL and almost certainly was estimated postmortem. The quantity of ethanol ingested can be calculated from the product of plasma level and volume of distribution (0.5–0.7 L/kg). In this case, the young man ingested 200 g of ethanol, the equivalent of over 20 fluid ounces of distilled 80 proof spirits. The answer is **(E)**.

5. Compared with those who abstain, individuals who regularly ingest modest quantities of ethanol (1–2 drinks daily) are reported to have a **decreased** risk of coronary heart disease. The chronic use of alcohol is a risk factor for the other items listed. The answer is **(B)**.

6. Behavioral disinhibition is a feature of early intoxication due to ethanol and most other alcohols but not of ingestion of the solvent hexane. Ocular dysfunction, including horizontal nystagmus and diplopia, is also a common finding in poisoning with alcohols, but the complaint of "flickering white spots before the eyes" or "being in a snowstorm" is highly suggestive of methanol intoxication. In some cases, the odor of formaldehyde may be present on the breath. In this patient, blood methanol levels should be determined as soon as possible. The answer is **(E)**.

7. In all poisoning situations, it is important to establish adequate respiration. Bicarbonate may be needed to counteract metabolic acidosis. In patients with suspected methanol intoxication, ethanol (10% solution) is often given intravenously before laboratory diagnosis is confirmed to block the formation of toxic products of ADH-catalyzed metabolism of methanol. Blood levels of methanol in excess of 50 mg/dL are an absolute indication for hemodialysis. Activated charcoal does not bind alcohols. The answer is **(B)**.

8. Alcohol dehydrogenase, a cytosolic enzyme that contains zinc, is the main enzyme involved in the oxidation of low to moderate doses of ethanol. NAD is required as a cofactor, and its concentration is rate-limiting. The enzyme also oxidizes methanol to formaldehyde and ethylene glycol to oxalic acid (Figure 23–1). Ethanol—as a preferred substrate for ADH—competitively decreases the metabolism of the other alcohols and is used clinically in the management of methanol and ethylene glycol toxicity. The answer is **(B)**.

9. Disulfiram is an inhibitor of aldehyde dehydrogenase, the enzyme that converts acetaldehyde (formed from ethanol) to acetate. Disulfiram is sometimes used adjunctively in alcoholic rehabilitation programs, since ethanol ingestion leads to toxic accumulation of acetaldehyde in the presence of the drug. Disulfiram does not inhibit alcohol dehydrogenase (ADH) and thus does not block the metabolism of methanol or ethylene glycol to their aldehydes. The answer is **(C)**.

10. MEOS is a mixed function oxidase enzyme that requires NADPH as a cofactor. It plays a significant role in ethanol oxidation to acetaldehyde only when blood alcohol levels are high. With chronic exposure to ethanol, the activity of MEOS may increase via enzyme induction, and this may play a role in metabolic tolerance. The answer is **(F)**.

11. Chronic use of ethanol causes induction of a cytochrome P450 isozyme that converts acetaminophen to a cytotoxic metabolite. This may explain the increased susceptibility of alcoholics to hepatotoxicity with overdoses of acetaminophen. The answer is **(D)**.

12. Pyruvate dehydrogenase plays an important role in energy metabolism to provide ATP, utilizing thiamine pyrophosphate as a cofactor in the reaction. In thiamin deficiency, the activity of pyruvate dehydrogenase is decreased, impairing the formation of ATP. The answer is **(I)**.

24

Antiepileptic Drugs

OBJECTIVES

You should be able to:

- List the major drugs used for partial seizures, generalized tonic-clonic seizures, absence and myoclonic seizures, and status epilepticus.
- Identify the mechanisms of anticonvulsant action.
- Describe the main pharmacokinetic features and the major adverse effects of each drug.
- Describe the factors that must be considered in designing a dosage regimen for an antiepileptic drug.

Learn the definitions that follow.

Table 24–1. Definitions.

Term	Definition
Seizure	Finite episodes of brain dysfunction resulting from abnormal discharge of cerebral neurons
Partial seizures, simple	Consciousness preserved; manifested variously as convulsive jerking, paresthesias, psychic symptoms (altered sensory perception, illusions, hallucinations, affect changes), and autonomic dysfunction
Partial seizures, complex	Impaired consciousness that is preceded, accompanied, or followed by psychic symptoms
Tonic-clonic seizures, generalized	Tonic phase (< 1 minute) involves abrupt loss of consciousness, muscle rigidity and respiratory arrest; clonic phase (2–3 minutes) involves jerking of body muscles, with lip or tongue biting, and fecal and urinary incontinence; formerly called grand mal
Absence seizures, generalized	Impaired consciousness (often abrupt onset and brief), sometimes with automatisms, loss of postural tone, or enuresis; begin in childhood (formerly called petit mal) and usually cease by age 20 years
Myoclonic seizures	Simple or multiple myoclonic muscle jerks
Status epilepticus	A series of seizures (usually tonic-clonic) without recovery of consciousness between attacks; it is a life-threatening emergency

CONCEPTS

A. Classification: Epilepsy comprises a group of chronic syndromes that involve the recurrence of seizures, ie, limited periods of abnormal discharge of cerebral neurons (see Table 24–1). Several chemical subgroups of antiepileptic drugs are structurally related; these include **hydantoins** (eg, phenytoin), **barbiturates** (eg, phenobarbital), and **succinimides** (eg, ethosuximide). There are several unrelated subgroups, including two tricyclic compounds, **carbamazepine** and **oxcarbazepine; valproic acid,** a carboxylic acid; **benzodiazepines** (eg, diazepam, clonazepam); **felbamate,** a carbamate; **GABA derivatives** (eg, gabapentin, vigabatrin); **lamotrigine,** a phenyltriazine; and **topiramate,** a substituted monosaccharide. Subgroups of antiepileptic drugs are selective in their therapeutic effects for specific types of seizures (see Figure 24–1).

B. Pharmacokinetics: Antiepileptic drugs are commonly used for long periods of time, and consideration of their pharmacokinetic properties is important for avoiding toxicity and drug interactions. For some of these drugs (eg, phenytoin), determination of plasma levels and clearance rates in individual patients may be necessary for optimal therapy. In general, antiepileptic drugs are well absorbed orally and have good bioavailability. Most are metabolized by hepatic enzymes, and in some cases (eg, primidone, trimethadione) active metabolites are formed.

Pharmacokinetic drug interactions are common in this drug group. In the presence of drugs that inhibit antiepileptic drug metabolism or displace anticonvulsants from plasma protein binding sites, plasma concentrations of the antiepileptic agents may reach toxic levels. On the other

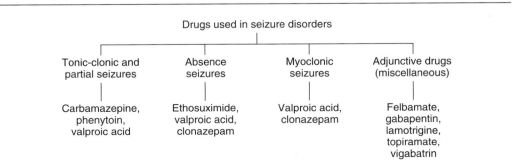

Figure 24–1. Subgroups of antiepileptic drugs.

hand, drugs that induce hepatic drug-metabolizing enzymes (eg, rifampin) may result in lowered plasma levels of the antiepileptic agents that are inadequate for seizure control.

1. **Phenytoin:** The oral bioavailability of phenytoin is variable because of differences in first-pass metabolism. Phenytoin metabolism is nonlinear; elimination kinetics shift from first-order to zero-order at moderate to high dosage levels. The drug binds extensively to plasma proteins (97–98%), and free (unbound) phenytoin levels in plasma are increased by drugs that compete for binding (eg, sulfonamides, valproic acid). The metabolism of phenytoin is enhanced in the presence of inducers of liver metabolism (eg, phenobarbital, rifampin) and inhibited by other drugs (eg, cimetidine, isoniazid). **Fosphenytoin** is a water-soluble prodrug form of phenytoin that is used parenterally.

2. **Carbamazepine:** Carbamazepine induces formation of liver drug-metabolizing enzymes that increase metabolism of the drug itself and may increase the clearance of many other anticonvulsant drugs. Carbamazepine metabolism can be inhibited by other drugs (eg, propoxyphene, valproic acid).

3. **Valproic acid:** In addition to competing for phenytoin plasma protein-binding sites, valproic acid inhibits the metabolism of phenytoin, phenobarbital, and lamotrigine. Hepatic biotransformation of valproic acid leads to formation of a toxic metabolite that has been implicated in the hepatotoxicity of the drug.

4. **Newer drugs:** Gabapentin and vigabatrin are unusual in that they are eliminated by the kidney, largely in unchanged form. Lamotrigine is eliminated via hepatic glucuronidation. Topiramate undergoes both hepatic metabolism and renal elimination of intact drug.

C. **Mechanisms of Action:** The general effect of antiepileptic drugs is to suppress repetitive action potentials in epileptic foci in the brain. Different mechanisms are involved in achieving this effect. In the case of some drugs, multiple mechanisms may contribute to their antiseizure activities. Some of the recognized mechanisms are listed below.

1. **Sodium channel blockade:** At therapeutic concentrations, phenytoin, carbamazepine, and lamotrigine block voltage-gated sodium channels in neuronal membranes. This action is rate-dependent (ie, dependent on the frequency of neuronal discharge) and results in prolongation of the inactivated state of the Na^+ channel and the refractory period of the neuron. Phenobarbital and valproic acid may exert similar effects at high doses.

2. **GABA-related targets:** As described in Chapter 22, benzodiazepines interact with specific receptors on the $GABA_A$ receptor-chloride ion channel macromolecular complex. In the presence of benzodiazepines, the *frequency* of chloride ion channel opening is increased; these drugs facilitate the inhibitory effects of GABA. Phenobarbital and other barbiturates also enhance the inhibitory actions of GABA but interact with a different receptor site on chloride ion channels that results in an increased *duration* of chloride ion channel opening.

   GABA transaminase is an important enzyme in the termination of action of GABA. The enzyme is irreversibly inactivated by vigabatrin at therapeutic plasma levels and can also be inhibited by valproic acid at very high concentrations. Inhibition of GABA transaminase is presumed to enhance the effects of GABA at synaptic sites. Gabapentin is a structural analog of GABA but it does not activate GABA receptors, and its mechanism of anticonvulsant action is unclear.

3. **Calcium channel blockade:** Ethosuximide inhibits low-threshold (T-type) Ca^{2+} currents, especially in thalamic neurons that act as pacemakers to generate rhythmic cortical discharge.

4. **Other mechanisms:** Valproic acid causes neuronal membrane hyperpolarization, possibly by enhancing K^+ channel permeability. In addition to its actions on sodium channels and GABA-chloride channels, phenobarbital also acts as an antagonist at some glutamate receptors. Topiramate appears to block sodium channels and potentiate the actions of GABA.

D. **Clinical Use:** Diagnosis of a specific seizure type is important for prescribing the most appropriate antiseizure drug (or combination of drugs). Drug choice is usually made on the basis of established efficacy in the specific seizure state that has been diagnosed, the prior responsiveness of the patient, and the anticipated toxicity of the drug. Treatment may involve combinations of drugs following the principle of adding known effective agents if the preceding drugs are not sufficient.

1. **Generalized tonic-clonic and partial seizures:** Valproic acid, carbamazepine, and phenytoin are the drugs of choice for generalized tonic-clonic (grand mal) seizures and for most cases of simple and complex partial seizures. Phenobarbital (or primidone) is now considered to be an alternative agent in adults but continues to be a primary drug in infants. Lamotrigine is also an alternative agent, but its usefulness is limited by its toxic potential (see below). Gabapentin may be used adjunctively in refractory cases. The new drug topiramate is approved for adjunctive use with other agents in partial seizures, and vigabatrin may also be useful as a backup drug.

2. **Absence seizures:** Ethosuximide and valproic acid are the preferred drugs for absence seizures since they cause minimal sedation. Ethosuximide is usually selected in uncomplicated absence seizures. Valproic acid is particularly useful in patients who have concomitant generalized tonic-clonic or myoclonic seizures. Clonazepam is effective as an alternative drug but has the disadvantages of causing sedation and tolerance. Though not currently approved for absence seizures, lamotrigine may also be useful.

3. **Myoclonic syndromes:** Myoclonic seizure syndromes are usually treated with valproic acid. Clonazepam can be effective, but the high doses required cause drowsiness. Lamotrigine is also reported to be effective in myoclonic syndromes in children. Felbamate has been used adjunctively with the primary drugs but has hematotoxic potential.

4. **Status epilepticus:** Intravenous diazepam, or lorazepam, is usually effective in terminating attacks and provides short-term control. For prolonged therapy, intravenous phenytoin is usually employed since it is highly effective and less sedating than benzodiazepines or barbiturates. However, phenytoin may cause cardiotoxicity (perhaps owing to its solvent, propylene glycol), and fosphenytoin (water soluble) may prove to be safer. Phenobarbital has also been used in status epilepticus, especially in children. In very severe status epilepticus that does not respond to these measures, general anesthesia may be employed.

5. **Infantile spasms:** Corticotropin and corticosteroids are commonly used but cause characteristic cushingoid side effects. Benzodiazepines and other anticonvulsants may also be used, but their efficacy is limited.

E. **Toxicity:** Chronic therapy with antiepileptic drugs is associated with specific toxic effects, the most important of which are listed in Table 24–2.

1. **Teratogenicity:** Children born of mothers taking anticonvulsant drugs have an increased risk of congenital malformations. Neural tube defects (eg, spina bifida) are associated with the use of valproic acid, and a fetal hydantoin syndrome has been described following phenytoin use by pregnant women.

2. **Overdosage toxicity:** Most of the commonly used anticonvulsants are CNS depressants, and respiratory depression may occur with overdosage. Management is primarily supportive (airway management, mechanical ventilation), and flumazenil may be used in benzodiazepine overdose.

Table 24–2. Adverse effects and complications of the use of antiepileptic drugs.

Antiepileptic Drug	Adverse Effects
Benzodiazepines	Sedation, tolerance, dependence
Carbamazepine	Diplopia, ataxia, enzyme induction, blood dyscrasias
Ethosuximide	Gastrointestinal distress, lethargy, headache
Felbamate	Aplastic anemia, hepatotoxicity
Gabapentin	Sedation, behavioral changes in children, movement disorders
Lamotrigine	Sedation, ataxia, life-threatening rash, Stevens-Johnson syndrome
Phenobarbital	Sedation, enzyme induction, tolerance, dependence
Phenytoin	Nystagmus, diplopia, ataxia, sedation, gingival hyperplasia, hirsutism, anemias, enzyme induction
Topiramate	Sedation, mental dulling, renal stones, weight loss
Valproic acid	Gastrointestinal distress, hepatotoxicity (rare but possibly fatal), inhibition of drug metabolism
Vigabatrin	Sedation, weight gain, agitation, confusion, psychosis

3. **Life-threatening toxicity:** Fatal hepatotoxicity has occurred with valproic acid, with greatest risk to children less than 2 years of age and patients taking multiple anticonvulsant drugs. Lamotrigine has caused skin rashes and life-threatening Stevens-Johnson syndrome or toxic epidermal necrolysis. Children are at higher risk (1–2% incidence), especially if they are also taking valproic acid. Reports of aplastic anemia and acute hepatic failure have limited the use of felbamate to severe, refractory seizure states.

4. **Withdrawal:** Withdrawal from antiepileptic drugs should be accomplished gradually to avoid increased seizure frequency and severity. In general, withdrawal from anti-absence drugs is more easily achieved than withdrawal from drugs used in partial or generalized tonic-clonic seizure states.

DRUG LIST

The following drugs are important members of the group discussed in this chapter. Prototypes should be learned in detail; features of the major variants should be known well enough so that the variants can be distinguished from prototypes and from each other; the other significant agents should be recognized as belonging to a specific subclass.

Subclass	Prototype	Major Variants	Other Significant Agents
Barbiturates	Phenobarbital	Primidone	Metharbital
Benzodiazepines	Diazepam	Lorazepam, clorazepate	Clonazepam, nitrazepam
Carboxylic acids	Valproic acid	Sodium valproate	
Hydantoins	Phenytoin	Fosphenytoin	Mephenytoin
Succinimides	Ethosuximide	Phensuximide	
Tricyclics	Carbamazepine	Oxcarbazepine	
Newer agents	Felbamate, gabapentin, lamotrigine, topiramate, vigabatrin		

QUESTIONS

DIRECTIONS: Each of the numbered items or incomplete statements in this section is followed by answers or by completions of the statement. Select the ONE lettered answer or completion that is BEST in each case.

1. A 26-year-old woman develops a seizure disorder characterized by recurrent contractions of the muscle in the right hand that then spread to the right arm and to the right side of the face ("jacksonian march"). Consciousness is not impaired, and the attacks usually last for only a minute or two. Which one of the following drugs is LEAST likely to be useful in the treatment of this patient?
   (A) Carbamazepine
   (B) Ethosuximide
   (C) Lamotrigine
   (D) Phenytoin
   (E) Primidone

2. A 9-year-old child is having learning difficulties at school. He has brief lapses of awareness, with eyelid fluttering, that occur every 5–10 minutes. EEG studies reveal brief 3-Hz spike-and-wave discharges appearing synchronously in all leads. Which one of the following drugs would be effective in this child but has the disadvantage of causing sedation and tolerance?
   (A) Clonazepam
   (B) Diazepam

   (C) Ethosuximide
   (D) Phenobarbital
   (E) Valproic acid

3. Which one of the following statements concerning proposed mechanisms of action of anticonvulsant drugs is FALSE?
   (A) Diazepam facilitates GABA-mediated inhibitory actions
   (B) Ethosuximide selectively blocks K^+ ion channels in thalamic neurons
   (C) Phenobarbital has multiple actions, including enhancement of the effects of GABA, antagonism of glutamate receptors, and blockade of Na^+ ion channels
   (D) Phenytoin prolongs the inactivated state of the Na^+ ion channel
   (E) Vigabatrin elevates brain GABA levels

4. Which of the following antiseizure drugs is most likely to elevate the plasma concentration of other drugs administered concomitantly?
   (A) Carbamazepine
   (B) Diazepam
   (C) Phenobarbital
   (D) Phenytoin
   (E) Valproic acid

Items 5–6: A young woman employed as a computer programmer suffers from myoclonic jerking with no overt signs of neurologic deficit. There is no history of generalized tonic-clonic seizures. You are considering drug therapy for this patient.

5. If the seizures are to be effectively controlled without excessive sedation, the most appropriate drug is
   (A) Acetazolamide
   (B) Carbamazepine
   (C) Clonazepam
   (D) Valproic acid
   (E) Vigabatrin

6. In the drug treatment of this woman, all of the following are important considerations EXCEPT
   (A) Liver enzymes should be monitored
   (B) The patient should be examined periodically for deep tendon reflex activity
   (C) Abdominal pain and heartburn are likely side effects
   (D) The patient should avoid barbiturates
   (E) She should contact her physician immediately if she becomes pregnant

7. Which one of the following statements concerning the pharmacokinetics of antiseizure drugs is FALSE?
   (A) At high doses, phenytoin elimination follows zero-order kinetics
   (B) Phenobarbital may increase the activity of hepatic ALA synthase and the synthesis of porphyrins
   (C) The administration of phenytoin to patients in methadone maintenance programs has led to symptoms of opioid overdose, including respiratory depression
   (D) Although ethosuximide has a half-life of approximately 40 hours, the drug is usually taken twice a day
   (E) Treatment with carbamazepine may reduce the effectiveness of oral contraceptives

DIRECTIONS (Items 8–12): Each set of matching questions in this section consists of a list of three to twenty-six lettered options (some of which may be figures) followed by several numbered items. For each numbered item, select the ONE lettered option that is MOST closely associated with it. Each lettered option may be selected once, more than once, or not at all.
   (A) Carbamazepine
   (B) Clonazepam
   (C) Ethosuximide
   (D) Fosphenytoin
   (E) Gabapentin
   (F) Lamotrigine
   (G) Lorazepam

      (H) Phenobarbital
      (I) Phenytoin
      (J) Primidone
      (K) Topiramate
      (L) Valproic acid
      (M) Vigabatrin

8. This drug is used for both partial and generalized tonic-clonic seizures. It should be used cautiously in pregnancy because of possible teratogenicity. Hirsutism and gingival hyperplasia are relatively common side effects

9. In addition to its uses in seizure states, this drug can be used in bipolar affective disorders in patients intolerant to lithium; chronic use increases hepatic cytochrome P450 isozymes

10. The risk of hepatotoxicity due to this drug is greatest in children under 2 years of age; most fatalities have occurred within 4 months after initiation of therapy

11. This drug is an inhibitor of GABA metabolism; its duration of action is much longer than its half-life in the plasma; the drug has caused psychiatric symptoms in some patients

12. In about 5% of adults this drug causes a rash, and a few patients develop the Stevens-Johnson syndrome

ANSWERS

1. Simple partial seizures can have the characteristics described in this patient. The jacksonian march is due to the progression of epileptiform discharges in the contralateral motor cortex. Phenytoin, carbamazepine, primidone, and lamotrigine are effective in partial seizures. The succinimides (ethosuximide, phensuximide) are not effective in partial seizures or in generalized tonic-clonic seizure states. The answer is **(B)**.

2. Three of the drugs listed are effective in absence seizures. Ethosuximide and valproic acid are not sedating, and tolerance does not develop to their antiseizure activity. Clonazepam is effective but exerts troublesome CNS depressant effects, and tolerance develops with chronic use. At high doses, the drug has a dependence liability like most benzodiazepines. The answer is **(A)**.

3. Though not completely understood, the mechanism of action of ethosuximide is thought to involve blockade of T-type Ca^{2+} ion channels in thalamic neurons. The drug does not block K^+ ion channels, which in any case would be likely to increase (rather than decrease) neuronal excitability. The answer is **(B)**.

4. With chronic use, the anticonvulsant barbiturates, carbamazepine, and phenytoin all induce the formation of hepatic drug-metabolizing enzymes. This action may lead to a *decrease* in the plasma concentration of other drugs used concomitantly. Valproic acid, an inhibitor of drug metabolism, can increase the plasma levels of many drugs, including carbamazepine, lamotrigine, phenobarbital, and phenytoin. Benzodiazepines have no major effects on the metabolism of other drugs. The answer is **(E)**.

5. Valproic acid is highly effective in specific myoclonic syndromes and is usually considered to be the drug of choice since it is nonsedating. Clonazepam is a backup drug since the high doses required cause excessive drowsiness. None of the other drugs listed are effective. Acetazolamide is rarely used in seizure states because tolerance develops rapidly; however, the drug may be useful in women who experience seizures at the time of menses. The answer is **(D)**.

6. Valproic acid often causes gastrointestinal distress and is potentially hepatotoxic. Use of this drug in pregnancy has been associated with teratogenicity (neural tube defects). Valproic acid inhibits the metabolism of barbiturates; marked CNS depression may result if such drugs are given concomitantly. Peripheral neuropathy—in the form of diminished deep tendon reflexes in the lower extremities—is associated with chronic use of phenytoin. The answer is **(B)**.

7. Monitoring of plasma concentration of phenytoin may be critical in establishing an effective dosage since the drug exhibits nonlinear elimination kinetics. Owing to possible induction of liver enzymes responsible for porphyrin synthesis—such as aminolevulinic acid synthase—barbiturates are contraindicated in patients with porphyrias; similarly, carbamazepine may enhance estrogen metabolism. The enzyme-inducing activity of phenytoin has led to symptoms of opioid *withdrawal,* presumably due to an increase in the rate of metabolism of methadone. Twice-daily dosage of ethosuximide is common because it reduces the severity of adverse gastrointestinal effects. The answer is **(C)**.

8. The use of antiseizure drugs in pregnancy is associated with an increased incidence of congenital abnormalities. Of the drugs listed, carbamazepine, phenytoin, and valproic acid are the most frequently implicated teratogens. The most frequent adverse effects of phenytoin are nystagmus, diplopia, and ataxia; gingival hyperplasia and hirsutism also occur to some degree in most patients. The answer is (I).

9. Carbamazepine, clonazepam, and valproic acid are alternative agents to lithium in bipolar affective disorders. Clonazepam and valproic acid do not increase the activity of liver drug-metabolizing enzymes. The answer is (A).

10. The idiosyncratic hepatotoxicity of valproic acid may be related to the formation of a reactive metabolite by a minor pathway of hepatic biotransformation of the drug. Careful monitoring of liver function is recommended; hepatotoxicity may be reversible if the drug is withdrawn immediately. The answer is (L).

11. Vigabatrin is an *irreversible* inhibitor of GABA transaminase. Its action in the CNS continues to increase GABA levels for several days, though the elimination half-life of the drug is 4–8 hours. The usefulness of vigabatrin in partial seizures may be limited by psychiatric symptoms, including major depression and psychosis. The answer is (M).

12. Lamotrigine is approved for use as an add-on drug in partial seizures, but it also effective as monotherapy. With the appearance of a rash, the drug should be discontinued since this may become life-threatening with toxic epidermal necrolysis. The answer is (F).

General Anesthetics

25

OBJECTIVES

You should be able to:

- Identify the main inhalation anesthetic agents and describe their pharmacodynamic properties.
- Describe the relationship of the blood:gas partition coefficient of an inhalation anesthetic to its speed of onset of anesthesia and its recovery time.
- List the factors that influence inhalation anesthetic biodisposition.
- Describe the main pharmacokinetic and pharmacodynamic characteristics of the intravenous anesthetics.

Learn the definitions that follow.

Table 25–1. Definitions.

Term	Definition
Balanced anesthesia	Anesthesia produced by a mixture of drugs, often including both inhaled and intravenous agents
Inhalation anesthesia	Anesthesia produced by inhalation of a drug
Minimum alveolar anesthetic concentration (MAC)	The alveolar concentration of an anesthetic that is required to prevent a response to a standardized painful stimulus in 50% of patients
Analgesia	A state of decreased awareness of pain, sometimes with amnesia
General anesthesia	A state of unconsciousness, analgesia, and amnesia, with skeletal muscle relaxation and loss of reflexes

CONCEPTS

A. General Anesthesia: General anesthesia is a state characterized by unconsciousness, analgesia, amnesia, skeletal muscle relaxation, and loss of reflexes. General anesthetics are CNS depressants with actions that can be induced and terminated more rapidly than those of sedative-hypnotics. Modern anesthetics act very rapidly and achieve deep anesthesia quickly. With older and more slowly acting anesthetics, the progressively greater depth of central depression associated with increasing dose or time of exposure is traditionally described as **four stages of anesthesia:**

1. **Analgesia:**   In stage 1, the patient has decreased awareness of pain, sometimes with amnesia. Consciousness may be impaired but is not lost.
2. **Disinhibition:**   In stage 2, the patient appears to be delirious and excited. Amnesia occurs, reflexes are enhanced, and respiration is typically irregular; retching and incontinence may occur.
3. **Surgical anesthesia:**   In stage 3, the patient is unconscious and has no pain reflexes; respiration is very regular and blood pressure is maintained.
4. **Medullary depression:**   In stage 4, the patient experiences severe respiratory and cardiovascular depression that requires mechanical and pharmacologic support.

B. Anesthesia Protocols: For minor procedures, **conscious sedation** techniques are often used that combine intravenous agents with local anesthetics. For more extensive procedures, **balanced anesthesia** regimens are used that employ short-acting intravenous agents with opioids and nitrous oxide. For major surgery, anesthesia protocols commonly include the use of intravenous drugs to induce the anesthetic state, inhaled anesthetics to maintain anesthesia, and neuromuscular blocking agents to effect muscle relaxation.

C. Mechanisms of Action: The mechanisms of action of general anesthetics are unclear, but these drugs usually increase the threshold for firing of CNS neurons. The potency of most inhaled anesthetics is proportionate to their lipid solubility. Possible mechanisms of action include effects on ion channels by interactions with membrane lipids or proteins and effects on central neurotransmitter mechanisms. CNS neurons in different regions of the brain have different sensitivities to general anesthetics; inhibition of neurons involved in pain pathways occurs before inhibition of neurons in the midbrain reticular formation.

INHALED ANESTHETICS

A. Classification and Pharmacokinetics: The agents currently used in inhalation anesthesia are nitrous oxide (a gas) and several easily vaporized liquid halogenated hydrocarbons, including halothane, desflurane, enflurane, isoflurane, sevoflurane, and methoxyflurane. They are administered as gases; their partial pressure, or "tension," in the inhaled air—or in blood or tissue—is a measure of their concentration. Since the standard pressure of the total inhaled mixture is atmospheric pressure (760 mm Hg at sea level), the partial pressure may also be expressed as a

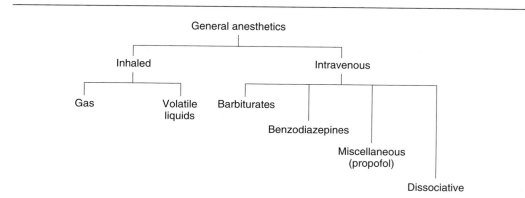

Figure 25–1. Subgroups of drugs discussed in this chapter.

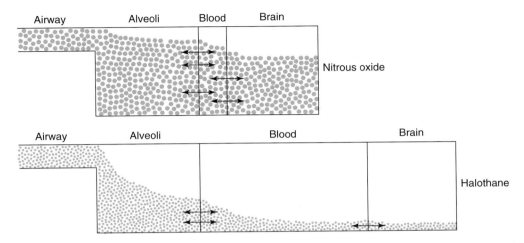

Figure 25–2. Why induction of anesthesia is slower with more soluble anesthetic gases and faster with less soluble ones. In this schematic diagram, solubility is represented by the size of the blood compartment (the more soluble, the larger the compartment). For a given concentration or partial pressure of the two anesthetic gases in the inspired air, it will take much longer with halothane than with nitrous oxide for the blood partial pressure to rise to the same partial pressure as in the alveoli. Since the concentration in the brain can rise no faster than the concentration in the blood, the onset of anesthesia will be much slower with halothane than with nitrous oxide. (Reproduced, with permission, from Katzung BG [editor]: *Basic & Clinical Pharmacology,* 7th ed. Appleton & Lange, 1998.)

percentage. Thus, 50% nitrous oxide in the inhaled air would have a partial pressure of 380 mm Hg. The speed of induction of anesthetic effects depends on several factors.

1. **Solubility:** The more rapidly a drug equilibrates with the blood, the more quickly the drug passes into the brain to produce anesthetic effects. Drugs with a low blood:gas partition coefficient (eg, nitrous oxide) equilibrate more rapidly than do drugs with a higher blood solubility (eg, halothane), as illustrated in Figure 25–2. Partition coefficients for inhalation anesthetics are shown in Table 25–2.

2. **Inspired gas partial pressure:** A high partial pressure of the gas in the lungs results in more rapid achievement of anesthetic levels in the blood. Advantage is taken of this effect by the initial administration of gas concentrations higher than those required for maintenance of anesthesia.

3. **Ventilation rate:** The greater the ventilation, the more rapid the rise in alveolar and blood partial pressure of the agent and the more rapid the onset of anesthesia (Figure 25–3). Advantage is taken of this effect in induction of the anesthetic state.

Table 25–2. Properties of inhalation anesthetics.*

Anesthetic	Blood:Gas Partition Coefficient	Minimum Alveolar Concentration (%)[1]	Metabolism
Nitrous oxide	0.47	> 100	None
Desflurane	0.42	6.5	< 0.1%
Sevoflurane	0.67	2.0	2–5% (fluoride released)
Isoflurane	1.40	1.4	< 2%
Enflurane	1.80	1.7	8%
Halothane	2.30	0.75	> 40%
Methoxyflurane	12	0.16	> 70% (fluoride released)

*Modified and reproduced, with permission, from Katzung BG (editor): *Basic & Clinical Pharmacology,* 7th ed. Appleton & Lange, 1998.
[1]Minimum alveolar concentration (MAC) is the anesthetic concentration that eliminates the response in 50% of patients exposed to a standardized painful stimulus. In this table, MAC is expressed as a percentage of the inspired gas mixture.

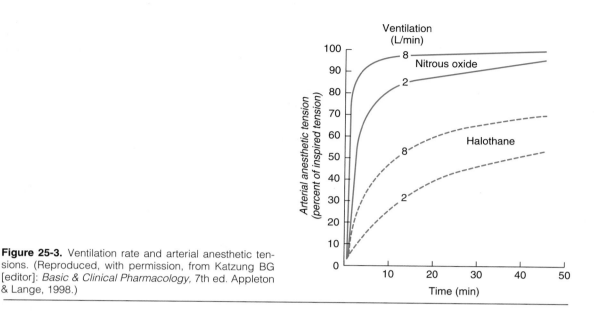

Figure 25-3. Ventilation rate and arterial anesthetic tensions. (Reproduced, with permission, from Katzung BG [editor]: *Basic & Clinical Pharmacology,* 7th ed. Appleton & Lange, 1998.)

    4. Pulmonary blood flow: At high pulmonary blood flows, the gas partial pressure rises at a slower rate; thus, the speed of onset of anesthesia is reduced. At low flow rates, onset is faster. In circulatory shock, this effect may accelerate the rate of onset of anesthesia with agents of high blood solubility.

    5. Arteriovenous concentration gradient: Uptake of soluble anesthetics into highly perfused tissues may decrease gas tension in mixed venous blood. This can influence the rate of onset of anesthesia, since achievement of equilibrium is dependent on the difference in anesthetic tension between arterial and venous blood.

B. Elimination: Anesthesia is terminated by redistribution of the drug from the brain to the blood and elimination of the drug through the lungs. The rate of recovery from anesthesia using agents with low blood:gas partition coefficients is faster than that of anesthetics with high blood solubility. Halothane and methoxyflurane are metabolized by liver enzymes to a significant extent (see Table 25–2). Metabolism of halothane and methoxyflurane has only a minor influence on the speed of recovery from their anesthetic effect but does play a role in the toxicity of these anesthetics.

C. Minimum Alveolar Anesthetic Concentration (MAC): The potency of inhaled anesthetics is best measured by the minimum alveolar anesthetic concentration, defined as the alveolar concentration required to eliminate the response to a standardized painful stimulus in 50% of patients. Each anesthetic has a defined MAC (see Table 25–2), but this value may vary among different patients depending on age, cardiovascular status, and use of adjuvant drugs. MACs for infants and elderly patients are lower than those for adolescents and young adults. When several anesthetic agents are used simultaneously, their MAC values are additive.

D. Effects of Inhaled Anesthetics:
    1. CNS effects: Inhaled anesthetics decrease brain metabolic rate. They reduce vascular resistance and thus increase cerebral blood flow. This may lead to an increase in intracranial pressure. High concentrations of enflurane may cause spike-and-wave activity and muscle twitching, but this effect is unique to this drug. Though nitrous oxide has low anesthetic potency (ie, a high MAC), it exerts marked analgesic and amnestic actions.

    2. Cardiovascular effects: Most inhaled anesthetics decrease arterial blood pressure moderately. Enflurane and halothane are myocardial depressants that decrease cardiac output, while isoflurane causes peripheral vasodilation. Nitrous oxide is less likely to lower blood pressure than are other inhaled anesthetics. Blood flow to the liver and kidney is decreased by most inhaled agents. Halothane may sensitize the myocardium to the arrhythmogenic effects of catecholamines.

3. **Respiratory effects:** Rate of respiration may be increased by inhaled anesthetics, but tidal volume and minute ventilation are decreased, leading to an increase in arterial CO_2 tension. Inhaled anesthetics decrease ventilatory response to hypoxia even at subanesthetic concentrations (eg, during recovery). Nitrous oxide has the smallest effect on respiration.

4. **Toxicity:** Postoperative hepatitis has occurred (rarely) following halothane anesthesia in patients experiencing hypovolemic shock or other severe stress. Fluoride released by metabolism of methoxyflurane (and possibly enflurane) may cause renal insufficiency after prolonged anesthesia. Prolonged exposure to nitrous oxide decreases methionine synthase activity and may lead to megaloblastic anemia. Susceptible patients may develop **malignant hyperthermia** when exposed to halogenated anesthetics. This rare condition of uncontrolled release of calcium by the sarcoplasmic reticulum of skeletal muscle leads to muscle spasm, hyperthermia, and autonomic lability. Dantrolene is indicated for the treatment of this life-threatening condition, along with management of hyperthermia and cardiovascular instability.

INTRAVENOUS ANESTHETICS

A. **Classification, Pharmacokinetics, and Pharmacodynamics:** Several chemical classes of drugs are used as intravenous agents in anesthesia.

1. **Barbiturates:** **Thiopental, thiamylal,** and **methohexital** have high lipid solubility, which promotes rapid entry into the brain and results in surgical anesthesia in one circulation time (less than 1 minute). These agents are used for induction of anesthesia and for short surgical procedures. Their anesthetic effects are terminated by redistribution from the brain to other tissues (Figure 25–4), but hepatic metabolism is required for their elimination from the body. They are respiratory and circulatory depressants; because they depress cerebral blood flow, they can also decrease intracranial pressure.

2. **Benzodiazepines:** **Midazolam** is used adjunctively with inhaled anesthetics and opioids. The onset of its CNS effects is slower than that of thiopental, and it has a longer duration of action. Cases of severe postoperative respiratory depression have occurred. The antagonist flumazenil accelerates recovery from midazolam and other benzodiazepines.

3. **Dissociative anesthetic:** **Ketamine** produces a state called "dissociative anesthesia" in which the patient remains conscious but has marked catatonia, analgesia, and amnesia. Ketamine is an antagonist of glutamic acid, blocking the actions of this excitatory transmitter at its NMDA receptor. The drug is a cardiovascular stimulant, and this action may lead to an increase in intracranial pressure. Disorientation and hallucinations, which commonly occur during recovery from ketamine anesthesia, can be reduced by the preoperative use of benzodiazepines.

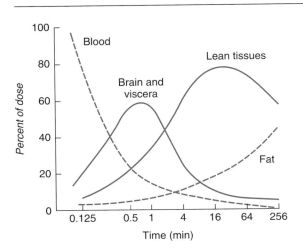

Figure 25-4. Redistribution of thiopental after an intravenous bolus administration. (Reproduced, with permission, from Katzung BG [editor]: *Basic & Clinical Pharmacology*, 7th ed. Appleton & Lange, 1998.)

4. **Opioids:** **Morphine** and **fentanyl** are used with other CNS depressants (nitrous oxide, benzodiazepines) in certain high-risk patients who might not survive a full general anesthetic. Intravenous opioids may cause chest wall rigidity that can impair ventilation. Respiratory depression with these drugs may be reversed postoperatively with naloxone. **Neuroleptanesthesia** is a state of analgesia and amnesia produced when fentanyl is used with droperidol and nitrous oxide.

5. **Propofol:** Propofol produces anesthesia at a rate similar to that achieved with the intravenous barbiturates, and recovery is more rapid. Propofol has antiemetic actions, and recovery is not delayed after prolonged infusion. The drug is commonly used as a component of balanced anesthesia and as an anesthetic in outpatient surgery. Propofol may cause marked hypotension during induction of anesthesia, primarily through decreased peripheral resistance. Total body clearance of propofol is greater than hepatic blood flow, suggesting that its elimination includes other mechanisms in addition to metabolism by liver enzymes.

DRUG LIST

The following drugs are important members of the group discussed in this chapter. Prototypes should be learned in detail; features of the major variants should be known well enough so that the variants can be distinguished from prototypes and from each other.

Subclass	Prototype	Major Variants
Inhaled anesthetics Volatile liquids	Halothane	Enflurane, desflurane, isoflurane, methoxyflurane, sevoflurane
Gas	Nitrous oxide	
Intravenous anesthetics Barbiturates	Thiopental	Thiamylal, methohexital
Opioids	Morphine	Fentanyl
Phenols	Propofol	
Benzodiazepines	Midazolam	
Dissociative agent	Ketamine	

QUESTIONS

DIRECTIONS: Each of the numbered items or incomplete statements in this section is followed by answers or by completions of the statement. Select the ONE lettered answer or completion that is BEST in each case.

1. A new halogenated gas anesthetic has a blood:gas partition coefficient of 0.5 and a MAC value of 1.0%. Which of the following predictions about this agent is MOST accurate? (Refer to Table 25–2 for comparison of agents.)
   (A) The new agent will be more potent than halothane
   (B) It will be metabolized by the liver to release fluoride ions
   (C) It will be more soluble in the blood than isoflurane
   (D) Its speed of onset of action will be similar to that of nitrous oxide
   (E) Equilibrium between arterial and venous gas tension will be achieved very slowly with this agent

2. Which of the following statements concerning the effects of anesthetic agents is LEAST accurate?
   (A) Relaxation of bronchiolar smooth muscle occurs during halothane anesthesia
   (B) Mild generalized muscle twitching occurs at high doses of enflurane
   (C) Chest muscle rigidity often follows the administration of fentanyl

    (D) Intraoperative use of midazolam with inhalation anesthetics may prolong the postanesthesia recovery period

    (E) Severe hepatitis has been reported following the use of isoflurane

3. A 23-year-old man has a pheochromocytoma, a blood pressure of 190/120 mm Hg, and a hematocrit of 50%. Pulmonary function and renal function are normal. His catecholamines are elevated, and he has a well-defined abdominal tumor on MRI. He has been scheduled for surgery. Of the agents listed below, which drug is LEAST suitable for inclusion in his anesthesia protocol?

    (A) Desflurane

    (B) Fentanyl

    (C) Halothane

    (D) Midazolam

    (E) Thiopental

4. Which one of the following statements concerning nitrous oxide is LEAST correct?

    (A) It continues to be a useful component of anesthesia protocols because of its lack of cardiovascular depression

    (B) Megaloblastic anemia is a common adverse effect in patients exposed to nitrous oxide for periods longer than 2 hours

    (C) It is the least potent of the inhaled anesthetics

    (D) There is no direct association between the use of nitrous oxide and malignant hyperthermia

    (E) More than 98% of nitrous oxide is eliminated through the lungs

5. Which one of the following statements concerning anesthetic MAC values is LEAST correct?

    (A) At a given level of anesthesia, measurement of alveolar concentrations of different anesthetics allows potency comparisons

    (B) MACs give information about the slope of the dose-response curve

    (C) Desflurane has the lowest blood:gas partition coefficient value of the currently available inhaled anesthetics

    (D) MAC values decrease in elderly patients

    (E) Simultaneous use of opioid analgesics lowers the MAC for inhaled anesthetics

6. Total intravenous anesthesia with opioids has been selected for a frail 72-year-old woman about to undergo cardiac surgery. Which one of the following statements about this anesthesia protocol is LEAST accurate?

    (A) High-dose intravenous opioids provide relatively stable hemodynamics

    (B) Opioids control the hypertensive response to surgical stimulation

    (C) Muscle rigidity may occur, especially with rapid administration of opioids

    (D) Patient awareness may occur during surgery, with recall after recovery

    (E) The patient is unlikely to experience pain during surgery

7. Which of the following inhalation anesthetics has a low blood:gas partition coefficient but is not used for induction of anesthesia because of its pungency, which causes patients to hold their breath?

    (A) Desflurane

    (B) Enflurane

    (C) Halothane

    (D) Isoflurane

    (E) Sevoflurane

8. A 22-year-old man in the operating room for hernia surgery is anesthetized with intravenous thiopental followed by halothane and nitrous oxide. Vecuronium, a peripherally acting skeletal muscle relaxant, is used adjunctively. If malignant hyperthermia occurs, he should be treated with

    (A) Baclofen

    (B) Dantrolene

    (C) Diazepam

    (D) Naloxone

    (E) Neostigmine

9. The inhalation anesthetic with the fastest onset of action is:

    (A) Enflurane

    (B) Isoflurane

    (C) Nitric oxide

    (D) Nitrogen dioxide
    (E) Nitrous oxide

DIRECTIONS (Items 10–15):   Each set of matching questions in this section consists of a list of three to twenty-six lettered options (some of which may be figures) followed by several numbered items. For each numbered item, select the ONE lettered option that is MOST closely associated with it. Each lettered option may be selected once, more than once, or not at all.

    (A) Desflurane
    (B) Fentanyl
    (C) Halothane
    (D) Isoflurane
    (E) Ketamine
    (F) Methoxyflurane
    (G) Midazolam
    (H) Morphine
    (I) Nitrous oxide
    (J) Propofol
    (K) Sevoflurane
    (L) Thiopental

10.   Vasopressin-resistant polyuric renal insufficiency has occurred after prolonged administration of this anesthetic

11.   Use of this agent is associated with a high incidence of disorientation, sensory and perceptual illusions, and vivid dreams during recovery from anesthesia

12.   Respiratory depression following use of this agent may be reversed by administration of flumazenil

13.   Postoperative vomiting is uncommon with this intravenous agent; patients are able to ambulate sooner than those who receive other anesthetics

14.   Heart rate, arterial blood pressure, and cardiac output are all increased following administration of this anesthetic agent

15.   This drug decreases cerebral blood flow; redistribution from the brain to other highly perfused tissues is responsible for termination of its anesthetic effects

ANSWERS

1.   Inhaled anesthetics with low blood:gas solubility characteristically have a fast onset of action and a short duration of recovery. The new agent described here resembles nitrous oxide but is much more potent, as indicated by its low MAC value. Not all halogenated anesthetics undergo hepatic metabolism. The answer is **(D).**

2.   Hepatitis following general anesthesia has been linked to use of *halothane,* though the incidence of severe hepatic necrosis is only about 1 out of 35,000 halothane administrations. The results of animal experiments suggest that halothane hepatotoxicity may be due to the formation of a toxic metabolite produced under anoxic conditions. Hepatotoxicity has not been reported following desflurane administration; it may be relevant that this agent is the least metabolized of the fluorinated hydrocarbons. All of the other statements are correct. The answer is **(E).**

3.   Halothane sensitizes the myocardium to catecholamines; arrhythmias may occur in patients with cardiac disease who have high circulating levels of epinephrine and norepinephrine (eg, patients with pheochromocytoma). Other modern anesthetics are considerably less arrhythmogenic. The answer is **(C).**

4.   Bone marrow depression by nitrous oxide has *not* been reported in patients exposed to nitrous oxide anesthesia for periods as long as 6 hours. However, megaloblastic anemia may be an occupational hazard for staff working in poorly ventilated dental operating rooms. AIDS patients may be more susceptible to the potential myelotoxicity of nitrous oxide. The answer is **(B).**

5.   *Tissue* dose-*tissue* response characteristics of inhaled anesthetics are difficult to estimate, since it is not possible to measure brain concentrations of such drugs at different stages of CNS depression. On the basis of *alveolar* gas concentration measurements, we can conclude that dose-

response relationships are steep. Whereas (by definition) a partial pressure of one MAC of any agent prevents movement in response to surgical stimulation in 50% of patients, individual patients may require from 0.5 to 1.5 MACs for adequate anesthesia. The MAC gives no information about the slope of the dose-response curve. The answer is **(B)**.

6. High-dose intravenous opioids (eg, fentanyl, morphine) are widely used in anesthesia for cardiac surgery because they cause less cardiac depression than inhalation anesthetic agents. One disadvantage of this technique is patient recall, though the likelihood of patient awareness can be decreased by use of a benzodiazepine. Another disadvantage is the occurrence of hypertensive responses to surgical stimulation. The addition of vasodilators (eg, nitroprusside) or a beta-blocker (eg, esmolol) may be needed to prevent intraoperative hypertension. The answer is **(B)**.

7. The pungency of desflurane leads to a high incidence of coughing and sometimes bronchospasm. Desflurane also causes a centrally mediated tachycardia and increase in blood pressure. Despite its low blood:gas partition coefficient, anesthesia with desflurane does not always lead to faster rates of recovery. The answer is **(A)**.

8. Malignant hyperthermia is a rare but life-threatening reaction that may occur during general anesthesia with halogenated anesthetics and skeletal muscle relaxants. The drug of choice is dantrolene, which blocks the release of calcium from the sarcoplasmic reticulum of skeletal muscle cells. The answer is **(B)**.

9. The purpose of this easy question is to remind the reader that there are *three* medically important oxides of nitrogen. Nitric oxide (NO) is a powerful vasodilator (see Chapter 19). Nitrogen dioxide (NO_2) is a pulmonary irritant generated in fermenting silage; it may cause lethal pulmonary damage in farm workers. Nitrous oxide (N_2O) is the inhalation anesthetic agent discussed in this chapter. The answer is **(E)**.

10. Methoxyflurane, the most potent halogenated inhalation anesthetic, undergoes extensive hepatic metabolism, releasing fluoride ions at levels that can be nephrotoxic. The answer is **(F)**.

11. The emergence phenomena described are adverse effects of ketamine. Administration of diazepam immediately prior to ketamine anesthesia reduces the incidence of these effects. The answer is **(E)**.

12. Flumazenil is a benzodiazepine receptor antagonist (see Chapter 22). It accelerates recovery from postoperative depression of the CNS caused by midazolam and other benzodiazepines used in anesthesia. The short duration of action of flumazenil may necessitate multiple doses. The sedative actions of benzodiazepines are more reliably reversed by flumazenil than is respiratory depression. Use of flumazenil does not obviate the need for adequate monitoring of respiration and provision of ventilatory support when needed. The answer is **(G)**.

13. Propofol is used extensively in balanced anesthesia protocols and is especially suitable for day surgery anesthesia. The favorable properties of the drug include an antiemetic effect and a rate of recovery that is more rapid than that following use of other intravenous drugs. Propofol does not cause cumulative effects, perhaps due to its short half-life (2–8 minutes) in the body. The drug is also used for prolonged sedation in critical care settings. The answer is **(J)**.

14. Ketamine is the only anesthetic that routinely causes cardiovascular stimulation. This results in part from central sympathetic stimulation and possibly from inhibition of norepinephrine reuptake at sympathetic nerve endings. The answer is **(E)**.

15. Drug redistribution from brain to other body tissues may play a role in termination of CNS effects of both ketamine and thiobarbiturates. In contrast to ketamine, however, thiopental decreases cerebral blood flow. This makes thiopental a more desirable drug than inhalation anesthetics in patients with cerebral swelling. The answer is **(L)**.

26

Local Anesthetics

OBJECTIVES

You should be able to:

- Describe the mechanism of blockade of the nerve impulse by local anesthetics and understand the rate dependency of their actions.
- Understand the relation between pH, pK_a, and the rate of onset of local anesthesia.
- List the factors that determine the susceptibility of nerve fibers to blockade.
- Identify the major toxic effects of the local anesthetics.

CONCEPTS

Local anesthesia is the condition that results when sensory transmission from a local area of the body to the CNS is blocked. The local anesthetics constitute a group of chemically similar agents that block the sodium channels of excitable membranes. Because these drugs can be administered locally by topical application or by injection in the target area, the anesthetic effect can be restricted to a localized area, eg, the cornea, or an arm. When given intravenously, these drugs have effects on other tissues. Many drugs classified in other groups, eg, antihistamines and beta-blockers, have significant local anesthetic effects.

A. Chemistry and Subclasses: Most local anesthetic drugs are esters or amides of simple benzene derivatives. Subgroups within the local anesthetics are based on this chemical characteristic and on duration of action (Figure 26–1). All of the commonly used local anesthetics carry at least one amine function and are therefore weak bases that become charged through the gain of a proton (H^+). As discussed in Chapter 1, the degree of ionization is a function of the pK_a of the drug and the pH of the medium. Because the pH of tissue may differ from the physiologic 7.4 (eg, it may be as low as 6.4 in infected tissue), the degree of ionization of the drug will vary. Because the pK_a of most local anesthetics is between 8.0 and 9.0 (benzocaine is an exception), variations in pH associated with infection can have significant effects on the proportion of ionized to nonionized drug.

B. Pharmacokinetics: Many shorter-acting local anesthetics are readily absorbed from the injection site after administration. The duration of local action is therefore limited unless blood flow to the area is reduced. This can be accomplished by administration of a vasoconstrictor (usually an alpha agonist sympathomimetic) with the local anesthetic agent. Cocaine is an important exception to this rule since it has intrinsic sympathomimetic action (because it inhibits norepinephrine reuptake into nerve terminals); cocaine does not require any additional vasocon-

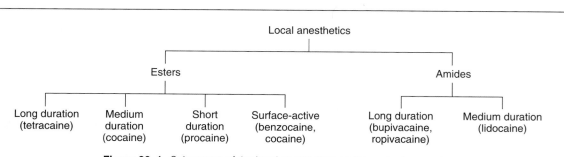

Figure 26–1. Subgroups of the local anesthetics and important examples.

strictor. The longer-acting agents (bupivacaine, ropivacaine, tetracaine) are also less dependent on the coadministration of epinephrine. Surface activity (ability to reach superficial nerves when applied to the surface of mucous membranes) is a property of only a few local anesthetics, including cocaine and benzocaine.

Metabolism of esters is by plasma and tissue cholinesterases and may be rapid. Procaine and chloroprocaine have half-lives of only 1–2 minutes. The amides are hydrolyzed in the liver by cytochrome P450 isozymes and have half-lives of 1.8–6 hours. Bupivacaine and ropivacaine are the longest-acting local anesthetics, reflecting their slower rates of hepatic metabolism. Liver dysfunction or decreases in hepatic blood flow may increase the elimination half-life of amide local anesthetics.

C. Mechanism of Action: Local anesthetics block voltage-dependent sodium channels and reduce the influx of sodium ions, thereby preventing depolarization of the membrane and blocking conduction of the action potential. Local anesthetics gain access to their receptors from the cytoplasm or the membrane (Figure 26–2). Since the drug molecule must cross the lipid membrane to reach the cytoplasm, the more lipid-soluble (nonionized, nonprotonated) form reaches effective intracellular concentrations more rapidly than the ionized form. On the other hand, once inside the axon, the ionized (protonated) form of the drug appears to be the more effective blocking entity. Thus, both the uncharged and the charged forms of the drug play important roles, the first in reaching the receptor site and the second in causing the effect. The affinity of the receptor site within the sodium channel for the local anesthetic is a function of the state of the channel—binding more readily to open or inactivated channels—and therefore follows the same rules of use-dependence and potential-dependence that were described for the sodium channel-blocking antiarrhythmic drugs (see Chapter 14).

D. Effects:
1. **Nerves:** Differential sensitivity of various types of nerve fibers to local anesthetics depends on fiber diameter, myelination, physiologic firing rate, and anatomic location (Table 26–1). In general, smaller fibers are blocked more easily than larger ones and myelinated fibers more easily than unmyelinated ones. Because activated pain fibers fire rapidly, pain sensation may be selectively blocked by these drugs. Fibers located in the periphery of a thick nerve bundle are blocked sooner than those in the core because they are exposed earlier to higher concentrations of the anesthetic. High concentrations of extracellular K^+ may enhance local anesthetic activity, while elevated extracellular Ca^{2+} may antagonize it.

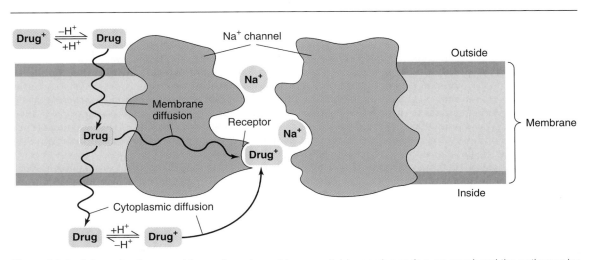

Figure 26–2. Schematic diagram of the sodium channel in an excitable membrane (eg, an axon) and the pathways by which a local anesthetic molecule *(Drug)* may reach its receptor. Sodium ions are not able to pass through the channel when the drug is bound to the receptor. The local anesthetic diffuses within the membrane in its uncharged form. In the aqueous extracellular and intracellular spaces, the charged form *(Drug⁺)* is also present.

Table 26–1. Susceptibility to block of types of nerve fibers.*

Fiber Type	Function	Diameter (μm)	Sensitivity to Block
Type A (myelinated)			
Alpha	Proprioception, motor	12–20	+
Beta	Touch, pressure	5–12	++
Gamma	Muscle spindles	3–6	++
Delta	Pain, temperature	2–5	+++
Type B (myelinated)	Preganglionic ANS	< 3	++++
Type C (unmyelinated)			
Dorsal root	Pain	0.4–1.2	++++
Sympathetic	Postganglionic	0.3–1.3	++++

*Modified and reproduced, with permission, from Katzung BG (editor): *Basic & Clinical Pharmacology,* 7th ed. Appleton & Lange, 1998.

2. **Other tissues:** The effects of these drugs on the heart are discussed in Chapter 14 (see class I antiarrhythmic agents). Most local anesthetics also have weak blocking effects on skeletal muscle neuromuscular transmission, but these actions have no clinical application. The mood elevation induced by cocaine reflects actions on dopamine- or norepinephrine-mediated synaptic transmission in the CNS.

E. **Clinical Use:** The local anesthetics are most commonly used for minor surgical procedures. They are also used in spinal anesthesia and to produce autonomic blockade in ischemic conditions. Slow epidural infusion at low concentrations has been used successfully for postoperative analgesia (in the same way as epidural opioid infusion). However, repeated epidural injection in anesthetic doses may lead to tachyphylaxis.

F. **Toxicity:**
  1. **CNS effects:** The most important toxic effects of the local anesthetics concern the CNS. All local anesthetics are capable of producing a spectrum of central effects, including light-headedness or sedation, restlessness, nystagmus, and tonic-clonic convulsions. Severe convulsions may be followed by coma with respiratory and cardiovascular depression. If large doses of a local anesthetic are needed, premedication with diazepam is prophylactic against seizures.
  2. **Cardiovascular effects:** With the exception of cocaine, all local anesthetics are vasodilators. Patients with preexisting cardiovascular disease may develop heart block and other disturbances of cardiac electrical function at high plasma concentrations of local anesthetics. Bupivacaine may produce severe cardiovascular toxicity, including arrhythmias and hypotension, if given intravenously. Ropivacaine, the other long-acting amide, is less cardiotoxic. The ability of cocaine to block norepinephrine reuptake at sympathetic neuroeffector junctions and its vasoconstricting actions contribute to cardiovascular toxicity. When used as a drug of abuse, the toxicity of cocaine includes severe hypertension with cerebral hemorrhage, cardiac arrhythmias, and myocardial infarction.
  3. **Other toxic effects:** Prilocaine is metabolized to *o*-toluidine, which is capable of causing methemoglobinemia. The ester-type local anesthetics are metabolized to products that can cause antibody formation in some patients. Allergic responses to local anesthetics are rare and can usually be avoided by using an agent from the amide subclass. In high concentrations, local anesthetics may cause a local neurotoxic action that includes histologic damage and permanent impairment of function.
  4. **Treatment of toxicity:** Severe toxicity is best treated symptomatically. Seizures are often treated with intravenous diazepam or a short-acting barbiturate such as thiopental. Hyperventilation with oxygen is helpful. Occasionally, a neuromuscular blocking drug may be used to control violent convulsive activity. The cardiovascular toxicity of bupivacaine overdose is difficult to treat and has caused fatalities in healthy young adults.

DRUG LIST

The following drugs are important members of the group discussed in this chapter. Prototypes should be learned in detail; features of the major variants should be known well enough so that the variants can be distinguished from prototypes and from each other; the other significant agents should be recognized as belonging to a specific subclass.

Subclass	Prototype	Major Variants	Other Significant Agents
Esters	Procaine	Cocaine, tetracaine	Benzocaine
Amides	Lidocaine	Bupivacaine	Etidocaine, mepivacaine, prilocaine, ropivacaine

QUESTIONS

DIRECTIONS: Each of the numbered items or incomplete statements in this section is followed by answers or by completions of the statement. Select the ONE lettered answer or completion that is BEST in each case.

1. Which one of the following statements concerning the properties of local anesthetics is FALSE?
   (A) They block voltage-dependent sodium channels
   (B) Preferential binding to resting channels is a key feature of their action
   (C) Local anesthetics slow axonal impulse conduction
   (D) Increases in membrane refractory period result from the action of local anesthetics
   (E) Most are esters or amides
2. The pK_a of lidocaine is 7.9. In infected tissue at pH 6.9, the fraction in the ionized form will be
   (A) 1%
   (B) 10%
   (C) 50%
   (D) 90%
   (E) 99%
3. Which one of the following statements about nerve blockade with local anesthetics is LEAST correct?
   (A) Speed of onset may be reduced when injected into infected tissues
   (B) Block is faster in onset with smaller-diameter fibers
   (C) Activity is use-dependent
   (D) Smaller diameter fibers recover faster
   (E) Fibers in the periphery of a nerve bundle are blocked sooner than fibers in the center of a bundle
4. The MOST important effect of inadvertent intravenous administration of a large dose of an amide local anesthetic is
   (A) Bronchoconstriction
   (B) Gangrene
   (C) Hepatic damage
   (D) Renal failure
   (E) Seizures
5. Which one of the following factors is LEAST likely to influence the action of local anesthetics?
   (A) Activity of acetylcholinesterase
   (B) Amount of local anesthetic injected
   (C) Blood flow through the tissue
   (D) Tissue pH
   (E) Use of vasoconstrictors
6. A vial contains 4 mL of a 2% solution of lidocaine. How much lidocaine is present in 1 mL?
   (A) 2 mg
   (B) 8 mg

    (C) 20 mg

    (D) 40 mg

    (E) 80 mg

7. Which one of the following statements about the toxicity of local anesthetics is LEAST accurate?

    (A) Cyanosis may occur following injection of large doses of prilocaine, especially in patients with pulmonary disease

    (B) In overdosage, hyperventilation (with oxygen) is helpful to correct acidosis and lower extracellular potassium

    (C) Intravenous injection of local anesthetics may depress cardiac pacemaker activity

    (D) Most local anesthetics cause vasodilation

    (E) Serious cardiovascular reactions are more likely to occur with tetracaine than with bupivacaine

8. Epinephrine added to a solution of lidocaine for a peripheral nerve block will

    (A) Increase the risk of convulsions

    (B) Prolong the duration of action of the local anesthetic

    (C) Prevent local ischemia

    (D) Both (A) and (B) are correct

    (E) (A), (B), and C are correct

DIRECTIONS (Items 9–12): Each set of matching questions in this section consists of a list of three to twenty-six lettered options (some of which may be figures) followed by several numbered items. For each numbered item, select the ONE lettered option that is MOST closely associated with it. Each lettered option may be selected once, more than once, or not at all.

    (A) Benzocaine

    (B) Bupivacaine

    (C) Cocaine

    (D) Lidocaine

    (E) Mepivacaine

    (F) Prilocaine

    (G) Procaine

    (H) Ropivacaine

    (I) Tetracaine

9. This drug is an ester and has high surface activity; the vasoconstrictor actions of the drug may be useful clinically

10. This long-acting drug is available as the pure *S*-enantiomer, which has a low affinity for the sodium channels in cardiac cells

11. This drug is poorly soluble in aqueous fluids, remains at the site of its application, and is not absorbed into the systemic circulation; it has good surface activity and a low toxic potential

12. This ester has very poor surface activity and a very short duration of action

ANSWERS

1. Local anesthetics bind preferentially to sodium channels in the open and inactivated states. Recovery from drug-induced block is 10–1000 times slower than recovery from normal inactivation. Resting channels have a lower affinity for local anesthetics. The answer is **(B).**

2. Since the drug is a weak base, it will be more ionized (protonated) at pH values lower than its pK_a. Since the stated pH is 1 log unit lower (more acid) than the pK_a, the ratio of ionized to nonionized drug will be approximately 90:10. The answer is **(D).** (Recall from Chapter 1 that at a pH equal to pK_a, the ratio is 1:1; at 1 log unit difference, the ratio is [approximately] 90:10; at 2 units difference, 99:1; etc.)

3. Smaller diameter nerve fibers are more sensitive to local anesthetics and are blocked more rapidly than those of larger size. As the local concentration of drug declines during recovery from local anesthesia, smaller fibers continue to be blocked and are the last to recover. The answer is **(D).**

4. Of the effects listed, the most important in local anesthetic overdose (of both amide and ester types) concern the CNS. Such effects can include sedation or restlessness, nystagmus, convulsions, coma, and respiratory depression. Diazepam is used for seizures caused by local anesthetics, usually without significant effects on ventilation or circulation. The answer is **(E)**.

5. The ester group of ester-type local anesthetics is hydrolyzed by plasma (and tissue) pseudocholinesterases. These drugs are poor substrates for acetylcholinesterase; the activity of this enzyme does not play a part in terminating the actions of local anesthetics. Individuals with genetically based defects in pseudocholinesterase activity are unusually sensitive to procaine and other esters. The answer is **(A)**.

6. The fact that you have 4 mL of the solution of lidocaine is irrelevant. A 2% solution of any drug contains 2 g per 100 mL. The amount of lidocaine in 1 mL of a 2% solution is 0.02 grams, or 20 mg. The answer is **(C)**.

7. Bupivacaine has the highest toxicity of the local anesthetics (other than cocaine, when used in substance abuse). Unlike that of most local anesthetics, the action of bupivacaine on cardiac cells occurs at normal heart rates. Accidental intravenous administration of bupivacaine may lead to arrhythmias and cardiovascular collapse. The answer is **(E)**.

8. Epinephrine will increase the duration of a nerve block when it is administered with short- and medium-duration local anesthetics. As a result of the vasoconstriction that prolongs the duration of this block, less local anesthetic is required, so the risk of systemic toxicity, eg, a convulsion, is reduced. However, local vasoconstriction can lead to ischemia. The answer is **(B)**.

9. Cocaine is the only local anesthetic with intrinsic vasoconstrictor activity. It also has significant surface activity and is favored for head, neck, and pharyngeal surgery. Cocaine is an ester. The answer is **(C)**.

10. Ropivacaine is the first amide local anesthetic to be made available as the pure *S*-enantiomer; other amides are used as racemic mixtures. Ropivacaine has been used mainly for epidural analgesia. It appears to be less cardiotoxic than bupivacaine. The answer is **(H)**.

11. Benzocaine is an ester that is used for topical anesthesia. Because of its low toxic potential, it has been used for anesthesia of large surface areas, including those within the oral cavity. The answer is **(A)**.

12. Procaine is an ester with short duration of action and negligible surface activity. The answer is **(G)**.

Skeletal Muscle Relaxants

27

OBJECTIVES

You should be able to:

- Describe the transmission process at the neuromuscular end plate and the points at which drugs can modify this process.
- Identify three nondepolarizing neuromuscular blockers and one depolarizing neuromuscular blocker; compare their pharmacokinetics.
- Describe the differences between depolarizing and nondepolarizing blockers from the standpoint of tetanic and posttetanic twitch strength.
- Describe the method of reversal of nondepolarizing blockade.
- List the major drugs used in the treatment of acute and chronic skeletal muscle spasticity and describe their mechanisms.

Learn the definitions that follow.

Table 27–1. Definitions.

Term	Definition
Depolarizing blockade	Neuromuscular paralysis that results from persistent depolarization of the end plate, eg, by succinylcholine
Desensitization	A phase of blockade by a depolarizing blocker during which the end plate repolarizes but is less than normally responsive to agonists (acetylcholine or succinylcholine)
Malignant hyperthermia	Hyperthermia that results from massive release of calcium from the sarcoplasmic reticulum, leading to uncontrolled contraction and stimulation of metabolism in skeletal muscle
Nondepolarizing blockade	Neuromuscular paralysis that results from pharmacologic antagonism at the acetylcholine receptor of the end plate, eg, by tubocurarine
Spasmolytic	A drug that reduces abnormally elevated muscle tone (spasm) without paralysis, eg, baclofen, dantrolene
Stabilizing blockade	Synonym for nondepolarizing blockade

CONCEPTS

The drugs in this chapter are divided into two dissimilar groups (Figure 27–1). The **neuromuscular blocking drugs** are used to produce muscle paralysis in order to facilitate surgery or artificial ventilation. The **spasmolytic drugs** are used to reduce abnormally elevated tone caused by neurologic or muscle disease.

NEUROMUSCULAR BLOCKING DRUGS

A. Classification and Prototypes: Skeletal muscle contraction is evoked by a nicotinic cholinergic transmission process. It is subject to the same types of pharmacologic modification as autonomic ganglionic transmission. Blockade of transmission at the end plate (the postsynaptic structure bearing the nicotinic receptors) is clinically useful in producing relaxation of muscle, a requirement for surgery. The neuromuscular blockers are structurally related to acetylcholine and are either antagonists (nondepolarizing type) or agonists (depolarizing type) at the nicotinic end plate receptor. The prototype nondepolarizing agent is **tubocurarine;** the prototype depolarizing drug is **succinylcholine.**

B. Nondepolarizing Neuromuscular Blocking Drugs:
   1. Pharmacokinetics: All agents are given parenterally. Drugs that are metabolized (eg, mivacurium, by plasma cholinesterase) or eliminated in the bile (eg, vecuronium) usually have shorter durations of action than those eliminated by the kidney (eg, doxacurium, pancuronium, tubocurarine). Atracurium clearance involves spontaneous breakdown (Hofmann elimination) to form laudanosine and is independent of hepatic or renal function.
   2. Mechanism of action: Nondepolarizing drugs act as surmountable blockers, ie, the blockade can be overcome by increasing the amount of agonist (acetylcholine) in the

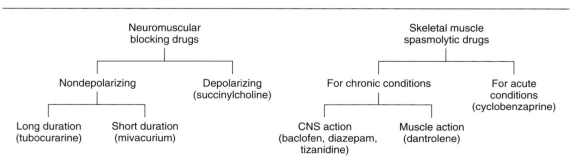

Figure 27–1. Subgroups and prototype drugs discussed in this chapter.

synaptic cleft. They behave as though they compete with acetylcholine at the receptor, and their effect is reversed by cholinesterase inhibitors. There is evidence, however, that some drugs in this group may also act directly to plug the ion channel operated by the acetylcholine receptor. Posttetanic potentiation is preserved in the presence of these agents, but tension during the tetanus fades rapidly. See Table 27–2 for additional details.

C. Depolarizing Neuromuscular Blocking Drugs:
    1. Pharmacokinetics: Succinylcholine is composed of two acetylcholine molecules linked end to end. Succinylcholine is metabolized by plasma cholinesterase (butyrylcholinesterase, or pseudocholinesterase), which determines the amount of drug reaching the end plate. It has a duration of action of only a few minutes if given as a single dose. Blockade may be prolonged in patients with a genetic variant of plasma cholinesterase that metabolizes succinylcholine very slowly. Succinylcholine is not rapidly hydrolyzed by acetylcholinesterase.

    2. Mechanism of action: Depolarizing blockers act like nicotinic agonists and depolarize the neuromuscular end plate. The initial depolarization is often accompanied by twitching and fasciculations. Because tension cannot be maintained in skeletal muscle without periodic repolarization and depolarization of the end plate, continuous depolarization results in muscle relaxation and paralysis. As with the nondepolarizing blockers, some evidence suggests that these drugs can also plug the end plate channels.

    When given by continuous infusion, the effect of succinylcholine changes from continuous depolarization (phase I) to gradual repolarization with resistance to depolarization (phase II), ie, a curare-like block (see Table 27–2).

D. Reversal of Blockade: The action of nondepolarizing blockers is readily reversed by increasing the concentration of normal transmitter at the receptors. This is best accomplished by administration of cholinesterase inhibitors such as neostigmine or pyridostigmine. In contrast, the paralysis produced by depolarizing blockers is increased by cholinesterase inhibitors during phase I. During phase II, the block produced by succinylcholine is usually reversed by cholinesterase inhibitors.

E. Toxicity:
    1. Respiratory paralysis: The action of full doses of neuromuscular blockers leads directly to respiratory paralysis. If mechanical ventilation is not provided, the patient will asphyxiate.

    2. Autonomic effects and histamine release: Autonomic ganglia are stimulated by succinylcholine and blocked by tubocurarine. Succinylcholine also stimulates cardiac muscarinic receptors, while vecuronium is a moderate blocking agent. Tubocurarine is the most likely of these agents to cause histamine release, but it may also occur to a slight extent

Table 27–2. Comparison of a typical nondepolarizing neuromuscular blocker (tubocurarine) and a depolarizing neuromuscular blocker (succinylcholine).*

Process	Tubocurarine	Succinylcholine	
		Phase I	Phase II
Administration of tubocurarine	Additive	Antagonistic	Augmented[1]
Administration of succinylcholine	Antagonistic	Additive	Augmented[1]
Effect of neostigmine	Antagonistic	Augmented[1]	Antagonistic
Initial excitatory effect on skeletal muscle	None	Fasciculations	Not applicable
Response to tetanic stimulus	Unsustained ("fade")	Sustained[2]	Unsustained
Posttetanic facilitation	Yes	No	Yes

*Reproduced, with permission, from Katzung BG (editor): *Basic & Clinical Pharmacology,* 7th ed. Appleton & Lange, 1998.
[1]It is not known whether this interaction is additive or synergistic (super-additive).
[2]The amplitude is decreased, but the response is sustained.

Table 27–3. Autonomic effects of neuromuscular blocking drugs.*

Drug	Effect on Autonomic Ganglia	Effect on Cardiac Muscarinic Receptors	Ability to Release Histamine
Nondepolarizing			
Atracurium	None	None	Slight
Mivacurium	None	None	Slight
Pancuronium	None	Blocks moderately	None
Tubocurarine	Blocks	None	Moderate
Vecuronium, pipecuronium, rocuronium	None	None	None
Depolarizing			
Succinylcholine	Stimulates	Stimulates	Slight

*Modified and reproduced, with permission, from Katzung BG (editor): *Basic & Clinical Pharmacology,* 7th ed. Appleton & Lange, 1998.

with atracurium, mivacurium, and succinylcholine. A summary of these autonomic effects is shown in Table 27–3.

3. **Specific effects of succinylcholine:** Muscle pain is a common postoperative complaint, and muscle damage has occurred. Succinylcholine may cause hyperkalemia, especially in patients with burn or spinal cord injury, peripheral nerve dysfunction, or muscular dystrophy. Increases in intragastric pressure may promote emesis.

4. **Interactions:** Inhaled anesthetics, especially isoflurane, strongly potentiate and prolong neuromuscular blockade. Aminoglycoside antibiotics and antiarrhythmic drugs potentiate and prolong the relaxant action of neuromuscular blockers to a lesser degree.

SPASMOLYTIC DRUGS

Certain chronic diseases of the CNS (eg, cerebral palsy, multiple sclerosis, stroke) are associated with abnormally high reflex activity in the neuronal pathways that control skeletal muscle; the result is painful spasm. Bladder and anal sphincter control are also affected in most cases and may require autonomic drugs for management. In other circumstances, acute injury or inflammation of muscle leads to spasm and pain. Such temporary spasm can sometimes be reduced with appropriate drug therapy.

The goal of spasmolytic therapy in both chronic and acute conditions is reduction of excessive skeletal muscle tone without reduction of strength. Reduced spasm results in reduction of pain and improved mobility.

A. **Drugs for Chronic Spasm:**
1. **Classification:** The spasmolytic drugs do not resemble acetylcholine in structure or effect. They act in the CNS or in the skeletal muscle cell rather than at the neuromuscular end plate. The spasmolytic drugs used in the treatment of the chronic conditions mentioned above include **diazepam,** a benzodiazepine (see Chapter 22); **baclofen,** a GABA agonist; **tizanidine,** a congener of clonidine; and **dantrolene,** an agent that acts on the sarcoplasmic reticulum of skeletal muscle. These agents are usually given by the oral route. Refractory cases may respond to chronic intrathecal administration of baclofen. Rarely, **botulinum toxin** is injected into selected muscles to reduce pain caused by severe spasm (see Chapter 6).

2. **Mechanism of action:** The spasmolytic drugs act by several different mechanisms. Three of the drugs act in the spinal cord. Diazepam facilitates GABA-mediated presynaptic inhibition, and baclofen acts as a $GABA_B$ agonist. Tizanidine reinforces both presynaptic and postsynaptic inhibition in the cord. All three drugs reduce the tonic output of the primary spinal motoneurons.

Dantrolene acts in the skeletal muscle cell to reduce the release of activator calcium from the sarcoplasmic reticulum. Dantrolene is also effective in the treatment of malignant hyperthermia, a genetically determined disorder characterized by massive calcium release from the sarcoplasmic reticulum of skeletal muscle. Malignant hyperthermia is most often triggered by general anesthesia or by succinylcholine. In this emergency condition, dantrolene is given intravenously.

3. **Toxicity:** The sedation produced by diazepam is significant but milder than that produced by other sedative-hypnotic drugs at doses that induce equivalent muscle relaxation. Baclofen produces less sedation than diazepam. Dantrolene causes significant muscle weakness but less sedation than either diazepam or baclofen. Tizanidine may cause drowsiness and hypotension.

B. **Drugs Used for Acute Muscle Spasm:** Many drugs are promoted for the treatment of acute spasm due to muscle injury. Most of these drugs are sedatives or act in the brain stem or spinal cord. **Cyclobenzaprine,** a typical member of this group, is believed to act in the brain stem, possibly by interfering with polysynaptic reflexes that maintain skeletal muscle tone. The drug is active by the oral route and has marked sedative and antimuscarinic actions. Cyclobenzaprine may cause confusion and visual hallucinations in some patients. It is not effective in muscle spasm due to cerebral palsy or spinal cord injury.

DRUG LIST

The following drugs are important members of the groups discussed in this chapter. Prototypes should be learned in detail; features of the major variants should be known well enough so that the variants can be distinguished from prototypes and from each other; the other significant agents should be recognized as belonging to a specific subclass.

Subclass	Prototype	Major Variants	Other Significant Agents
Nondepolarizing neuromuscular blockers Renal elimination, long duration	Tubocurarine		Pancuronium
Hepatic elimination, intermediate duration	Vecuronium		Rocuronium
Spontaneous or plasma ChE,[1] intermediate-short duration	Atracurium	Mivacurium	Cisatracurium
Depolarizing blockers	Succinylcholine		
Spasmolytic drugs	Diazepam, baclofen, dantrolene, tizanidine, botulinum toxin	Cyclobenzaprine	

[1]ChE, cholinesterase. (Atracurium breaks down spontaneously; mivacurium is metabolized by plasma ChE.)

QUESTIONS

DIRECTIONS: Each of the numbered items or incomplete statements in this section is followed by answers or by completions of the statement. Select the ONE lettered answer or completion that is BEST in each case.

1. Characteristics of phase I depolarizing neuromuscular blockade include which one of the following?
    (A) Easy reversibility with pharmacologic antagonists
    (B) Marked muscarinic blockade
    (C) Muscle fasciculations in the later stages of block
    (D) Reversible by pyridostigmine
    (E) Well-sustained tension during a period of tetanic stimulation

Items 2–3: A patient underwent a surgical procedure lasting 2 hours. Anesthesia was provided by isoflurane, supplemented by intravenous midazolam and a nondepolarizing muscle relaxant. At the end of the procedure, glycopyrrolate was administered followed by pyridostigmine.

2. The main reason for administering glycopyrrolate is to
   (A) Dry secretions induced by isoflurane
   (B) Reverse the effects of the muscle relaxant
   (C) Provide postoperative analgesia
   (D) Prevent activation of cardiac muscarinic receptors
   (E) Enhance the action of pyridostigmine

3. Glycopyrrolate would be LEAST likely to be needed during reversal of the effects of a nonde-polarizing relaxant if the agent used was
   (A) Atracurium
   (B) Mivacurium
   (C) Pancuronium
   (D) Tubocurarine
   (E) Vecuronium

4. Characteristics of nondepolarizing neuromuscular blockade include which one of the following?
   (A) Block of posttetanic potentiation
   (B) Histamine-blocking action
   (C) Poorly sustained tetanic tension
   (D) Significant muscle fasciculations during onset of block
   (E) Stimulation of autonomic ganglia

5. Which one of the following does not cause skeletal muscle contractions or twitching?
   (A) Acetylcholine
   (B) Nicotine
   (C) Strychnine
   (D) Succinylcholine
   (E) Vecuronium

6. Which one of the following is most effective in the management of malignant hyperthermia?
   (A) Baclofen
   (B) Dantrolene
   (C) Haloperidol
   (D) Succinylcholine
   (E) Vecuronium

7. Succinylcholine is associated with
   (A) Antagonism by pyridostigmine during the early phase of blockade
   (B) Blockade of autonomic ganglia
   (C) Elevated serum enzymes indicative of muscle damage
   (D) Histamine release in a genetically determined population
   (E) Metabolism by acetylcholinesterase at the neuromuscular junction

8. A 22-year-old patient was given a bolus intravenous dose of a drug for muscle relaxation that should have lasted only 5–10 minutes. Instead, the patient required mechanical ventilation for over 8 hours. Which one of the following statements about this problem is LEAST accurate?
   (A) The agent administered was succinylcholine
   (B) Fewer than 1:2500 persons have the homozygous trait responsible for this type of problem
   (C) Pseudocholinesterase in this patient is resistant to the inhibitory action of dibucaine
   (D) About 1:500 persons may experience a slight prolongation of neuromuscular blockade when given this agent ie, have the heterozygous trait
   (E) Neostigmine should be administered to establish the nature of the problem

9. Which one of the following drugs is most often associated with hypotension caused by his-tamine release?
   (A) Diazepam
   (B) Pancuronium
   (C) Tizanidine
   (D) Tubocurarine
   (E) Vecuronium

10. Regarding the spasmolytic drugs, which one of the following statements is LEAST accurate?
    (A) Baclofen acts on neurons in the spinal cord to increase chloride ion conductance
    (B) Cyclobenzaprine is likely to dry oropharyngeal secretions and to decrease gut motility
    (C) Dantrolene has little effect on calcium release in cardiac muscle
    (D) Diazepam causes sedation at most doses required to reduce muscle spasms
    (E) Intrathecal use of baclofen is effective in some refractory cases of muscle spasticity

DIRECTIONS (Items 11–16): Each set of matching questions in this section consists of a list of three to twenty-six lettered options (some of which may be figures) followed by several numbered items. For each numbered item, select the ONE lettered option that is MOST closely associated with it. Each lettered option may be selected once, more than once, or not at all.

(A) Atracurium
(B) Baclofen
(C) Cyclobenzaprine
(D) Dantrolene
(E) Diazepam
(F) Edrophonium
(G) Isoflurane
(H) Mivacurium
(I) Pancuronium
(J) Succinylcholine
(K) Tubocurarine
(L) Vecuronium

11. This agent has caused hyperkalemia leading to cardiac arrest in patients with neurologic disorders

12. The elimination of this drug is due to its spontaneous breakdown in the plasma; no enzymes are involved in its degradation

13. A spasmolytic drug that is also useful in treatment of convulsions caused by local anesthetics

14. A nondepolarizing neuromuscular blocker that is hydrolyzed by plasma cholinesterase

15. A volatile liquid that, when inhaled, potentiates nondepolarizing neuromuscular blockers

16. Contraction of the jaw musculature (trismus) following administration of this drug is often a premonitory sign of malignant hyperthermia

ANSWERS

1. Phase I depolarizing blockade is not associated with muscarinic blockade nor is it reversible with cholinesterase inhibitors. Muscle fasciculations occur at the start of the action of succinylcholine. The answer is **(E)**.

2. Acetylcholinesterase inhibitors used for reversing the effects of nondepolarizing muscle relaxants cause increases in ACh at all sites where it acts as a neurotransmitter. To offset the resulting side effects, including bradycardia, a muscarinic blocking agent is used concomitantly. The answer is **(D)**.

3. One of the unusual characteristics of pancuronium is that it can block muscarinic receptors. It has sometimes caused tachycardia and hypertension and may cause dysrhythmias in predisposed individuals. The answer is **(C)**.

4. Nondepolarizing blockers result in poorly sustained tetanic tension. They do not cause ganglionic stimulation or fasciculations at any time during their action. The answer is **(C)**.

5. Nicotine, succinylcholine, and acetylcholine cause end plate depolarization and skeletal muscle contractions (they are nicotinic receptor agonists). Strychnine causes skeletal muscle contractions (convulsions) by blocking glycine receptors in the spinal cord. Vecuronium, a nondepolarizing blocker, does not cause contractions at any dose. The answer is **(E)**.

6. Prompt treatment is essential in malignant hyperthermia to control body temperature, correct acidosis, and prevent calcium release. Dantrolene blocks the release of activator calcium from its stores in the sarcoplasmic reticulum, preventing the tension-generating interaction of actin with myosin. The answer is **(B)**.

7. Succinylcholine use is associated with a rise in serum enzyme levels when muscle twitching and fasciculations are marked. The answer is **(C)**.

8. Cholinesterase inhibitors (eg, neostigmine) markedly prolong the neuromuscular blockade caused by succinylcholine. They increase ACh at the end plate, which intensifies depolarization, and they also inhibit succinylcholine metabolism by pseudocholinesterase. About one in 500 persons have a single abnormal gene for pseudocholinesterase. Fewer than one in 2500 persons have two abnormal genes (homozygous atypical) that produce an enzyme with only 1% of the normal affinity for succinylcholine. The atypical enzyme is resistant to the inhibitory action of dibucaine. The answer is **(E)**.

9. Hypotension may occur with tubocurarine and with the spasmolytic drug tizanidine. In the case of tubocurarine, the decrease in blood pressure may be due partly to histamine release and also

to ganglionic blockade. Tizanidine causes hypotension via an interaction with adrenoceptors similar to that of its congener clonidine. The answer is **(D)**.

10. Baclofen does activate GABA$_B$ receptors in the spinal cord. However, these receptors are coupled to K$^+$ ion channels. The answer is **(A)**.

11. Muscle depolarization by succinylcholine releases potassium, and the ensuing hyperkalemia can be life-threatening. Patients most susceptible include those with extensive burns, spinal cord injuries, neurologic dysfunction, or intra-abdominal infection. The answer is **(J)**.

12. Atracurium breaks down spontaneously in the plasma (Hofmann elimination) to form laudanosine. The answer is **(A)**.

13. Diazepam is useful in treating convulsions and in reducing spasm of skeletal muscle. The answer is **(E)**.

14. Mivacurium is the only nondepolarizing neuromuscular blocking drug that is eliminated by plasma cholinesterase. The answer is **(H)**.

15. Isoflurane, an inhalation anesthetic, strongly potentiates most nondepolarizing blocking drugs. The answer is **(G)**.

16. Succinylcholine is a potent triggering agent in patients with hereditary impairment of the sarcoplasmic reticulum. This impairment renders them susceptible to malignant hyperthermia, with massive muscle contraction and lactic acidosis. The answer is **(J)**.

28

Drugs Used in Parkinsonism & Other Movement Disorders

OBJECTIVES

You should be able to:

- Describe the mechanisms by which levodopa, bromocriptine, amantadine, selegiline, and muscarinic blocking drugs alleviate parkinsonism.
- Describe the therapeutic and toxic effects of the antiparkinsonism agents.
- List the chemical agents and drugs that cause parkinsonism symptoms.
- Identify the drugs used in management of tremor, Huntington's disease, drug-induced dyskinesias, and Wilson's disease.

CONCEPTS

Movement disorders constitute a number of heterogeneous neurologic conditions with very different therapies (Figure 28–1).

PARKINSONISM

A. **Pathophysiology:** Parkinsonism is a common movement disorder that involves dysfunction in the basal ganglia and associated brain structures. Signs (mnemonic **RAFT**) include rigidity of skeletal muscles, akinesia (or bradykinesia), flat facies, and tremor at rest.

1. **Naturally occurring parkinsonism:** The naturally occurring disease is of uncertain etiology and occurs with increasing frequency during aging from the fifth or sixth decade of life onward. Pathologic characteristics include decrease in the levels of striatal dopamine and degeneration of dopaminergic neurons in the nigrostriatal tract that normally *inhibit* the

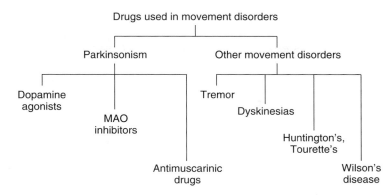

Figure 28–1. Some of the movement disorders and subgroups of drugs discussed in this chapter.

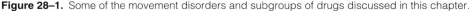

activity of striatal GABAergic neurons (Figure 28–2). Most of the postsynaptic dopamine receptors on GABAergic neurons are of the D_2 subclass (negatively coupled to adenylyl cyclase). The reduction of normal dopaminergic neurotransmission leads to excessive *excitatory* actions of cholinergic neurons on striatal GABAergic neurons; thus, dopamine and acetylcholine activities are out of balance in parkinsonism. (Figure 28–2).

2. **Drug-induced parkinsonism:** Many drugs can cause parkinsonian symptoms (usually reversible). The most important ones are the butyrophenone and phenothiazine **antipsychotic drugs,** which block brain dopamine receptors. At high doses, **reserpine** causes similar symptoms, presumably by depleting brain dopamine. **MPTP** (1-methyl-4-phenyl-1,2,3,6-tetrahydropyridine), a by-product of the attempted synthesis of an illicit meperidine analog, causes irreversible parkinsonism through destruction of dopaminergic neurons in the nigrostriatal tract. Treatment with inhibitors of monoamine oxidase (MAO) type B protects against MPTP neurotoxicity in animals.

DRUG THERAPY OF PARKINSONISM

Strategies of drug treatment of parkinsonism involve increasing dopamine activity in the brain or decreasing muscarinic cholinergic activity in the brain (or both).

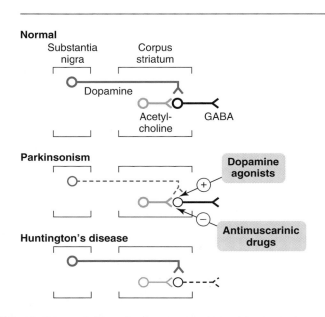

Figure 28–2. Schematic representation of the sequence of neurons involved in parkinsonism and Huntington's chorea. **Top:** Neurons in the normal brain. **Middle:** Neurons in parkinsonism. The dopaminergic neuron is lost. **Bottom:** Neurons in Huntington's disease. The GABAergic neuron is lost. (Reproduced, with permission, from Katzung BG [editor]: *Basic & Clinical Pharmacology,* 7th ed. Appleton & Lange, 1998.)

A. Levodopa:
  1. **Mechanisms of action:** Because dopamine has low bioavailability and does not readily cross the blood-brain barrier, its precursor, L-dopa (levodopa), is used. This amino acid is converted to dopamine by the enzyme aromatic L-amino acid decarboxylase (DOPA decarboxylase), which is present in many body tissues, including the brain. Levodopa is usually given with carbidopa, a drug that does not cross the blood-brain barrier but inhibits DOPA decarboxylase in peripheral tissues. With this combination, lower doses of levodopa are effective and there are fewer peripheral side effects.
  2. **Pharmacologic effects:** Levodopa ameliorates the signs of parkinsonism, particularly bradykinesia; moreover, the mortality rate is decreased. However, the drug does not cure parkinsonism, and responsiveness decreases with time, which may reflect progression of the disease. Clinical response to the drug may fluctuate quite rapidly, changing from akinesia to dyskinesia over a few hours. These so-called **on-off phenomena** may be related partly to changes in levodopa levels in plasma. Drug holidays—periods of a few weeks during which the drug is not taken—are sometimes used to reduce response fluctuations and toxic effects.
  3. **Toxicity:** Most adverse effects are dose-dependent.
      a. **Gastrointestinal effects:** Anorexia, nausea, and vomiting can be reduced by taking the drug in divided doses. Tolerance to the emetogenic action of levodopa usually occurs after several months.
      b. **Cardiovascular effects:** Postural hypotension is common, especially in the early stage of treatment. Other cardiac effects include tachycardia, asystole, and cardiac arrhythmias (rare).
      c. **Dyskinesias:** Choreoathetosis of the face and distal extremities occurs frequently. Some patients may exhibit chorea, ballismus, myoclonus, tics, and tremor.
      d. **Behavioral effects:** Behavioral effects may include anxiety, agitation, confusion, delusions, hallucinations, and depression.

B. Bromocriptine and Other Dopamine Agonists:
  1. **Mechanism of action:** Bromocriptine is an ergot alkaloid that acts as a partial agonist at certain dopamine D_2 receptors in the brain; the drug increases the functional activity of dopamine neurotransmitter pathways, including those involved in extrapyramidal functions. **Pergolide** is another ergot derivative that activates dopamine receptors. Pergolide may decrease response fluctuations and prolong the effectiveness of levodopa, but the drug loses its efficacy with time.
  2. **Clinical use:** Bromocriptine or pergolide may be used in conjunction with levodopa (and with anticholinergic drugs) and in patients who are refractory to or cannot tolerate levodopa.
  3. **Toxicity:** **Gastrointestinal effects** include anorexia, nausea, and vomiting. **Cardiovascular effects** commonly include postural hypotension; cardiac arrhythmias may also occur. **Dyskinesias** may occur with abnormal movements similar to those caused by levodopa. **Behavioral effects** include confusion, hallucinations, and delusions; these occur more commonly than with levodopa. Like levodopa, bromocriptine and pergolide are contraindicated in patients with a history of psychosis. **Miscellaneous effects** with bromocriptine include pulmonary infiltrates and erythromelalgia.
  4. **Pramipexole and ropinirole:** Pramipexole and ropinirole are recently introduced dopamine receptor agonists; they are not ergot derivatives. These drugs are as effective as bromocriptine and appear to cause fewer side effects.

C. Amantadine:
  1. **Mechanism of action:** Amantadine enhances dopaminergic neurotransmission by mechanisms that may involve increasing synthesis or release of dopamine or inhibition of reuptake of dopamine.
  2. **Pharmacologic effects:** Amantadine may improve bradykinesia, rigidity, and tremor but is usually effective for only a few weeks. Amantadine also has antiviral effects.
  3. **Toxicity:** **Behavioral effects** include restlessness, agitation, insomnia, confusion, hallucinations, and acute toxic psychosis. **Dermatologic reactions** include livedo reticularis. **Miscellaneous effects** may include gastrointestinal disturbances, urinary retention, and postural hypotension. Amantadine also causes peripheral edema that responds to diuretics.

D. **Selegiline:**
 1. **Mechanism of action:** Selegiline is a selective inhibitor of MAO type B, the enzyme iso-form that metabolizes dopamine in preference to norepinephrine and serotonin. Selegiline may increase brain dopamine levels.
 2. **Pharmacologic effects:** The drug is used as an adjunct to levodopa in parkinsonism and has also been used as the sole agent in newly diagnosed patients. Hepatic metabolism of selegiline results in the formation of amphetamine.
 3. **Toxicity:** Adverse effects include insomnia, mood changes, dyskinesias, gastrointestinal distress, and hypotension. Meperidine in combination with selegiline has caused agitation, delirium, and death.

E. **Acetylcholine-Blocking (Antimuscarinic) Drugs:**
 1. **Mechanism of action:** These drugs decrease the excitatory actions of cholinergic neu-rons on cells in the striatum by blocking muscarinic receptors.
 2. **Pharmacologic effects:** Drugs like benztropine or trihexyphenidyl may improve the tremor and rigidity of parkinsonism but have little effect on bradykinesia. They are used adjunctively in parkinsonism and also alleviate the reversible extrapyramidal symptoms caused by antipsychotic drugs.
 3. **Toxicity:** CNS toxicity includes drowsiness, inattention, confusion, delusions, and hallu-cinations. Peripheral adverse effects are typical of atropine-like drugs. These agents exacer-bate tardive dyskinesias that result from prolonged use of antipsychotic drugs.

DRUG THERAPY OF OTHER MOVEMENT DISORDERS

A. **Tremor:** Physiologic and essential tremor are clinically similar conditions characterized by postural tremor. They may be alleviated by beta-blocking drugs such as **propranolol.** Beta-blockers should be used with caution in patients with congestive heart failure, asthma, diabetes, or hypoglycemia.

B. **Huntington's Disease and Gilles de la Tourette's Syndrome:** Huntington's disease, an in-herited disorder, results from a brain neurotransmitter imbalance such that GABA functions are diminished and dopaminergic functions are enhanced (Figure 28–2). There may also be a cholinergic deficit, since choline acetyltransferase is decreased in the basal ganglia of patients with this disease. Drug therapy involves the use of amine-depleting drugs (eg, **tetrabenazine**) or antipsychotic agents (eg, **haloperidol** or a **phenothiazine**) that block dopamine receptors. Pharmacologic attempts to enhance brain GABA and acetylcholine activities have not been successful in patients with this disease.
   Tourette's syndrome is a disorder of unknown cause that responds to haloperidol and similar dopamine D_2 receptor blockers.

C. **Drug-Induced Dyskinesias:** Parkinsonism symptoms caused by antipsychotic agents are usually reversible by lowering drug dosage, by switching to a drug that is less toxic to ex-trapyramidal function, or by adding muscarinic blockers. Levodopa and bromocriptine are not useful because dopamine receptors are blocked by the antipsychotic drugs. **Tardive dyskine-sias** that develop from neuroleptic therapy may be a form of denervation supersensitivity. They are not readily reversed; no specific drug therapy is available.

D. **Wilson's Disease:** This recessively inherited disorder of copper metabolism results in deposi-tion of copper salts in the liver and other tissues. Hepatic and neurologic damage may be se-vere, even fatal. Treatment involves use of the chelating agent penicillamine (dimethylcys-teine), which removes excess copper. Toxic effects of penicillamine include gastrointestinal distress, myasthenia, optic neuropathy, and blood dyscrasias.

DRUG LIST

The following drugs are important members of the group discussed in this chapter. Prototypes should be learned in detail; features of the major variants should be known well enough so that the variants can be distinguished from prototypes and from each other.

Subclass	Prototype	Major Variants
Drugs used in parkinsonism Dopamine prodrug	Levodopa	
Levodopa adjunct (DOPA decarboxylase inhibitor)	Carbidopa	
Dopamine agonist	Bromocriptine	Pergolide, pramipexole, ropinirole
Indirect dopamine agonist	Amantadine	
MAO inhibitor	Selegiline	
Antimuscarinic	Benztropine	Biperiden, orphenadrine, trihexyphenidyl
Drugs used in tremor	Propranolol	
Drugs used in Huntington's disease, Tourette's syndrome	Haloperidol	Phenothiazines
Drugs used in Wilson's disease	Penicillamine	

QUESTIONS

DIRECTIONS: Each of the numbered items or incomplete statements in this section is followed by answers or by completions of the statement. Select the ONE lettered answer or completion that is BEST in each case.

Items 1–2: Bradykinesia has now made drug treatment necessary in a 60-year-old male patient with Parkinson's disease. You decide to initiate therapy with levodopa.

1. As the physician, you could tell the patient (and his close family members) all of the following things about levodopa EXCEPT
   (A) Taking the drug in divided doses will decrease nausea and vomiting
   (B) He should be careful when he stands up because he may get dizzy
   (C) Uncontrollable muscle jerks may occur
   (D) A net-like reddish to blue discoloration of the skin is a likely side effect of the medication
   (E) The drug will probably improve his symptoms for a period of time but not indefinitely

2. As the physician who is prescribing levodopa, you will note that the drug
   (A) Has less severe behavioral side effects if given with carbidopa
   (B) Fluctuates in its effectiveness with increasing frequency as treatment continues
   (C) Effectively antagonizes the extrapyramidal adverse effects of antipsychotic drugs
   (D) Has anticancer effects in patients with melanoma
   (E) Causes irreversible tardive dyskinesias

3. The major reason why carbidopa is of value in parkinsonism is that the compound
   (A) Crosses the blood-brain barrier
   (B) Inhibits monoamine oxidase type A
   (C) Inhibits aromatic L-amino acid decarboxylase
   (D) Is converted to the false neurotransmitter, carbidopamine
   (E) Inhibits monoamine oxidase type B

4. Which one of the following statements about bromocriptine is LEAST accurate?
   (A) It should not be administered to patients taking antimuscarinic drugs
   (B) It may cause pulmonary infiltrates
   (C) It is contraindicated in patients with a history of psychosis
   (D) It is a direct-acting dopamine receptor agonist
   (E) Mental disturbances occur more commonly with bromocriptine than with levodopa

5. A 72-year-old patient with parkinsonism presents with swollen feet. They are red, tender, and very painful. You could clear up these symptoms within a few days if you told the patient to stop taking
   (A) Amantadine
   (B) Benztropine
   (C) Bromocriptine
   (D) Levodopa
   (E) Selegiline

6. A patient with parkinsonism is being treated with levodopa. He suffers from irregular, involuntary muscle jerks that affect the proximal muscles of the limbs. Which one of the following statements about these symptoms is LEAST accurate?

(A) The symptoms will usually be decreased if the dose of levodopa is reduced

(B) Administration of other drugs that activate dopamine receptors will exacerbate dyskinesias

(C) The symptoms are unlikely to be alleviated by continued treatment with levodopa

(D) Dyskinesias are less likely to occur if levodopa is administered with carbidopa

(E) Coadministration of muscarinic blockers does not prevent the occurrence of dyskinesias during treatment with levodopa

7. A 51-year-old patient with parkinsonism is being maintained on levodopa-carbidopa with adjunctive use of selegiline. He presents with symptoms of severe depression, and treatment with antidepressants is appropriate. Which of the following is contraindicated?

(A) Amitriptyline

(B) Doxepin

(C) Fluoxetine

(D) Phenelzine

(E) Trazodone

8. Concerning the drugs used in parkinsonism, which of the following statements is LEAST accurate?

(A) Levodopa causes mydriasis and can precipitate an attack of acute glaucoma

(B) Useful therapeutic effects of amantadine may disappear after only a few weeks of treatment

(C) The primary therapeutic benefit of antimuscarinic drugs in parkinsonism is their ability to relieve bradykinesia

(D) The limited efficacy of pergolide may be due to down-regulation of dopamine receptors

(E) The concomitant use of selegiline may increase the adverse effects of levodopa

9. A previously healthy 50-year-old woman begins to suffer from slowed mentation and develops writhing movements of her tongue and hands. In addition, she has delusions of being persecuted. She has no past history of psychiatric or neurologic disorders. The most appropriate drug for treatment is

(A) Amantadine

(B) Bromocriptine

(C) Haloperidol

(D) Levodopa

(E) Trihexyphenidyl

DIRECTIONS (Items 10–12): Each set of matching questions in this section consists of a list of three to twenty-six lettered options (some of which may be figures) followed by several numbered items. For each numbered item, select the ONE lettered option that is MOST closely associated with it. Each lettered option may be selected once, more than once, or not at all.

(A) Amantadine

(B) Biperiden

(C) Bromocriptine

(D) Carbidopa

(E) Clonazepam

(F) Haloperidol

(G) Levodopa

(H) MPTP

(I) Pramipexole

(J) Propranolol

(K) Reserpine

(L) Selegiline

10. Contraindicated in patients with prostatic hypertrophy or obstructive gastrointestinal disease

11. Recently approved for the treatment of parkinsonism, this drug directly activates dopamine receptors but is not an ergot alkaloid

12. Causes akinesia, rigidity, and tremor; in animal experiments, the prior administration of an inhibitor of MAO type B protects against these effects

ANSWERS

1. In prescribing levodopa, the physician should inform the patient about side effects, including gastrointestinal distress, postural hypotension, and dyskinesias. It would be reasonable to advise the patient that therapeutic benefits cannot be expected to continue indefinitely. Livedo reticularis is an adverse effect of amantadine. The answer is **(D).**

2. Levodopa causes less peripheral toxicity but more behavioral side effects when used with carbidopa. The drug is not effective in antagonizing the akinesia, rigidity, and tremor caused by treatment with antipsychotic agents. Dyskinesias are common but are not of the type caused by antipsychotic drugs. Levodopa is a precursor of melanin and may *activate* malignant melanoma. The answer is **(B).**

3. Carbidopa is an inhibitor of aromatic L-amino acid decarboxylase, the enzyme that converts levodopa to dopamine. Since it does not enter the CNS, the drug acts only on the enzyme present in peripheral tissues (eg, liver). The use of carbidopa in combination with levodopa decreases the dose requirement and reduces peripheral side effects of levodopa. The answer is **(C).**

4. The use of dopaminergic agents in combination with antimuscarinic drugs is common in the treatment of parkinsonism. Bromocriptine does not complicate treatment with antimuscarinic drugs or amantadine. If combined with levodopa, bromocriptine should be used at reduced doses to avoid intolerable adverse effects. Confusion, delusions, and hallucinations occur more frequently with bromocriptine than with levodopa. The answer is **(A).**

5. The signs and symptoms described are those of *erythromelalgia,* an adverse effect of bromocriptine. The distal extremities (feet and hands) are usually involved. Arthralgia may occur along with the signs described. The answer is **(C).**

6. The form and severity of dyskinesias due to levodopa may vary widely in different patients. Dyskinesias occur in up to 80% of patients receiving levodopa for long periods. With continued treatment, dyskinesias may develop at a dose of levodopa that was previously well tolerated. They occur more commonly in patients treated with levodopa in combination with carbidopa. The answer is **(D).**

7. Remember that levodopa is a precursor of norepinephrine and epinephrine as well as dopamine and that norepinephrine and epinephrine are metabolized primarily by monoamine oxidase type A. In the presence of nonselective inhibitors of monoamine oxidases, levodopa may cause a hypertensive crisis. The answer is **(D).**

8. The drug most effective in relieving the bradykinesia of parkinsonism—and the disabilities arising from bradykinesia—is levodopa. Antimuscarinic drugs may improve the tremor and rigidity of parkinsonism but have little effect on bradykinesia. The answer is **(C).**

9. Choreoathetosis with decreased mental abilities and psychosis (paranoia) suggest that this patient has Huntington's disease. Drugs that are partly ameliorative include agents (such as the antipsychotics) that decrease dopaminergic activity. The answer is **(C).**

10. Biperiden may cause urinary retention and gastrointestinal effects and should be used with caution in patients with prostatic hypertrophy or obstructive gastrointestinal disease and in those with angle-closure glaucoma. The contraindications listed are typical for drugs that block acetylcholine at muscarinic receptors. The answer is **(B).**

11. Pramipexole is an agonist at dopamine receptors and may have greater selectivity for D_2 receptors in the striatum. It is not an ergot and appears to be less toxic than bromocriptine and pergolide. The answer is **(I).**

12. MPTP causes parkinsonism-like extrapyramidal dysfunction by destroying dopaminergic neurons in the nigrostriatal tract. This neurotoxic action requires the formation of toxic metabolites from the metabolism of MPTP by monoamine oxidase type B. MPTP is used as an experimental tool in animal models of parkinsonism. Antipsychotic drugs (eg, haloperidol) and reserpine also cause parkinsonism-like adverse effects, but these are not prevented by the administration of inhibitors of MAO type B. The answer is **(H).**

Antipsychotic Drugs & Lithium **29**

OBJECTIVES

You should be able to:

- Describe the dopamine hypothesis of schizophrenia.
- List the major receptors blocked by antipsychotic drugs.
- Describe the pharmacodynamics of older antipsychotic drugs and relate these characteristics to their clinical uses.
- Identify the main characteristics of newer atypical antipsychotic drugs.
- List the adverse effects of the major antipsychotic drugs.
- Describe the pharmacokinetics and pharmacodynamics of lithium.

CONCEPTS

ANTIPSYCHOTIC DRUGS

The antipsychotic drugs (**neuroleptics**) are effective in controlling many manifestations of psychotic illness. Though the disease is not cured by drug therapy, the symptoms of schizophrenia, including thought disorder, emotional withdrawal, and hallucinations or delusions, may be attenuated by antipsychotic drugs. Unfortunately, protracted therapy (years) is often needed and can result in severe toxicity in some patients.

A. Classification: The major chemical subgroups of antipsychotic drugs are the **phenothiazines** (eg, chlorpromazine, thioridazine, fluphenazine), the **thioxanthenes** (eg, thiothixene), and the **butyrophenones** (eg, haloperidol).

Several newer drugs of varied **heterocyclic structure** are also effective in schizophrenia, including clozapine, loxapine, olanzapine, molindone, pimozide, risperidone, quetiapine, and sertindole. In some cases, these atypical antipsychotic drugs have proved to be more effective and less toxic than the older drugs. However, they are much more costly than standard drugs, most of which are prescribed generically.

B. Pharmacokinetics: The antipsychotic drugs are well absorbed when given orally and, because they are lipid-soluble, readily enter the CNS and most other body tissues. Many are bound extensively to plasma proteins. These drugs require metabolism by liver enzymes prior to excretion and have long plasma half-lives that permit once-daily dosing. Parenteral forms of several agents, including fluphenazine, thioridazine, and haloperidol, are available for rapid initiation of therapy.

C. Mechanism of Action:
1. **The dopamine hypothesis:** The dopamine hypothesis of schizophrenia proposes that the disorder is caused by a relative excess of functional activity of the neurotransmitter dopamine in specific neuronal tracts in the brain. This hypothesis is based on the following observations. (1) Most antipsychotic drugs block brain dopamine receptors (especially D_2 receptors). (2) Dopamine agonist drugs (eg, amphetamine, levodopa) exacerbate schizophrenia. (3) An increased density of dopamine receptors has been detected in certain brain regions of untreated schizophrenics. The dopamine hypothesis of schizophrenia is not fully satisfactory because antipsychotic drugs are only partly effective in most patients and because some effective drugs have a much higher affinity for other receptors than for D_2 receptors.
2. **Dopamine receptors:** Five different dopamine receptors (D_1–D_5) have been characterized. Each is G protein-coupled and is composed of seven transmembrane domains. The D_2 receptor, found in the caudate-putamen, nucleus accumbens, cerebral cortex, and hypothal-

amus, is negatively coupled to adenylyl cyclase. The therapeutic efficacy of most of the older antipsychotic drugs correlates with their relative affinity for the D_2 receptor. Unfortunately, there is also a correlation between blockade of D_2 receptors and extrapyramidal dysfunction.

3. **Other receptors:** Several newer antipsychotic agents have higher affinities for other receptors than for the D_2 receptor. For example, alpha adrenoceptor-blocking action correlates well with antipsychotic effect for many of the drugs (see Table 29–1). Clozapine, a drug with significant D_4 and 5-HT$_2$ receptor-blocking actions, has low affinity for D_2 receptors. Most of the newer atypical drugs (olanzapine, quetiapine, risperidone, and sertindole) have high affinity for 5-HT$_{2a}$ receptors, though they may also interact with D_2 and other receptors. Some (not all) of these atypical drugs are much less likely to cause extrapyramidal dysfunction than standard agents.

D. Effects: Dopamine receptor blockade is the major effect that correlates with therapeutic benefit for most of the older antipsychotic drugs. Dopaminergic tracts in the brain include the mesocortical-mesolimbic pathways (regulating mentation and mood), the nigrostriatal tract (extrapyramidal function), the tuberoinfundibular pathways (control of prolactin release), and the chemoreceptor trigger zone (emesis). Mesocortical-mesolimbic dopamine receptor blockade presumably underlies antipsychotic effects, and a similar action on the chemoreceptor trigger zone leads to the useful antiemetic properties of some antipsychotic drugs. Adverse effects resulting from receptor blockade in the other dopaminergic tracts include extrapyramidal dysfunction and hyperprolactinemia (see below). The relative receptor-blocking actions of different antipsychotic drugs are shown in Table 29–1.

E. Clinical Use:

1. **Treatment of schizophrenia:** Most antipsychotic drugs reduce some of the positive symptoms of schizophrenia, including hyperactivity, bizarre ideation, hallucinations, and delusions. Consequently, they can facilitate functioning in both inpatient and outpatient environments. Beneficial effects may take several weeks to develop. Overall efficacy of the older antipsychotic drugs is equivalent, though individual patients may respond best to a specific drug. None of the traditional drugs have much effect on negative symptoms of schizophrenia. Among the newer atypical drugs, olanzapine and sertindole are reported to improve some of the negative symptoms of schizophrenia, including emotional blunting and social withdrawal, and clozapine and risperidone are often effective in patients refractory to standard drugs.

2. **Other psychiatric and neurologic indications:** Antipsychotic drugs may be useful in the initial treatment of mania, in the management of psychotic symptoms of schizoaffective disorders, in Tourette's syndrome, and for management of toxic psychoses caused by overdosage of certain CNS stimulants. Molindone is used mainly in Tourette's syndrome; it is rarely used in schizophrenia.

Table 29–1. Relative receptor-blocking actions of neuroleptic drugs.

Drug	D_2 Block	D_4 Block	Alpha$_1$ Block	5-HT$_2$ Block	M Block	H$_1$ Block
Most phenothiazines and thioxanthines	++	–	++	+	+	+
Thioridazine	++	–	++	+	+++	+
Haloperidol	+++	–	+	–	–	–
Clozapine	–	++	++	++	++	+
Molindone	++	–	+	–	+	+
Olanzapine	+	–	+	++	+	+
Quetiapine	+	–	+	++	+	+
Risperidone	++	–	+	++	+	+
Sertindole	++	–	+	+++	–	–

+, blockade; –, no effect. The number of plus signs indicates the intensity of receptor blockade.

3. **Nonpsychiatric indications:** With the exception of thioridazine, most phenothiazines have antiemetic actions; prochlorperazine is promoted solely for this indication. H₁ receptor blockade, most often present in short side chain phenothiazines, provides the basis for their use as antipruritics and sedatives and contributes to their antiemetic effects.

F. **Toxicity:**
   1. **Reversible neurologic effects:** Dose-dependent extrapyramidal effects include a parkinsonismlike syndrome with bradykinesia, rigidity, and tremor. This toxicity may be reversed by a decrease in dose and may be antagonized by concomitant use of muscarinic blocking agents. Extrapyramidal toxicity occurs most frequently with haloperidol (Figure 29–1) and the more potent piperazine side-chain phenothiazines (eg, fluphenazine, trifluoperazine). Parkinsonism occurs infrequently with clozapine and is less common with several newer drugs, including olanzapine, risperidone, and sertindole. Other reversible neurologic dysfunctions include akathisia and dystonias; these usually respond to treatment with diphenhydramine or muscarinic blocking agents.
   2. **Tardive dyskinesias:** This important toxicity includes choreoathetoid movements of muscles of the mouth and tongue and may be irreversible. Tardive dyskinesias tend to develop after several years of antipsychotic drug therapy but have appeared as early as 6 months. Antimuscarinic drugs that usually ameliorate other extrapyramidal effects generally *increase* the severity of tardive dyskinesia. There is no effective drug treatment for tardive dyskinesia. Switching to clozapine does not exacerbate the condition. Tardive dyskinesia may be attenuated *temporarily* by increasing neuroleptic dosage; this suggests that tardive dyskinesia may be caused by dopamine receptor sensitization.
   3. **Autonomic effects:** Autonomic effects result from blockade of peripheral muscarinic receptors and alpha adrenoceptors and are more difficult to manage in elderly patients. Tolerance to some of the autonomic effects occurs with continued therapy. As shown in Figure 29–1, thioridazine has the strongest autonomic effects and haloperidol the weakest. Clozapine and most of the atypical drugs have intermediate autonomic effects.
      a. **Muscarinic receptor blockade:** Atropine-like effects (dry mouth, constipation, urinary retention, and visual problems) are often pronounced during use of thioridazine and phenothiazines with aliphatic side chains (eg, chlorpromazine). These effects also occur with clozapine and most of the atypical drugs but not with sertindole. Antimuscarinic CNS effects may include a toxic confusional state similar to that produced by atropine and the tricyclic antidepressants.
      b. **Alpha receptor blockade:** Postural hypotension caused by alpha blockade is a common manifestation of many of these drugs, especially phenothiazines. In the elderly,

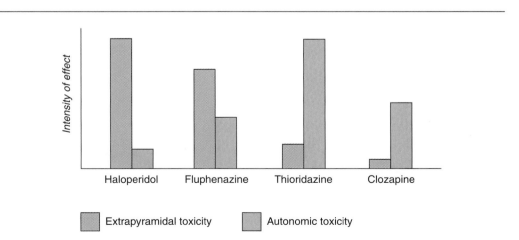

Figure 29–1. Relative extrapyramidal and autonomic toxicities of representative antipsychotic drugs. Extrapyramidal toxicities take the form of parkinsonism, akathisias, and dystonias. Autonomic toxicities are manifest as alpha-adrenoceptor blockade (orthostatic hypotension) or muscarinic blockade (dry mouth, blurred vision, urinary retention).

measures must be taken to avoid falls due to postural fainting. All of the atypical drugs can cause orthostatic hypotension. Failure to ejaculate is common in men taking phenothiazines.

4. **Endocrine and metabolic effects:** Endocrine and metabolic effects include hyperprolactinemia, weight gain, gynecomastia, the amenorrhea-galactorrhea syndrome, and infertility. These effects are predictable manifestations of dopamine receptor blockade in the pituitary; dopamine is the normal inhibitory regulator of prolactin secretion.

5. **Neuroleptic malignant syndrome:** Patients who are particularly sensitive to the extrapyramidal effects of antipsychotic drugs may develop a malignant hyperthermic syndrome. The symptoms include muscle rigidity, impairment of sweating, hyperpyrexia, and autonomic instability that may be life-threatening. Drug treatment involves the prompt use of dantrolene and perhaps dopamine agonists.

6. **Sedation:** Sedation is more marked with phenothiazines than with other antipsychotics; this effect is normally perceived as unpleasant by nonpsychotic individuals. With the exception of sertindole, the atypical drugs all block histamine receptors, an action that contributes to sedation.

7. **Miscellaneous toxicities:** Visual impairment caused by retinal deposits has occurred with **thioridazine;** at high doses, this drug may also cause severe conduction defects in the heart that result in fatal ventricular arrhythmias. **Sertindole** prolongs the QT interval of the ECG; the underlying myocardial effect may lead to cardiac arrhythmias. **Clozapine** causes a small but important (1–2%) incidence of agranulocytosis and at high doses has caused seizures.

8. **Overdosage toxicity:** Poisoning with antipsychotics other than thioridazine is not usually fatal. Hypotension often responds to fluid replacement. Neuroleptics lower the convulsive threshold and may cause seizures, which are usually managed with diazepam or phenytoin. Thioridazine overdose, because of cardiotoxicity, is more difficult to treat.

LITHIUM & OTHER DRUGS USED IN BIPOLAR (MANIC-DEPRESSIVE) DISORDER

A. **Pharmacokinetics:** Lithium is absorbed rapidly and completely from the gut. The drug is distributed throughout the body water and excreted by the kidneys with a half-life of about 20 hours. Plasma levels should be monitored, especially during the first weeks of therapy, to establish an effective and safe dosage regimen. The therapeutic plasma concentration is 0.6–1.4 meq/L. Plasma levels of the drug may be altered by changes in body water. Thus, dehydration or treatment with diuretics (thiazides) may result in an increase of lithium in the blood to toxic levels. Theophylline increases the renal clearance of lithium.

B. **Mechanism of Action:** The mechanism of action of lithium is not well defined. The drug inhibits the recycling of neuronal membrane phosphoinositides involved in the generation of inositol trisphosphate (IP_3) and diacylglycerol (DAG). These second messengers are important in amine neurotransmission, including that mediated by central adrenoceptors and muscarinic receptors (Figure 29–2).

Figure 29–2. Postulated effect of lithium on the IP_3 and DAG second messenger system. The schematic diagram shows the synaptic membrane of a neuron in the brain. PLC, phospholipase-C; G, coupling protein; R, receptor; PI, PIP, PIP_2, IP_2, IP_1, intermediates in the production of IP_3. By interfering with this cycle, lithium may cause a use-dependent reduction of synaptic transmission. (Modified and reproduced, with permission, from Katzung BG [editor]: *Basic & Clinical Pharmacology,* 7th ed. Appleton & Lange, 1998.)

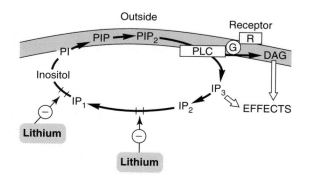

C. **Clinical Use:** Lithium carbonate is used in the treatment of bipolar affective disorder (manic-depressive disease). Maintenance therapy with lithium decreases manic behavior and reduces both the frequency and the magnitude of mood swings. Drug therapy with neuroleptics or benzodiazepines may also be required at the initiation of lithium treatment. Antidepressant drugs may be required adjunctively during maintenance. Alternative drugs of value in bipolar affective disorder include **carbamazepine, clonazepam,** and **valproic acid.**

D. **Toxicity:** Adverse neurologic effects of lithium include tremor, sedation, ataxia, and aphasia. Thyroid enlargement may occur, but thyroid dysfunction is rare. Reversible nephrogenic diabetes insipidus occurs commonly at therapeutic drug levels. Edema is a frequent adverse effect of lithium therapy, and leukocytosis is always present. The use of lithium during pregnancy may increase the incidence of congenital cardiac anomalies.

DRUG LIST

The following drugs are important members of the group discussed in this chapter. Prototypes should be learned in detail; the other significant agents should be recognized as belonging to a specific subclass.

Subclass	Prototype	Other Significant Agents
Phenothiazines Aliphatic	Chlorpromazine[1]	
Piperidine	Thioridazine	Mesoridazine
Piperazine	Trifluoperazine	Perphenazine, fluphenazine
Thioxanthenes	Thiothixene	
Butyrophenones	Haloperidol	
Heterocyclics	Clozapine, molindone, pimozide	Loxapine, olanzapine, risperidone, sertindole
Antimanic drugs	Lithium	Carbamazepine, clonazepam

[1]Some authorities consider chlorpromazine obsolete because of its high incidence of toxic effects.

QUESTIONS

DIRECTIONS: Each of the numbered items or incomplete statements in this section is followed by answers or by completions of the statement. Select the ONE lettered answer or completion that is BEST in each case.

1. Concerning hypotheses for the pathophysiologic basis of schizophrenia, which one of the following statements is LEAST accurate?
   (A) Positron emission tomography has shown increased dopamine receptors in the brains of both untreated and drug-treated schizophrenics
   (B) In a patient with parkinsonism, psychotic effects may occur during treatment with dopamine receptor agonists
   (C) The clinical potency of many antipsychotic drugs correlates well with their alpha adrenoceptor-blocking actions
   (D) Drug treatment of schizophrenics sometimes results in changes in the cerebrospinal fluid levels of the dopamine metabolite, homovanillic acid
   (E) All effective antipsychotic drugs have high affinity for dopamine D_2 receptors

2. Fluphenazine has been prescribed for a 20-year-old male patient. His schizophrenic symptoms have improved enough for him to reside in a halfway house in the community. He visits his physician with a list of complaints about his medication. Which one of the following is LEAST likely to be on his list?
   (A) Constipation
   (B) Dizziness if he stands up too quickly

    (C)   He has become disinterested in sex

    (D)   He salivates excessively

    (E)   Newspaper print is hard to read

3. A 50-year-old woman has been receiving antipsychotic medication for 27 years. Which one of the following statements concerning adverse effects of antipsychotic drugs is LEAST accurate?

    (A)   The late-occurring choreoathetoid movements caused by conventional antipsychotic drugs are exacerbated by antimuscarinic agents

    (B)   Retinal pigmentation is a dose-dependent toxic effect of thioridazine

    (C)   Uncontrollable restlessness in a patient receiving antipsychotic medications is usually alleviated by increasing the drug dose

    (D)   Acute dystonic reactions usually respond to diphenhydramine

    (E)   Blurring of vision and urinary retention are likely side effects of chlorpromazine

4. Conventional antipsychotic drugs would NOT be indicated for

    (A)   Acute management of mania

    (B)   The amenorrhea-galactorrhea syndrome

    (C)   Psychosis caused by phencyclidine intoxication

    (D)   Schizoaffective disorders

    (E)   Tourette's syndrome

5. A schizophrenic patient developed bradykinesia, rigidity, and tremor during treatment with haloperidol. His drug therapy was changed to thioridazine, which was just as effective in reducing his psychiatric symptoms. However, thioridazine did not cause extrapyramidal dysfunction in this patient. The most likely explanation is that

    (A)   Haloperidol has a low affinity for D_2 receptors

    (B)   Thioridazine has greater alpha adrenoceptor-blocking actions

    (C)   Haloperidol activates GABAergic neurons in the striatum

    (D)   Thioridazine has greater blocking actions on brain muscarinic receptors

    (E)   Haloperidol acts presynaptically to block dopamine release

6. Which one of the following statements concerning the treatment of bipolar affective disorder is LEAST accurate?

    (A)   Lithium is usually effective at plasma levels between 0.6 and 1.4 meq/L

    (B)   Excessive intake of sodium chloride enhances the toxicity of lithium

    (C)   Lithium dosage may need to be decreased in patients taking thiazides

    (D)   Elimination of lithium is proportionate to creatinine clearance

    (E)   Lack of compliance is a significant cause of treatment failure with lithium

7. A 30-year-old male patient is on drug therapy for a psychiatric problem. He complains that he feels "flat" and that he gets confused at times. He has been gaining weight and has lost his sex drive. As he moves his hands, you notice a slight tremor. He tells you that since he has been on medication he is always thirsty and frequently has to urinate. The drug he is most likely to be taking is:

    (A)   Clonazepam

    (B)   Clozapine

    (C)   Haloperidol

    (D)   Lithium

    (E)   Trifluoperazine

8. A young male patient diagnosed as schizophrenic develops severe muscle cramps with torticollis a short time after drug therapy is initiated with haloperidol. The best course of action would be to

    (A)   Add clozapine to the drug regimen

    (B)   Discontinue haloperidol and observe the patient

    (C)   Give oral diphenhydramine

    (D)   Switch the patient to fluphenazine

    (E)   Inject benztropine

9. A patient diagnosed as suffering from bipolar affective disorder has been effectively treated with lithium at doses achieving a mean plasma level of approximately 1.4 meq/L. Lately he has begun to suffer from increased motor activity, aphasia, and mental confusion. The best course of action would be to

    (A)   Add amitriptyline to the drug regimen

    (B)   Continue lithium and add haloperidol

    (C)   Discontinue lithium and start valproic acid

    (D)   Discontinue lithium and start clozapine

    (E)   Increase the dose of lithium

DIRECTIONS (Items 10–14): Each set of matching questions in this section consists of a list of three to twenty-six lettered options (some of which may be figures) followed by several numbered items. For each numbered item, select the ONE lettered option that is MOST closely associated with it. Each lettered option may be selected once, more than once, or not at all.

- **(A)** Bromocriptine
- **(B)** Carbamazepine
- **(C)** Clonazepam
- **(D)** Clozapine
- **(E)** Diphenhydramine
- **(F)** Haloperidol
- **(G)** Lithium
- **(H)** Olanzapine
- **(I)** Promethazine
- **(J)** Risperidone
- **(K)** Thioridazine
- **(L)** Valproic acid

10. The calming and antiemetic properties of this phenothiazine, together with its atropine-like properties, form the basis for its use in preoperative sedation
11. Weekly blood counts are mandatory for patients who are taking this drug
12. This drug is notable for causing retinal deposits, marked atropine-like effects, and abnormal electrocardiograms
13. Although it can exacerbate the symptoms of schizophrenia, this drug may be useful in the management of the neuroleptic malignant syndrome
14. Useful as a mood stabilizer in patients with bipolar affective disorders who are intolerant of lithium, this drug induces the formation of liver drug-metabolizing enzymes

ANSWERS

1. Although positive correlations have been made between antipsychotic efficacy and the abilities of drugs to block D_2 receptors, similar correlations have also been made with respect to their alpha adrenoceptor-blocking actions. Most conventional antipsychotic drugs block D_2 receptors. However, such an action does not appear to be an absolute requirement for antipsychotic action, since clozapine and newer drugs have a very low affinity for such receptors. All of the other statements are accurate. The answer is **(E)**.

2. Sedative effects occur with most of the phenothiazines; these drugs also act as antagonists at muscarinic and alpha adrenoceptors. Postural hypotension, blurring of vision, and constipation are common autonomic side effects, as is *dry* mouth. Effects on the male libido may result from increases in prolactin or from increased peripheral conversion of androgens to estrogens. The answer is **(D)**.

3. Uncontrollable restlessness (akathisia) is an extrapyramidal adverse effect of antipsychotic medications. In some patients, akathisias may be difficult to distinguish from the expression of the positive symptoms of schizophrenia. Akathisias are managed by *decreasing* the antipsychotic drug dose or by treatment with drugs that have anticholinergic actions. The answer is **(C)**.

4. Hyperprolactinemia and the amenorrhea-galactorrhea syndrome may occur as an adverse effect during treatment with antipsychotic drugs that block dopamine receptors in the tuberoinfundibular tract. This prevents the normal inhibitory action of dopamine on release of prolactin from the anterior pituitary gland. The answer is **(B)**.

5. Parkinsonian adverse effects occur more commonly with haloperidol than with thioridazine. One possible explanation is that thioridazine exerts more pronounced blocking actions at brain muscarinic receptors. This action partly compensates for dopamine receptor blockade in the nigrostriatal tract, so that extrapyramidal function is more effectively maintained. A second possibility (not listed) is that haloperidol has a higher affinity for dopamine D_2 receptors than does thioridazine. The answer is **(D)**.

6. Reliance is placed on measurements of serum lithium concentrations for optimal dosage regimens. Lithium clearance is influenced by many factors, including renal function, serum sodium concentration, hydration state, pregnancy, and the presence of other drugs. High urinary levels of sodium inhibit renal tubular reabsorption of lithium, thus *decreasing* its plasma levels. By decreasing blood volume, thiazides may increase lithium plasma levels. The answer is **(B)**.

7. Confusion, mood changes, decreased sexual interest, and weight gain are symptoms that may be unrelated to drug administration. On the other hand, psychiatric drugs, including those used in the treatment of psychotic and affective disorders, may be responsible for such symptoms. Tremor and symptoms of nephrogenic diabetes insipidus are characteristic adverse effects of lithium that may occur at therapeutic blood levels of the drug. The answer is **(D)**.

8. Acute dystonic reactions are usually very painful and should be treated immediately with parenteral administration of a muscarinic blocking agent. Adding clozapine will not be protective, and fluphenazine is as likely as haloperidol to cause acute dystonia. Oral administration of diphenhydramine is a possibility, but the patient may find it difficult to swallow and it would take a longer time to act. The answer is **(E)**.

9. The symptoms described in this patient are toxic effects of lithium. Increasing the dose of lithium will increase blood levels and exacerbate these symptoms. Adding amitriptyline or haloperidol to the regimen would not alleviate the problem. A trial of an alternative drug (eg, carbamazepine, clonazepam, or valproic acid) is appropriate. Clozapine as a single agent has minimal efficacy in bipolar disorder. The answer is **(C)**.

10. With the exception of thioridazine, phenothiazines exert strong antiemetic effects. Phenothiazines with short side chains have marked histamine H_1 receptor-blocking actions and are used for relief of pruritus or, in the case of promethazine, as preoperative sedatives. The answer is **(I)**.

11. Agranulocytosis occurs in a small percentage of patients taking clozapine. This potentially fatal abnormality can develop rapidly, usually between the sixth and eighteenth weeks of therapy. Hematotoxicity is reversible if clozapine is discontinued immediately following a significant decrease in leukocyte count. The answer is **(D)**.

12. Atropine-like side effects are more prominent with thioridazine than with other phenothiazines, but the drug is less likely to cause extrapyramidal dysfunction. At high doses, thioridazine causes retinal deposits that in advanced cases resemble retinitis pigmentosa. The patient may complain of browning of vision. The drug has quinidine-like actions on the heart and, in overdose, may cause arrhythmias and cardiac conduction block. The answer is **(K)**.

13. Neuroleptic malignant syndrome is characterized by muscle rigidity, high fever, and autonomic instability. The syndrome may result from a too-rapid block of dopamine receptors in patients who are highly sensitive to the extrapyramidal effects of antipsychotic drugs. Management involves control of fever, the use of muscle relaxants (eg, dantrolene or diazepam), and administration of the dopamine receptor agonist bromocriptine. Like most drugs that increase brain dopaminergic activity, bromocriptine may exacerbate psychotic symptoms. The answer is **(A)**.

14. Carbamazepine can be used to treat mania and for prophylaxis in patients with bipolar affective disorders. The drug is also used in seizure disorders and for trigeminal neuralgia. Its chronic administration increases drug-metabolizing enzymes, including cytochrome P450 isozymes. The answer is **(B)**.

30

Antidepressants

OBJECTIVES

You should be able to:

- Describe the probable mechanisms of action and the major properties of tricyclic antidepressants.
- List the toxic effects that occur during chronic therapy and with an acute overdose of tricyclic antidepressants.
- Identify the second- and third-generation heterocyclic antidepressants and their distinctive properties.

- Identify the selective serotonin reuptake inhibitors and list their major characteristics.
- Describe the therapeutic use and toxic effects of MAO inhibitors.
- Identify the major drug interactions associated with antidepressant drugs.

Learn the definitions that follow.

Table 30–1. Definitions.

Term	Definition
Amine hypothesis of mood	The hypothesis that major depressive disorders result from a functional deficiency of norepinephrine or serotonin at synapses in the central nervous system
Tricyclics	A group of structurally related drugs resembling phenothiazines chemically; block reuptake of both norepinephrine and serotonin
MAO inhibitors	Drugs that inhibit monoamine oxidase type A, which metabolizes norepinephrine and serotonin; or monoamine oxidase type B, which metabolizes dopamine
Selective serotonin reuptake inhibitors	A group of drugs that selectively inhibit the serotonin transporters of the nerve ending membrane
Heterocyclics (second- and third-generation antidepressants)	Drugs of varied chemical structures; several have actions different from those of tricyclic antidepressants or selective serotonin reuptake inhibitors

CONCEPTS

Depression is a common condition with both psychologic and physical manifestations. The three major types of depression are (1) **reactive depression,** a response to external events; (2) **bipolar affective (manic-depressive) disorder,** discussed in Chapter 29; and (3) **major depressive disorder,** or **endogenous depression,** a depression of mood without any obvious medical or situational causes. The drugs used in endogenous depression are the subject of this chapter.

The **amine hypothesis of mood** postulates that brain amines, particularly norepinephrine (NE) and serotonin (5-HT), are neurotransmitters in pathways that function in the expression of mood. According to the amine hypothesis, a functional decrease in the activity of such amines would result in depression; a functional increase of activity would result in mood elevation. Difficulties with this hypothesis are that (1) antidepressant drugs cause changes in amine activity within hours, but weeks may be required for them to achieve clinical effects; and (2) most antidepressants ultimately cause a *down*-regulation of amine receptors.

A. **Classification and Pharmacokinetics:** Four groups of drugs are used to treat endogenous depression (Figure 30–1): **tricyclic antidepressants, heterocyclic antidepressants, selective serotonin reuptake inhibitors,** and **monoamine oxidase inhibitors.**

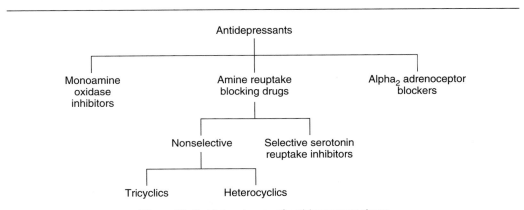

Figure 30–1. Major classes of antidepressant drugs.

1. **Tricyclics (TCAs):** Tricyclic antidepressant drugs (eg, **imipramine, amitriptyline**) are structurally related to the phenothiazine antipsychotics and share certain of their pharmacologic effects. The tricyclics are well absorbed orally but may undergo first-pass metabolism. They have high volumes of distribution and are not readily dialyzable. Extensive hepatic metabolism is required prior to their excretion; plasma half-lives of 8–36 hours usually permit once-daily dosing. Some tricyclics form active metabolites.

2. **Heterocyclics:** These drugs have varied structures and include second-generation antidepressants (eg, **amoxapine, bupropion, maprotiline, trazodone**) and newer, third-generation drugs **(mirtazapine, nefazodone, venlafaxine).** The pharmacokinetics of most of these agents are similar to those of the tricyclic drugs. Nefazodone and trazodone are exceptions; their half-lives are quite short and usually require administration two or three times daily.

3. **Selective serotonin reuptake inhibitors (SSRIs):** **Fluoxetine** is the prototype of a group of drugs that selectively inhibit the reuptake of serotonin. All of them require hepatic metabolism and have half-lives of 18–24 hours. However, fluoxetine forms an active metabolite with a half-life of several days. Other members of this group (eg, **sertraline, paroxetine**) do not form long-acting metabolites.

4. **MAO inhibitors (MAOIs):** These drugs (eg, **phenelzine, tranylcypromine, isocarboxazid**) are structurally related to amphetamines and are orally active. They inhibit both MAO-A (which metabolizes norepinephrine, serotonin, and tyramine) and MAO-B (which metabolizes dopamine). Tranylcypromine is the fastest in onset of effect, but it has a shorter duration of action (about a week) than that of other MAO inhibitors (with durations of 2–3 weeks). In spite of these prolonged actions, the MAO inhibitors are given daily. These drugs are inhibitors of hepatic drug-metabolizing enzymes and cause many drug interactions.

   Moclobemide is a *reversible* inhibitor of MAO-A, the form that metabolizes serotonin and norepinephrine. The drug is readily displaced from the enzyme by tyramine and has a much shorter duration of action than other drugs in this group.

B. **Mechanisms of Antidepressant Action:** Potential sites of action of antidepressants at central nervous system synapses are shown in Figure 30–2. By means of several mechanisms, almost

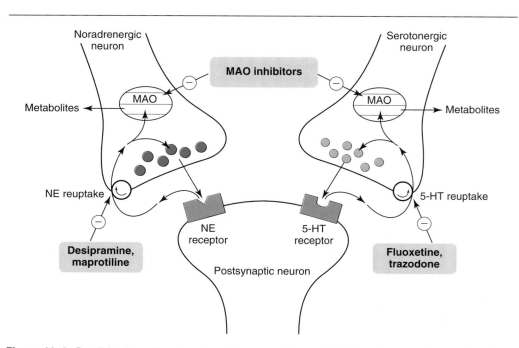

Figure 30–2. Possible sites of action of antidepressant drugs. Inhibition of neuronal reuptake of norepinephrine and serotonin increases the synaptic activities of these neurotransmitters. Inhibition of MAO increases the presynaptic stores of both norepinephrine and serotonin, which leads to increased neurotransmitter effects. *Note:* These are acute actions of antidepressants.

all antidepressants result in potentiation of the neurotransmitter actions of norepinephrine, serotonin, or both. The only exception is bupropion, which has an unknown mechanism of action.

1. **Tricyclic antidepressants:** The acute effect of tricyclic drugs is to inhibit the reuptake mechanisms (transporters) responsible for the termination of the synaptic actions of both NE and 5-HT in the brain. This results in potentiation of their neurotransmitter actions at postsynaptic receptors.

2. **Heterocyclic antidepressants:** The acute actions of heterocyclics are varied. Some second-generation drugs inhibit the reuptake of NE (eg, maprotiline); others have more action on serotonin reuptake (eg, trazodone, see Table 30–2). The third-generation drug venlafaxine, though not a tricyclic, is a potent inhibitor of both NE and 5-HT transporters. Mirtazapine appears to increase amine release from nerve endings by antagonism of presynaptic α_2 adrenoceptors involved in feedback inhibition.

3. **Selective serotonin reuptake inhibitors:** The acute effect of the selective serotonin reuptake inhibitors is a highly selective inhibition of the 5-HT transporter.

4. **Monoamine oxidase inhibitors:** The MAO inhibitors increase brain amine levels by interfering with their metabolism in the nerve endings, resulting in an increase in the vesicular stores of norepinephrine and serotonin. When neuronal activity discharges the vesicles, increased amounts of the amines are released, enhancing the actions of the neurotransmitters.

C. Pharmacologic Effects:

1. **Amine uptake blockade:** The drugs that block norepinephrine transporters in the CNS (eg, tricyclics) also inhibit the reuptake of norepinephrine at nerve endings in the autonomic nervous system. Likewise, MAO inhibitors increase NE in sympathetic nerve terminals. In both cases this can lead to peripheral autonomic sympathomimetic effects.

2. **Sedation:** Sedation is a common CNS effect of tricyclic drugs (though less so with protriptyline and desipramine) and of most heterocyclic agents (Table 30–2). MAO inhibitors, selective serotonin reuptake inhibitors, and bupropion are more likely to cause CNS-stimulating effects.

Table 30–2. Pharmacodynamics of common tricyclic antidepressants, heterocyclic agents, and selective serotonin reuptake inhibitors (SSRIs).[1,2]

Drug	Sedation	Muscarinic Receptor Block	NE Reuptake Block	5-HT Reuptake Block
Tricyclics				
Amitriptyline, doxepin	+++	+++	++	+++
Desipramine, protriptyline	+	+	+++	−
Imipramine, nortriptyline	++	+	+	++
Heterocyclics (second-generation)				
Amoxapine	++	+	++	+
Bupropion	−	−	−	−
Trazodone	+++	−	−	++
Maprotiline	++	+	+++	−
Heterocyclics (third-generation)				
Mirtazapine	+++	−	−	−
Nefazodone	+	−	+	++
Venlafaxine	−	−	+++	++
SSRIs				
Fluoxetine, paroxetine, sertraline	−	+	−	+++

[1]Similar drugs have been grouped together for study purposes even though they may not be identical in their actions.
[2]Key: − = none; + = slight; ++ = moderate; +++ = marked. NE, neuroepinephrine; 5-HT, serotonin.

3. **Muscarinic receptor blockade:** Antagonism of muscarinic receptors occurs with all tricyclics and is particularly marked with amitriptyline and doxepin (Table 30–2). The newer agents appear to be less potent antimuscarinics; atropine-like effects are minimal with selective serotonin reuptake inhibitors, bupropion, and trazodone.

4. **Cardiovascular effects:** Cardiovascular effects include hypotension—from alpha-adrenoceptor blockade—and depression of cardiac conduction. The latter effect may lead to arrhythmias.

5. **Seizures:** Because the convulsive threshold is lowered by tricyclic drugs and by MAO inhibitors, seizures may occur with overdoses of these agents. Overdoses of maprotiline and the SSRIs have also caused seizures.

D. **Clinical Use:**

1. **Major depressive disorders:** Endogenous depression is the major clinical indication for the antidepressant drugs. Patients typically vary in their responsiveness to individual agents. Because of more tolerable side effects and safety in overdose (see below), the newer drugs (SSRIs, certain heterocyclics) are now the most widely prescribed agents. They are sometimes effective in patients refractory to tricyclics or MAO inhibitors. As alternative agents, tricyclic drugs continue to be most useful in patients with psychomotor retardation, sleep disturbances, poor appetite, and weight loss. MAO inhibitors may be most useful in patients with significant anxiety, phobic features, and hypochondriasis. Selective serotonin reuptake inhibitors may decrease appetite; overweight patients often lose weight on these drugs.

2. **Other clinical uses:** Tricyclic drugs are also used in the treatment of bipolar affective disorders, acute panic attacks, phobic disorders (compare with alprazolam, Chapter 22), enuresis, and chronic pain states. Clomipramine and the selective serotonin reuptake inhibitors are effective in obsessive-compulsive disorders. SSRIs are also effective in patients who suffer from panic attacks or from bulimia and may be useful in the treatment of alcohol dependence. Bupropion was recently approved for management of patients with nicotine dependence.

E. **Toxicity:**

1. **Tricyclics:** The adverse effects of tricyclic antidepressants are largely predictable from their pharmacodynamic actions. These include (1) excessive sedation, lassitude, fatigue, and occasionally confusion; (2) sympathomimetic effects, including tachycardia, agitation, sweating, and insomnia; (3) atropine-like effects; (4) orthostatic hypotension, ECG abnormalities, and cardiomyopathies; and (5) tremor and paresthesias. Overdosage with tricyclics is extremely hazardous, and the ingestion of as little as a 2-week supply has been lethal. Manifestations include (1) agitation, delirium, neuromuscular irritability, convulsions, and coma; (2) respiratory depression and circulatory collapse; (3) hyperpyrexia; and (4) cardiac conduction defects and severe arrhythmias. The "three Cs" of coma, convulsions, and cardiotoxicity are characteristic.

    Tricyclic drug interactions (Table 30–3) include additive depression of the CNS with other central depressants, including ethanol, barbiturates, benzodiazepines, and opioids. Tricyclics may also cause reversal of the antihypertensive action of guanethidine by blockade of active guanethidine accumulation into sympathetic nerve endings. Less commonly, tricyclics may interfere with the antihypertensive actions of methylnorepinephrine (the active metabolite of methyldopa) and clonidine.

2. **Heterocyclic drug toxicity:** Mirtazapine and trazodone cause sedative effects. Amoxapine, maprotiline, mirtazapine, and trazodone cause some autonomic effects. Amoxapine is also a dopamine receptor blocker and may cause akathisia, parkinsonism, and the amenorrhea-galactorrhea syndrome. Adverse effects of bupropion include dizziness, dry mouth, aggravation of psychosis, and, at high doses, seizures. Seizures and cardiotoxicity are prominent features of overdosage with amoxapine and maprotiline. Venlafaxine has stimulant effects similar to those of the SSRIs. Both nefazodone and venlafaxine are inhibitors of cytochrome P450 isozymes. Through this action, nefazodone inhibits the metabolism of alprazolam and triazolam, and venlafaxine inhibits the metabolism of haloperidol (see Table 30–3).

3. **SSRI toxicity:** Fluoxetine and the other SSRIs may cause nausea, headache, anxiety, agitation, insomnia, and sexual dysfunction. Jitteriness can be alleviated by starting with low doses or by adjunctive use of benzodiazepines. Extrapyramidal effects early in treatment may include akathisia, dyskinesias, and dystonic reactions. Seizures are a consequence of

Table 30–3. Drug interactions observed with antidepressant medications.

Antidepressant	Taken With	Consequence
Fluoxetine	Lithium, tricyclics, warfarin	Increased blood levels of the second drug; doses may need to be decreased
Fluvoxamine	Alprazolam, theophylline, tricyclics, warfarin	Increased blood levels of the second drug; doses may need to be decreased
MAO inhibitors	Sympathomimetics, tyramine, SSRIs	Hypertensive crisis; "serotonin syndrome"
Nefazodone	Alprazolam, triazolam	Increased blood levels of the second drug; doses may need to be decreased
Paroxetine	Procyclidine, theophylline, tricyclics, warfarin	Increased blood levels of the second drug; doses may need to be decreased
Sertraline	Tricyclics, warfarin	Increased effects of tricyclic drug or warfarin; doses may need to be decreased
Tricyclics	CNS depressants (ethanol, sedative-hypnotics, etc)	Additive CNS depression[1]
	Clonidine, guanethidine, methyldopa	Decreased antihypertensive effects

[1]Includes tricyclics and heterocyclics with sedative actions (eg, mirtazapine, nefazodone, and trazodone).

gross overdosage. A withdrawal syndrome has been described for SSRIs that includes nausea, dizziness, anxiety, tremor, and palpitations. The SSRIs are potent inhibitors of hepatic cytochrome P450 isozymes, an action that has led to increased activity of other drugs, including tricyclic antidepressants and warfarin. Fluvoxamine inhibits the metabolism of astemizole, cisapride, and terfenadine, which may lead to cardiotoxicity (see Table 30–3). Dexfenfluramine, a drug related to the SSRIs, was recently withdrawn from the market in the USA because of reports of cardiac valve damage that occurred during treatment with dexfenfluramine and phentermine ("fen-phen").

4. **MAO inhibitor toxicity:** Adverse effects of the MAO inhibitors include hypertensive reactions in response to indirectly acting sympathomimetics, hyperthermia, and CNS stimulation leading to agitation and convulsions. Hypertensive crisis may occur in patients taking MAO inhibitors who consume food that contains high concentrations of the indirect sympathomimetic tyramine (see Table 30–3). In the absence of indirect sympathomimetics, MAO inhibitors typically *lower* blood pressure; overdosage with these drugs may result in shock, hyperthermia, and seizures. MAO inhibitors should not be administered together with fluoxetine or other selective serotonin reuptake inhibitors because their combined use has caused a life-threatening **"serotonin syndrome"** characterized by hyperthermia, muscle rigidity, myoclonus, and rapid changes in mental status and vital signs.

DRUG LIST

The following drugs are important members of the group discussed in this chapter. Prototypes should be learned in detail; features of the major variants should be known well enough so that the variants can be distinguished from prototypes and from each other; the other significant agents should be recognized as belonging to a specific subclass.

Subclass	Prototype	Major Variants	Other Significant Agents
Tricyclic drugs	Amitriptyline, imipramine	Desipramine, nortriptyline	Clomipramine, doxepin, protriptyline
Heterocyclics (second-generation)	Amoxapine, bupropion, maprotiline, trazodone		
Heterocyclics (third-generation)	Mirtazapine, nefazodone, venlafaxine		
Selective serotonin reuptake inhibitors	Fluoxetine	Fluvoxamine	Paroxetine, sertraline
MAO inhibitors	Phenelzine, moclobemide	Tranylcypromine	Isocarboxazid

QUESTIONS

DIRECTIONS: Each of the numbered items or incomplete statements in this section is followed by answers or by completions of the statement. Select the ONE lettered answer or completion that is BEST in each case.

1. A 28-year-old woman presents with symptoms of major depression that are unrelated to a general medical condition, bereavement, or substance abuse. She is not currently taking any prescription or over-the-counter medications. Drug treatment is to be initiated with a selective serotonin reuptake inhibitor. In your instructions to the patient, you would NOT tell her that
   (A) Divided doses may help to reduce nausea and gastrointestinal distress
   (B) Muscle cramps and twitches sometimes occur
   (C) She must inform you if she anticipates using other medications
   (D) Taking the drug in the evening will ensure a good night's sleep
   (E) The drug may require 2 weeks or more to become effective

2. Concerning the proposed mechanisms of action of antidepressant drugs, which one of the following statements is LEAST accurate?
   (A) Bupropion is not an effective inhibitor of NE or 5-HT transporters
   (B) Chronic treatment with an antidepressant often leads to the down-regulation of adrenoceptors
   (C) Elevation of amine metabolites in cerebrospinal fluid may be noted in most depressed patients prior to drug therapy
   (D) MAO inhibitors used as antidepressants decrease the metabolism of norepinephrine, serotonin, and dopamine
   (E) The acute effect of most tricyclics is to block the neuronal reuptake of both norepinephrine and serotonin in the CNS

3. Which one of the following effects does NOT occur with amitriptyline?
   (A) Alpha-adrenoceptor blockade
   (B) Elevation of the seizure threshold
   (C) Mydriasis
   (D) Sedation
   (E) Urinary retention

4. A 54-year-old male patient was using fluoxetine for depression but decided to stop taking the drug. When questioned he said that it affected his sexual performance and that "he wasn't getting any younger." If you decide to reinstitute drug therapy in this patient, the best choice would be
   (A) Amoxapine
   (B) Bupropion
   (C) Imipramine
   (D) Sertraline
   (E) Venlafaxine

5. Regarding the clinical use of antidepressant drugs, which one of the following statements is LEAST accurate?
   (A) Patients should be advised not to abruptly discontinue antidepressant medications
   (B) In selecting an appropriate drug for treatment of depression, the past history of patient response to specific drugs is a valuable guide
   (C) In the treatment of major depressive disorders, sertraline is usually more effective than fluoxetine
   (D) MAO inhibitors are sometimes effective in depressions with attendant anxiety, phobic features, and hypochondriasis
   (E) Weight loss often occurs in patients taking SSRIs

Items 6–7: A patient under treatment for a major depressive disorder is brought to the emergency room after ingesting 30 times the normal daily therapeutic dose of amitriptyline.

6. Of the possible signs and symptoms in this patient, which one of the following is LEAST likely to be observed?
   (A) Acidosis
   (B) Coma and shock
   (C) Hot, dry skin
   (D) Hypotension
   (E) Pinpoint pupils

7. During the course of treatment of this patient, it would be reasonable to institute all of the following measures EXCEPT

    (A) The administration of lidocaine (to control cardiac arrhythmias)
    (B) Hemodialysis (to hasten drug elimination)
    (C) The administration of bicarbonate and KCl (to correct acidosis and hypokalemia)
    (D) Intravenous administration of diazepam (to control seizures)
    (E) Electrical pacing (to maintain the rhythm of the heart)

8. Drug interactions involving antidepressants include all of the following EXCEPT
    (A) Additive impairment of driving ability in patients taking trazodone when ethanol is ingested
    (B) Behavioral excitation and hypertension in patients taking MAO inhibitors with meperidine
    (C) Elevated plasma levels of lithium if fluoxetine is administered
    (D) Increased antihypertensive effects of methyldopa when tricyclics are administered
    (E) Prolongation of tricyclic drug half-life if cimetidine is administered

9. A recently bereaved 74-year-old woman was treated with a benzodiazepine for several weeks after the death of her husband but did not like the daytime sedation it caused. She has no major medical problems but appears rather infirm for her age and has poor eyesight. Because her depressive symptoms are not abating, you decide on a trial of an antidepressant medication. Which one of the following drugs would be the most appropriate choice for this patient?
    (A) Amitriptyline
    (B) Mirtazapine
    (C) Paroxetine
    (D) Phenelzine
    (E) Trazodone

DIRECTIONS (Items 10–15): Each set of matching questions in this section consists of a list of three to twenty-six lettered options (some of which may be figures) followed by several numbered items. For each numbered item, select the ONE lettered option that is MOST closely associated with it. Each lettered option may be selected once, more than once, or not at all.

    (A) Amoxapine
    (B) Amitriptyline
    (C) Bupropion
    (D) Clomipramine
    (E) Desipramine
    (F) Fluoxetine
    (G) Fluvoxamine
    (H) Maprotiline
    (I) Mirtazapine
    (J) Moclobemide
    (K) Phenelzine
    (L) Sertraline
    (M) Trazodone
    (N) Venlafaxine

10. This is a heterocyclic selective inhibitor of norepinephrine reuptake with four rings in its structure; despite the fact that it has sedative effects, seizures may occur in overdose

11. This tricyclic antidepressant is used primarily in the management of obsessive-compulsive disorder; it is an effective blocker of the reuptake of serotonin

12. This second-generation antidepressant drug may block dopamine receptors and has caused the amenorrhea-galactorrhea syndrome

13. This is a selective inhibitor of monoamine oxidase type A with a short half-life of less than 12 hours

14. The antidepressant actions of this drug do not appear to occur via effects on MAO or on the reuptake systems for norepinephrine or serotonin; it blocks histamine receptors

15. This is a heterocyclic drug that has limited use as an antidepressant because of its marked sedative effects; it has caused priapism, necessitating operative management

ANSWERS

    1. The SSRIs have CNS-stimulating effects. They may cause agitation, anxiety, "the jitters," and insomnia. The evening is not the best time to take such drugs. Anorexia and nausea, akathisia, dyskinesias, and dystonic reactions may occur. Because of the possibility of drug interactions, the physician needs to be informed of changes in drug regimens when maintaining a patient on antidepressants. The answer is **(D)**.

2. Levels of norepinephrine and serotonin metabolites in the cerebrospinal fluid of depressed patients prior to drug treatment are not higher than normal. Some studies have reported *decreased* levels of these metabolites. Down-regulation of adrenoceptors appears to be a common feature of all modes of chronic drug treatment of depression, including the use of drugs that have no direct actions on catecholamine receptors. The answer is **(C)**.

3. Tricyclics modify peripheral sympathetic effects in two ways: through blockade of norepinephrine reuptake at neuroeffector junctions and through alpha-adrenoceptor blockade. Sedation and atropine-like side effects are common with tricyclics, especially amitriptyline. In contrast to sedative-hypnotics, tricyclics lower the threshold to seizures. The answer is **(B)**.

4. Selective serotonin reuptake inhibitors cause sexual dysfunction in some patients, with changes in libido or erectile function. Tricyclic antidepressants may also decrease libido or prevent ejaculation. Of the heterocyclic antidepressants, bupropion is least likely to affect sexual performance. The answer is **(B)**.

5. There is no evidence that any SSRI is more effective than another in its antidepressant efficacy. While an individual patient may respond more favorably to a specific drug, several controlled studies have shown equivalent effectiveness of these agents. However, SSRIs may be more effective than tricyclic antidepressants in some patients. The answer is **(C)**.

6. Anticholinergic effects common in tricyclic drug overdosage include hot dry skin, decreased bowel sounds, tachycardia, and *dilated* pupils. Hypotension occurs frequently owing to marked blockade at alpha adrenoceptors. The answer is **(E)**.

7. Tricyclic antidepressant overdose is a medical emergency. The "three Cs"—coma, convulsions, and cardiac problems—are the most common causes of death. Widening of the QRS complex on the ECG is a major diagnostic feature of cardiac toxicity. Arrhythmias resulting from cardiac toxicity are difficult to manage; they require the use of drugs with the least effect on cardiac conduction (eg, lidocaine, phenytoin). There is no evidence that hemodialysis (or hemoperfusion) increases the rate of elimination of tricyclic antidepressants, presumably because of their large volume of distribution and their binding to tissue components. The answer is **(B)**.

8. Tricyclic drugs block the uptake of guanethidine into sympathetic nerve endings, thus *reversing* its beneficial effects on blood pressure. While the precise mechanism is not defined, the tricyclics may also block the antihypertensive effects of clonidine and methyldopa. All of the other drug interactions have been reported. The answer is **(D)**.

9. The elderly patient may be especially sensitive to antidepressant drugs that cause sedation, atropine-like side effects, or postural hypotension. Paroxetine (or another SSRI) is the best choice for this patient because of all the drugs listed it is the least likely to exert such actions. The answer is **(C)**.

10. Maprotiline is chemically similar to the tricyclic drug desipramine except that it has a tetracyclic structure. Maprotiline is almost equivalent to desipramine in terms of its sedative and muscarinic receptor blocking actions, but it has caused seizures at the top of its recommended dose range. Both drugs act selectively to block the reuptake of norepinephrine. The answer is **(H)**.

11. Clomipramine appears to have selective activity in the treatment of obsessive-compulsive disorder. Clomipramine may act via blockade of serotonin reuptake, since obsessive-compulsive disorder is also responsive to sertraline and other selective serotonin reuptake inhibitors. The answer is **(D)**.

12. Amoxapine, a metabolite of the antipsychotic drug loxapine, retains dopamine receptor-blocking action. This results in some of the adverse effects commonly associated with antipsychotic drug use, including akathisia, parkinsonism symptoms, and hyperprolactinemia. The answer is **(A)**.

13. Older MAO inhibitors have very long durations of action (weeks). Moclobemide is almost completely excreted within 12 hours and acts selectively on MAO-A, the form of the enzyme that metabolizes norepinephrine and serotonin. The drug is readily displaced from MAO by tyramine and is less likely than the older drugs to contribute to a tyramine-induced hypertensive crisis. The answer is **(J)**.

14. Mirtazapine is the first of a new subclass of antidepressants—the α_2 antagonists. The drug also blocks histamine H_1 receptors (it is quite sedating), 5-HT$_2$, and 5-HT$_3$ receptors. The answer is **(I)**.

15. Trazodone has few anticholinergic effects but is strongly sedating. The drug is sometimes used at low doses to offset the "jitters" caused by SSRIs. The patient is warned to report any prolonged or painful erections because trazodone may cause priapism. Generic trazodone is usually prescribed—the drug is 10–20 times more costly when prescribed by trade name. The answer is **(M)**.

Opioid Analgesics & Antagonists

31

OBJECTIVES

You should be able to:

- List the receptors activated by opioid analgesics and the endogenous opioid peptides.
- Given a list of major opioid agonists, rank them in order of analgesic efficacy.
- Identify opioid receptor antagonists and mixed agonist-antagonists.
- Describe the main pharmacodynamic and pharmacokinetic properties of agonist opioid analgesics and list their clinical uses.
- List the main adverse effects of acute and chronic use of opioid analgesics.
- Describe the clinical uses of the opioid receptor antagonists.
- List two opioids used for antitussive effects and one used for antidiarrheal effects.

Learn the definitions that follow.

Table 31–1. Definitions.

Term	Definition
Opiate	A drug derived from alkaloids of the opium poppy
Opioid	The class of drugs that includes opiates, opiopeptins, and all synthetic and semisynthetic drugs that mimic the actions of the opiates
Opiopeptins	Endogeneous peptides that act on opioid receptors
Opioid agonist	A drug that activates some or all opioid receptor subtypes and does not block any
Opioid antagonist	A drug that blocks some or all opioid receptor subtypes
Mixed agonist-antagonist	A drug that activates some opioid receptor subtypes and blocks others

CONCEPTS

A. Classification: Morphine and other natural derivatives of the opium poppy are **opiates.** Opiates, synthetic drugs, and the endogenous compounds that produce morphine-like effects comprise the **opioids.** The opioids are derived from several chemical subgroups, including phenanthrenes, phenylheptylamines, phenylpiperidines, morphinans, and benzomorphans. A useful subdivision of the opioids is presented in Figure 31–1.

   1. Spectrum of clinical uses: Opioid drugs can be subdivided on the basis of their major therapeutic uses (eg, as analgesics, antitussives, or antidiarrheal drugs).

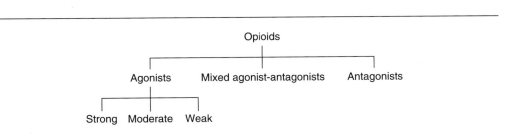

Figure 31–1. Subdivisions of drugs that act on opioid receptors.

2. **Strength of analgesia:** On the basis of their relative abilities to relieve pain, the analgesic opioids may be classified as strong, moderate, and weak agonists.
3. **Ratio of agonist to antagonist effects:** Opioid drugs may be classified as agonists (receptor activators), antagonists (receptor blockers), or mixed agonist-antagonists (drugs that activate some opioid receptors and block others).

B. **Pharmacokinetics:** Most drugs in this class are well absorbed, but morphine, hydromorphone, and oxymorphone undergo extensive first-pass metabolism when taken orally. Opioid drugs cross the placental barrier and exert effects on the fetus that can result in both respiratory depression and (with protracted exposure) physical dependence in neonates. Most opioids undergo metabolism by hepatic enzymes, usually to glucuronide conjugates, prior to their excretion by the kidney. Depending on the specific drug, the duration of their analgesic effects ranges from 1 to 2 hours (eg, fentanyl) to 6 to 8 hours (eg, buprenorphine); this may increase in patients with liver disease. One exception is remifentanil, a congener of fentanyl, which is metabolized by tissue esterases and has a very short half-life.

C. **Mechanism of Action:**
1. **Receptor mechanisms:** Some of the effects of opioid analgesics have been interpreted in terms of their interactions with specific opioid receptors in the CNS and peripheral tissues. Certain opioid receptors are located on primary afferents and spinal cord pain *transmission* neurons (ascending pathways) and on neurons in the midbrain and medulla (descending pathways) that function in pain *modulation* (Figure 31–2). Other opioid receptors that may be involved in altering *reactivity* to pain are located on neurons in the basal ganglia, the hypothalamus, the limbic structures, and the cerebral cortex. Several opioid receptor types have been cloned and characterized pharmacologically.
   a. **Mu (μ) and delta (δ) receptors:** Activation of mu and delta receptors contributes to analgesia at both spinal and supraspinal levels, to respiratory depression, and to physical dependence that can result from chronic use of some opioid analgesics.
   b. **Kappa (κ) receptors:** Kappa receptor activation contributes to spinal analgesia and plays a role in the sedative effects of opioid drugs.
2. **Opioid peptides:** Opioid receptors are thought to be activated by endogenous chemicals under physiologic conditions. Several naturally occurring peptides (opiopeptins) that produce morphine-like effects have been identified; these include two pentapeptides (leu-enkephalin and met-enkephalin), a 17-amino-acid peptide (dynorphin), and a 31-amino-acid peptide (beta-endorphin). These peptides bind to opioid receptors and can be displaced from binding by opioid antagonists. Although it remains unclear if these peptides function as classic neurotransmitters, they appear to modulate transmission at many sites in the brain and spinal cord and in primary afferents.
3. **Second messengers:** Opioid analgesics *inhibit* synaptic activity, partly through direct activation of opioid receptors and partly through release of the endogenous opiopeptins, which are themselves inhibitory to neurons. All three major opioid receptors are coupled to their effectors by G proteins and activate phospholipase C or inhibit adenylyl cyclase. Activation of these receptors either opens K^+ channels to cause membrane hyperpolarization or closes voltage-gated Ca^{2+} channels to inhibit neurotransmitter release.

D. **Acute Effects:** The acute effects of opioids include the following:
1. **Analgesia:** The opioids are the most powerful drugs available for the relief of pain. Strong agonists (ie, those with the highest analgesic efficacy) include morphine, methadone, meperidine, and fentanyl. Codeine, hydrocodone, and oxycodone are mild to moderate agonists. Propoxyphene is a very weak agonist drug.
2. **Sedation and euphoria:** These central effects may occur at doses below those required for maximum analgesia. Some patients experience dysphoria. At higher doses, the drugs may cause mental clouding and result in a stuporous state called narcosis.
3. **Respiratory depression:** Opioid actions in the medulla lead to inhibition of the respiratory center, with decreased response to carbon dioxide challenge. Increased P_{CO_2} may cause cerebrovascular dilation, resulting in increased blood flow and increased intracranial pressure.
4. **Antitussive actions:** Suppression of the cough reflex (by unknown mechanisms) is the basis for the clinical use of opioids as antitussives.

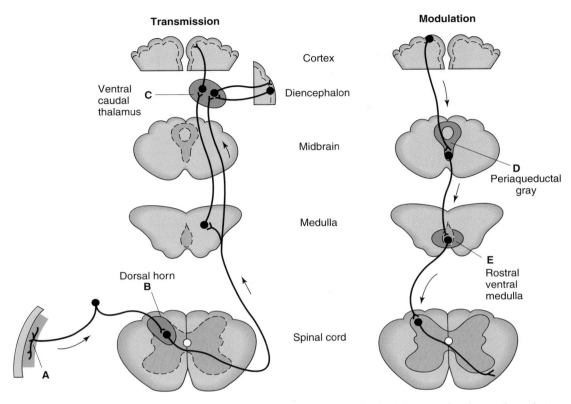

Transmission

Modulation

Cortex

Ventral caudal thalamus

C

Diencephalon

Midbrain

D
Periaqueductal gray

Medulla

E
Rostral ventral medulla

Dorsal horn
B

Spinal cord

A

Figure 31–2. Putative sites of action (darker color) of opioid analgesics. On the left, sites of action on the pain transmission pathway from the periphery to the higher centers are shown. At **A,** possible direct action of opioids on painful peripheral tissues. **B:** Inhibition occurs in the spinal cord. **C:** Possible site of action in the thalamus. On the right, actions on pain-modulating neurons in the midbrain (site **D**) and the medulla (site **E**); these actions secondarily affect pain transmission pathways. (Reproduced, with permission, from Katzung BG [editor]: *Basic & Clinical Pharmacology,* 7th ed. Appleton & Lange, 1998.)

5. **Nausea and vomiting:**   Nausea and vomiting are caused by activation of the chemoreceptor trigger zone and are increased by ambulation.
6. **Gastrointestinal effects:**   Constipation occurs through decreased intestinal peristalsis, which is probably mediated by effects on opioid receptors in the enteric nervous system. This powerful action is the basis for the clinical use of these drugs as antidiarrheal agents.
7. **Smooth muscle:**   Opioids cause contraction of biliary tract smooth muscle (which may cause biliary spasm), increased ureteral and bladder sphincter tone, and a reduction in uterine tone that may contribute to prolongation of labor.
8. **Miosis:**   Pupillary constriction is a characteristic effect of all opioids except meperidine, which has a muscarinic blocking action.

E. **Chronic Effects:**
1. **Tolerance:**   Marked tolerance develops to the above acute pharmacologic effects with the exception of miosis and constipation. There is **cross-tolerance** between different opioid agonists.
2. **Dependence:**   Psychologic and physical dependence is part of the basis for the abuse liability of many drugs in this group, particularly the strong agonists. Physical dependence is revealed on abrupt discontinuance as an **abstinence syndrome,** which includes rhinorrhea, lacrimation, chills, gooseflesh, muscle aches, diarrhea, anxiety, and hostility. A more intense state of **precipitated withdrawal** results when an opioid antagonist is administered to a physically dependent individual.

F. Clinical Use:

1. **Analgesia:** Treatment of relatively constant moderate to severe pain is the major indication. (See the Drug List for examples in each category.) In the acute setting, strong agonists are usually given parenterally. Prolonged analgesia, with some reduction in adverse effects, can be achieved with epidural administration of certain strong agonist drugs, eg, morphine. Fentanyl has been used by the transdermal route for analgesia. For more moderate pain— and in the chronic setting—moderate agonists are given by the oral route.

2. **Cough suppression:** Useful antitussive drugs include codeine and dextromethorphan. They are given orally.

3. **Treatment of diarrhea:** Selective antidiarrheal opioids include diphenoxylate and loperamide. They are given orally.

4. **Management of acute pulmonary edema:** Morphine is useful in acute pulmonary edema because of its hemodynamic actions; its calming effects probably also contribute to relief of the pulmonary symptoms. It is given parenterally.

5. **Anesthesia:** Opioids are used as preoperative medications and as intraoperative adjunctive agents in balanced anesthesia protocols. High-dose intravenous opioids (eg, morphine, fentanyl) are often the major component of anesthesia for cardiac surgery.

6. **Opioid dependence:** Methadone, one of the longer-acting opioids, is used in the management of opioid withdrawal states and in maintenance programs for addicts. In withdrawal states, methadone permits a slow tapering of opioid effect, which diminishes the intensity of abstinence symptoms. Buprenorphine (see below) has an even longer duration of action and is sometimes used in withdrawal states. In maintenance programs, the prolonged action of methadone blocks the euphoria-inducing effects of doses of shorter-acting opioids (eg, heroin, morphine).

G. Toxicity: Most of the adverse effects of the opioid analgesics (eg, constipation) are predictable extensions of their pharmacologic effects. In addition, overdose and drug interaction toxicities are very important.

1. **Overdose:** Coma with marked respiratory depression and hypotension are common and may be fatal if untreated. Diagnosis of overdosage is confirmed if intravenous injection of naloxone, an antagonist drug, results in prompt signs of recovery. Treatment of overdose involves the use of antagonists such as naloxone and other therapeutic measures, especially respiratory support.

2. **Drug interactions:** The most important drug interactions involving opioid analgesics are additive CNS depression with ethanol, sedative-hypnotics, anesthetics, antipsychotic drugs, tricyclic antidepressants, and antihistamines. Concomitant use of certain opioids (eg, meperidine) with MAO inhibitors increases the risk of hyperpyrexic coma.

H. Agonist-Antagonist and Partial Agonist Drugs:

1. **Analgesic activity:** The analgesic activity of some mixed agonist-antagonists (eg, butorphanol, nalbuphine) may be close to that of strong agonist drugs; others (eg, pentazocine) have only moderate efficacy. Buprenorphine, a partial agonist at mu receptors, is considered to be a strong analgesic.

2. **Receptors:** Butorphanol, nalbuphine, and pentazocine are kappa agonists, with weak mu receptor antagonist activity. This can lead to unpredictable results if these mixed agonist-antagonist drugs are used together with pure agonists. Buprenorphine has a long duration of effect since it binds strongly to mu receptors; this property renders its effects resistant to naloxone reversal.

3. **Effects:** The mixed agonist-antagonist drugs usually cause sedation at analgesic doses. Dizziness, sweating, and nausea may also occur, and anxiety, hallucinations, and nightmares are possible adverse effects. Respiratory depression may be less intense than with pure agonists but is not as predictably reversed by naloxone. Tolerance develops with chronic use but is less than the tolerance that develops to the pure agonists; there is minimal cross-tolerance. Physical dependence occurs, but the abuse liability of mixed agonist-antagonist drugs is less than that of the full agonists (eg, fentanyl, morphine, meperidine).

I. Opioid Antagonists: Naloxone and naltrexone are pure opioid receptor antagonists that have few other effects at doses that produce marked antagonism of agonist opioids. The major clinical use of the opioid antagonists is in the management of acute opioid overdose. Naloxone is given intravenously. Because it has a short duration of action (1–2 hours), multiple doses of naloxone may be required in opioid analgesic overdose. Naltrexone decreases the craving for ethanol and is approved for adjunctive use in alcohol dependency programs. It has a duration of action of 24–48 hours following oral use.

DRUG LIST

The following drugs are important members of the group discussed in this chapter. Prototypes should be learned in detail; features of the major variants should be known well enough so that the variants can be distinguished from prototypes and from each other; the other significant agents should be recognized as belonging to a specific subclass.

Subclass	Prototypes	Major Variants	Other Significant Agents
Strong agonists	Morphine	Heroin, meperidine, methadone	Fentanyl, levorphanol
Moderate agonists	Codeine		Oxycodone, hydrocodone
Weak agonists	Propoxyphene		
Partial agonists	Buprenorphine		
Mixed agonist-antagonists	Pentazocine	Nalbuphine	Butorphanol
Antagonists	Naloxone	Naltrexone	
Antitussives	Dextromethorphan		Codeine
Antidiarrheals	Diphenoxylate		Loperamide

QUESTIONS

DIRECTIONS: Each of the numbered items or incomplete statements in this section is followed by answers or by completions of the statement. Select the ONE lettered answer or completion that is BEST in each case.

Items 1–2: Following surgery for prostatic carcinoma, a 63-year-old man is undergoing radiation treatment as an outpatient because the tumor has metastasized to bone. He has pain in his right hip that is exacerbated when he sits down and backache when he moves about. The pain has been managed with a fixed combination of oxycodone plus acetaminophen taken orally. Despite increasing doses of the analgesic combination, the pain is getting worse.

1. If you decide to continue oral medication for the increasing pain, the best choice of drug for this patient would be
   (A) Butorphanol
   (B) Codeine plus aspirin
   (C) Levorphanol
   (D) Pentazocine
   (E) Propoxyphene

2. If the appropriate oral drug is prescribed, the patient will experience more pain relief (at least initially) and, possibly, some euphoria. However, he may have problems with nausea and sedation. Because of tolerance, it is possible that this patient will have to increase the dose of the analgesic as his condition progresses. One can anticipate that tolerance to the drug will reduce each of the following effects EXCEPT
   (A) Constipation
   (B) Euphoria
   (C) Nausea and vomiting
   (D) Sedation
   (E) Urinary retention

3. Which one of the following actions of opioid analgesics is mediated via activation of kappa receptors?
   (A) Cerebrovascular dilation

    (B) Decreased uterine tone
    (C) Euphoria
    (D) Spinal analgesia
    (E) Psychologic dependence

4. You are on your way to take an examination and you suddenly get an attack of diarrhea. If you stop at a nearby drugstore for an over-the-counter opioid with antidiarrheal action, you will be asking for
    (A) Codeine
    (B) Dextromethorphan
    (C) Diphenoxylate
    (D) Loperamide
    (E) Nalbuphine

5. Fentanyl transdermal patches have been used postoperatively to provide transdermal analgesia. The most dangerous adverse effect of this mode of administration is
    (A) Cutaneous reactions
    (B) Diarrhea
    (C) Hypertension
    (D) Relaxation of skeletal muscle
    (E) Respiratory depression

6. A patient injured in an auto accident received an intramuscular injection of 80 mg of meperidine. He subsequently developed a severe reaction characterized by tachycardia, hypertension, hyperpyrexia, and seizures. When questioned, the uninjured spouse revealed that the patient has been taking a drug for a psychiatric condition. Which of the following psychiatric drugs is most likely to be responsible for this untoward interaction with meperidine?
    (A) Alprazolam
    (B) Fluoxetine
    (C) Lithium
    (D) Paroxetine
    (E) Phenelzine

7. A patient (weight 50 kg) with moderate pain was given a high dose (60 mg) of pentazocine intramuscularly at 10 AM. At 10:15 AM, the pain intensified and then continued to get worse. At 10:30 AM, 10 mg of morphine was given intramuscularly. Unfortunately, the addition of morphine provided little additional analgesia for a further period of 90 minutes. The most plausible explanation for this type of drug interaction is that pentazocine is
    (A) An agonist at kappa receptors
    (B) An inhibitor of bioactivation of morphine
    (C) An inducer of hepatic cytochrome P450
    (D) An antagonist or partial agonist at mu and delta receptors
    (E) Interfering with the systemic absorption of morphine

8. Opioid analgesics are either contraindicated or must be used with extreme caution in several clinical situations. For morphine, such situations include all of the following EXCEPT
    (A) Adrenal insufficiency
    (B) Biliary tract surgery
    (C) Hypothyroidism
    (D) Late stage of labor
    (E) Pulmonary edema

Items 9–10: A heroin addict comes to the emergency room in an anxious and agitated state. He complains of chills, muscle aches, and diarrhea; he has also been vomiting. His symptoms include hyperventilation and hyperthermia. He claims to have had an intravenous "fix" approximately 12 hours ago. The physician notes that pupil size is greater than normal.

9. What is the most likely cause of these signs and symptoms?
    (A) The patient has overdosed with an opioid
    (B) These are early signs of the toxicity of MPTP, a contaminant in "street heroin"
    (C) The signs and symptoms are those of the abstinence syndrome
    (D) In addition to opioids, the patient has been taking barbiturates
    (E) The patient has hepatitis B

10. Which one of the following will be most effective in alleviating the symptoms experienced by this patient?

(A) Acetaminophen
(B) Buprenorphine
(C) Codeine
(D) Diazepam
(E) Naltrexone

DIRECTIONS (Items 11–15): Each set of matching questions in this section consists of a list of three to twenty-six lettered options (some of which may be figures) followed by several numbered items. For each numbered item, select the ONE lettered option that is MOST closely associated with it. Each lettered option may be selected once, more than once, or not at all.

(A) Buprenorphine
(B) Butorphanol
(C) Codeine
(D) Dextromethorphan
(E) Diphenoxylate
(F) Fentanyl
(G) Meperidine
(H) Methadone
(I) Morphine
(J) Nalbuphine
(K) Naloxone
(L) Naltrexone
(M) Oxycodone
(N) Propoxyphene

11. This drug has analgesic efficacy equivalent to that of morphine; the agent is an antagonist at mu receptors

12. This antagonist drug has been proposed as a maintenance drug in treatment programs for opioid addicts; a single oral dose will block the effects of injected heroin for up to 48 hours

13. This drug is an effective antitussive; it is free of analgesic and addictive properties and only rarely causes constipation

14. This drug is a full agonist at opioid receptors. It has excellent oral bioavailability, analgesic activity equivalent to that of morphine, and a longer duration of action. Withdrawal signs on abrupt discontinuance are milder than those associated with withdrawal from morphine

15. In some studies, this opioid agonist is reported to have analgesic efficacy no greater than that of a placebo; the drug may cause seizures in overdosage

ANSWERS

1. In most situations, pain associated with metastatic carcinoma will ultimately necessitate the use of an opioid analgesic that is equivalent in strength to morphine, so levorphanol would be indicated. Pentazocine or the combination of codeine plus salicylate are unlikely to be as effective as the original drug combination. Propoxyphene is less active than codeine alone. Butorphanol is a strong agent but is only available for parenteral injection. The answer is **(C).**

2. Chronic use of strong opioid analgesics leads to the development of tolerance to their analgesic, euphoric, and sedative actions. Tolerance also develops to their emetic effects and to effects on some smooth muscle, including the urethral sphincter muscle. However, tolerance does not develop to the constipating or miotic actions of the opioid analgesics. The answer is **(A).**

3. Kappa receptor activation does not appear to be responsible for dependence, euphoria, or effects on smooth muscle. Increases in cerebral blood flow and (possibly) increased intracranial pressure result from the respiratory depressant actions of opioid analgesics. The latter effects are due to increased arterial P_{CO_2}, which results from mu receptor inhibition of the medullary respiratory center. However, the activation of kappa receptors contributes to analgesia at the spinal level and is probably responsible for sedative actions of the opioids. The answer is **(D).**

4. Codeine and possibly nalbuphine could decrease gastrointestinal peristalsis but not without marked side effects (and a prescription). Dextromethorphan is a cough suppressant. The other two drugs listed are opioids with antidiarrheal actions. Diphenoxylate is not available over-the-

counter since it is a constituent of a proprietary combination that includes atropine sulfate (Lomotil, others). Loperamide is available over-the-counter. The answer is **(D)**.

5. The fentanyl transdermal patch releases the drug over 72 hours. The blood levels achieved will often provide analgesia for postoperative pain but at the same time will increase arterial P_{CO_2} because of depression of the brain stem respiratory center. This effect has contributed to severe respiratory depression with occasional fatalities. The answer is **(E)**.

6. Concomitant administration of meperidine and MAO inhibitors has resulted in life-threatening hyperpyrexic reactions that may culminate in seizures or coma. Such reactions have even occurred when phenelzine was administered 14 days after a patient had been treated with meperidine! The answer is **(E)**.

7. Pentazocine is either a partial agonist or a weak agonist at mu and delta receptors. Its occupancy of these receptors can block the binding of pure agonists such as morphine. The result can be antagonism of morphine analgesia or a delay in its onset. The answer is **(D)**.

8. Intravenous morphine relieves the dyspnea of pulmonary edema associated with left ventricular failure. The mechanism may involve a decrease in perception of shortness of breath, relief of anxiety, and reductions in cardiac preload (decreased venous tone) and afterload (decreased peripheral resistance). Opioids cause exaggerated effects in Addison's disease and hypothyroidism, are contraindicated in head injury because they increase intracranial pressure, and may cause biliary muscle spasm. If given during labor, they may cause respiratory depression in the newborn. The answer is **(E)**.

9. The signs and symptoms are those of withdrawal in a patient physically dependent on an opioid agonist. Such signs and symptoms usually start within 6–10 hours after the last dose; their intensity depends on the degree of physical dependence that has developed. Effects usually peak at 36–48 hours. Mydriasis is a prominent feature of the abstinence syndrome; other symptoms include rhinorrhea, lacrimation, piloerection, and yawning. The answer is **(C)**.

10. Prevention of signs and symptoms of withdrawal after chronic use of a strong opiate like heroin usually requires replacement with another strong opioid analgesic drug such as methadone. However, the partial agonist drug buprenorphine is also effective and has an even longer duration of action than methadone. Acetaminophen and codeine will not be effective. Beneficial effects of diazepam are restricted to relief of anxiety and agitation. The answer is **(B)**.

11. Mixed agonist-antagonist drugs may have analgesic efficacy almost equivalent to that of strong agonists. This is true for nalbuphine despite its antagonist action at mu receptors. Use of drugs in the agonist-antagonist subclass may lead to unpredictable results if combined with full agonists; agonist-antagonist drugs may precipitate an abstinence syndrome by blocking opioid receptors. While these drugs are less likely to cause respiratory depression, reversal with opioid antagonists is unpredictable if respiratory depression does occur. The answer is **(J)**.

12. The opioid antagonist naltrexone has a much longer half-life than naloxone, and effects may last 2 days. A high degree of client compliance would be required for naltrexone to be of value in opioid dependence treatment programs. The same reservation is applicable with regard to the use of naltrexone in alcoholism. The answer is **(L)**.

13. Dextromethorphan, an effective antitussive drug, is the dextrorotatory stereoisomer of levorphanol. Dextromethorphan has no appreciable analgesic activity and minimal abuse liability. In comparison with codeine, also an effective antitussive, dextromethorphan causes less constipation. The answer is **(D)**.

14. The other full agonists—fentanyl, hydromorphone, levorphanol, meperidine, methadone, and oxymorphone—are all equivalent to morphine in analgesic efficacy. Methadone has the greatest bioavailability of the drugs used orally, and its effects are more prolonged. Tolerance and physical dependence develop and dissipate more slowly with methadone than with morphine. Levorphanol also has high bioavailability. These properties underlie the use of methadone for detoxification and maintenance programs. The answer is **(H)**.

15. Propoxyphene is chemically related to methadone but has very low analgesic activity. Propoxyphene causes a small additive analgesic effect when used in combination with aspirin or acetaminophen. Overdosage of propoxyphene results in severe toxicity, including respiratory depression, circulatory collapse, pulmonary edema, and seizures. The answer is **(N)**.

Drugs of Abuse

32

OBJECTIVES

You should be able to:

- Describe the major actions of drugs that are commonly abused.
- Describe the major signs and symptoms of overdose with, and withdrawal from, CNS stimulants, opioid analgesics, and sedative-hypnotics, including ethanol.
- Identify the most likely causes of death from commonly abused agents.

Learn the definitions that follow.

Table 32–1. Definitions.	
Term	**Definition**
Tolerance	A decreased response to a drug, necessitating larger doses to achieve the same effect. This can result from increased disposition of the drug (metabolic tolerance), an ability to compensate for the effects of a drug (behavioral tolerance), or changes in receptor or effector systems involved in drug actions (functional tolerance)
Psychologic dependence	Compulsive drug-using behavior in which the individual uses the drug for personal satisfaction, often in spite of known risks to health
Physiologic dependence	A state characterized by signs and symptoms, frequently the opposite of those *caused* by a drug, when it is withdrawn from chronic use or when the dose is abruptly lowered. Psychologic dependence usually precedes physiologic dependence
Abstinence syndrome	A term used to describe the signs and symptoms that occur on withdrawal of a drug in a physiologically dependent person
Controlled substance	A drug deemed to have abuse liability that is listed on governmental Schedules of Controlled Drugs.[1] Such schedules categorize illicit drugs, control prescribing practices, and mandate penalties for illegal possession, manufacture, and sale of listed drugs. Controlled substance schedules are presumed to reflect current attitudes toward substance abuse; therefore, which drugs are regulated depends on a social judgment
Designer drug	A synthetic derivative of a drug, with slightly modified structure but no major change in pharmacodynamic action. Circumvention of the Schedules of Controlled Drugs is a motivation for the illicit synthesis of designer drugs

[1] An example of such a schedule promulgated by the United States Drug Enforcement Agency is shown in Table 32–2. Note that the criteria given by the agency do not always reflect the actual pharmacologic properties of the drugs.

CONCEPTS

Drug abuse is usually taken to mean the use of an illicit drug, or the excessive or nonmedical use of a licit drug. It also denotes the deliberate use of chemicals that generally are not considered drugs by the lay public but may be harmful to the user. The motivation for drug abuse appears to be the anticipated feeling of pleasure derived from the CNS effects of the drug. If physiologic dependence is present, prevention of an abstinence syndrome acts as reinforcement to continued drug abuse.

MAJOR CATEGORIES OF DRUGS OF ABUSE

A. Sedative-Hypnotics: The sedative-hypnotic drugs are responsible for many cases of drug abuse in the United States, Europe, and Japan. The group includes **ethanol, barbiturates,** and **benzodiazepines,** all of which are more readily available to the general public than are opioids, cocaine, or hallucinogens. Benzodiazepines are the most commonly prescribed drugs for anxiety and, as Schedule IV drugs, are judged by the United States government to have low abuse liability (Table 32–2). Ethanol is not listed in schedules of controlled substances with abuse liability.

1. **Effects:** Sedative-hypnotics reduce inhibitions, suppress anxiety, and produce relaxation. All of these actions are thought to encourage repetitive use and the development of psychologic dependence. The drugs are CNS depressants, and their depressant effects are enhanced by concomitant use of opioid analgesics, antipsychotic agents, marijuana, and any other drug with sedative properties. Acute overdoses commonly result in death through depression of the medullary respiratory and cardiovascular centers (see Table 32–3). Flunitrazepam (Rohypnol), a potent rapid-onset benzodiazepine with marked amnestic properties, has been used in "date rape."

2. **Withdrawal:** Physiologic dependence occurs with continued use of sedative-hypnotics; the signs and symptoms of the withdrawal (abstinence) syndrome are most pronounced with drugs that have a half-life of less than 24 hours (eg, ethanol, secobarbital, methaqualone). However, physiologic dependence may occur with any sedative-hypnotic, including the longer-acting benzodiazepines. The most important signs of withdrawal derive from excessive **CNS stimulation,** and include anxiety, tremor, nausea and vomiting, delirium, and hallucinations (see Table 32–3). **Seizures** are not uncommon and may be life-threatening.

    Treatment of sedative-hypnotic withdrawal involves administration of a long-acting sedative-hypnotic (eg, chlordiazepoxide or diazepam) to suppress the acute withdrawal syndrome, followed by a gradual reduction of the dose. Clonidine or propranolol may also be of value to suppress sympathetic overactivity.

    A syndrome of **therapeutic withdrawal** has occurred on discontinuance of sedative-hypnotics after long-term treatment. In addition to the symptoms of classic withdrawal listed above, this syndrome includes weight loss, paresthesias, and headache. (See Chapters 22 and 23 for additional details.)

B. **Opioid Analgesics:**

1. **Effects:** The most commonly abused drugs in this group are **heroin, morphine, oxycodone,** and—among health professionals—**meperidine** and **fentanyl.** The effects of intravenous heroin are described by abusers as a "rush" or orgasmic feeling followed by euphoria and then sedation. Intravenous administration of opioids is associated with rapid development of tolerance and psychologic and physiologic dependence. Oral administration or smoking of opioids causes milder effects, with a slower onset of tolerance and dependence. Overdose of opioids leads to respiratory depression progressing to coma and death (see Table 32–3). Overdose is managed with intravenous naloxone and ventilatory support.

2. **Withdrawal:** Deprivation of opioids in physiologically dependent individuals leads to an abstinence syndrome that includes lacrimation, rhinorrhea, yawning, sweating, weakness, gooseflesh ("cold turkey"), nausea and vomiting, tremor, and hyperpnea. Although extremely unpleasant, withdrawal from opioids is rarely fatal (unlike withdrawal from sedative-hypnotics). Treatment involves replacement of the illicit drug with a pharmacologically equivalent agent (eg, methadone), followed by slow dose reduction.

Table 32–2. Schedules of Controlled Drugs.*

Schedule	Criteria	Examples
I	No medical use; high addiction potential	Heroin, LSD, mescaline, methaqualone, PCP, DOM, MDMA
II	Medical use; high addiction potential	Strong opioid agonists, cocaine, short-half-life barbiturates, amphetamines, cannabinols
III	Medical use; moderate potential for dependence	Moderate opioid agonists (codeine), thiopental
IV	Medical use; low abuse potential	Benzodiazepines, chloral hydrate, meprobamate, weak opioid agonists

*Adapted, with permission, from Katzung BG (editor): *Basic & Clinical Pharmacology,* 7th ed. Appleton & Lange, 1998.

Table 32–3. Signs and symptoms of overdose and withdrawal for selected drugs of abuse.

Drug	Overdose Effects	Withdrawal Symptoms
Amphetamines, methylphenidate, cocaine[1]	Agitation, hypertension, tachycardia, delusions, hallucinations, hyperthermia, seizures, death	Apathy, irritability, increased sleep time, disorientation, depression
Barbiturates, benzodiazepines, ethanol[2]	Slurred speech, "drunken" behavior, dilated pupils, weak and rapid pulse, clammy skin, shallow respiration, coma, death	Anxiety, insomnia, delirium, tremors, seizures, death
Heroin, other opioid analgesics	Constricted pupils, clammy skin, nausea, drowsiness, respiratory depression, coma, death	Nausea, chills, sweats, cramps, lacrimation, rhinorrhea, yawning, hyperpnea, tremor

[1]Cardiac arrhythmias, myocardial infarction, and stroke occur more frequently in cocaine overdose than with other CNS stimulants.
[2]Ethanol withdrawal includes the excited hallucinatory state of delirium tremens.

C. **Stimulants:**   A chemically heterogeneous group, the stimulants include caffeine, nicotine, amphetamines, and cocaine.
   1. **Caffeine and nicotine:**
       a. **Effects:**   Caffeine (in beverages) and nicotine (in tobacco products) are legal in most Western cultures even though they have adverse medical effects. In the USA, cigarette smoking is now the major preventable cause of death; tobacco use is associated with a high incidence of cardiovascular, respiratory, and neoplastic disease. Psychologic dependence on caffeine and nicotine has been recognized for some time. More recently, demonstration of abstinence signs and symptoms has provided evidence for physiologic dependence.
       b. **Withdrawal:**   Withdrawal from caffeine is accompanied by lethargy, irritability, and headache. The anxiety, craving, and mental discomfort experienced on discontinuing nicotine are major impediments to discontinuing its use.
       c. **Toxicity:**   Acute toxicity from overdosage of caffeine or nicotine includes excessive CNS stimulation with tremor, insomnia, and nervousness; cardiac stimulation and arrhythmias; and, in the case of nicotine, respiratory paralysis (Chapters 6 and 7), although the latter probably never occurs from the use of tobacco products.
   2. **Amphetamines:**
       a. **Effects:**   Amphetamines cause a feeling of euphoria and self-confidence that contributes to the rapid development of psychologic dependence. Drugs in this class include **dextroamphetamine** and **methamphetamine** ("speed"), a crystal form of which ("ice") can be smoked. Chronic high-dose abuse leads to a psychotic state (with delusions and paranoia) that is difficult to differentiate from schizophrenia.
       b. **Tolerance and withdrawal:**   Tolerance can be marked, and an abstinence syndrome, characterized by increased appetite, sleepiness, exhaustion, and mental depression, can occur upon withdrawal.
       c. **Congeners of amphetamines:**   Several chemical congeners of amphetamines have hallucinogenic properties. These include 2,5-dimethoxy-4-methylamphetamine (**DOM, STP**), methylene dioxyamphetamine (**MDA**), and methylene dioxymethamphetamine (**MDMA, "ecstasy"**). The last compound is purported to facilitate communication in psychotherapy, a claim made for many failed psychotherapeutic adjunct drugs in the past. These derivatives have been reported to be toxic to serotonergic neurons in the brains of animals, with uncertain toxic consequences in humans.
   3. **Cocaine:**   Cocaine has marked amphetamine-like effects ("super-speed"). Its abuse continues to be widespread in the USA, partly because of the availability of a freebase form ("crack") that can be smoked. The euphoria, self-confidence, and mental alertness produced by cocaine are short-lasting and positively reinforce its continued use.
       a. **Effects:**   Overdoses with cocaine commonly result in fatalities from arrhythmias, seizures, or respiratory depression. Cardiac toxicity is due partly to blockade of norepinephrine reuptake by cocaine; its local anesthetic action contributes to the production of seizures. In addition, the powerful vasoconstrictive action of cocaine may lead to severe hypertensive episodes, resulting in myocardial infarcts and strokes.

b. **Withdrawal:** The abstinence syndrome following withdrawal from cocaine is similar to that following amphetamine discontinuance. Severe depression of mood is common and strongly reinforces the compulsion to use the drug. Infants born to mothers who abuse cocaine (or amphetamines) have possible teratogenic abnormalities (cystic cortical lesions), increased morbidity and mortality, and may be "cocaine-dependent." The signs and symptoms of CNS stimulant overdose and withdrawal are listed in Table 32–3.

D. **Hallucinogens:**
1. **Phencyclidine:** The arylcyclohexylamine drug phencyclidine (PCP, "angel dust") is probably the most dangerous of the currently popular hallucinogenic agents. Psychotic reactions are common with PCP, and impaired judgment often leads to reckless behavior. This drug should be classified as a **psychotomimetic.** Effects of overdosage with PCP include nystagmus, marked hypertension, and seizures, which may be fatal.
2. **Miscellaneous hallucinogenic agents:** Several drugs with hallucinogenic effects have been classified as having abuse liability; these drugs include **lysergic acid diethylamide** (LSD), **mescaline,** and **psilocybin.** Hallucinogenic effects may also occur with scopolamine and other antimuscarinic agents. Terms used to describe the CNS effects of such drugs include "psychedelic" and "mind-revealing." The perceptual and psychologic effects of such drugs are usually accompanied by marked somatic effects, especially nausea, weakness, and paresthesias. Panic reactions ("bad trips") may also occur. There is little evidence that use of these agents leads to the development of physiologic dependence.

E. **Marijuana:**
1. **Classification:** Marijuana ("grass") is a collective term for the psychoactive constituents present in crude extracts of *Cannabis sativa* (hemp), the active principles of which include the compounds **tetrahydrocannabinol** (THC), cannabidiol (CBD), and cannabinol (CBN). **Hashish** is a partially purified form that is more potent.
2. **Effects:** CNS effects of marijuana include a feeling of being "high," with euphoria, disinhibition, uncontrollable laughter, changes in perception, and achievement of a dreamlike state. Mental concentration may be difficult. Vasodilation occurs, and the pulse rate is characteristically increased. Habitual users show reddened conjunctivae. A mild withdrawal state has been noted only in long-term heavy users of marijuana. The dangers of marijuana use concern its impairment of judgment and reflexes, effects that are potentiated by concomitant use of sedative-hypnotics, including ethanol. The specific hazards of long-term use are unknown. Potential therapeutic effects of marijuana include its ability to decrease intraocular pressure and its antiemetic actions. **Dronabinol** (a controlled-substance formulation of THC) is used to combat nausea in cancer chemotherapy.

F. **Inhalants:** Certain gases or volatile liquids are abused because they provide a feeling of euphoria or disinhibition. This class includes the following agents:
1. **Anesthetics:** This group includes nitrous oxide, chloroform, and diethylether. These agents are hazardous because they affect judgment and induce loss of consciousness. Inhalation of nitrous oxide as the pure gas (with no oxygen) has caused asphyxia and death. Ether is highly flammable.
2. **Industrial solvents:** Solvents and a wide range of volatile compounds are present in commercial products such as gasoline, paint thinners, aerosol propellants, glues, rubber cements, and shoe polish. Because of their ready availability, these substances are most frequently abused by children in early adolescence. Active ingredients that have been identified include benzene, hexane, methylethylketone, toluene, and trichloroethylene. Many of these are toxic to the liver, kidneys, lungs, bone marrow, and peripheral nerves and cause brain damage in animals.
3. **Organic nitrites:** Amyl nitrite, isobutyl nitrite, and other organic nitrites are referred to as "poppers" and are alleged to be sex enhancers. Inhalation of the nitrites causes dizziness, tachycardia, hypotension, and flushing. With the exception of methemoglobinemia, few serious adverse effects have been reported.

DRUG LIST

The following drugs are important members of the group discussed in this chapter. Prototypes should be learned in detail; features of the major variants should be known well enough so that the variants can be distinguished from prototypes and from each other; the other significant agents should be recognized as belonging to a specific subclass.

Subclass	Prototype	Major Variants	Other Significant Agents
Sedative-hypnotics	Ethanol, phenobarbital, chlordiazepoxide	Secobarbital, diazepam	Methaqualone, meprobamate
Opioids	Heroin	Meperidine	Strong agonist opioid analgesics
Stimulants	Amphetamine	Methamphetamine, phenmetrazine	DOM, MDA, MDMA
	Cocaine, caffeine, nicotine		
Hallucinogens	LSD, phencyclidine	Mescaline	Scopolamine
Marijuana	"Grass"	Hashish	Dronabinol
Inhalants	Nitrous oxide, toluene	Ether	Chloroform, benzene
	Amyl nitrite	Isobutyl nitrite	

QUESTIONS

DIRECTIONS: Each of the numbered items or incomplete statements in this section is followed by answers or by completions of the statement. Select the ONE lettered answer or completion that is BEST in each case.

Items 1–3:   A 42-year-old homemaker with two school-age children suffers from anxiety with phobic symptoms and occasional panic attacks. No specific medical, financial, or domestic cause can be identified. Her prescription drugs include oral contraceptives and low-dose thyroxine. She also uses over-the-counter antihistamines for allergic rhinitis. She claims that ethanol use is restricted to a glass or two of wine with dinner. After several sessions with her psychiatrist, alprazolam is prescribed. The patient continues monthly sessions with her psychiatrist and is maintained on alprazolam for 3 years with several dose increments over that time period. Her family notices that she does not seem to be improving and that her speech is often slurred in the evenings. She is finally hospitalized with severe withdrawal signs one weekend while attempting to end her dependence on drugs.

1. Which one of the following statements about the use of alprazolam in this patient is LEAST accurate?
    (A)   Additive CNS depression will occur with ethanol and with over-the-counter antihistamines
    (B)   Alternative nondrug treatments should have been tried long before 3 years had elapsed
    (C)   Tolerance can be anticipated with chronic use of any benzodiazepine
    (D)   The anxiolytic effects of sedative-hypnotic drugs encourage dependence
    (E)   If she had discontinued alprazolam after 1 month she would not have experienced any withdrawal signs at that time

2. The main reason for hospitalization of this patient was to be able to effectively control
    (A)   Anxiety
    (B)   Cardiac arrhythmias
    (C)   Respiratory depression
    (D)   Seizures
    (E)   Thyroid dysfunction

3. The symptoms being experienced by this hospitalized patient can best be ameliorated by the administration of
    (A)   Amphetamine
    (B)   Chlordiazepoxide
    (C)   Oxycodone
    (D)   Propranolol
    (E)   Secobarbital

4. Which one of the following statements about abuse of the opioid analgesics is LEAST accurate?
    (A)   A patient experiencing withdrawal from heroin is free of the symptoms of abstinence in 6–8 days

    (B)   In withdrawal from opioids, clonidine may be useful in reducing symptoms caused by sympathetic overactivity

    (C)   Lacrimation, rhinorrhea, yawning, and sweating are early signs of withdrawal from opioid analgesics

    (D)   Naloxone may precipitate a severe withdrawal state in abusers of opioid analgesics, with symptoms starting within 15–30 minutes

    (E)   Methadone alleviates most of the symptoms of heroin withdrawal

5.   A young male patient is brought to the emergency room of a hospital suffering from an overdose of cocaine following intravenous administration. His symptoms are NOT likely to include

    (A)   Agitation

    (B)   Bradycardia

    (C)   Hyperthermia

    (D)   Myocardial infarct

    (E)   Seizures

6.   Which one of the following statements about central nervous system stimulants is LEAST accurate?

    (A)   "Herbal Ecstasy" causes amphetamine-like effects

    (B)   Withdrawal from caffeine may lead to severe headaches

    (C)   MDMA ("ecstasy") is reported to be neurotoxic to brain serotonergic systems

    (D)   While psychologic dependence to amphetamines is strong, physiologic dependence does not occur

    (E)   Treatment of cocaine overdose may include the use of diazepam and propranolol

7.   Which one of the following statements about hallucinogens is LEAST accurate?

    (A)   Mescaline and related hallucinogens are thought to exert their CNS actions through serotonergic systems in the brain

    (B)   Teratogenic effects are known to occur with the use of LSD during pregnancy

    (C)   Phencyclidine is unique among hallucinogens in that animals will self-administer it

    (D)   Dilated pupils, tachycardia, tremor, and increased alertness are characteristic effects of psilocybin

    (E)   Scopolamine can be anticipated to cause blurred vision, dry mouth, and urinary retention

8.   Which one of the following statements about inhalants is LEAST accurate?

    (A)   Solvent inhalation is mainly a drug abuse problem in boys aged 8–12 years from lower socioeconomic classes

    (B)   Euphoria, numbness, and tingling sensations with visual and auditory disturbances occur in most persons who inhale 35% nitrous oxide

    (C)   Methemoglobinemia is a common toxicologic problem following repetitive inhalation of industrial solvents

    (D)   Fluorocarbons may cause sudden death due to cardiac arrhythmias

    (E)   The use of isobutyl nitrite is likely to cause headache

9.   Which one of the following signs or symptoms is LEAST likely to occur with marijuana?

    (A)   Conjunctival reddening

    (B)   Decreased psychomotor performance

    (C)   Hypotension

    (D)   Increased pulse rate

    (E)   Pupillary constriction

Items 10–11:   A college student is brought to the emergency room by friends. The physician is informed that he had taken a drug and that he "went crazy." The patient is agitated and delirious. Several persons are required to hold him down. His skin is warm and sweaty, and his pupils are dilated. Bowel sounds are normal. Signs and symptoms include tachycardia, marked hypertension, hyperthermia, increased muscle tone, and both horizontal and vertical nystagmus.

10.   The most likely cause of these signs and symptoms is intoxication due to

    (A)   Hashish

    (B)   LSD

    (C)   Mescaline

    (D)   Phencyclidine

    (E)   Scopolamine

11.   The management of this patient is LEAST likely to include

    (A)   Activated charcoal

     (B)   Benzodiazepine administration
     (C)   Haloperidol if psychosis ensues
     (D)   Nasogastric suction
     (E)   Urinary alkalinization to increase drug elimination

12. This agent has sedative and amnestic properties. Small doses added to alcoholic beverages are not readily detected by taste and have been used in "date-rape" behavior. The drug is chemically related to the brain inhibitory neurotransmitter GABA. Which one of the following MOST closely resembles the description given?
     (A)   Amyl nitrite
     (B)   Flunitrazepam
     (C)   Gamma-hydroxybutyrate
     (D)   Hashish
     (E)   Metcathinone

ANSWERS

1. Even normal therapeutic doses of benzodiazepines may lead to physiologic dependence with withdrawal symptoms. These can include increases in REM sleep (REM rebound), increased anxiety, agitation, and insomnia. The severity of withdrawal symptoms depends on the dose used and on the concomitant use of other sedative-hypnotics, including ethanol. In general, withdrawal symptoms are more severe with use of shorter-acting sedative-hypnotics. The answer is **(E)**.

2. In addition to the symptoms described above, abrupt withdrawal from sedative-hypnotic dependence may include hyperreflexia progressing to seizures, with ensuing coma and possibly death. The risk of a convulsion is increased if the patient abruptly withdraws from ethanol use at the same time. The answer is **(D)**.

3. The standard approach to detoxification during withdrawal from physiologic dependence on barbiturates, benzodiazepines, or ethanol is the use of a long-acting sedative hypnotic with dose tapering. Chlordiazepoxide or diazepam is used most frequently. The answer is **(B)**.

4. Symptoms of opioid withdrawal usually begin within 6–8 hours, and the acute course may last 6–8 days. However, a secondary phase of heroin withdrawal, characterized by bradycardia, hypotension, hypothermia, and mydriasis, may last 26–30 weeks. Methadone is commonly used in detoxification of the heroin addict because it is a strong agonist, has high oral bioavailability, and has a relatively long half-life. The answer is **(A)**.

5. Overdoses with amphetamines or cocaine have many signs and symptoms in common. However, the ability of cocaine to block the reuptake of norepinephrine at sympathetic nerve terminals results in greater cardiotoxicity. Tachycardia is the rule, with the possibility of an arrhythmia, infarct, or stroke. The answer is **(B)**.

6. Abuse of amphetamines results in marked tolerance and both psychologic and physiologic dependence. Withdrawal is manifested by signs and symptoms opposite to those produced by such drugs, including apathy and depression. "Herbal Ecstasy" is a plant extract that causes CNS stimulation, decreased appetite, insomnia, and sympathomimetic effects; its primary ingredient is ephedrine. The answer is **(D)**.

7. Psilocybin, mescaline, and LSD have similar central and peripheral effects. None of these agents have been shown to have teratogenic potential. Contrast this with the established potential for teratogenicity or other fetal toxicity with abuse of ethanol, amphetamines, and cocaine. Unlike most hallucinogens, phencyclidine acts as a positive reinforcer of self-administration in animals. The answer is **(B)**.

8. Toxic inhalants, including heptane, hexane, methylethylketone, toluene, and trichloroethylene, may result in central and peripheral neurotoxicity, liver and kidney damage, and pulmonary disease. Industrial solvents rarely cause methemoglobinemia, but this (and headaches) may occur following excessive use of nitrites. The answer is **(C)**.

9. Two of the most characteristic signs of marijuana use are increased pulse rate and reddening of the conjunctiva. Pupil size is *not* changed by marijuana. The answer is **(E)**.

10. The signs and symptoms point to phencyclidine intoxication. The presence of both horizontal and vertical nystagmus is pathognomonic. The answer is **(D)**.

11. Overdose with phencyclidine is dangerous. The basic principles of treatment are to maintain ventilation and to control seizures, blood pressure, and hyperthermia. Phencyclidine is secreted into the stomach, so removal of the drug may be hastened by activated charcoal or continual nasogastric suction. Phencyclidine is a weak base, and its renal elimination may be accelerated by urinary *acidification.* Treatment with antipsychotic drugs may be appropriate if psychotic symptoms follow the acute intoxication. The answer is **(E).**

12. Flunitrazepam fits part of the description of this "date rape" drug, but it is not chemically related to GABA. Gamma-hydroxybutyrate (GHB, "liquid ecstasy") is a popular street drug that causes amnesia and in overdose has resulted in seizures, coma, and death. Metcathinone ("cat") is a natural plant alkaloid with CNS-stimulating properties similar to amphetamine. The answer is **(C).**

Part VI: Drugs With Important Actions on Blood, Inflammation, & Gout

Agents Used in Anemias

33

OBJECTIVES

You should be able to:

- Describe the normal mechanism of regulation of iron storage in the body.
- List the major forms of iron used in the therapy of anemias.
- List the anemias for which iron supplementation is indicated and those for which it is contraindicated.
- Describe the acute and chronic toxicity of iron.
- Describe the clinical applications of vitamin B_{12} and folic acid.
- Describe the major hazard involved in the use of folic acid as sole therapy for megaloblastic anemia.
- Describe the major bone marrow colony-stimulating factors.

CONCEPTS

TYPES OF ANEMIAS

A. **Iron and Vitamin Deficiency Anemias:** Microcytic hypochromic anemia, caused by iron deficiency, is the most common type of anemia. Megaloblastic anemias are caused by a deficiency of vitamin B_{12} or folic acid, cofactors required for the normal maturation of red blood cells. Pernicious anemia, the most common type of vitamin B_{12}-deficiency anemia, is caused by a defect in the synthesis of intrinsic factor, a protein required for efficient absorption of dietary vitamin B_{12}.

B. **Other Anemias:** Anemias caused by radiation or cancer chemotherapy involve suppression of bone marrow stem cells. Development of techniques for recombinant DNA-directed synthesis of marrow growth factors (erythropoietin [epoetin alfa] and the white cell colony-stimulating factors filgrastim and sargramostim) now make possible the treatment of more patients with depressed marrow activity. Complete marrow eradication—used in the treatment of certain neoplasms—must be treated by marrow transplantation.

C. **Prototypes:** Figure 33–1 illustrates the major drugs discussed in this chapter.

IRON

A. **Role of Iron:** Iron is the essential metallic component of heme, the molecule responsible for the bulk of oxygen transport in the blood. Although most of the iron in the body is present in hemoglobin (heme plus globin), an important fraction is bound to transferrin, a transport protein, and to ferritin and hemosiderin, two storage proteins. Deficiency of iron occurs most often in women because of menstrual blood loss and in vegetarians or malnourished individuals because of inadequate dietary iron intake.

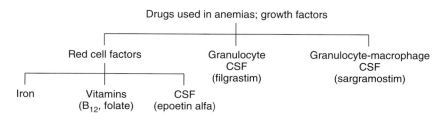

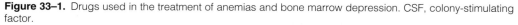

Figure 33–1. Drugs used in the treatment of anemias and bone marrow depression. CSF, colony-stimulating factor.

B. **Regulation of Iron Stores:** Regulation of body iron content occurs through modulation of absorption in the intestine. There is no mechanism for the efficient excretion of iron. As a result, failure of gastrointestinal regulation of iron absorption is one cause of diseases associated with excess iron stores, eg, hemochromatosis.

1. **Absorption:** Iron is absorbed as the ferrous ion and oxidized in the mucosal cell to the ferric form.

2. **Storage:** Trivalent (ferric) iron can be stored in the mucosa (bound to ferritin) or carried elsewhere in the body (bound to transferrin). Excess iron is stored in protein-bound form as hemosiderin in the reticuloendothelial system. An accumulation of hemosiderin occurs in hemolytic anemias (anemias caused by excess destruction of red blood cells) and in hemochromatosis.

3. **Elimination:** Minimal amounts of iron are lost from the body with sweat and saliva and in exfoliated skin and intestinal mucosal cells. As noted above, there is no efficient method for excretion of excess iron.

C. **Clinical Use:** Iron deficiency anemia is the only indication for the use of iron. Iron deficiency can be diagnosed from red blood cell changes (microcytosis, diminished hemoglobin content of blood) and from measurements of serum and bone marrow iron stores. The disease is treated by dietary ferrous iron supplementation and, in special cases, by parenteral administration of the metal (see Drug List). Iron should *not* be given in hemolytic anemia because iron stores are elevated, not depressed, in this type of anemia.

D. **Toxicity of Iron:** (See also Chapter 58.)

1. **Signs and symptoms:** Acute iron intoxication is most common in children and usually occurs as a result of accidental ingestion of iron supplementation tablets. Depending on the amount ingested and absorbed, necrotizing gastroenteritis, shock, metabolic acidosis, coma, and death may result. Chronic toxicity occurs most often in individuals who must receive frequent transfusions (eg, patients with sickle cell anemia) and in those with hemochromatosis, an inherited abnormality of iron absorption.

2. **Treatment of acute iron intoxication:** Immediate treatment is necessary and usually consists of removal of unabsorbed tablets from the gut, correction of acid-base and electrolyte abnormalities, and administration of iron-complexing agents. The latter agents include oral phosphate or carbonate salts (to precipitate unabsorbed iron) and parenteral deferoxamine, which chelates circulating iron.

3. **Treatment of chronic iron toxicity:** Treatment of hemochromatosis is usually by phlebotomy, which efficiently removes approximately 250 mg iron with each unit of blood withdrawn.

VITAMIN B$_{12}$

A. **Role of Vitamin B$_{12}$:** Vitamin B$_{12}$ (cobalamin), a cobalt-containing molecule, is (along with folic acid) a cofactor in the transfer of one-carbon units, a step necessary for the synthesis of DNA. Impairment of DNA synthesis affects all cells, but because red blood cells must be produced continuously, deficiency of either B$_{12}$ or folic acid usually is manifested first as anemia.

B. **Pharmacokinetics:**   Vitamin B_{12} is produced only by bacteria; this vitamin cannot be synthesized by multicellular organisms. It is absorbed from the gastrointestinal tract in the presence of intrinsic factor, a product of the parietal cells of the stomach. Vitamin B_{12} is stored in the liver in large amounts; a normal individual has enough to last 5 years. Plasma transport is accomplished by binding to transcobalamin II, a glycoprotein. When parenteral vitamin B_{12} is given, any in excess of the transport protein binding capacity (about 50–100 µg) is excreted. The two available forms of vitamin B_{12}, cyanocobalamin and hydroxocobalamin, have similar pharmacokinetics, but hydroxocobalamin is somewhat more firmly bound to plasma proteins and has a longer circulating half-life.

C. **Pharmacodynamics:**   Vitamin B_{12} is essential in two reactions: conversion of methylmalonyl-CoA to succinyl-CoA and conversion of homocysteine to methionine. The first of these reactions appears to be essential for lipid metabolism; a deficiency of vitamin B_{12} results in abnormalities of the lipids essential for normal neuronal function. The second reaction, conversion of homocysteine to methionine, is linked to folic acid metabolism and DNA synthesis. This reaction is essential for normal production of red blood cells.

D. **Clinical Use and Toxicity:**   Vitamin B_{12} is available as hydroxocobalamin and cyanocobalamin, which have equivalent effects. The major application is in the treatment of naturally occurring pernicious anemia and anemia caused by gastric resection. Because B_{12}-deficiency anemia is almost always caused by inadequate absorption, therapy should be parenteral. Although oral therapy may suffice for maintenance, massive doses must be used. In addition to anemia, an important manifestation of vitamin B_{12} deficiency is the development of neurologic defects, which may become irreversible if not treated promptly. Treatment is by parenteral replacement of vitamin B_{12}.

   Because hydroxocobalamin avidly binds cyanide ion to form cyanocobalamin, hydroxocobalamin has also been used successfully to treat cyanide toxicity caused by nitroprusside. Neither form of vitamin B_{12} has significant toxicity.

FOLIC ACID

A. **Role of Folic Acid:**   Folic acid is necessary for the synthesis of purines and for the formation of thymidylic acid. Because of the need for continuous production of red cells, anemia is usually the first sign of folic acid deficiency. In addition, deficiency of folic acid during pregnancy increases the risk of neural tube defects in the fetus.

B. **Pharmacokinetics:**   Folic acid is also known as pteroylglutamic acid. It is readily absorbed from the gastrointestinal tract. Only modest amounts are stored in the body, so a decrease in dietary intake is followed by anemia within a few months.

C. **Pharmacodynamics:**   Folic acid is necessary for the transfer of one-carbon fragments in the synthesis of purine and pyrimidine bases. Therefore, it is most important for the health of rapidly dividing cells, in which DNA must be rapidly synthesized. (For the same reason, *antifolate drugs* are useful in the treatment of various infections and neoplasms.)

D. **Clinical Use and Toxicity:**   Folic acid deficiency is most often caused by dietary insufficiency or by malabsorption. Anemia due to folic acid deficiency is readily treated by oral folic acid supplementation. Folic acid supplements will also correct the anemia but not the neurologic deficits of vitamin B_{12} deficiency. Therefore, vitamin B_{12} deficiency *must* be ruled out before folic acid can be chosen as the sole therapeutic agent in megaloblastic anemia. Folic acid has no recognized toxicity.

BONE MARROW COLONY-STIMULATING FACTORS

Almost a dozen glycoprotein hormones have been discovered that regulate the differentiation and maturation of stem cells within the bone marrow. Three substances are now available, through recombinant DNA technology, for the treatment of various conditions associated with bone marrow depression. Other members of this group are under study.

A. **Erythropoietin:**   Erythropoietin is produced by the kidney; reduction in its synthesis is responsible for the anemia of renal failure. The substance stimulates the production of red cells by combination with specific receptors on erythroid progenitors in the bone marrow.

Erythropoietin (epoetin alfa) is used for treatment of anemias associated with renal failure and with bone marrow failure, eg, following transplantation or treatment with drugs that are toxic to bone marrow. The drug has also been used to accelerate the replacement of red cells removed by phlebotomy. Toxicity is minimal and usually results from excessive increase in hematocrit.

B. **Sargramostim:**   Sargramostim (granulocyte-macrophage colony-stimulating factor, GM-CSF) stimulates the production of granulocytes and macrophages. The drug is used to accelerate the recovery of granulocytes after cancer chemotherapy and other marrow-suppressing therapies. This agent reduces the incidence of infection following bone marrow suppression, presumably by strengthening natural defense mechanisms. Sargramostim also stimulates production of red cells and platelets, though these effects are of far less importance. Toxicities include fever, arthralgias, and capillary damage with edema.

C. **Filgrastim:**   Filgrastim (granulocyte colony-stimulating factor, G-CSF) stimulates the production of neutrophils. This agent is much more selective than sargramostim, having no detectable effect on cell lines other than granulocytes. However, filgrastim's clinical applications duplicate those of sargramostim. Toxicity is minimal but can include bone pain.

D. **Other Hematopoietic Growth Factors:**   Other growth factors include monocyte colony stimulating factor (M-CSF), stem cell factor (SCF), and interleukins 3, 6, 9, and 11. SCF and interleukin-3 have the broadest progenitor cell line effects, including red cell, granulocyte, monocyte-macrophage, megakaryocyte, eosinophil, and basophil cell lines. None of these growth factors are currently available for clinical use.

DRUG LIST

The following drugs are important members of the group discussed in this chapter. Prototypes should be learned in detail; features of the major variants should be known well enough so that the variants can be distinguished from prototypes and from each other; the other significant agents should be recognized as belonging to a specific subclass.

Subclass	Prototype	Major Variants	Other Significant Agents
Oral iron supplements	Ferrous sulfate		Ferrous gluconate, ferrous fumarate
Parenteral iron	Iron dextran		
Vitamin B_{12}	Cyanocobalamin	Hydroxocobalamin	
Folic acid	Pteroylglutamic acid		
Red cell colony–stimulating factor	Erythropoietin (epoetin alfa)		
Granulocyte-macrophage colony-stimulating factor	Sargramostim		
Granulocyte colony-stimulating factor	Filgrastim		

QUESTIONS

DIRECTIONS: Each of the numbered items or incomplete statements in this section is followed by answers or by completions of the statement. Select the ONE lettered answer or completion that is BEST in each case.

Items 1–2: A 23-year-old pregnant woman is referred by her obstetrician for evaluation of anemia. She is in her fourth month of pregnancy and has no prior history of anemia; her grandfather had pernicious anemia. Her hemoglobin is 10 g/dL.

1. Each of the following statements about factors important in anemias is correct EXCEPT
    - (A) Pernicious anemia is associated with both neurologic abnormalities and anemia; only the anemia of pernicious anemia responds to folic acid
    - (B) Efficient absorption of vitamin B_{12} requires binding with a protein that is secreted by the stomach
    - (C) Megaloblastic anemias usually respond to folic acid or vitamin B_{12}
    - (D) Vitamin B_{12} supplements are important in pregnancy to reduce the risk of neural tube defects
    - (E) Ordinary nutritional iron deficiencies should be treated with oral iron supplements

2. The laboratory data for your pregnant patient indicate that she does not have a macrocytic anemia but instead has a typical microcytic anemia of pregnancy. Optimal treatment of normocytic or mild microcytic anemia associated with pregnancy utilizes
    - (A) A high-fiber diet
    - (B) Parenteral iron dextran injections
    - (C) Iron dextran tablets
    - (D) Ferrous sulfate tablets
    - (E) Folic acid supplements

3. Syndromes of toxicity associated with iron include all of the following EXCEPT
    - (A) Acute oral ingestion of a large overdose causes constipation due to fecal impaction
    - (B) Chronic iron overload, as in hemochromatosis, causes liver disease
    - (C) Acute overdose may cause metabolic acidosis
    - (D) Hemolytic anemia is often associated with chronic iron toxicity
    - (E) Overdoses of iron are usually treated medically, since the body does not have a natural means of excreting this element

DIRECTIONS (Items 4–12): Each set of matching questions in this section consists of a list of three to twenty-six lettered options (some of which may be figures) followed by several numbered items. For each numbered item, select the ONE lettered option that is MOST closely associated with it. Each lettered option may be selected once, more than once, or not at all.

Items 4–7:
    - (A) Cyanocobalamin
    - (B) Deferoxamine
    - (C) Ferrous sulfate
    - (D) Folic acid
    - (E) Iron dextran

4. Essential for the therapy of neurologic defects in pernicious anemia
5. Used parenterally in severe iron deficiency and iron malabsorption syndromes
6. Used in the emergency treatment of acute iron intoxication
7. Stored in the liver in an amount sufficient for approximately 5 years

Items 8–12:
    - (A) Erythropoietin
    - (B) Filgrastim
    - (C) Folic acid
    - (D) Hemosiderin
    - (E) Interleukin-9
    - (F) Sargramostim
    - (G) Transferrin

8. Greatly increased in tissues of patients with hemochromatosis
9. Granulocyte-macrophage colony-stimulating factor
10. Most useful in patients with red cell deficiency caused by renal disease or depression of the bone marrow
11. Essential for the endocytosis of iron into red cell progenitors
12. Deficiency during pregnancy increases the risk of neural tube defects in the newborn

ANSWERS

1. Folic acid deficiency in pregnancy, not vitamin B_{12} deficiency, is associated with neural tube defects. The answer is **(D)**.
2. The anemia usually associated with pregnancy is a simple iron deficiency anemia. In this condition, only oral iron supplementation is indicated. The answer is **(D)**.
3. Intolerance to normal oral doses of iron is sometimes associated with constipation. Acute iron overdose, however, causes severe necrotizing gastroenteritis, including diarrhea, not constipation. The answer is **(A)**.
4. Only vitamin B_{12} reverses the neurologic deficits of pernicious anemia—and only if used early in the course of the disease. The answer is **(A)**.
5. Iron dextran, which can be given parenterally, is useful if iron stores must be replenished rapidly. The answer is **(E)**.
6. Deferoxamine, a chelator of iron, is useful in acute iron intoxication. The answer is **(B)**.
7. Vitamin B_{12} is stored in the liver in amounts sufficient for about 5 years of red cell production. The answer is **(A)**.
8. Hemosiderin is one of the major storage forms of iron. Deposits in the liver, heart, and other tissues cause clinical abnormalities in hemochromatosis. The answer is **(D)**.
9. Sargramostim is GM-CSF. The answer is **(F)**.
10. Erythropoietin is now used in patients with severe anemia caused by renal disease (in which erythropoietin is reduced) and by other causes of marrow depression, eg, chemotherapy or radiation. The answer is **(A)**.
11. Iron must be complexed with transferrin for endocytosis into red cell progenitors. The answer is **(G)**.
12. In adults, folic acid deficiency does not have major neurologic consequences, whereas B_{12} deficiency does. On the other hand, deficiency of folic acid during pregnancy has been recognized as a teratogenic factor in neural tube defects in the fetus. The answer is **(C)**.

34 Drugs Used in Coagulation Disorders

OBJECTIVES

You should be able to:

- Compare the oral anticoagulants with heparin in terms of their pharmacokinetics, mechanisms, and toxicities.
- Compare the four thrombolytic preparations.
- Compare the antiplatelet drugs.
- List three different drugs used to treat disorders of excessive bleeding.

Learn the definitions that follow.

Table 34–1. Definitions.

Term	Definition
Clotting cascade	System of serine proteases and substrates in the plasma and tissues that provides for very rapid generation of clotting factors to prevent loss of blood when damage occurs to a vessel
Extrinsic pathway	Factors in tissues that are important in triggering the clotting process
Intrinsic pathway	Factors in the plasma that are activated for clotting, eg, VII, IX, X, II
Low-molecular-weight heparin	Preparation of heparin fractions of MW 2000–6000. Regular heparin has a molecular weight range of 5000–30,000
Partial thromboplastin time (PTT)	Laboratory test for heparin effect; prolonged when drug effect is adequate
Prothrombin time test (PT)	Laboratory test for warfarin (and other oral anticoagulant) effect; prolonged when drug effect is adequate

CONCEPTS

The drugs used in clotting and bleeding disorders fall into two primary groups: drugs used to decrease clotting (or dissolve clots already present) in patients at risk of vascular occlusion and drugs used to increase clotting in patients with clotting deficiencies (Figure 34–1). All of these drugs interact at some point with the clotting process or cascade (as shown in Figure 34–2), a series of enzyme activation steps that originate within the blood itself (intrinsic system) or in tissues (extrinsic system).

ANTICOAGULANTS

A. Classification and Prototypes: Anticoagulants reduce the formation of fibrin clots. Two major types of anticoagulants are available: heparin and its derivatives, which must be used parenterally, and the orally active coumarin derivatives. The two groups differ in their chemistry, pharmacokinetics, and pharmacodynamics (Table 34–2).

B. Heparin:
1. Chemistry: Heparin is a large sulfated polysaccharide polymer obtained from animal sources. Each batch contains molecules of varying size with a molecular weight range (in the regular, high-molecular-weight formulation) of 5,000–30,000. Heparin is highly acidic and can be neutralized by basic molecules (eg, protamine). The drug must be given intravenously or subcutaneously. Intramuscular injection is avoided because of the risk of hematoma formation.

Low-molecular-weight depolymerized fractions of heparin have been developed. These—an example is **enoxaparin**—have molecular weights of 2000–6000. Like regular heparin, they are given intravenously or subcutaneously. Low-molecular-weight heparins have greater bioavailability and longer durations of action than regular heparin; thus, doses can be given less frequently, eg, once or twice a day. The aPTT test does not reliably measure the anticoagulant effect of the low-molecular-weight heparins. **Hirudin,** an anticoagulant protein extracted from the saliva of the leech, is a powerful and selective thrombin in-

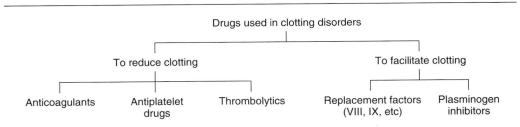

Figure 34–1. Subclasses of drugs used in the treatment of clotting disorders.

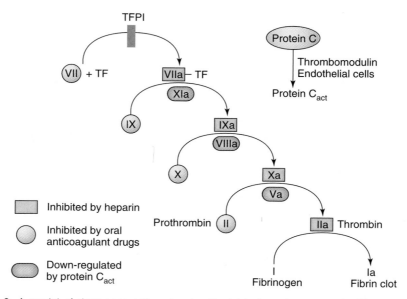

Figure 34–2. A model of drug coagulation showing the intrinsic system cascade. The extrinsic system generates tissue factor (TF), which is important in maintaining the velocity of the intrinsic system cascade. (Reproduced, with permission, from Katzung BG [editor]: *Basic & Clinical Pharmacology,* 7th ed. Appleton & Lange, 1998.)

hibitor that can inactivate thrombin within a developing clot. This drug is relatively free of effects on bleeding time and platelets. A recombinant preparation is in clinical trials.

2. **Mechanism and effects:** Regular (high-molecular-weight) heparin binds to and activates **antithrombin III (ATIII).** The heparin-ATIII complex combines with and inactivates thrombin (activated factor II) and several other factors, especially factor X. In the presence of heparin, antithrombin III inhibits the coagulation factors approximately 1000-fold faster than in its absence. Low doses of heparin also coat the endothelial wall of vessels and reduce the activation of clotting elements by these cells. Because it acts on preformed blood components, heparin is active in vitro—almost instantaneously. The action of heparin is monitored with the activated partial thromboplastin time (aPTT or PTT).

Low-molecular-weight heparin fractions, like regular heparin, bind ATIII, and this complex has the same inhibitory effect on factor X as the regular heparin-ATIII complex. However, the short chain heparin-ATIII complex has a smaller effect on thrombin.

3. **Clinical use:** Because of its rapid effect, heparin is used when anticoagulation is needed immediately (eg, when starting therapy). The drug is often used for 1–2 weeks immediately following myocardial infarction. Because it does not pass the placenta, it is the drug of choice when an anticoagulant must be used in pregnancy. Low-molecular-weight heparins are approved for prevention of deep vein thrombosis after surgery.

Table 34–2. Properties of heparin and warfarin.

Property	Heparin	Warfarin
Structure	Large polymer, acidic	Small lipid-soluble molecule
Route of administration	Parenteral	Oral
Site of action	Blood (in vivo and in vitro)	Liver
Onset of action	Rapid (seconds)	Slow, limited by half-lives of factors being replaced
Mechanism of action	Activates antithrombin III	Impairs synthesis of factors II, VII, IX, X
Antidote	Protamine	Vitamin K, plasma
Use	Acute, over days	Chronic, over weeks to months

4. **Toxicity:** Increased bleeding is the most common adverse effect of regular and low-molecular-weight heparins and may result in hemorrhagic stroke. Additive interactions with other anticoagulants often occur. Regular heparin causes moderate transient thrombocytopenia in many patients and severe thrombocytopenia in a few. Prolonged use is associated with osteoporosis. Toxicities of long-term use of low-molecular-weight heparins are not yet known.

C. **Coumarin Anticoagulants:**
   1. **Chemistry and pharmacokinetics:** The coumarin anticoagulants are small, lipid-soluble molecules. They are readily absorbed after oral administration (and therefore are commonly called "oral anticoagulants" to distinguish them from heparin). They also pass the placental barrier readily and are therefore potentially dangerous to the fetus. Warfarin is the only member of this group that is of clinical importance in the USA.
   2. **Mechanism and effects:** Coumarins interfere with the normal synthesis of clotting factors in the liver, a process that depends on vitamin K. These vitamin K-dependent factors include II, VII, IX, and X. Because these factors have half-lives of 8–60 hours in the plasma, an anticoagulant effect is observed only after sufficient time has passed for the preformed normal factors to be eliminated. Because it acts in the liver, warfarin has no effect on blood clotting in vitro. The action of warfarin can be reversed with vitamin K, but recovery requires the synthesis of new normal clotting factors and is therefore slow (2–3 days). More rapid reversal can be achieved by transfusion with fresh or frozen plasma that contains normal clotting factors. The effect of warfarin is monitored by means of the prothrombin time (PT, or "pro time") test.
   3. **Clinical use:** Warfarin is used for chronic anticoagulation except in pregnant women (heparin must be used during pregnancy). Warfarin is indicated in established venous thrombosis and is often used for 2–6 months following a myocardial infarction.
   4. **Toxicity:** Bleeding is the most important adverse effect of warfarin. Like heparin, it interacts with other anticlotting drugs. Warfarin also causes bone defects in the developing fetus and therefore is contraindicated in pregnancy. Because it acts in and is metabolized in the liver, warfarin interacts with drugs that influence hepatic drug metabolism.

ANTIPLATELET DRUGS

Platelet aggregation plays a central role in the clotting process and is especially important in clots that form in the arterial circulation. Therefore, platelets are believed to be especially important in coronary and cerebral artery occlusion. Platelet aggregation is facilitated by thromboxane, adenosine, fibrin, serotonin, and other substances. Prostacyclin and cAMP inhibit platelet aggregation.

A. **Classification and Prototypes:** Antiplatelet drugs include **aspirin** and other nonsteroidal anti-inflammatory drugs (NSAIDs), **ticlopidine, abciximab,** and **dipyridamole.** These drugs increase bleeding time, a test used to monitor their effects.

B. **Mechanism of Action:** Aspirin and other NSAIDs inhibit thromboxane synthesis by blocking the enzyme cyclooxygenase. Aspirin is particularly effective because it irreversibly inactivates the enzyme. Because the platelet lacks the machinery for synthesis of new protein, inhibition by aspirin persists until new platelets are formed (several days). Other NSAIDs cause a less persistent antiplatelet effect (hours).

Ticlopidine's mechanism of action involves a reduction in fibrin binding to platelets, a process important in normal platelet aggregation. The effect, which may involve the platelet fibrin receptor—a glycoprotein called glycoprotein IIb/IIIa—occurs in vivo but not in vitro. It is irreversible and of long duration (several days).

Abciximab is a monoclonal antibody that reversibly inhibits fibrin binding to its receptor, glycoprotein IIb/IIIa, on platelets, thereby inhibiting platelet aggregation. Its action is of short duration (hours).

The mechanism of dipyridamole is not well understood. Some evidence suggests that dipyridamole increases the concentration of cAMP in the platelet by inhibiting phosphodiesterase.

C. Clinical Use: Aspirin is used in individuals who have had one or more myocardial infarcts to prevent further infarcts. A large recent study suggested that the drug also reduces the incidence of first infarcts. Aspirin is also being used extensively to prevent transient ischemic attacks ("TIAs") and other thrombotic events.

Ticlopidine is effective in preventing transient ischemic attacks and is particularly valuable for patients who cannot tolerate aspirin. Abciximab is approved for the prevention of restenosis after coronary angioplasty. Dipyridamole alone is rarely used, but in the past it was combined with warfarin to prevent thrombosis on artificial heart valves.

D. Toxicity: All antiplatelet drugs significantly enhance the effects of other anticlotting agents. Aspirin and other NSAIDs cause gastrointestinal and CNS effects (see Chapter 35). The toxicity of ticlopidine includes gastrointestinal upset, bleeding in up to 5% of patients, and leukopenia in about 1%. The major toxicity of abciximab is bleeding.

THROMBOLYTIC AGENTS

A. Classification and Prototypes (Table 34–3): The thrombolytic drugs currently available are alteplase and reteplase (forms of tissue plasminogen activator, t-PA), anistreplase, urokinase, and streptokinase. All are given intravenously.

B. Mechanism of Action: Plasmin is the normal endogenous fibrinolytic enzyme. It splits fibrin into fragments, promoting the breakdown and dissolution of the clot (Figure 34–3). The thrombolytic enzymes catalyze the activation of the inactive precursor, plasminogen, to plasmin.

1. Tissue plasminogen activator: t-PA is a large human protein (MW > 50,000) produced in bacteria through recombinant DNA techniques. t-PA directly converts fibrin-bound plasminogen to plasmin. In theory, the drug's selectivity for plasminogen that has already bound to fibrin (ie, a clot) should result in greater selectivity and less danger of spontaneous bleeding. In fact, t-PA's selectivity appears to be quite limited. Alteplase is a normal human plasminogen activator. Reteplase is a mutated form of human t-PA with identical effects but a slightly longer duration of action.

2. Anistreplase: This anisoylated plasminogen-streptokinase activator complex (APSAC) is a prodrug. As the anisoyl group is hydrolyzed in vivo (a slow, spontaneous process), the streptokinase-activated plasminogen is released and converts endogenous plasminogen to plasmin. This slow release provides for the relatively long half-life of this drug. The human plasminogen in this product is obtained through recombinant bacterial synthesis.

Table 34–3. Properties of thrombolytic enzymes.

Agent	Source	Duration of Action	Comments
Alteplase, reteplase	Recombinant human protein	2–10 minutes	Active tissue plasminogen activator, (t-PA); converts plasminogen to plasmin; IV infusion (alteplase) or bolus doses (reteplase) required. Most expensive (> $2000 per treatment). Reteplase is somewhat longer-acting than alteplase
Anistreplase	Prodrug: streptokinase plus recombinant human plasminogen	1–2 hours	Slowly releases streptokinase-activated plasminogen; single bolus administration provides long duration of action. Second most expensive (> $1800 per treatment)
Streptokinase	Bacterial product	20–25 minutes	Streptokinase combines with plasminogen; the combination activates plasminogen to plasmin; IV infusion required. Least expensive ($200 per treatment)
Urokinase	Human kidney cell culture	< 20 minutes	Active plasminogen activator

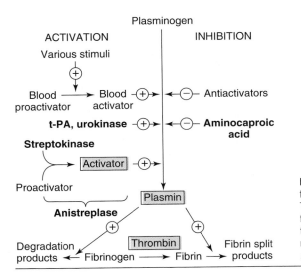

Figure 34–3. Diagram of the fibrinolytic system. The useful thrombolytic drugs are shown on the left in **bold** type. These drugs increase the formation of plasmin, the major fibrinolytic enzyme. Aminocaproic acid, a useful inhibitor of fibrinolysis, is shown on the right. (Reproduced, with permission, from Katzung BG [editor]: *Basic & Clinical Pharmacology,* 7th ed. Appleton & Lange, 1998.)

3. Streptokinase: Streptokinase is obtained from bacterial cultures. Though not an enzyme itself, it forms a complex with endogenous plasminogen that catalyzes the rapid conversion of plasminogen to plasmin.

4. Urokinase: Urokinase is extracted from cultured human kidney cells. This enzyme directly converts plasminogen to plasmin.

C. Clinical Use: The major application of the thrombolytic agents is in the emergency treatment of coronary artery thrombosis. Under ideal conditions (ie, treatment within 1–4 hours), these agents may cause prompt recanalization of the occluded vessel. They have been used by the intra-arterial route in coronary thrombosis, but results are no better by this route than by the intravenous route. Although initial trials of these agents in occlusive stroke were disappointing, recent evidence suggests that very prompt use (ie, within 2 hours of the first symptoms) may result in a significantly better clinical outcome. Hemorrhage must be positively ruled out before such use. The thrombolytic agents are also used in cases of multiple pulmonary emboli and deep venous thrombosis.

D. Toxicity: Bleeding is the most important hazard and has about the same frequency with all of these drugs. Cerebral hemorrhage is the most serious manifestation. Because it is a foreign protein, streptokinase may evoke the production of antibodies and lose its effectiveness or even induce severe allergic reactions upon subsequent therapy. Patients who have had streptococcal infections may have preformed antibodies to the drug. Because they are human proteins, urokinase and t-PA are not subject to this problem. However, they (and anistreplase) are much more expensive than streptokinase and not much more effective.

DRUGS USED IN BLEEDING DISORDERS

Inadequate blood clotting may result from vitamin K deficiency, genetically determined errors of clotting factor synthesis (eg, hemophilia), a variety of drug-induced conditions, and thrombocytopenia. Treatment, therefore, involves administration of vitamin K, preformed clotting factors, or antiplasmin drugs. Thrombocytopenia is usually treated by administration of platelets.

A. Vitamin K: Vitamin K deficiency is particularly common in newborns and in older individuals with abnormalities of fat absorption. The deficiency is readily treated with oral or parenteral vitamin K supplements using phytonadione (K_1) or menadione (K_2).

B. Clotting Factors: The most important agents used to treat hemophilia are fresh plasma and purified human blood clotting factors, especially **factor VIII** and **factor IX**. These products are extremely expensive and carry a risk of infection and immunologic reactions. The factors have been produced by recombinant synthesis, but this process is more expensive than purifying them from whole blood.

C. Antiplasmin Agents: Antiplasmin agents are valuable for the management of acute bleeding episodes in hemophiliacs and others with bleeding disorders. **Aminocaproic acid** and **tranexamic acid** are orally active drugs that inhibit fibrinolysis by inhibiting plasminogen activation (Figure 34–3). **Aprotinin** is a direct inhibitor of plasmin and may be useful in patients with a variety of bleeding disorders and in patients bleeding from excessive effect of thrombolytic enzymes.

DRUG LIST

The following drugs are important members of the group discussed in this chapter. Prototypes should be learned in detail; features of the major variants should be known well enough so that the variants can be distinguished from prototypes and from each other; the other significant agents should be recognized as belonging to a specific subclass.

Subclass	Prototype	Major Variants	Other Significant Agents
Anticoagulants Parenteral	Heparin	Enoxaparin	Dalteparin, danaparoid
Oral	Warfarin		
Antiplatelet drugs	Aspirin	Ticlopidine, abciximab	Dipyridamole
Thrombolytic drugs	Streptokinase, alteplase		Anistreplase, urokinase
Clotting factors	Factor VIII	Factor IX	
Vitamin K	Phytonadione (K_1)		Menadione (K_2)
Antiplasmin drugs	Aminocaproic acid, aprotinin		Tranexamic acid

QUESTIONS

DIRECTIONS: Each of the numbered items or incomplete statements in this section is followed by answers or by completions of the statement. Select the ONE lettered answer or completion that is BEST in each case.

Items 1–3: A 58-year-old business executive is brought to the emergency room two hours after the onset of severe chest pain during a vigorous tennis game. He has a history of poorly controlled mild hypertension and elevated blood cholesterol but does not smoke. ECG changes confirm the diagnosis of myocardial infarction. The decision is made to reduce clotting and attempt to open his occluded artery.

1. Activation of plasminogen to plasmin
   (A) Is brought about by heparin
   (B) Is brought about by warfarin
   (C) Is brought about by anistreplase
   (D) Is used preoperatively and during surgery in patients at risk of deep vein thromboses
   (E) Can be reversed by administration of vitamin K_1 oxide
2. Concerning antithrombotic drugs
   (A) Aspirin's antiplatelet activity is due to the inhibition of prostacyclin production
   (B) Abciximab blocks adenosine receptors on platelets
   (C) Ticlopidine produces a brief, reversible antiplatelet action
   (D) Newer nonsteroidal anti-inflammatory drugs (eg, ibuprofen) produce an irreversible inhibition of platelet cyclooxygenase
   (E) Thromboxane is the primary platelet-active agent produced in platelets
3. Aspirin should be used cautiously in a patient receiving heparin because aspirin
   (A) Inhibits vitamin K absorption

    (B) Has antithrombin activity
    (C) Inhibits metabolism of heparin
    (D) Inhibits platelet aggregation
    (E) All of the above

4. The following changes in plasma concentration of warfarin were observed in a patient when two other agents, drugs B and C, were given on a daily basis at constant dosage starting at the times shown. Which of the following statements most accurately describes what is shown in the graph below?
    (A) Drug B displaces warfarin from plasma proteins; drug C displaces warfarin from tissue binding sites
    (B) Drug B stimulates hepatic metabolism of warfarin; drug C displaces warfarin from plasma protein
    (C) Drug B stimulates renal clearance of warfarin; drug C inhibits hepatic metabolism of drug B
    (D) Drug B stimulates hepatic metabolism of warfarin; drug C displaces drug B from tissue binding sites
    (E) None of the above

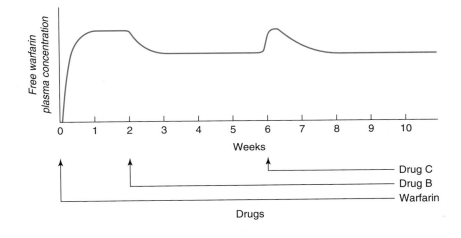

5. Which of the following may be of value in the treatment of multiple small pulmonary emboli?
    (A) Heparin
    (B) Warfarin
    (C) Urokinase
    (D) Streptokinase
    (E) All of the above

6. Concerning anticoagulants, all of the following are correct EXCEPT
    (A) Parenteral administration of heparin provides immediate anticoagulation
    (B) Oral administration of warfarin provides delayed anticoagulation
    (C) The anticoagulant action of regular heparin requires the presence of antithrombin III
    (D) Warfarin is the preferred anticoagulant in pregnant women
    (E) Heparin overdosage can be reversed with the basic protein, protamine

DIRECTIONS (Items 7–15): Each set of matching questions in this section consists of a list of three to twenty-six lettered options (some of which may be figures) followed by several numbered items. For each numbered item, select the ONE lettered option that is MOST closely associated with it. Each lettered option may be selected once, more than once, or not at all.
    (A) Abciximab
    (B) Alteplase
    (C) Aminocaproic acid
    (D) Anistreplase
    (E) Enoxaparin

    (F)   Factor IX
    (G) Heparin
    (H) Protamine
    (I)   Ticlopidine
    (J)   Warfarin
    (K) Whole plasma

7. Used for rapid reversal of effects of warfarin

8. Small synthetic nonprotein chemical used for the treatment of an acute bleeding episode in a hemophiliac

9. Polymer of MW 2000–6000 that inhibits activated factor X

10. Small lipid-soluble molecule that acts in the liver to inhibit synthesis of vitamin K-dependent factors

11. Used for the treatment of bleeding due to excess heparin

12. Human protein used in hemophiliacs to prevent or treat bleeding

13. A long-acting thrombolytic agent composed of a bacterial protein complexed with a recombinant human protein

14. A monoclonal antibody that blocks platelet receptors

15. An antiplatelet drug that requires several days for full effect; it is active in vivo but not in vitro and has no effect on cyclooxygenase

ANSWERS

1. Thrombolytic drugs are not used in patients scheduled for surgery or in those with neoplasms because of the risk of drug-induced bleeding in surgical incisions. The answer is **(C)**, anistreplase.

2. Prostacyclin is the major *antiaggregation* platelet-active product of the endothelium. Abciximab is an antibody that blocks the fibrin receptor, glycoprotein IIb/IIIa. Ticlopidine produces a long-lasting, irreversible inhibition of platelet aggregation. Unlike aspirin, which irreversibly inhibits cyclooxygenase, the newer NSAIDs such as ibuprofen cause reversible inhibition. Thromboxane, an important contributor to the platelet aggregation process, is produced mainly in platelets. The answer is **(E)**.

3. In very high overdosage, aspirin may inhibit hepatic prothrombin synthesis. In ordinary dosage, aspirin interferes with clotting by a different mechanism (inhibition of platelet aggregation). At all doses, the drug has the potential to interact synergistically with heparin (and other anticlotting drugs). The answer is **(D)**.

4. A drug that increases metabolism (clearance) of the anticoagulant will lower the steady state plasma concentration (both free and bound forms), whereas one that displaces the anticoagulant will increase the plasma level of the free form only until elimination of the drug has again lowered it to the steady state level. The answer is **(B)**.

5. Urokinase and streptokinase may be useful in the removal of a clot that is already present; heparin (immediately) and warfarin (more slowly) act to prevent extension of the clot and the formation of new ones. The answer is **(E)**.

6. Warfarin is avoided in pregnant women because it crosses the placental barrier and causes teratogenic effects. The answer is **(D)**.

7. Only a full complement of normal clotting factors can reverse warfarin's effects rapidly. The answer is **(K)**.

8. Aminocaproic acid is a small nonprotein molecule that inhibits thrombolysis (Figure 34–3) and is useful in bleeding episodes in hemophilia. The answer is **(C)**.

9. Enoxaparin, dalteparin, and danaparoid are smaller polymers of heparin with more effect on factor X than on factor II. The answer is **(E)**.

10. Warfarin is the small lipid-soluble agent that acts in the liver to inhibit the synthesis of clotting factors II, VII, IX, and X. The answer is **(J)**.

11. Heparin is a very acidic molecule that binds firmly to basic polymers such as protamine. Such binding prevents the action of heparin. The answer is **(H)**.

12. Factor VIII and factor IX are human proteins used to treat hemophilia. The answer is **(F)**.

13. Anistreplase consists of bacterial streptokinase complexed with human plasminogen. The answer is **(D)**.

14. Abciximab is a monoclonal antibody. The answer is **(A)**.

15. Ticlopidine has an irreversible effect of slow onset in vivo. The answer is **(I)**.

Drugs Used in the Treatment of Hyperlipidemias

35

OBJECTIVES

You should be able to:

- Describe the dietary management of hyperlipoproteinemia.
- Describe the mechanism of action and toxic effects of nicotinic acid, HMG-CoA reductase inhibitors, gemfibrozil, probucol, and bile acid-binding resins.

Learn the definitions that follow.

Table 35–1. Definitions.

Term	Definition
Chylomicrons	Largest of the lipoproteins; carry fat from the gut to the other tissues
FFA	Free fatty acids; products of triglyceride hydrolysis
HDL	High-density lipoproteins; formed in the tissues, a mechanism for cholesterol transport *from* the periphery *to* the liver
HMG-CoA	3-Hydroxy-3-methylglutaryl-coenzyme A; a precursor of cholesterol
IDL	Intermediate-density lipoproteins; remnants of LDL particles that have been depleted of FFA by lipoprotein lipase
LDL	Low-density lipoproteins; major form in which lipid is recaptured by the liver; requires functional LDL receptors for normal endocytosis in hepatocytes
Lipoproteins	Macromolecular complexes in which lipids are transported in the blood
LPL	Lipoprotein lipase; an enzyme found in the peripheral tissue that hydrolyzes lipoproteins and depletes triglycerides in the lipoprotein complexes
Triglyceride	Ester of three fatty acids with glycerol; a major form of fat storage
VLDL	Very-low-density lipoproteins; secreted by the liver; the initial transporter of cholesterol and other lipids *from* the liver *to* the periphery

CONCEPTS

HYPERLIPOPROTEINEMIA

A. Pathogenesis: Premature or accelerated development of atherosclerosis is strongly associated with elevated levels (above 200 mg/dL) of certain plasma lipoproteins. Elevations of low-density lipoproteins (LDL), intermediate-density lipoproteins (IDL), or very-low-density lipoproteins (VLDL) constitute hyperlipoproteinemias. Such elevations are usually present in families with high frequencies of cardiovascular disease. A *depressed* level of high-density lipoproteins (HDL) is also associated with an increased risk of atherosclerosis. In some families, hyperlipemia, an elevation of triglycerides, is similarly correlated with atherosclerosis. Chylomicronemia, the occurrence of chylomicrons in the serum while fasting, is a recessive trait correlated with a high incidence of acute pancreatitis and can be managed by restriction of total fat intake. (See Table 35–2.)

Regulation of plasma lipoprotein levels involves a balance between dietary fat intake, hepatic processing, and utilization in peripheral tissues. Primary disturbances in regulation occur in various familial diseases. Secondary disturbances are associated with many endocrine conditions and diseases of the liver or kidneys.

Table 35–2. The primary hyperlipoproteinemias and their drug treatment.*

Condition	Single Drug	Drug Combination
Primary chylomicronemia (familial lipoprotein lipase or cofactor deficiency)	Dietary management	Niacin plus gemfibrozil
Familial hypertriglyceridemia		
Severe	Niacin, gemfibrozil	Niacin plus gemfibrozil
Moderate	Gemfibrozil, niacin	
Familial combined hyperlipidemia		
VLDL increased	Niacin, gemfibrozil	
LDL increased	Resin, niacin, reductase inhibitor	Niacin plus resin or reductase inhibitor
VLDL, LDL increased	Niacin, reductase inhibitor	Niacin plus resin or reductase inhibitor
Familial dysbetalipopro-teinemia	Niacin, gemfibrozil	Gemfibrozil plus niacin or niacin plus reductase inhibitor
Familial hypercholesterolemia		
Heterozygous	Resin, reductase inhibitor, niacin	Two or three of the individual drugs
Homozygous	Niacin	Resin plus niacin plus reductase inhibitor
LP(a) hyperlipoproteinemia	Niacin	Niacin plus reductase inhibitor
Unclassified hyperchole-sterolemia	Resin, niacin, reductase inhibitor, gemfibrozil	

*Reproduced, with permission, from Katzung BG (editor): *Basic & Clinical Pharmacology,* 7th ed. Appleton & Lange, 1998.

Major enzymes involved in lipoprotein regulation include the following: (1) acyl-CoA:cholesterol acyltransferase (ACAT), which esterifies some cholesterol in the core of chylomicrons; (2) lecithin:cholesterol acyltransferase (LCAT), which esterifies cholesterol and helps transfer it to LDL; (3) lipoprotein lipase (LPL), which hydrolyzes triglycerides to free fatty acids (FFA) and glycerol; and (4) 3-hydroxy-3-methylglutaryl-coenzyme A (HMG-CoA) reductase, which is essential for the synthesis of cholesterol and other steroids in the liver.

B. Treatment Strategies: Treatment always includes dietary management. Drug therapy is added if necessary.

  1. Diet: Dietary measures are the first method of management and may be sufficient to reduce lipoprotein levels to a safe range. Cholesterol and saturated fats are the primary dietary factors that contribute to elevated levels of plasma lipoproteins. Diets are designed to reduce the total intake of these substances. Alcohol intake raises VLDL levels.

  2. Drugs: Drug therapy can reduce fat absorption from the intestine (resins), modify hepatic cholesterol synthesis (HMG-CoA reductase inhibitors), decrease secretion of lipoproteins (niacin), increase peripheral clearance of lipoproteins (gemfibrozil group), and perhaps exert other effects (probucol). These drugs are all given orally. (See Figure 35–1.)

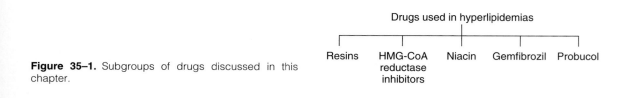

Figure 35–1. Subgroups of drugs discussed in this chapter.

RESINS

    A.   **Mechanism and Effects:**   Bile acid-binding resins (**cholestyramine** and **colestipol**) are large nonabsorbable polymers that bind bile acids and similar steroids in the intestine. Neomycin, though not a resin, also causes a reduction in bile acid reabsorption.

        By preventing absorption of dietary cholesterol and reducing reabsorption of bile acids secreted by the liver, these agents greatly enhance the diversion of hepatic cholesterol synthesis to new bile acids, thereby reducing the availability of cholesterol for the production of plasma lipids (Figure 35–2). A compensatory increase in high-affinity LDL receptors, which increases the removal of LDL cholesterol from the blood, often occurs in the liver.

    B.   **Clinical Use:**   See Table 35–2.

    C.   **Toxicity:**   Adverse effects include bloating, constipation, and impaired absorption of some cationic or neutral drugs. Neomycin is rarely used because it is associated with a higher incidence of adverse effects than are the resins.

HMG-CoA REDUCTASE INHIBITORS

    A.   **Mechanism and Effects:**   **Lovastatin** (mevinolin) and **simvastatin** are prodrug lactones. **Pravastatin, fluvastatin,** and **atorvastatin** are active as given. In the body, the active drugs are

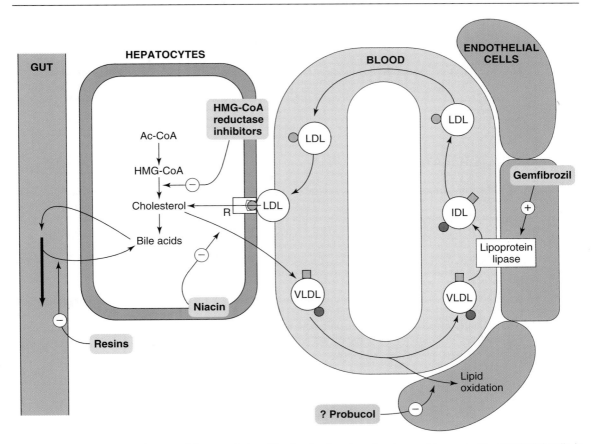

Figure 35–2. Schematic diagram of lipoprotein handling by the liver hepatocytes and by vascular endothelial cells in vessels in peripheral tissues. Shaded squares and circles associated with VLDL, IDL, and LDL particles represent apoproteins, eg, ApoA-I, ApoB-100, ApoC-II. These proteins serve as cofactors in some enzyme reactions and as ligands for receptors that bind lipoprotein particles. R = LDL receptor.

structural analogs that competitively inhibit mevalonate synthesis by HMG-CoA reductase, a process essential for cholesterol biosynthesis in the liver (Figure 35–2). The liver compensates by increasing the number of high-affinity LDL receptors, and this results in increased clearance of VLDL remnants (IDL) and LDL from the blood.

B. **Clinical Use:**   (See Table 35–2.) These drugs often reduce LDL levels dramatically, especially when used in combination with other drugs. Early evidence suggests that atorvastatin may have higher efficacy than the other reductase inhibitors, and it appears to reduce triglycerides more than the older drugs in this group.

C. **Toxicity:**   Mild elevations of aminotransferases are common but are not often associated with hepatic damage. Patients with preexisting liver disease may have more severe reactions. An increase in creatine kinase (released from skeletal muscle) is noted in about 10% of patients; in a few, severe muscle pain and even rhabdomyolysis may occur. Progression of cataracts was reported in a few patients in early studies but has not been found in more extensive trials.

NIACIN (NICOTINIC ACID)

A. **Mechanism and Effects:**   Niacin (but not nicotinamide) directly reduces the secretion of VLDL from the liver (Figure 35–2) or inhibits hepatic synthesis of apolipoproteins or cholesterol. Consequently, LDL formation is reduced. Increased clearance of VLDL by lipoprotein lipase in the periphery has also been demonstrated. In addition, the levels of HDL may increase. Finally, niacin decreases circulating fibrinogen and increases tissue plasminogen activator.

B. **Clinical Use:**   See Table 35–2.

C. **Toxicity:**   Cutaneous flushing is a common adverse effect. Aspirin may reduce the intensity of this flushing, suggesting that it is mediated by prostaglandin release. Tolerance usually develops within a few days. Pruritus and other skin conditions are reported. Moderate elevations of liver enzymes may occur.

GEMFIBROZIL & RELATED DRUGS

A. **Mechanism and Effects:**   Gemfibrozil, fenofibrate, and clofibrate cause a decrease in VLDL levels through a peripheral effect. This effect is probably stimulation of lipoprotein lipase (Figure 35–2), resulting in an increase in the clearance of triglyceride-rich lipoproteins. Cholesterol biosynthesis in the liver is secondarily reduced. There may be an increase in HDL levels.

B. **Clinical Use:**   (See Table 35–2.) Clofibrate is less widely used than gemfibrozil and other newer analogs because of the greater toxicity associated with clofibrate.

C. **Toxicity:**   Nausea is the most common adverse effect with all members of this subgroup. Skin rashes are common with gemfibrozil. Myalgia is reported in patients taking clofibrate; an antiplatelet effect may cause an interaction between this drug and anticoagulants. Most importantly, clofibrate has been associated with an increase in the incidence of gallstones and hepatobiliary neoplasms.

PROBUCOL

A. **Mechanism and Effects:**   Probucol reduces LDL cholesterol levels by an unknown mechanism. Unfortunately, this drug often reduces HDL levels as well, which limits its usefulness. However, some evidence suggests that the drug may inhibit atherogenesis by other mechanisms in addition to its effect on plasma lipids, possibly by an antioxidant effect (Figure 35–2). Probucol distributes into adipose tissue and has a very long half-life. Because of decreasing use, probucol was withdrawn from the market in 1996. However, a recent (1997) large double-blind study reported that use of probucol before and after coronary artery angioplasty markedly reduced restenosis of dilated coronaries. If these results are confirmed, probucol may be reintroduced.

B. Clinical Use: (See Table 35–2.) Probucol is not currently in clinical use.

C. Toxicity: Probucol frequently caused gastrointestinal symptoms. The drug also caused ECG changes and precipitated dangerous cardiac arrhythmias in some patients.

COMBINATION THERAPY

All patients with hyperlipidemia are treated first with dietary modification, but this is often insufficient and drugs must be added. Because of the difficulty of lowering serum lipids with a single drug, combinations of drugs are often required to achieve the maximum lowering possible with minimum toxicity. The most common combinations are listed in Table 35–2.

DRUG LIST

The following drugs are important members of the group discussed in this chapter. Prototypes should be learned in detail; features of the major variants should be known well enough so that the variants can be distinguished from prototypes and from each other; the other significant agents should be recognized as belonging to a specific subclass.

Subclass	Prototype	Major Variants	Other Significant Agents
Bile acid-binding resins	Cholestyramine		Colestipol
Cholesterol synthesis inhibitor	Lovastatin	Atorvastatin	Pravastatin, simvastatin, fluvastatin
VLDL secretion inhibitor	Niacin		
Lipoprotein lipase stimulants	Gemfibrozil		Fenofibrate, clofibrate
Mechanism uncertain	Probucol		

QUESTIONS

DIRECTIONS: Each of the numbered items or incomplete statements in this section is followed by answers or by completions of the statement. Select the ONE lettered answer or completion that is BEST in each case.

1. Increased levels of which of the following may be associated with a *decreased* risk of atherosclerosis?
   (A) Very-low-density lipoproteins (VLDL)
   (B) Low-density lipoproteins (LDL)
   (C) Intermediate-density lipoproteins (IDL)
   (D) High-density lipoproteins (HDL)
   (E) Cholesterol

2. Lovastatin has all of the following effects EXCEPT
   (A) Increased synthesis of high affinity LDL receptors
   (B) Decreased LDL and VLDL plasma levels
   (C) Increased serum aminotransferase levels
   (D) Skeletal muscle pain and rhabdomyolysis
   (E) Increased lipoprotein lipase activity

3. Which of the following cause a reduction in absorption of bile acids from the gastrointestinal tract?
    (A) HMG-CoA reductase inhibitors
    (B) Colestipol
    (C) Niacin
    (D) Probucol
    (E) All of the above

4. The major recognized mechanism of action of niacin is
    (A) Increased endocytosis of HDL by the liver
    (B) Decreased secretion of VLDL by the liver
    (C) Increased lipid hydrolysis by lipoprotein lipase
    (D) Decreased lipid synthesis in adipose tissue
    (E) Decreased oxidation of lipids in endothelial cells

5. The major mechanism of action of gemfibrozil is
    (A) Reduction of secretion of HDL by the liver
    (B) Reduction of secretion of VLDL by the liver
    (C) Increased lipid hydrolysis by lipoprotein lipase
    (D) Decreased lipid hydrolysis by lipoprotein lipase
    (E) Reduced oxidation of lipids in endothelial cells

6. The major toxicity of HMG-CoA reductase inhibitors is
    (A) Severe cardiac arrhythmias
    (B) Tissue injury with elevated liver and muscle enzymes
    (C) Gallstones
    (D) Acute pancreatitis
    (E) Gastrointestinal and hepatobiliary neoplasms

7. The major toxicity of gemfibrozil is
    (A) Liver damage
    (B) Severe cardiac arrhythmias
    (C) Nausea, vomiting, and skin rashes
    (D) Flushing of the skin
    (E) Gastrointestinal and hepatobiliary neoplasms

DIRECTIONS (Items 8–15): Each set of matching questions in this section consists of a list of three to twenty-six lettered options (some of which may be figures) followed by several numbered items. For each numbered item, select the ONE lettered option that is MOST closely associated with it. Each lettered option may be selected once, more than once, or not at all.
    (A) Atorvastatin
    (B) Cholestyramine
    (C) Clofibrate
    (D) Gemfibrozil
    (E) Lovastatin
    (F) Neomycin
    (G) Nicotinic acid
    (H) Probucol

8. Associated with cardiac arrhythmias
9. Causes cutaneous vasodilation that may be prevented by aspirin
10. Nonabsorbable synthetic polymer; acts entirely within the intestine
11. Prodrug analog of a steroid precursor that competitively inhibits cholesterol synthesis in the liver
12. Activates lipoprotein lipase and increases hydrolysis of triglycerides
13. Reduces secretion of VLDL particles from the liver and possibly synthesis of cholesterol
14. Newer reductase inhibitor with ability to lower triglycerides as well as cholesterol
15. Older drug associated with production of biliary stones and hepatic neoplasms

ANSWERS

1. Increase of most of the lipoproteins is associated with increased risk of atherosclerosis. HDL ("good cholesterol"), however, is associated with a decrease in risk. The answer is **(D)**.

2. Lovastatin can cause all of the effects except stimulation of lipoprotein lipase, a peripheral (not hepatic) enzyme. The answer is **(E)**.
3. Colestipol (a resin) reduces absorption of bile acids (see Figure 35–2). The answer is **(B)**.
4. The major recognized effect of niacin is reduction of VLDL secretion by the liver (Figure 35–2). The answer is **(B)**.
5. The major mechanism recognized for gemfibrozil is stimulation of lipoprotein lipase. The answer is **(C)**.
6. The major toxicity of the HMG-CoA reductase inhibitors is tissue damage with resulting elevation of enzymes of liver and muscle. The answer is **(B)**.
7. The major toxicities of gemfibrozil (and fenofibrate) are gastrointestinal upset and skin rash. The answer is **(C)**.
8. Probucol has been associated with serious arrhythmias. Nicotinic acid may also cause arrhythmias, but this is uncommon. The answer is **(H)**.
9. The answer is **(G)**, nicotinic acid (niacin).
10. Cholestyramine and neomycin both slow the absorption of bile acids from the gut. However, neomycin is a natural product and not a polymer (see Chapter 45). The answer is **(B)**.
11. HMG-CoA reductase inhibitors are structural analogs. Atorvastatin is active as given; it is not a prodrug. The answer is **(E)**, lovastatin.
12. Gemfibrozil activates lipoprotein lipase. The answer is **(D)**.
13. Nicotinic acid reduces VLDL particle secretion into the blood. It appears to also reduce cholesterol synthesis. The answer is **(G)**.
14. Atorvastatin is the newest HMG-CoA reductase inhibitor and is of considerable interest because of its high efficacy in reducing cholesterol and triglycerides in the blood. The answer is **(A)**.
15. Clofibrate, though still available, is rarely used because of its association with neoplasms. The answer is **(C)**.

Nonsteroidal Anti-inflammatory Drugs, Acetaminophen, & Drugs Used in Gout   36

OBJECTIVES

You should be able to:

- Describe the effects of aspirin on prostaglandin synthesis.
- List the toxic effects of aspirin.
- Contrast the actions of aspirin and the newer NSAIDs.
- Describe the mechanisms of action of three different drug groups used in gout.
- Describe the effects and the major toxicity of acetaminophen.

CONCEPTS

ANTI-INFLAMMATORY DRUGS

Inflammation is a common and nonspecific manifestation of many diseases. It may be acute or chronic, and the two forms may occur independently. The immune response is involved in most types of inflammation; thus many of the treatment strategies for reduction of inflammation are targeted at immune processes and the mediators involved in the immune system (Figure 36–1).

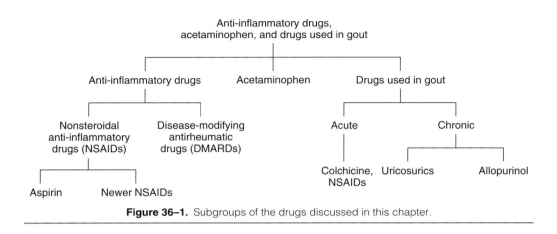

Figure 36–1. Subgroups of the drugs discussed in this chapter.

ASPIRIN & NEWER NONSTEROIDAL ANTI-INFLAMMATORY DRUGS (NSAIDs)

A. **Classification and Prototypes:** Aspirin (acetylsalicylic acid) and the salicylates are traditionally used in the treatment of pain, inflammation, and fever. Aspirin is the prototypical salicylate. The newer NSAIDs (ibuprofen, indomethacin, many others) vary mainly in their potency
and duration of action. Ibuprofen is the lower-potency, shorter-acting NSAID prototype.
Naproxen is a longer-acting agent. Indomethacin is the prototypical high-potency NSAID.

B. **Mechanism of Action:** As noted in Chapter 18, cyclooxygenase, the enzyme that converts
arachidonic acid into the endoperoxide precursors of prostaglandin, has been found to have at
least two different isoforms: COX I and COX II (Figure 18–1). COX I is present in noninflam-
matory cells, whereas COX II is present in lymphocytes, polymorphonuclear cells, and other
inflammatory cells.
　　Aspirin and all newer NSAIDs inhibit cyclooxygenase. As a result, synthesis of prostaglandins
and thromboxane is reduced. Because available NSAIDs inhibit COX I as much as or more than
COX II, these drugs deplete prostaglandins necessary for normal cell function (eg, cytoprotection
in the stomach) as well as prostaglandins involved in inflammation. The major difference between
the mechanisms of aspirin and the newer NSAIDs is that aspirin (but not its active metabolite, salicylate) acetylates and thereby irreversibly inhibits cyclooxygenase, whereas the inhibition produced by newer agents is reversible. The irreversible action of aspirin results in a longer duration
of its antiplatelet effect.

C. **Effects:** Arachidonic acid derivatives are important mediators of inflammation; cyclooxygenase inhibitors reduce the manifestations of inflammation, although they have no effect on underlying tissue damage or immunologic reactions. Prostaglandin synthesis in the CNS in response to pyrogenic substances is similarly suppressed by NSAIDs, resulting in reduction of
fever (antipyretic action). The analgesic mechanism of these agents is less well understood. Activation of peripheral pain sensors may be diminished as a result of reduced production of
prostaglandins in injured tissue; in addition, a central mechanism is operative.

D. **Pharmacokinetics and Clinical Use:**
1. **Aspirin:** Aspirin has three therapeutic dose ranges: the low range (< 300 mg/d) is effective in reducing platelet aggregation; intermediate doses (300–2400 mg/d) have antipyretic
and analgesic effects; and high doses (2400–4000 mg/d) are used for their anti-inflammatory effect. Aspirin is readily absorbed and is hydrolyzed in blood and tissues to acetate and
salicylic acid. Salicylate is probably the major active molecule in the anti-inflammatory action of aspirin. Elimination of salicylate is first-order at low doses, with a half-life of 3–5
hours. At high (anti-inflammatory) doses, half-life increases to 15 hours or more and elimination becomes zero-order. Excretion is via the kidney.
2. **Newer NSAIDs:** The newer cyclooxygenase inhibitors are well absorbed after oral administration and are excreted via the kidney. Ibuprofen has a half-life of about 2 hours, is

relatively safe, and is the least expensive of the newer NSAIDs. Indomethacin is a potent NSAID with increased toxicity. Naproxen and piroxicam are noteworthy because of their longer half-lives (12–24 hours), which permit less frequent dosing. Newer NSAIDs are used for pain of dysmenorrhea, inflammation (especially that of rheumatoid arthritis and gout), and patent ductus arteriosus in premature infants. Both ibuprofen and naproxen are now available in low-dose over-the-counter formulations.

E. Toxicity:

    1. Aspirin: Possible adverse effects from therapeutic anti-inflammatory doses of aspirin are gastrointestinal disturbances and increased risk of bleeding. Chronic aspirin overdosage is associated with reduced synthesis of prothrombin. When prostaglandin synthesis is inhibited by even small doses of aspirin, persons with aspirin hypersensitivity (especially associated with nasal polyps) may experience asthma from the increased synthesis of leukotrienes. At higher doses, tinnitus, vertigo, hyperventilation, and respiratory alkalosis are observed. At very high doses, the drug causes metabolic acidosis, dehydration, hyperthermia, collapse, coma, and death. Children with viral infections are at increased risk of developing Reye's syndrome (hepatic fatty degeneration and encephalopathy) if given aspirin. Dialysis is effective in removing salicylates.

    2. Newer NSAIDs: Like aspirin, these agents may cause significant gastrointestinal disturbance, but the incidence is lower than with aspirin. At high therapeutic dosage, however, there is a significant risk of renal damage with all the newer NSAIDs, especially in patients with preexisting renal disease. Since these drugs are cleared by the kidney, renal damage results in higher, more toxic serum concentrations. Phenylbutazone should not be used chronically because it causes aplastic anemia and agranulocytosis.

DISEASE-MODIFYING, SLOW-ACTING ANTIRHEUMATIC DRUGS (DMARDs, SAARDs)

A. Classification and Prototypes: This heterogeneous group of agents has anti-inflammatory actions in several connective tissue diseases. These agents are called "disease-modifying" because some evidence shows slowing or even reversal of joint damage, an effect never seen with NSAIDs. They are also called "slow-acting" because it may take 6 weeks to 6 months for their benefits to become apparent. The major members of the group are cytotoxic agents, especially **methotrexate;** the **gold compounds,** which are used only as anti-inflammatory agents; **hydroxychloroquine** (an antimalarial drug); **penicillamine,** which is also used as a chelating agent; and **sulfasalazine,** a drug used in ulcerative colitis. **Corticosteroids** may be considered anti-inflammatory drugs with an intermediate rate of action, ie, slower than NSAIDs but faster than the DMARDs. However, the corticosteroids are too toxic for chronic use (see Chapter 39) and are reserved for temporary control of severe exacerbations.

B. Mechanisms of Action: The mechanisms of these drugs are poorly understood. Methotrexate, a cytotoxic immunosuppressant drug, probably acts by reducing the numbers of immune cells available to maintain the inflammatory response. Organic gold compounds alter the activity of macrophages, cells that play a central role in inflammation, especially that of arthritis. Gold compounds also inhibit lysosomal enzyme activity, reduce histamine release, and suppress phagocytic activity by polymorphonuclear leukocytes. Hydroxychloroquine may interfere with the activity of T lymphocytes, decrease leukocyte chemotaxis, stabilize lysosomal membranes, interfere with DNA and RNA synthesis, and trap free radicals. Penicillamine appears to have anti-inflammatory effects similar to those of hydroxychloroquine. The mechanism of sulfasalazine's anti-inflammatory action is poorly understood but appears to differ from its mechanism in ulcerative colitis: sulfapyridine alone or sulfapyridine plus the parent drug (sulfasalazine is a compound of sulfapyridine and 5-aminosalicylic acid) appears to be more important than the 5-aminosalicylic acid component. Controlled trials indicate that sulfasalazine has definite benefits in rheumatoid arthritis.

C. Effects: These agents have a very slow onset of anti-inflammatory action in patients with rheumatoid or other immune complexes in their serum. Benefits may require several months to become manifest. It has been claimed that these drugs may slow or arrest the underlying joint destruction in rheumatoid arthritis.

D. Pharmacokinetics and Clinical Use: Disease-modifying anti-inflammatory drugs are used in patients with rheumatoid arthritis that does not respond to other agents. Methotrexate, hydroxychloroquine, penicillamine, and sulfasalazine are given orally. Gold compounds are available for parenteral use (gold sodium thiomalate and aurothioglucose) and for oral administration (auranofin). Many patients do not respond to the DMARDs (especially gold), and there is continuing controversy about the efficacy of these drugs in the therapy of arthritis.

E. Toxicity: All disease-modifying agents can cause severe or fatal toxicities. Careful monitoring of patients who take these drugs is mandatory. Methotrexate causes bone marrow depression, hepatotoxicity, and teratogenic fetal damage or abortion. The major toxicities of gold include potentially fatal dermatitis and bone marrow depression. Oral gold causes a high incidence of severe gastrointestinal disturbances. Hydroxychloroquine causes dermatitis, bone marrow depression, and retinal degeneration. Penicillamine causes renal damage and aplastic anemia. Sulfasalazine is somewhat more toxic in rheumatoid arthritis than in ulcerative colitis, but life-threatening toxicity is rare.

ACETAMINOPHEN

A. Classification and Prototype: Acetaminophen is the only over-the-counter non-anti-inflammatory analgesic commonly available in the USA. Phenacetin, a toxic prodrug that is metabolized to acetaminophen, is still available in some other countries.

B. Mechanism of Action: The mechanism of analgesic action of acetaminophen is unclear. The drug is a weak cyclooxygenase inhibitor in peripheral tissues, thus accounting for its lack of anti-inflammatory effect. Acetaminophen may be a more effective inhibitor of prostaglandin synthesis in the CNS, resulting in analgesic and antipyretic action.

C. Effects: As noted above, acetaminophen is an analgesic and antipyretic agent that lacks the anti-inflammatory effects of NSAIDs. This drug does not have significant antiplatelet effects.

D. Pharmacokinetics and Clinical Use: Acetaminophen is effective for the same indications as intermediate-dose aspirin. Acetaminophen is therefore useful as an aspirin substitute, especially in children with viral infections (who are at risk for Reye's syndrome if they take aspirin) and in individuals with any type of aspirin intolerance. Acetaminophen is well absorbed and metabolized in the liver. Its half-life, which is 2–3 hours in persons with normal hepatic function, is unaffected by renal disease.

E. Toxicity: In therapeutic dosages, acetaminophen has negligible toxicity in most individuals. However, when taken in overdose—or by patients with severe liver impairment—the drug is a very dangerous hepatotoxin. The mechanism of toxicity requires oxidation to cytotoxic intermediates by phase I P450 enzymes. This occurs if substrates for phase II conjugation reactions (acetate and glucuronide) are lacking (see Chapter 4).

DRUGS USED IN GOUT

A. Classification and Prototypes: Gout is associated with increased body stores of uric acid. Acute attacks involve joint inflammation caused by precipitation of uric acid crystals. Treatment strategies include (1) reducing inflammation during acute attacks (with colchicine or NSAIDs; Figure 36–2); (2) accelerating renal excretion of uric acid with uricosuric drugs (probenecid or sulfinpyrazone); and (3) reducing the conversion of purines to uric acid by xanthine oxidase (with allopurinol).

B. Colchicine and Other Drugs Used for Acute Gout:
    1. Mechanism: Colchicine, a selective inhibitor of microtubule assembly, reduces leukocyte migration and phagocytosis; the drug may also reduce production of leukotriene B$_4$. Potent NSAIDs such as indomethacin are also effective (but not as selective) in inhibiting the inflammation of acute gouty arthritis. These agents act through reduction of prostaglandin for-

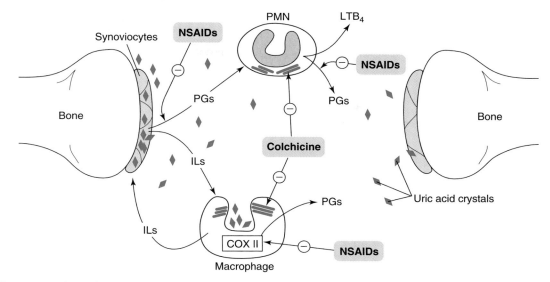

Figure 36–2. Sites of action of some anti-inflammatory drugs in a gouty joint. Synoviocytes damaged by uric acid crystals release prostaglandins (PGs), interleukins (ILs), and other mediators of inflammation. Polymorphonuclear leukocytes (PMNs), macrophages, and other inflammatory cells enter the joint and also release inflammatory substances, including leukotrienes (eg, LTB$_4$) that attract additional inflammatory cells. Colchicine acts on microtubules in the inflammatory cells. NSAIDs act on cyclooxygenase II in all of the cells of the joint.

mation (see the discussion at the beginning of this chapter and Chapter 18) and through inhibition of crystal phagocytosis by macrophages (Figure 36–2).

2. **Effects:** Because it reacts with tubulin and interferes with microtubule assembly, colchicine is a general mitotic poison. Tubulin is necessary for normal cell division, motility, and many other processes; therefore, colchicine has systemic toxicity if used in excess. NSAIDs reduce the synthesis of mediators of inflammation by inflammatory cells in the gouty joint.

3. **Pharmacokinetics and clinical use:** Indomethacin or colchicine is preferred for the treatment of acute gouty arthritis. Colchicine is also of value in the management of "Mediterranean fever," a disease of unknown cause characterized by fever, hepatitis, peritonitis, pleuritis, arthritis, and, occasionally, amyloidosis. Phenylbutazone, a dangerous NSAID when used chronically, is still sometimes used for short-term management of gouty arthritis. Indomethacin and colchicine are used orally; a parenteral preparation of colchicine is also available.

4. **Toxicity:** Because colchicine can severely damage the liver and kidney, dosage must be carefully limited and monitored. Therapeutic doses are often associated with gastrointestinal upset, especially diarrhea. Indomethacin may cause renal damage or bone marrow depression. Phenylbutazone has caused many cases of aplastic anemia.

C. **Uricosuric Agents:**
1. **Mechanism:** Uricosuric agents **(probenecid, sulfinpyrazone)** are weak acids that compete with uric acid in the S$_2$ segment of the proximal renal tubule for reabsorption by the weak acid transport mechanism. At low doses, these agents may also compete with uric acid for *secretion* by the tubule and (occasionally) can even elevate serum uric acid concentration. Elevation of uric acid levels by this mechanism occurs with aspirin (another weak acid) over much of its dose range.

2. **Effects:** Uricosuric drugs act primarily in the kidney and inhibit the secretion of other weak acids (eg, penicillin) in addition to inhibiting the reabsorption of uric acid.

3. **Pharmacokinetics and clinical use:** Chronic gout is treated orally with a uricosuric agent or allopurinol. These drugs are of no value in acute gouty arthritis and are best withheld for 1–2 weeks after an episode of that disorder.

4. **Toxicity:**   Uricosuric drugs may precipitate an attack of acute gouty arthritis during the early phase of their action. This can be avoided by simultaneously administering colchicine or indomethacin. Because they are sulfonamides, the uricosuric drugs share allergenicity with other classes of sulfonamide drugs (diuretics, antimicrobials, oral hypoglycemic drugs).

D. Allopurinol:
1. **Mechanism:**   Allopurinol is converted to oxipurinol (alloxanthine) by xanthine oxidase, the enzyme that converts hypoxanthine to xanthine and xanthine to uric acid. Allopurinol and oxipurinol are inhibitors of this enzyme. Allopurinol is relatively selective in humans but can severely impair purine metabolism of some protozoa; the drug has also been used in the treatment of leishmaniasis.
2. **Effects:**   Inhibition of conversion to uric acid increases the concentrations of the more soluble hypoxanthine and xanthine and decreases the concentration of the less soluble uric acid. As a result, there is less likelihood of precipitation of uric acid crystals in joints and tissues.
3. **Pharmacokinetics and clinical use:**   Allopurinol is given orally in the management of chronic gout. It is usually withheld for 1–2 weeks after an acute episode of gouty arthritis.
4. **Toxicity:**   Allopurinol causes gastrointestinal upset and, rarely, peripheral neuritis and vasculitis.

DRUG LIST

The following drugs are important members of the group discussed in this chapter. Prototypes should be learned in detail; features of the major variants should be known well enough so that the variants can be distinguished from prototypes and from each other; the other significant agents should be recognized as belonging to a specific subclass.

Subclass	Prototype	Major Variants	Other Significant Agents
Anti-inflammatory drugs Salicylates	Aspirin		Sodium salicylate

Newer nonsteroidal anti-
  inflammatory drugs
	Ibuprofen	Indomethacin	Naproxen, piroxicam, many
			  others

Slow-acting antirheumatic drugs	Methotrexate	Gold, hydroxychloroquine, penicillamine, sulfasalazine	
Acetaminophen class	Acetaminophen		Phenacetin
Drugs used in gout Anti-inflammatory drugs	Colchicine		NSAIDs, eg, indomethacin
Uricosurics	Probenecid		Sulfinpyrazone
Xanthine oxidase inhibitors	Allopurinol		

QUESTIONS

DIRECTIONS: Each of the numbered items or incomplete statements in this section is followed by answers or by completions of the statement. Select the ONE lettered answer or completion that is BEST in each case.

1. Important effects of aspirin include all of the following EXCEPT
    (A) Reduction of fever
    (B) Reduction of prostaglandin synthesis in inflamed tissues
    (C) Respiratory stimulation when taken in toxic dosage
    (D) Reduction of bleeding tendency
    (E) Tinnitus and vertigo
2. Important effects of ibuprofen include all of the following EXCEPT
    (A) Reversal of joint destruction in rheumatoid arthritis

   (B) Reduction of uterine contractions in dysmenorrhea
   (C) Reduction of fever
   (D) Analgesic action in headache
   (E) Reduction of thromboxane synthesis in platelets

3. Drugs that are useful in dysmenorrhea include all of the following EXCEPT
   (A) Aspirin
   (B) Colchicine
   (C) Ibuprofen
   (D) Naproxen
   (E) Piroxicam

4. Drugs that are useful in the treatment of gout include all of the following EXCEPT
   (A) Allopurinol
   (B) Aspirin
   (C) Colchicine
   (D) Indomethacin
   (E) Probenecid

5. Which of the following drug effects is linked with a FALSE statement about its mechanism of action?
   (A) Allopurinol action in gout: Inhibits oxidation of hypoxanthine
   (B) Aspirin antiplatelet action: Inhibits cyclooxygenase
   (C) Hydroxychloroquine antirheumatic action: Interferes with T lymphocyte action
   (D) Probenecid uricosuric action: Increases secretion of uric acid by the loop of Henle
   (E) Indomethacin closure of patent ductus arteriosus: Blocks PGE production in the ductus of the newborn

6. Salicylate intoxication is characterized by all of the following EXCEPT
   (A) Hyperventilation
   (B) Hypoprothrombinemia
   (C) Hypothermia
   (D) Metabolic acidosis
   (E) Respiratory alkalosis

DIRECTIONS (Items 7–16): Each set of matching questions in this section consists of a list of three to twenty-six lettered options (some of which may be figures) followed by several numbered items. For each numbered item, select the ONE lettered option that is most closely associated with it. Each lettered option may be selected once, more than once, or not at all.

   (A) Acetaminophen
   (B) Allopurinol
   (C) Aspirin
   (D) Colchicine
   (E) Hydroxychloroquine
   (F) Indomethacin
   (G) Methotrexate
   (H) Penicillamine
   (I) Phenacetin
   (J) Probenecid
   (K) Sulfasalazine

7. A potent inhibitor of cyclooxygenase; used to accelerate closure of a patent ductus arteriosus
8. A relatively safe antipyretic drug with no anti-inflammatory action
9. A drug that has anti-inflammatory effects only in gout and "Mediterranean fever"
10. An antimalarial agent with a slow, disease-modifying anti-inflammatory effect in rheumatoid arthritis
11. A drug that may be metabolized to a hepatotoxic product; the antidote is acetylcysteine
12. A slow-acting antirheumatic drug that is cytotoxic and reduces the number of inflammatory cells in rheumatoid joints; also used in leukemia
13. A drug that is metabolized to a product that inhibits the enzyme that produced it
14. A highly selective inhibitor of microtubule assembly
15. A compound of a sulfonamide with 5-aminosalicylic acid
16. A drug that is metabolized to acetaminophen; it was withdrawn from the United States market because of its high incidence of renal damage

ANSWERS

1. Aspirin clearly *increases* bleeding tendency (by its antiplatelet effects). The answer is **(D).**
2. It is not clear that any drug actually reverses the joint damage of rheumatoid arthritis, though it has been claimed that disease-modifying antirheumatic drugs may do so. The answer is **(A).**
3. Primary dysmenorrhea is caused by excessive production of prostaglandin $F_{2\alpha}$; NSAIDs that inhibit cyclooxygenase are far more effective in relieving symptoms than other analgesics. Colchicine, which is not analgesic and is anti-inflammatory only in gout and "Mediterranean fever," would never be used in this condition. The answer is **(B).**
4. Aspirin should not be used in gout because the drug slows renal secretion of uric acid and raises uric acid blood levels over a large part of the dose range. The answer is **(B).**
5. Probenecid inhibits the reabsorption of uric acid in the S_2 segment of the proximal tubule. (Both secretion and reabsorption of weak acids occur in the proximal tubule, not the loop of Henle.) The answer is **(D).**
6. Salicylate intoxication is associated with **hyperthermia,** not hypothermia, because the drug causes uncoupling of oxidative phosphorylation, resulting in increased metabolism. The answer is **(C).**
7. The answer is **(F),** indomethacin.
8. The answer is **(A),** acetaminophen.
9. Colchicine has a highly selective effect on leukocytes that are partially responsible for the inflammation associated with urate crystal deposition. The drug's mechanism in Mediterranean fever, a familial inflammatory disease of the liver, is unknown. The answer is **(D).**
10. The answer is **(E),** hydroxychloroquine.
11. Acetaminophen toxicity, a common source of questions on board exams, has been discussed in this chapter and in Chapter 4. Acetaminophen toxicity is more difficult to treat than aspirin toxicity, but acetylcysteine is effective if given early. The answer is **(A).**
12. Methotrexate is cytotoxic (it is an important cancer chemotherapeutic drug) and has become one of the most popular slow-acting antirheumatic drugs. The answer is **(G).**
13. Allopurinol is metabolized to oxipurinol (alloxanthine) by xanthine oxidase; both allopurinol and its metabolite inhibit this enzyme. The answer is **(B).**
14. Colchicine is highly selective in its ability to inhibit microtubule assembly and is a standard agent used in research on these cellular organelles. The answer is **(D).**
15. Sulfasalazine breaks down in the colon to release sulfapyridine and 5-aminosalicylic acid. It is one of the primary drugs used in the treatment of ulcerative colitis. The answer is **(K).**
16. Phenacetin is a prodrug of acetaminophen and has been shown in very large epidemiologic studies to cause renal damage in large numbers of patients. The answer is **(I).**

Part VII: Endocrine Drugs

Hypothalamic & Pituitary Hormones

37

OBJECTIVES

You should be able to:

- Describe the major hypothalamic-releasing hormones.
- Describe the major anterior pituitary hormones and their effects.
- Describe the major posterior pituitary hormones and their effects.
- Describe the major drugs used as substitutes for the natural hypothalamic and pituitary hormones.

CONCEPTS

The hypothalamus and pituitary gland synthesize several hormones that regulate other glands and tissues throughout the body. One group of hypothalamic hormones (releasing hormones) regulates the release of anterior pituitary hormones. The other hypothalamic hormones (oxytocin and vasopressin) are transported to the posterior pituitary are released from the pituitary into the general circulation, and act directly on distant tissues. The hormones currently recognized as most important (and their targets) are listed in Table 37–1. Except for prolactin-inhibiting hormone (dopamine), all of these endocrine agents are peptides.

Table 37–1. Links between hypothalamic, pituitary, and target organ hormones.

Hypothalamic Hormone	Pituitary Hormone	Target Organ	Target Organ Hormone
Growth hormone-releasing hormone (GHRH)	Growth hormone (GH)	Liver	Somatomedins
Somatostatin			
Thyrotropin-releasing hormone (TRH)	Thyroid-stimulating hormone (TSH)	Thyroid	Thyroxine, triiodothyronine
Corticotropin-releasing hormone (CRH)	Adrenocorticotropin (ACTH)	Adrenal cortex	Glucocorticoids, mineralocorticoids, androgens
Gonadotropin-releasing hormone (GnRH or LHRH)	Follicle-stimulating hormone (FSH)	Gonads	Estrogen, progesterone, testosterone
	Luteinizing hormone (LH)		
Prolactin-releasing hormone (PRH)	Prolactin (PRL)	Lymphocytes	Lymphokines
Prolactin-inhibiting hormone (PIH, dopamine)		Breast	
Oxytocin	None	Smooth muscle, especially uterus	
Vasopressin	None	Renal tubule, smooth muscle	

HYPOTHALAMIC HORMONES

A.   Growth Hormone-Releasing Hormone (GHRH):   GHRH (also called somatocrinin) consists of several large peptides with releasing activity; two shorter synthetic peptides with similar activity are available for clinical use. In normal individuals, they produce a rapid increase in plasma growth hormone levels; they are effective in increasing growth in some patients with short stature. However, most patients with short stature suffer from pituitary insufficiency, not GHRH deficiency. Therefore, the primary use of GHRH preparations is to determine the cause of growth hormone deficiency.

B.   Somatostatin (Somatotropin Release–Inhibiting Hormone, SRIH):   Somatostatin, a 14-amino-acid peptide, has been isolated, sequenced, and synthesized. It is found in the pancreas and other parts of the gastrointestinal system as well as in the CNS. In addition to inhibiting the release of growth hormone, somatostatin inhibits the release of thyrotropin, glucagon, insulin, and gastrin. Although it can decrease the release of growth hormone in acromegaly, somatostatin is of no clinical value because of its short duration of action. **Octreotide,** a synthetic octapeptide somatostatin analog with a longer duration of action, has been found useful in the management of acromegaly, carcinoid, gastrinoma, glucagonoma, and other endocrine tumors.

C.   Thyrotropin-Releasing Hormone (TRH):   TRH is a tripeptide that stimulates release of thyrotropin from the anterior pituitary, possibly through the stimulation of adenylyl cyclase. TRH also increases prolactin production but has no effect on the release of growth hormone or ACTH.

D.   Corticotropin-Releasing Hormone (CRH):   This 41-amino-acid peptide stimulates secretion of both ACTH and beta-endorphin (a closely related peptide) from the pituitary. This effect is associated with increased cAMP levels in the gland. CRH can be used in the diagnosis of abnormalities of ACTH secretion because ACTH secretion by nonpituitary tumors (eg, of the lung) rarely increases in response to stimulation by CRH, whereas secretion by the pituitary in Cushing's disease consistently increases after CRH stimulation.

E.   Gonadotropin-Releasing Hormone (GnRH or LHRH; Gonadorelin):   GnRH is a decapeptide; **leuprolide** is a synthetic nonapeptide with similar activity. Several other synthetic peptides with GnRH activity are available. When given in pulsatile doses (resembling physiologic cycling), these agents stimulate gonadotropin release. In contrast, steady dosing causes a marked inhibition of gonadotropin release—in effect, reversible medical castration. GnRH is used in the diagnosis and treatment (by pulsatile administration) of hypogonadal states. Leuprolide and several analogs (nafarelin, gosarelin, buserelin) are used to suppress gonadotropin secretion (by administration in steady dosage) in patients with prostatic carcinoma or other gonadal steroid-sensitive tumors.

F.   Prolactin-Inhibiting Hormone (PIH, Dopamine):   Dopamine is the physiologic inhibitor of prolactin release. Because of its peripheral effects and the need for parenteral administration, dopamine is not useful in the control of hyperprolactinemia, but **bromocriptine,** an orally active ergot derivative, is effective in reducing prolactin secretion from the normal gland as well as from pituitary tumors. Bromocriptine may reduce the secretion of other hormones from such tumors; sometimes regression of the tumor may also result. **Pergolide** is another ergot derivative with similar effects.

ANTERIOR PITUITARY HORMONES

A.   Growth Hormone (Somatotropin):   Growth hormone is a large (191-amino-acid) peptide. In the past it was obtained from the pituitaries of human cadavers. This use was abolished when it was reported that several patients treated with growth hormone from this source developed Creutzfeld-Jakob disease, apparently from slow infectious prion agents contained in the extracts. Human growth hormone is now available in two forms through recombinant DNA technology: **somatrem** (somatotropin with an extra methionine) and **somatotropin.** These products, which are identical in their biologic properties, are useful in the treatment of growth hormone deficiency in children.

B. Thyroid-Stimulating Hormone (TSH): This peptide stimulates adenylyl cyclase in thyroid cells and increases iodine uptake and production of thyroid hormones. TSH has been used as a diagnostic tool to distinguish primary from secondary hypothyroidism. The hormone is still used occasionally to increase ^{131}I uptake (and tumoricidal effect) in metastatic thyroid carcinoma.

C. Adrenocorticotropin (ACTH): This peptide is formed from a large precursor peptide, proopiomelanocortin. This precursor is also the source of melanocyte-stimulating hormone, beta-endorphin, and met-enkephalin. Although it has been used therapeutically to increase corticosteroid levels, ACTH is now used almost exclusively for diagnostic purposes in patients with abnormal corticosteroid production. **Cosyntropin,** a synthetic analog consisting of the first 24 amino acids of ACTH, is most commonly used for this purpose rather than ACTH itself.

D. Follicle-Stimulating Hormone (FSH): FSH is a glycoprotein that stimulates gametogenesis and follicle development in women and spermatogenesis in men. The preparation most often used is urofollitropin, a product extracted from the urine of postmenopausal women.

E. Luteinizing Hormone (LH): LH is the major stimulant of gonadal steroid production. In women, LH also regulates follicular development and ovulation. No pure preparation of LH is currently in use. **Human chorionic gonadotropin (hCG)** has significant LH effect, is synthesized by the placenta, and is available for use (see below).

F. Menotropins (hMG): Menotropins is a preparation of human menopausal gonadotropins that consists of human FSH and LH from postmenopausal urine. The product is often combined with human chorionic gonadotropin in the treatment of hypogonadal states in both men and women.

G. Prolactin: Prolactin, a glycoprotein hormone responsible for lactation, is not used in therapy.

POSTERIOR PITUITARY HORMONES

A. Oxytocin: Oxytocin is a nonapeptide synthesized in cell bodies in the paraventricular nuclei of the hypothalamus and transported through the axons of these cells to the posterior pituitary, where the peptide is released into the circulation. Oxytocin is an effective stimulant of uterine contraction and is sometimes used intravenously to induce or reinforce labor. Because it causes contraction of smooth muscle in the myoepithelial cells of the breast, oxytocin also can be used by lactating women as a nasal spray to stimulate milk letdown.

B. Vasopressin (Antidiuretic Hormone, ADH): Vasopressin is synthesized in the supraoptic nuclei of the hypothalamus and released from the posterior pituitary. As discussed in Chapter 15, vasopressin acts on V_2 receptors and increases the synthesis or insertion of water channels by a cAMP-dependent mechanism, resulting in an increase in water permeability in the collecting tubules of the kidney. The increased water permeability permits water reabsorption into the hypertonic renal papilla, thus causing the antidiuretic effect. Vasopressin also causes smooth muscle contraction (a V_1 effect). The primary use of vasopressin is in the treatment of pituitary diabetes insipidus.

DRUG LIST

The drugs listed in Table 37–2 are pituitary hormone analogs or agents used for their effects on pituitary-related endocrine function. Many of the natural hormones described in Table 37–1 are also used as drugs.

Table 37–2. The following drugs are pituitary hormone analogs or agents used for their effects on pituitary-related endocrine function. Many of the natural hormones described in Table 37–1 are also used as drugs.

Drug	Actions	Clinical Use	Comment
Somatrem	Growth hormone	Pituitary deficiency	Protein from recombinant synthesis; has one additional methionine; recombinant somatotropin is also available
Octreotide	Somatostatin analog	Multiple uses to inhibit glandular secretion	Longer-acting than natural somatostatin
Cosyntropin	ACTH analog, stimulates adrenal cortex	Corticosteroid substitute; diagnosis; infantile spasms (seizures)	Cosyntropin is a 1–24 amino acid active fragment of ACTH
Leuprolide, goserelin, nafarelin	GnRH analogs	Infertility; cancer	Stimulate gonads if given in pulses; inhibit if given continuously
Urofollitropin	FSH-like activity	Infertility	Isolated from human urine
Human chorionic gonadotropin (hCG)	LH-like activity	Infertility	Isolated from human urine
Menotropins	FSH plus LH activity	Infertility	Isolated from human urine
Bromocriptine	Inhibits prolactin release	Stops lactation; inhibits growth of pituitary tumors	An ergot alkaloid with potent dopamine agonist activity
Desmopressin	Antidiuretic hormone analog	Pituitary diabetes insipidus	A V_2 receptor agonist; longer-acting than ADH

QUESTIONS

DIRECTIONS: Each of the numbered items or incomplete statements in this section is followed by answers or by completions of the statement. Select the ONE lettered answer or completion that is BEST in each case.

1. All of the following are hormones EXCEPT
   (A) Bromocriptine
   (B) Somatomedin
   (C) Somatotropin
   (D) Thyroxine
   (E) Vasopressin
2. Drugs useful in the treatment of infertility include all of the following EXCEPT
   (A) Bromocriptine
   (B) Clomiphene
   (C) Gonadotropin-releasing hormone
   (D) Human chorionic gonadotropin
   (E) Prolactin
3. Hormones that increase cAMP in the target organs include
   (A) Growth hormone
   (B) Luteinizing hormone
   (C) Oxytocin
   (D) Prolactin
   (E) Vasopressin
4. Hormones that are synthesized in the hypothalamus include all of the following EXCEPT
   (A) Corticotropin-releasing hormone
   (B) Luteinizing hormone
   (C) Oxytocin
   (D) Thyrotropin-releasing hormone
   (E) Vasopressin
5. Hormones that are useful in the diagnosis of endocrine insufficiency include
   (A) Corticotropin-releasing hormone
   (B) Cosyntropin

    (C)   Gonadotropin-releasing hormone
    (D)   Thyrotropin-releasing hormone
    (E)   All of the above

DIRECTIONS (Items 6–10): Each set of matching questions in this section consists of a list of three to twenty-six lettered options (some of which may be figures) followed by several numbered items. For each numbered item, select the ONE lettered option that is most closely associated with it. Each lettered option may be selected once, more than once, or not at all.

    (A)   Bromocriptine
    (B)   Cosyntropin
    (C)   Desmopressin
    (D)   Human chorionic gonadotropin
    (E)   Leuprolide
    (F)   Menotropins
    (G)   Octreotide
    (H)   Somatomedin
    (I)   Somatrem
    (J)   Thyroid-stimulating hormone

   6. A 24-amino-acid peptide with ACTH-like properties
   7. A substance derived from the urine of pregnant women; useful for its LH-like activity
   8. A substance produced in the liver under the control of growth hormone
   9. A recombinant form of growth hormone with one additional amino acid
 10. A peptide with GnRH activity but longer duration of action than the naturally occurring hormone

ANSWERS

   1. Bromocriptine, an ergot alkaloid with central dopamine agonist activity, is not produced in the body. The answer is **(A)**.
   2. Clomiphene is an ovulation-stimulating partial agonist estrogen (see Chapter 39). Prolactin has inhibitory effects on fertility and is never used in infertility. The answer is **(E)**.
   3. Vasopressin acts by increasing cAMP. The other hormones act by other mechanisms. The answer is **(E)**.
   4. Luteinizing hormone is synthesized in the anterior pituitary. The answer is **(B)**.
   5. All are correct. The answer is **(E)**.
   6. Cosyntropin is the form of ACTH most commonly used. ACTH is now rarely used; cosyntropin is used mainly for diagnostic procedures. The answer is **(B)**.
   7. Human chorionic gonadotropin (hCG) is produced by the placenta in pregnant women and has potent LH activity. The answer is **(D)**.
   8. The somatomedins are synthesized in the liver under growth hormone control. The answer is **(H)**.
   9. Somatrem is recombinant growth hormone with an extra methionine. True somatotropin is also available through recombinant synthesis. The answer is **(I)**.
 10. Leuprolide is a longer-acting GnRH analog. The answer is **(E)**.

Thyroid & Antithyroid Drugs

38

OBJECTIVES

You should be able to:

- List the principal drugs used in the treatment of hypothyroidism.
- List the principal drugs used in the treatment of hyperthyroidism.
- Describe the major toxicities of thyroxine and the antithyroid drugs.

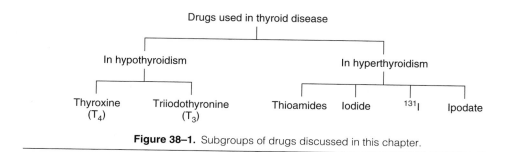

Figure 38–1. Subgroups of drugs discussed in this chapter.

CONCEPTS

The thyroid secretes two types of hormones: iodine-containing amino acids (thyroxine and tri-iodothyronine) and a peptide (calcitonin). Thyroxine and triiodothyronine have very general effects on growth, development, and metabolism. Calcitonin is important in calcium metabolism and is discussed in Chapter 41.

This chapter describes the drugs used in the treatment of hypo- and hyperthyroidism (Figure 38–1).

THYROID HORMONES

A. Synthesis and Transport of Thyroid Hormones: The thyroid secretes two primary iodine-containing hormones, **triiodothyronine (T_3)** and **thyroxine (T_4).** The iodine necessary for the synthesis of these molecules is derived from food or iodine supplements given orally. The up-take of iodine is an active process, and the iodide ion is highly concentrated in the thyroid gland. The tyrosine residues of a protein, thyroglobulin, are iodinated in the gland to form monoiodotyrosine (MIT) or diiodotyrosine (DIT). Thyroxine (T_4) is formed from the combination of two molecules of DIT, while triiodothyronine (T_3) contains one molecule of MIT and one of DIT. Some T_3 is released from the thyroid, but much of the circulating T_3 is formed by the deiodination of T_4 in the tissues. After release from the gland, both T_3 and T_4 are bound to thyroxine-binding globulin, a transport protein in the blood.

Thyroid function is controlled by the pituitary through the release of thyrotropin and by the availability of iodide. High levels of thyroid hormones inhibit the release of TRH and TSH, providing an effective negative feedback control mechanism. In Graves' disease, lymphocytes release a thyroid-stimulating immunoglobulin (TSI, also called TSH receptor-stimulating antibody, TSH-R Ab[stim]) that causes thyrotoxicosis. Since these lymphocytes are not susceptible to negative feedback, blood concentrations of thyroid hormone may become very high.

Iodide concentrations higher than normal inhibit iodination of tyrosine, an effect that is useful in the treatment of thyroid disease. Inadequate iodine intake results in diffuse enlargement of the thyroid (goiter).

B. Mechanisms of Action of Thyroxine and Triiodothyronine: T_3 is about ten times more potent than T_4; since T_4 is converted to T_3 in target cells, the liver, and the kidneys, most of the effect of circulating T_4 is probably due to T_3.

Thyroid hormone binds to receptors in the nucleus that control the expression of genes responsible for many metabolic processes. Like many other intracellular hormone receptors, the T_3 receptor exists in two monomeric forms, alpha and beta; they are synthesized in different amounts and different forms ($\alpha1$, $\alpha2$, $\beta1$, $\beta2$) in a developmentally specific way. When activated by T_3, the α and β monomers combine to form $\alpha\alpha$, $\beta\beta$, or $\alpha\beta$ dimers. These T_3-activated dimers bind to DNA response elements and control the synthesis of RNA that codes for specific proteins which mediate the actions of thyroid hormones.

The proteins synthesized under T_3 control differ depending upon the tissue involved; these proteins include Na^+/K^+ ATPase, specific contractile proteins in smooth muscle and the heart, enzymes involved in lipid metabolism, important developmental components in the brain, etc. T_3 may also have a separate membrane receptor-mediated effect in some tissues.

1. **Effects of thyroid hormone:** The organ level actions of the thyroid drugs include normal growth and development of nervous, skeletal, and reproductive systems and control of metabolism of fats, carbohydrates, proteins, and vitamins. The results of excess thyroid activity (thyrotoxicosis) and hypothyroidism (myxedema) are summarized in Table 38–1. A case of thyrotoxicosis is presented in Case 9 (Appendix IV).

2. **Clinical use:** Thyroid hormone therapy can be accomplished with either thyroxine or triiodothyronine. Synthetic levothyroxine (T_4) is used for most cases. T_3 is faster-acting but has a shorter half-life and higher cost.

3. **Toxicity:** Toxicity is that of thyrotoxicosis (Table 38–1).

ANTITHYROID DRUGS

A. **Thioamides:** Propylthiouracil and methimazole are small sulfur-containing molecules that inhibit thyroid hormone production by several mechanisms. The most important effect is to block iodination of the tyrosine residues of thyroglobulin (Figure 38–2). In addition, these drugs may

Table 38–1. Summary of thyroid hormone effects.*

System	Thyrotoxicosis	Hypothyroidism
Skin and appendages	Warm, moist skin; sweating; heat intolerance; fine, thin hair; Plummer's nails; pretibial dermopathy (Graves' disease)	Pale, cool, puffy skin; dry and brittle hair; brittle nails
Eyes, face	Retraction of upper lid with wide stare; periorbital edema; exophthalmos; diplopia (Graves' disease)	Drooping of eyelids; periorbital edema; loss of temporal aspects of eyebrows; puffy, nonpitting facies; large tongue
Cardiovascular system	Decreased peripheral vascular resistance; increased heart rate, stroke volume, cardiac output, pulse pressure; high-output congestive heart failure; increased inotropic and chronotropic effects; arrhythmias; angina	Increased peripheral vascular resistance, decreased heart rate, stroke volume, cardiac output, pulse pressure; low-output congestive heart failure; ECG: bradycardia, prolonged PR interval, flat T wave, low voltage; pericardial effusion
Respiratory system	Dyspnea; decreased vital capacity	Pleural effusions; hypoventilation and CO_2 retention
Gastrointestinal system	Increased appetite; increased frequency of bowel movements; hypoproteinemia	Decreased appetite; decreased frequency of bowel movements; ascites
Central nervous system	Nervousness; hyperkinesia; emotional lability	Lethargy; general slowing of mental processes; neuropathies
Musculoskeletal system	Weakness and muscle fatigue; increased deep tendon reflexes; hypercalcemia; osteoporosis	Stiffness and muscle fatigue; decreased deep tendon reflexes; increased alkaline phosphatase, LDH, AST
Renal system	Mild polyuria; increased renal blood flow; increased glomerular filtration rate	Impaired water excretion; decreased renal blood flow; decreased glomerular filtration rate
Hematopoietic system	Increased erythropoiesis; anemia[1]	Decreased erythropoiesis; anemia[1]
Reproductive system	Menstrual irregularities; decreased fertility; increased gonadal steroid metabolism	Hypermenorrhea; infertility; decreased libido; impotence; oligospermia; decreased gonadal steroid metabolism
Metabolic system	Increased basal metabolic rate; negative nitrogen balance; hyperglycemia; increased free fatty acids; decreased cholesterol and triglycerides; increased hormone degradation; increased requirements for fat- and water-soluble vitamins; increased drug detoxification	Decreased basal metabolic rate; slight positive nitrogen balance; delayed degradation of insulin, with increased sensitivity; increased cholesterol and triglycerides; decreased hormone degradation; decreased requirements for fat- and water-soluble vitamins; decreased drug detoxification

*Reproduced, with permission, from Katzung BG (editor): *Basic & Clinical Pharmacology*, 7th ed. Appleton & Lange, 1998.
[1]The anemia of hyperthyroidism is usually normochromic and caused by increased red blood cell turnover. The anemia of hypothyroidism may be normochromic, hyperchromic, or hypochromic and may be due to decreased production rate, decreased iron absorption, decreased folic acid absorption, or to autoimmune pernicious anemia.

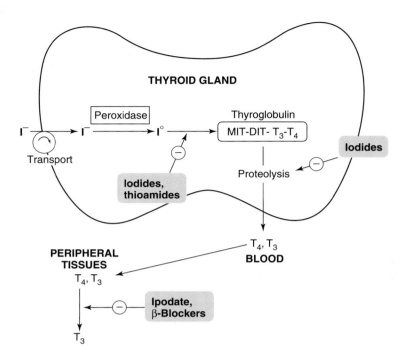

Figure 38–2. Sites of action of some antithyroid drugs. I⁻, iodide ion; I°, elemental iodine. Not shown: radioactive iodine (^{131}I), which destroys the gland through radiation.

block coupling of DIT and MIT. The thioamides can be used by the oral route and are effective in most patients with uncomplicated hyperthyroidism. Toxic effects include skin rash (common) and severe immune reactions (rare) such as vasculitis, hypoprothrombinemia, and agranulocytosis. These effects are usually reversible.

B.   Iodide Salts and Iodine: Iodide salts inhibit organification (iodination of tyrosine) and thyroid hormone release (Figure 38–2); these salts also decrease the size and vascularity of the hyperplastic thyroid gland. These effects of iodide are especially desirable if surgical resection of a hyperactive thyroid is planned. The usual forms of this drug are Lugol's solution (iodine and potassium iodide) and saturated solution of potassium iodide.

C.   Radioactive Iodine: Radioactive iodine (^{131}I) is taken up and concentrated in the thyroid gland so avidly that a dose large enough to severely damage the gland can be given without endangering other tissues. Unlike the thioamides and iodide salts, an effective dose of ^{131}I can produce a permanent cure of thyrotoxicosis without surgery.

D.   Iodinated Radiocontrast Media: Certain iodinated radiocontrast media, eg, ipodate, effectively suppress the conversion of T_4 to T_3 in the liver, kidney, and other peripheral tissues (Figure 38–2). Inhibition of hormone release from the thyroid may also play a part. Ipodate has proved to be very useful in rapidly reducing T_3 concentrations in thyrotoxicosis.

E.   Other Drugs: Other agents used in the treatment of thyrotoxicosis include the sympatholytic drugs, especially beta-blockers. These agents are particularly useful in controlling the tachycardia and other cardiac abnormalities of severe thyrotoxicosis.

DRUG LIST

The following drugs are important members of the group discussed in this chapter. Prototypes should be learned in detail; the other significant agents should be recognized as belonging to a specific subclass.

Subclass	Prototype	Other Significant Agents
Thyroid hormones	Thyroxine (T_4), triiodothyronine (T_3)	
Antithyroid drugs	Propylthiouracil, iodide salts, ^{131}I, ipodate	Methimazole
Miscellaneous	Propranolol	

QUESTIONS

DIRECTIONS: Each of the numbered items or incomplete statements in this section is followed by answers or by completions of the sentence. Select the ONE lettered answer or completion that is BEST in each case.

1. Important drugs used in the treatment of thyrotoxicosis include all of the following EXCEPT
   (A) Propylthiouracil
   (B) Potassium iodide
   (C) Thyroglobulin
   (D) Radioactive iodine
   (E) Methimazole

2. Actions of thyroxine include all of the following EXCEPT
   (A) Stimulation of oxygen consumption
   (B) Acceleration of cardiac rate
   (C) Fine tremor of skeletal muscles
   (D) Decreased glomerular filtration rate
   (E) Increased appetite

3. Effects of iodide salts given in large doses include all of the following EXCEPT
   (A) Decreased size of the thyroid gland
   (B) Decreased vascularity of the thyroid gland
   (C) Decreased hormone release
   (D) Decreased iodination of tyrosine
   (E) Increased ^{131}I uptake

4. Symptoms of hypothyroidism (myxedema) include all of the following EXCEPT
   (A) Slow heart rate
   (B) Dry, puffy skin
   (C) Lethargy, sleepiness
   (D) Increased appetite
   (E) Large tongue and drooping of the eyelids

Items 5–6: A 24-year-old woman is found to have thyrotoxicosis. She appears to be in good health otherwise.

5. It is decided to begin antithyroid drug therapy. Toxicities of possible therapies that would be considered in this case include all of the following EXCEPT
   (A) Ipodate: Skin rash
   (B) Iodide ion: Acne-like rash
   (C) Methimazole: Agranulocytosis
   (D) Propylthiouracil: Lupus erythematosus-like syndrome
   (E) Radioactive iodine: Radiation damage to the ovaries

6. The patient is lost to follow-up before therapy is begun, but she returns 6 months later for a prenatal workup. Although 3 months pregnant, she has lost weight, she has a marked tremor, and her resting heart rate is 120/min. Her thyrotoxicosis is obviously worse, and the gland is larger and more vascular. It is decided to correct her thyroid abnormality surgically. Before surgery can be done, however, her gland should be reduced in size and vascularity by administering
   (A) Radioactive iodine
   (B) Propylthiouracil
   (C) Ipodate
   (D) Iodide ion
   (E) Propranolol

DIRECTIONS (Items 7–10):   Each set of matching questions in this section consists of a list of three to twenty-six lettered options (some of which may be figures) followed by several numbered items. For each numbered item, select the ONE lettered option that is most closely associated with it. Each lettered option may be selected once, more than once, or not at all.

    (A) ^{131}I
    (B)   Ipodate
    (C)   Propranolol
    (D)   Propylthiouracil
    (E)   Triiodothyronine

  7.   Produced in the peripheral tissues when thyroxine is administered
  8.   Useful in "thyroid storm" to control cardiac manifestations
  9.   Radiocontrast medium that is also useful in thyrotoxicosis
10.   Produces a permanent reduction in thyroid activity

ANSWERS

  1.   Thyroglobulin contains thyroxine in its protein-bound form. This compound would never be used in thyrotoxicosis. Formerly used in hypothyroidism, thyroglobulin is now obsolete. The answer is **(C)**.
  2.   Thyroid hormone increases glomerular filtration rate. The answer is **(D)**.
  3.   Iodide has a negative feedback effect on the thyroid. The answer is **(E)**.
  4.   Appetite decreases in myxedema as the metabolic rate decreases. The answer is **(D)**.
  5.   The toxicities listed are all possible except radiation damage to the ovaries. Iodine is so avidly taken up by the thyroid that large doses of radioactive iodide can be given without damage to other tissues. The answer is **(E)**.
  6.   Surgical treatment is often preferred in hyperthyroidism that occurs during pregnancy because it offers minimal risk to the fetus and the fetal thyroid. Before surgical removal, a large, highly vascular thyroid gland should be prepared by administration of iodide ion. This treatment reduces the gland's size and vascularity and makes surgery much safer. Propylthiouracil may be considered for less severe thyrotoxicosis occurring during pregnancy. The answer is **(E)**.
  7. T_4 is converted into T_3 in the periphery. The answer is **(E)**.
  8.   Beta-blockers are particularly useful in controlling cardiac manifestations of severe thyrotoxicosis ("storm"). The answer is **(C)**.
  9.   Ipodate is a radiocontrast agent. The answer is **(B)**.
10.   Radioactive iodine is the only medical therapy that produces a permanent reduction of thyroid activity. The answer is **(A)**.

39

Corticosteroids & Antagonists

OBJECTIVES

You should be able to:

- Describe the major naturally occurring glucocorticoid and its actions.
- List several synthetic glucocorticoids and the differences between these agents and the naturally occurring hormone.
- Describe the actions of the naturally occurring mineralocorticoid and one synthetic agent in this subgroup.
- List the indications for the use of corticosteroids in adrenal and nonadrenal disorders.
- Describe the toxic effects of chronic glucocorticoid therapy.

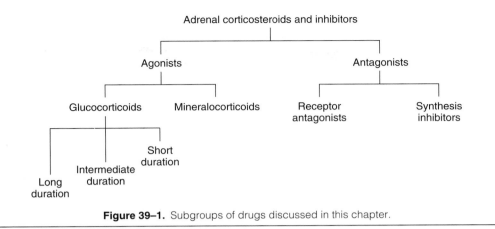

Figure 39–1. Subgroups of drugs discussed in this chapter.

CONCEPTS

The corticosteroids are steroid hormones produced by the adrenal cortex. They consist of two major physiologic and pharmacologic groups: (1) glucocorticoids, which have important effects on intermediary metabolism, catabolism, immune responses, and inflammation; and (2) mineralocorticoids, which regulate sodium and potassium reabsorption in the collecting tubules of the kidney. In addition, some androgenic and estrogenic steroids are also synthesized in the adrenal gland. This chapter reviews the glucocorticoids, the mineralocorticoids, and the adrenocorticosteroid antagonists (Figure 39–1).

GLUCOCORTICOIDS

A. **Mechanism of Action:** Corticosteroids enter the cell and bind to cytosolic receptors that transport the steroid into the nucleus. The steroid-receptor complex alters gene expression by binding to glucocorticoid response elements (GREs) or equivalent mineralocorticoid-specific elements (Figure 39–2). Tissue-specific responses to steroids are made possible by the presence in each tissue of different protein regulators that control the interaction between the hormone-receptor complex and particular response elements.

B. **Organ and Tissue Effects:**
1. **Metabolic effects:** Glucocorticoids stimulate gluconeogenesis. As a result, blood sugar rises, muscle protein is catabolized, and insulin secretion is stimulated. Both lipolysis and lipogenesis are stimulated, with a net increase of fat deposition in certain areas, eg, face (moon facies) and shoulders and back (buffalo hump).
2. **Catabolic effects:** As noted above, glucocorticoids cause muscle protein catabolism. In addition, lymphoid and connective tissue, fat, and skin undergo wasting under the influence of high concentrations of these steroids. Catabolic effects on bone can lead to osteoporosis. In children, growth is inhibited.
3. **Immunosuppressive effects:** Glucocorticoids inhibit some of the mechanisms involved in cell-mediated immunologic functions, especially those dependent on lymphocytes. These agents are actively lymphotoxic and are important in the treatment of lymphocytic leukemias. The drugs do not interfere with the development of normal acquired immunity but delay rejection reactions in patients with organ transplants.
4. **Anti-inflammatory effects:** Glucocorticoids have a dramatic effect on the distribution and function of leukocytes. These drugs increase neutrophils and decrease lymphocytes, eosinophils, basophils, and monocytes. The migration of leukocytes is also inhibited. The mechanism of these effects probably involves synthesis of inhibitors that suppress the production of prostaglandins and leukotrienes in the damaged tissue through inhibition of phospholipase (see Chapter 18).
5. **Other effects:** Glucocorticoids such as cortisol are required for normal renal excretion of water loads. The glucocorticoids also have effects on the CNS. When given in large doses

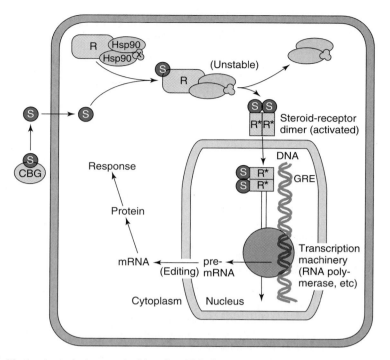

Figure 39–2. Mechanism of glucocorticoid action. This figure models the interaction of a steroid, S (eg, cortisol), with its receptor, R, and the subsequent events in a target cell. The steroid is present in the blood bound to the corticosteroid-binding globulin, CBG, but enters the cell as the free molecule. The intracellular receptor is bound to stabilizing proteins, including heat shock protein 90 (Hsp90) and several others, denoted as "X" in the figure. When the complex binds a molecule of steroid, the Hsp90 and associated molecules are released. The steroid-receptor complex enters the nucleus, binds to the glucocorticoid response element (GRE) on the gene, and regulates gene transcription by RNA polymerase II and associated transcription factors. The resulting mRNA is edited and exported to the cytoplasm for the production of protein that brings about the final hormone response. (Reproduced, with permission, from Katzung BG [editor]: *Basic & Clinical Pharmacology,* 7th ed. Appleton & Lange, 1998.)

(especially if given for long periods), these drugs may cause profound behavioral disturbances. Large doses stimulate gastric acid secretion and may decrease resistance to ulcer formation.

C. **Important Glucocorticoids:**   Many glucocorticoids have been developed in an effort to obtain longer duration of action, less mineralocorticoid activity, or better topical activity (Table 39–1).

1. **Cortisol:**   The major natural glucocorticoid is cortisol (hydrocortisone), a steroid synthesized in the adrenal cortex from 17-hydroxypregnenolone. The physiologic secretion of cortisol is regulated by ACTH and varies during the day (circadian rhythm), with the peak occurring in the morning and the trough around midnight. In the plasma, cortisol is 95% bound to corticosteroid-binding globulin. Given as a drug, cortisol is well absorbed from the gastrointestinal tract, is cleared by the liver, and has a short duration of action compared with its synthetic congeners (Table 39–1). Although it diffuses poorly across normal skin, cortisol is readily absorbed across inflamed skin and mucous membranes.

   The cortisol molecule also has a small but significant salt-retaining (mineralocorticoid) effect. This is an important cause of hypertension in patients with a cortisol-secreting adrenal tumor or a pituitary ACTH-secreting tumor (Cushing's syndrome).

2. **Synthetic glucocorticoids:**   The mechanism of action of these agents is identical to that of cortisol. A very large number have been synthesized and are available for use; prednisone and its active metabolite, prednisolone, dexamethasone, and triamcinolone are representative compounds. Their properties (when compared with cortisol) include longer

Table 39–1. Properties of representative corticosteroids.

Agent	Duration of Action (hours)	Anti-Inflammatory Potency[1]	Salt-Retaining Potency[1]	Topical Activity
Primarily glucocorticoid				
Cortisol	8–12	1	1	0
Prednisone	12–24	4	0.3	(+)
Triamcinolone	15–24	5	0	+++
Dexamethasone	24–36	30	0	+++++
Primarily mineralocorticoid				
Aldosterone	1–2	0.3	3000	0
Fludrocortisone	8–12	10	125–250	0

[1]Relative to cortisol.

half-life and duration of action, reduced salt-retaining effect, and better penetration of lipid barriers for topical activity (Table 39–1). Even greater surface activity can be achieved by adding acetonide or similar groups to the C-17 of the steroid ring.

Special glucocorticoids have been developed for use in asthma and other conditions in which good surface activity on mucous membranes is needed and systemic effects are to be avoided. **Beclomethasone** and **budesonide** readily penetrate the airway mucosa but have very short half-lives after they enter the blood, so that systemic effects and toxicity are greatly reduced.

D. Clinical Uses:

1. **Adrenal disorders:** Glucocorticoids are essential to preserve life in patients with chronic adrenal cortical insufficiency (Addison's disease). These drugs are also necessary in acute adrenal insufficiency associated with life-threatening shock, infection, or trauma. Glucocorticoids are also used in certain types of congenital adrenal hyperplasia, in which synthesis of abnormal forms of corticosteroids is stimulated by ACTH. Administration of a potent synthetic glucocorticoid suppresses ACTH secretion sufficiently to reduce the synthesis of the abnormal steroids.

2. **Nonadrenal disorders:** Many disorders respond to corticosteroid therapy. Some of these are inflammatory or immunologic in nature, eg, asthma, organ transplant rejection, and collagen diseases. Other applications include the treatment of leukemias, neurologic disorders, chemotherapy-induced vomiting, exophthalmos, hypercalcemia, and mountain sickness. The degree of benefit differs considerably in different disorders, however, and the toxicity of corticosteroids given chronically limits their use. Treatment of one patient with rheumatoid arthritis is described in Case 11 (Appendix IV).

E. Toxicity: Most of the toxic effects of the glucocorticoids are predictable from the effects already described. Some are life-threatening and include adrenal suppression (from suppression of ACTH secretion), metabolic effects (growth inhibition, diabetes, muscle wasting, osteoporosis), salt retention, and psychosis. Methods for minimizing these toxicities include local application (eg, aerosols for asthma), alternate-day therapy (to reduce pituitary suppression), and tapering the dose soon after achieving a therapeutic response.

MINERALOCORTICOIDS

A. Aldosterone: The major natural mineralocorticoid in humans is aldosterone, which has already been mentioned in connection with hypertension (see Chapter 11) and with control of its secretion by angiotensin II (see Chapter 17). Pregnenolone and progesterone are intermediates in the synthesis of this mineralocorticoid. The secretion of aldosterone is regulated by ACTH and by the renin-angiotensin system and is very important in the regulation of blood volume and pressure (see Figure 6–4). Aldosterone has a short half-life and little glucocorticoid activity (Table 39–1). Its mechanism of action is the same as that of the glucocorticoids.

B. **Other Mineralocorticoids:**   Other mineralocorticoids include deoxycorticosterone, the naturally occurring precursor of aldosterone, and **fludrocortisone.** The latter has significant glucocorticoid activity. Because of its long duration of action (Table 39–1), fludrocortisone is favored for replacement therapy after adrenalectomy and in other conditions in which mineralocorticoid therapy is needed.

CORTICOSTEROID ANTAGONISTS

A. **Receptor Antagonists:**   **Spironolactone,** an antagonist of aldosterone at its receptor, has been discussed in connection with the diuretics (see Chapter 15). **Mifepristone (RU 486)** is an inhibitor at glucocorticoid receptors as well as progesterone receptors (see Chapter 39) and has been used in the treatment of Cushing's syndrome.

B. **Synthesis Inhibitors:**   Several drugs are used in the treatment of adrenal cancer when surgical therapy is impractical or unsuccessful because of metastases. The most important of these drugs are **aminoglutethimide, metyrapone,** and **ketoconazole.** The drugs mitotane (a DDT analog) and amphenone B also reduce steroid synthesis in the adrenals but are considered toxic.

Aminoglutethimide is used in the treatment of advanced breast cancer to suppress adrenal secretion of estrogenic steroids. Ketoconazole (an antifungal drug) inhibits the P450 enzymes necessary for the synthesis of all steroids and has been studied in a number of conditions in which reduced steroid levels are desirable, eg, hirsutism and breast cancer. Metyrapone inhibits the normal synthesis of cortisol but not that of cortisol precursors; the drug can be used in diagnostic tests of adrenal function. A normal response to a test dose of metyrapone (increased levels of cortisol precursors) is evidence that the adrenal cortex is functioning.

DRUG LIST

The following drugs are important members of the group discussed in this chapter. Prototypes should be learned in detail; features of the major variants should be known well enough so that the variants can be distinguished from prototypes and from each other; the other significant agents should be recognized as belonging to a specific subclass.

Subclass	Prototype	Major Variants	Other Significant Agents
Agonists			
Glucocorticoids	Cortisol (hydrocortisone), prednisone	Dexamethasone, triamcinolone, beclomethasone	Triamcinolone acetonide
Mineralocorticoids	Aldosterone	Fludrocortisone	
Antagonists			
Receptor antagonists	Spironolactone	Mifepristone	
Synthesis inhibitors	Aminoglutethimide, metyrapone	Ketoconazole	

QUESTIONS

DIRECTIONS: Each of the numbered items or incomplete statements in this section is followed by answers or by completions of the statement. Select the ONE lettered answer or completion that is BEST in each case.

1. Effects of the glucocorticoids include all of the following EXCEPT
    (A) Altered fat deposition
    (B) Increased blood glucose
    (C) Increased skin protein synthesis

     (D) Inhibition of leukotriene synthesis
     (E) Reduction in circulating lymphocytes
  2. Toxic effects of the corticosteroids include all of the following EXCEPT
     (A) Growth inhibition
     (B) Hypoglycemia
     (C) Osteoporosis
     (D) Psychosis
     (E) Salt retention

Items 3–4: A 54-year-old man with miliary tuberculosis has developed signs of severe acute adrenal insufficiency.

  3. This patient will probably have all of the following manifestations EXCEPT
     (A) Moon facies
     (B) Reduced ability to excrete a water load
     (C) Reduced ability to combat infection
     (D) Hypoglycemia if food is withheld
     (E) Reduced blood volume
  4. The patient should be treated immediately. Which of the following combinations is most rational?
     (A) Aldosterone and fludrocortisone
     (B) Cortisol and fludrocortisone
     (C) Dexamethasone and metyrapone
     (D) Fludrocortisone and metyrapone
     (E) Triamcinolone and dexamethasone

DIRECTIONS (Items 5–12): Each set of matching questions in this section consists of a list of three to twenty-six lettered options (some of which may be figures) followed by several numbered items. For each numbered item, select the ONE lettered option that is most closely associated with it. Each lettered option may be selected once, more than once, or not at all.

     (A) Aldosterone
     (B) Aminoglutethimide
     (C) Beclomethasone
     (D) Cortisol
     (E) Fludrocortisone
     (F) Ketoconazole
     (G) Metyrapone
     (H) Prednisolone
     (I) Spironolactone
     (J) Triamcinolone acetonide

  5. Naturally occurring mineralocorticoid
  6. Corticosteroid with high salt-retaining potency, some glucocorticoid effect, and long duration of action
  7. Glucocorticoid with very low mineralocorticoid activity and very high topical activity; used for dermatologic conditions
  8. Endogenous substance that causes salt retention and buffalo hump in patients with Cushing's syndrome
  9. Active metabolite of a synthetic glucocorticoid; has an intermediate duration of action and low topical activity
  10. Antifungal agent that inhibits P450 enzymes required for steroid synthesis
  11. A drug used by aerosol in the treatment of asthma
  12. A drug used to suppress adrenal synthesis of steroid hormones (especially estrogens) in patients with breast cancer; not a diuretic or antifungal drug

ANSWERS

  1. Glucocorticoids stimulate protein breakdown, not synthesis (except in the liver). The answer is **(C).**
  2. Corticosteroids may induce hyperglycemia of sufficient magnitude to require insulin therapy. The answer is **(B).**

3. Moon facies is a manifestation of hypercortisolism, not adrenal insufficiency. The answer is **(A)**.
4. A rational combination of drugs should include agents with complementary effects, ie, a gluco-corticoid and a mineralocorticoid. The combination with these characteristics is cortisol and fludrocortisone. (Note that while fludrocortisone may have sufficient glucocorticoid activity for a patient with mild disease, a patient in severe acute adrenal insufficiency needs a full glu-cocorticoid such as cortisol.) The answer is **(B)**.
5. The answer is **(A)**, aldosterone.
6. Fludrocortisone has a much longer duration of action than the naturally occurring mineralocor-ticoids and has some glucocorticoid activity (Table 39–1). The answer is **(E)**.
7. The answer is **(J)**, triamcinolone acetonide.
8. Cortisol causes buffalo hump. It also has sufficient salt-retaining activity to cause hyperten-sion. Prednisolone would have the same effects (it has some salt-retaining action), but this drug is not an endogenous substance. Aldosterone is not a satisfactory answer because it has insufficient glucocorticoid activity to cause fat redistribution. The answer is **(D)**.
9. Prednisolone is the active metabolite of prednisone. The answer is **(H)**.
10. Ketoconazole is an antifungal agent that inhibits P450 enzymes in the adrenal gland (and else-where). The answer is **(F)**.
11. Beclomethasone has good ability to reduce inflammation in the airways when administered by aerosol. The answer is **(C)**.
12. Aminoglutethimide inhibits the conversion of cholesterol to pregnenolone, the first step in the synthesis of steroid hormones. The answer is **(B)**.

40 Gonadal Hormones & Inhibitors

OBJECTIVES

You should be able to:

- Describe the hormonal changes that occur during the menstrual cycle.
- List the benefits and hazards of oral contraceptives.
- Describe the status of pharmacologic contraception in the male.
- List the benefits and hazards of postmenopausal estrogen therapy.
- Describe the use of sex hormones and their antagonists in the treatment of cancer in women and men.
- List or describe the toxic effects of anabolic steroids used to build muscle mass.

CONCEPTS

The gonadal hormones include the steroids of the ovary (estrogens and progestins) and testis (chiefly testosterone) and a few other hormones (eg, peptides) of lesser importance. Sex steroids are also synthesized in the adrenal cortex. Because of their importance in oral contraceptive agents, many synthetic estrogens and progestins have been produced. In the course of development, several partial agonist analogs of the natural hormones have been discovered. Testosterone, partial agonist andro-gens, and androgen antagonists are of similar importance. This group is outlined in Figure 40–1.

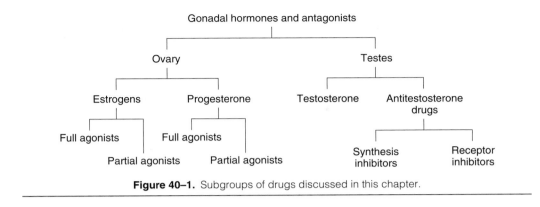

Figure 40–1. Subgroups of drugs discussed in this chapter.

OVARIAN HORMONES

The ovary is the primary source of sex hormones in women during the childbearing years, ie, between puberty and menopause. When properly regulated by FSH and LH from the pituitary, each menstrual cycle consists of the following events: a follicle in the ovary matures, secretes increasing amounts of estrogen, releases an ovum, and is transformed into a progesterone-secreting corpus luteum. If the ovum is not fertilized and implanted, the corpus luteum degenerates; the uterine endometrium (which has proliferated under the stimulation of estrogen and progesterone) is shed as part of the menstrual flow, and the cycle repeats. The mechanism of action of both estrogen and progesterone involves entry into cells, binding to cytosolic receptors that transport the hormones into the nucleus, and there causing modulation of gene expression (see Figure 39–2).

A. **Estrogens:** The major ovarian estrogen in women is estradiol. Other estrogens include estrone and estriol, which are produced in other tissues. Almost all of the estrogen in the blood is bound to a sex hormone-binding globulin (SHBG). Estradiol is active by the oral route as replacement therapy but has low bioavailability because of hepatic metabolism. Therefore, semisynthetic derivatives (especially ethinyl estradiol) or other estrogens are usually used (see Drug List).

1. **Effects:** Estrogen is essential for normal female sexual development. It is responsible for the growth of the genital structures (vagina, uterus, and uterine tubes) during childhood and for the appearance of secondary sexual characteristics and the growth spurt associated with puberty. Estrogen has many metabolic effects: it modifies serum protein levels, reduces bone resorption, and enhances nutrient absorption in the gastrointestinal tract. It enhances the coagulability of blood and increases plasma triglyceride levels while reducing LDL cholesterol. Estrogen is also an effective feedback suppressant of pituitary FSH (Figure 40–2).

2. **Clinical use:** An important therapeutic use of estrogens is in the treatment of hypogonadism in girls (Table 40–1). Another use is in the management of postmenopausal changes in women. Although the hormone is very effective in reducing or preventing the effects of estrogen deprivation after menopause (especially genital changes and osteoporosis), estrogen toxicities are such that use in postmenopausal women is not routine. The estrogens are very important as a component of oral contraceptives. A special use of brief, high-dose therapy is as a "morning after" contraceptive, ie, to prevent conception as a result of intercourse the night before. Estrogens are sometimes used in the palliative treatment of carcinoma of the prostate.

3. **Toxicity:** The primary toxicity of the estrogens relates to their stimulatory effects on vaginal, uterine, and breast tissue. Moderate doses may cause breast tenderness, endometrial hyperplasia, and breakthrough bleeding. Months-long treatment of pregnant women with diethylstilbestrol (DES), a practice long-since abandoned, may have caused vaginal adenocarcinoma in their daughters. Estrogen use is also associated with an increased incidence of gallbladder disease.

   Toxicity of long-term estrogen treatment is discussed below (see Oral Contraceptives).

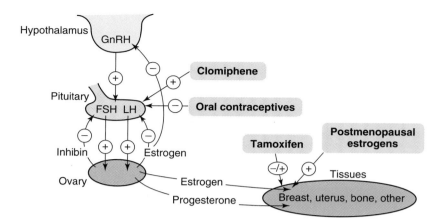

Figure 40–2. Sites of action of several ovarian hormones and their analogs. Clomiphene, a partial agonist, is mainly an antagonist at pituitary estrogen receptors; this prevents negative feedback and increases the output of the pituitary gonadotropic hormones. Tamoxifen is mainly an antagonist at estrogen receptors in the breast but apparently acts as an agonist in bone. Contraceptives reduce FSH and LH output from the pituitary by activating feedback receptors.

B. Progestins: Progesterone is the major progestin in humans. It is synthesized in the ovary, testis, and adrenal. It is rapidly metabolized in the liver and therefore has a very low bioavailability and a short half-life. Synthetic agents are used for replacement therapy and in oral and implantable contraceptives.

1. **Effects:** Progestins cause development of secretory tissue in the breast and maturation of the uterine endometrium. They have much less effect than the estrogens on plasma proteins but significantly affect carbohydrate metabolism and stimulate the deposition of fat.

2. **Clinical use:** The major clinical use of the progestins is as a component of oral or implantable contraceptives. The progestins are occasionally used to produce long-lasting ovarian suppression, eg, in endometriosis. They are of no value in threatened abortion, an indication promoted in the past.

Table 40–1. Representative applications for the gonadal hormones and hormone antagonists.

Clinical Application	Drugs
Hypogonadism in females	Conjugated equine estrogens, ethinyl estradiol
Postmenopausal estrogen replacement	Conjugated equine estrogens, ethinyl estradiol
Intractable dysmenorrhea or uterine bleeding	Ethinyl estradiol, oral contraceptive
"Morning after" contraception	Diethylstilbestrol; quadruple dose of oral contraceptive
Oral contraception	Estrogen: ethinyl estradiol or mestranol; progestin: norethindrone or norgestrel
Implanted or depot injection contraception	Norgestrel (implant); medroxyprogesterone (IM depot injection)
Infertility	Clomiphene; hMG and hCG; GnRH analogs (pulsatile administration); bromocriptine
Breast cancer	Tamoxifen
Abortifacient	Mifepristone (RU 486) and prostaglandin; methotrexate and prostaglandin
Endometriosis	Danazol
Hypogonadism in males; replacement therapy	Testosterone enanthate or cypionate; methyltestosterone; fluoxymesterone
Anabolic protein synthesis	Oxandrolone, stanozolol
Prostate hyperplasia (benign)	Finasteride
Prostate carcinoma	Flutamide, cyproterone; diethylstilbestrol

3. **Toxicity:** The toxicity of progestins is low. However, they may increase the blood pressure and decrease high-density plasma lipoproteins (HDL).

C. **Oral and Implantable Contraceptives:** Three different types of oral contraceptives for women are in use in the USA: combination estrogen-progestin tablets that are taken in constant dosage throughout the menstrual cycle (monophasic preparations); combination preparations (biphasic and triphasic) in which the progestin dosage is increased during the month (to mimic the natural cycle); and progestin-only preparations. Two parenteral progestin preparations are used: norgestrel implants, which prevent conception for up to 5 years; and medroxyprogesterone acetate depot injections, which provide contraceptive action for approximately 3 months.

1. **Mechanism of action:** The combination oral contraceptives have several actions, including inhibition of ovulation (the primary action) and effects on the uterine tubes and endometrium that decrease the likelihood of fertilization and implantation. Oral progestin-only agents do not always inhibit ovulation and may act through the other mechanisms. However, implantable and injected progestin-only contraceptives appear to act mainly through inhibition of ovulation.

2. **Toxicity:** Toxicity is an extremely important consideration in the use of contraceptives because they are commonly used over the course of many years.

   a. **Thromboembolism:** The major toxic effects of oral contraceptives relate to their actions on blood coagulation. There is a well-documented increase in the risk of thromboembolic phenomena (myocardial infarction, stroke, pulmonary embolism) in older women, in smokers, and in women with a family history of such problems. However, the risk incurred by the use of these drugs is usually less than the other risks associated with pregnancy.

   b. **Carcinogenesis:** Numerous studies have evaluated the effect of oral contraceptives on the incidence of cancer. Convincing evidence indicates that these agents *reduce* the incidence of endometrial and ovarian carcinoma. Cervical carcinoma incidence is probably unchanged. Evidence regarding the effects on breast cancer is still confusing. A few studies indicate that women who took the pill for many years after it first became available (ie, in high-dose formulations) may have an increased incidence of breast carcinoma. Most studies show no increase.

   c. **Other toxicities:** The other toxicities of the oral contraceptives are much less ominous and include nausea, breast tenderness, headache, skin pigmentation, acne, and hirsutism. All adverse effects appear to be considerably reduced by the use of modern preparations containing low doses of estrogen, ie, less than 50 µg/d.

D. **Partial Agonist Estrogens and Progestins; Aromatase Inhibitors; Miscellaneous Hormones:**

1. **Tamoxifen:** Tamoxifen is an extremely important nonsteroidal partial agonist estrogen that has been used successfully in the treatment of hormone-sensitive breast cancer. In this tissue, tamoxifen's antagonist properties dominate, so that endogenous estrogen is prevented from activating receptors in the tumor (Figure 40–2). Major trials are now under way to determine whether tamoxifen can *prevent* breast cancer in women who are at very high risk. The drug has little toxicity and appears to have more agonist than antagonist action on bone, so that it actually prevents osteoporosis in women taking the drug for breast cancer.

2. **Clomiphene:** Clomiphene is a nonsteroidal partial agonist estrogen that is used in anovulatory women who wish to become pregnant. Clomiphene blocks estrogen receptors in the pituitary, reducing negative feedback and increasing FSH and LH output. The increase in gonadotropins stimulates ovulation.

3. **Mifepristone (RU 486):** Mifepristone is an orally active steroid antagonist of progesterone and glucocorticoids. The drug binds to the cytosolic steroid receptors for these hormones and alters expression of the appropriate genes. Its major use thus far (restricted to a few European countries) has been as an abortifacient. When mifepristone is given in a single oral dose followed by administration of a prostaglandin E or F analog, complete abortion is achieved in a very high percentage of cases with a low incidence of serious toxicity. This drug also may have applications in the treatment of several malignancies.

4. **Danazol:** Danazol is a weak partial agonist that binds to progestin, androgen, and glucocorticoid receptors in cells and to steroid transport proteins in the blood. Danazol also in-

hibits several P450 enzymes involved in gonadal steroid synthesis. The drug is used in the treatment of endometriosis and fibrocystic disease of the breast.

5. **Aromatase inhibitors:** **Anastrozole** is a nonsteroidal inhibitor of aromatase, the enzyme required for estrogen synthesis. This new drug has been shown to be effective in some patients with breast cancer. Investigational agents with similar effects include letrozole and fedrozole.

6. **Relaxin:** Relaxin is an ovarian *peptide* hormone that causes relaxation of the pelvic ligaments and softening of the cervix. It may play a physiologic role in parturition but has no documented clinical applications at present.

ANDROGENS

Testosterone and related androgens are produced in the testis, the adrenal, and, to a small extent, in the ovary. Testosterone is synthesized from progesterone and dehydroepiandrosterone. In the plasma, testosterone is partly bound to sex hormone-binding globulin (SHBG), a transport protein. The hormone is converted in several organs (eg, prostate) to **dihydrotestosterone,** which is the active hormone in those tissues. Because of rapid hepatic metabolism, testosterone given by mouth has little effect. It may be given parenterally, or orally active variants may be used. (See Table 40–1 and the Drug List.)

Many androgens have been synthesized in an effort to increase the anabolic effect (see Effects, below) without increasing androgenic action. **Oxandrolone** and **stanozolol** are examples of drugs that, in laboratory testing, have an increased ratio of anabolic to androgenic action. However, none of these agents are devoid of androgenic effect in clinical use.

A. **Mechanism of Action:** Like other steroid hormones, androgens enter cells and bind to cytosolic receptors (Figure 39–2). The hormone-receptor complex enters the nucleus and modulates the expression of certain genes.

B. **Effects:** Testosterone is necessary for the normal development of the male fetus and infant and is responsible for the major changes in the male at puberty (growth of penis, larynx, and skeleton; development of facial, pubic, and axillary hair; darkening of skin; enlargement of muscle mass). Testosterone causes masculinization of the female.

The major effect of androgenic hormones—other than the development and maintenance of normal male characteristics—is an anabolic action that involves increased muscle size and strength and increased red blood cell production. Excretion of urea nitrogen is reduced, and nitrogen balance becomes more positive. As noted above, the ratio of androgenic to anabolic potency varies somewhat among the synthetic compounds available, but all retain considerable androgenic effect. Therefore, the use of these hormones by athletes to increase muscle strength is attended by the hazards of unwanted androgenic effects.

C. **Clinical Use:** The clinical uses of the androgens include replacement therapy in hypogonadism, stimulation of red blood cell production in certain anemias (largely obsolete), and, rarely, the suppression of estrogen secretion or function in women with severe endometriosis (Table 40–1). The anabolic effects have been exploited illicitly by athletes, especially weight lifters, to increase muscle bulk and strength. The availability of recombinant erythropoietin and other marrow growth factors has rendered obsolete the use of androgens in anemias and agranulocytosis.

D. **Toxicity:** The toxicity of the androgens is largely a result of their masculinizing effects. In addition, they have caused cholestatic jaundice, elevation of liver enzyme levels, and in a few cases hepatocellular carcinoma. Excessive use by athletes and muscle builders is sometimes associated with behavioral changes, including unpredictable rage and hostility. Development of dependence and a withdrawal syndrome have been reported.

ANTIANDROGENS

Reduction of androgen effects is an important mode of therapy for both benign and malignant prostate disease. Drugs are available that act at several different sites in the androgen pathway (Figure 40–3).

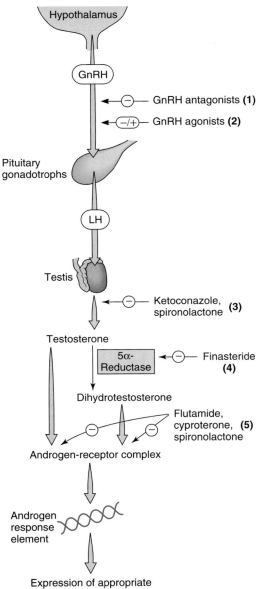

Figure 40–3. Control of androgen secretion and activity and some sites of action of antiandrogens. (1) Competitive inhibition of GnRH receptors; (2) stimulation (+) or inhibition (–) by GnRH analogs; (3) inhibition of testosterone synthesis by ketoconazole or spironolactone; (4) inhibition of dihydrotestosterone production by finasteride; (5) inhibition of androgen binding at its receptor by flutamide and other drugs. (Modified and reproduced, with permission, from Katzung BG [editor]: *Basic & Clinical Pharmacology,* 7th ed. Appleton & Lange, 1998.)

A. GnRH Analogs: Reduction of trophic hormones, especially LH, reduces the production of testosterone. This can be effectively accomplished with long-acting depot preparations of **leuprolide** or similar agonist GnRH analogs (Chapter 37). These analogs are used in prostatic carcinoma. GnRH antagonists are investigational at present.

B. Inhibitors of Steroid Synthesis: **Ketoconazole,** an antifungal agent, inhibits steroid synthesis. The drug has been used to suppress adrenal steroid synthesis in patients with steroid-dependent metastatic tumors. Spironolactone may have a similar but smaller effect.

C. 5α-Reductase Inhibitors: Testosterone is converted to dihydrotestosterone by the enzyme 5α-reductase. This enzyme can be inhibited by **finasteride,** a heterocyclic steroid. Finasteride has not proved effective in prostatic carcinoma but may be useful in benign prostatic hyperplasia.

D. Receptor Inhibitors: **Cyproterone** and its acetate derivative are steroidal competitive inhibitors of androgens at the testosterone receptor. Cyproterone also has progestational activity that provides negative feedback to the pituitary. **Flutamide** and **bicalutamide** are nonsteroidal androgen antagonists with the same action. These drugs have been used to decrease the action of endogenous hormone in prostate carcinoma. **Spironolactone** inhibits dihydrotestosterone receptors and has been used in the treatment of women with hirsutism.

CONTRACEPTION IN THE MALE

Gossypol is a cottonseed oil derivative that was serendipitously discovered to reduce spermatogenesis. It reduces fertility in most males by destroying seminiferous cells. However, gossypol is not nearly as reliable as the oral contraceptives used by women. It causes hypokalemia, and the weakness associated with this side effect may limit its use. Androgenic and estrogenic hormones also reduce spermatogenesis, primarily by suppressing pituitary LH and FSH production. However, the low efficacy of these agents and their other hormonal effects prevent serious consideration of their use as contraceptives.

DRUG LIST

The following drugs are important members of the group discussed in this chapter. Prototypes should be learned in detail; features of the major variants should be known well enough so that the variants can be distinguished from prototypes and from each other; the other significant agents should be recognized as belonging to a specific subclass.

Subclass	Prototype	Major Variants	Other Significant Agents
Estrogens Natural	Estradiol	Conjugated equine estrogens	Estrone, estriol
Synthetic	Ethinyl estradiol	Mestranol	Diethylstilbestrol
Estrogen partial agonists	Tamoxifen, clomiphene		
Aromatase inhibitors	Anastrozole		Letrozole, fadrozole
Progestins Natural	Progesterone		
Synthetic	Norgestrel, medroxyprogesterone		Norethindrone
Partial agonist	Danazol		
Antiprogestin	Mifepristone (RU 486)		
Androgens Natural	Testosterone		
Synthetic	Methyltestosterone	Fluoxymesterone	
Anabolic steroid	Oxandrolone		Stanozolol
Antiandrogens Synthesis inhibitor	Finasteride		
Receptor antagonist	Flutamide	Cyproterone	Bicalutamide

QUESTIONS

DIRECTIONS: Each of the numbered items or incomplete statements in this section is followed by answers or by completions of the statement. Select the ONE lettered answer or completion that is BEST in each case.

1. All of the following agents are useful in oral or implantable contraceptives EXCEPT
   (A) Clomiphene
   (B) Ethinyl estradiol
   (C) Mestranol
   (D) Norethindrone
   (E) Norgestrel

2. All of the following are recognized effects of oral contraceptives EXCEPT
   (A) Increased risk of myocardial infarction
   (B) Nausea
   (C) Edema
   (D) Increased risk of endometrial cancer
   (E) Decreased risk of ovarian cancer

3. All of the following are recognized effects of natural androgens or androgenic steroids EXCEPT
   (A) Growth of facial hair
   (B) Increased muscle bulk
   (C) Increased milk production in nursing women
   (D) Induction of a growth spurt in pubertal boys
   (E) Cholestatic jaundice and elevation of AST levels in the blood

4. A 50-year-old woman with a positive mammogram undergoes lumpectomy, and a small carcinoma is removed. After this procedure, she will probably receive
   (A) Danazol
   (B) Flutamide
   (C) Ketoconazole
   (D) Leuprolide
   (E) Tamoxifen

5. A 60-year-old man is found to have a prostate lump and an elevated PSA (prostate-specific antigen) blood test. MRI examination suggests several enlarged lymph nodes in the lower abdomen, and x-ray reveals two radiolucent lesions in the bony pelvis. This patient might benefit from any of the following EXCEPT
   (A) Cyproterone
   (B) Flutamide
   (C) Ketoconazole
   (D) Leuprolide
   (E) Mifepristone

6. A young woman complains of severe abdominal pain at the time of menstruation. Careful evaluation indicates the presence of significant endometrial deposits on the pelvic peritoneum. The most appropriate therapy for this patient would be
   (A) Danazol
   (B) Estradiol
   (C) Flutamide
   (D) Mestranol
   (E) Norgestrel

DIRECTIONS (Items 7–15): Each set of matching questions in this section consists of a list of three to twenty-six lettered options (some of which may be figures) followed by several numbered items. For each numbered item, select the ONE lettered option that is most closely associated with it. Each lettered option may be selected once, more than once, or not at all.
   (A) Anastrozole
   (B) Clomiphene
   (C) Cyproterone
   (D) Danazol
   (E) Finasteride
   (F) Flutamide
   (G) Goserelin
   (H) Ketoconazole
   (I) Leuprolide

   (J)   Mestranol
   (K)   Norgestrel
   (L)   Tamoxifen

   7.   A partial agonist estrogen that stimulates ovulation
   8.   A synthetic estrogen that is useful in oral contraceptives of the combined type
   9.   A synthetic progestin used in both combination and progestin-only contraceptives
   10. A steroid drug that competes with testosterone for its receptor
   11. A competitive partial agonist estrogen that is an antagonist in advanced breast cancer tissue but an agonist in bone
   12. An antifungal drug that inhibits P450 enzymes required for steroid hormone synthesis
   13. A nonsteroidal androgen receptor antagonist used in management of metastatic prostatic carcinoma
   14. An inhibitor of 5α-reductase in the prostate
   15. An inhibitor of aromatase; reduces synthesis of estrogen

ANSWERS

   1.   Clomiphene, an antiestrogen that stimulates ovulation, would be of no value in an oral contraceptive. The answer is **(A).**
   2.   The oral contraceptives are associated with a decreased risk of both endometrial and ovarian cancer. The answer is **(D).**
   3.   Androgens, like estrogens, reduce the pituitary release of prolactin and suppress lactation. The answer is **(C).**
   4.   Tamoxifen has proved useful in adjunctive therapy of breast cancer after apparently complete removal; the drug decreases the rate of recurrence of cancer. The answer is **(E).**
   5.   Most antiandrogenic drugs are potentially useful in this androgen-dependent type of tumor. Mifepristone (RU 486) has effects at glucocorticoid and progestin receptors but not at androgen receptors. The answer is **(E).**
   6.   In endometriosis, a partial agonist at progesterone and testosterone receptors is useful. Danazol reduces progesterone effects on the ectopic endometrial tissue while causing feedback inhibition of gonadotropin output from the pituitary. The answer is **(A).**
   7.   Clomiphene apparently reduces the feedback inhibition by estrogens of the hypothalamus and pituitary, resulting in an increased production of gonadotropins. The answer is **(B).**
   8.   The answer is **(J),** mestranol.
   9.   The answer is **(K),** norgestrel.
   10. The answer is **(C),** cyproterone.
   11. Tamoxifen, a competitive partial agonist estrogen, is useful in the treatment of estrogen-dependent breast carcinoma and appears to reduce osteoporosis. The answer is **(L).**
   12. Ketoconazole inhibits P450 enzymes preferentially in fungi, but in high doses it has been shown to have similar effects on mammalian enzymes. The answer is **(H).**
   13. Flutamide is a nonsteroid with strong affinity for the cytosolic androgen receptor. The answer is **(F).**
   14. Finasteride is an effective inhibitor of the enzyme that converts testosterone to dihydrotestosterone. The answer is **(E).**
   15. Anastrozole is a new drug that inhibits aromatase and reduces synthesis of estrogens; it is useful in women with breast cancer no longer responsive to tamoxifen. The answer is **(A).**

Pancreatic Hormones, Antidiabetic Agents, & Hyperglycemic Drugs

41

OBJECTIVES

You should be able to:

- List the sources of insulin in clinical use.
- List the types of insulin preparations and their durations of action.
- Describe the effects of insulin on the liver, on muscle, and on adipose tissue.
- Describe the major hazards of insulin therapy.
- List the prototypes and describe the mechanisms of action of the two major classes of oral hypoglycemic agents.
- Describe the clinical uses of acarbose, troglitazone, glucagon, and diazoxide.

CONCEPTS

The islets of Langerhans (the endocrine pancreas) contain at least four different types of endocrine cells, including A (alpha, glucagon-producing), B (beta, insulin-producing), D (delta, somatostatin-producing), and F (PP, pancreatic polypeptide-producing). Of these, the B (insulin-producing) cells are the most numerous.

The most common pancreatic disease requiring pharmacologic therapy is diabetes mellitus, a disorder due to deficiency of insulin production or effect. Diabetes is treated with several formulations of insulin (all administered parenterally at present) and with two different types of oral hypoglycemic agents (Figure 41–1). Two newer types of drugs for the treatment of diabetes have been introduced.

The treatment of hypoglycemia, which is usually due to excess insulin activity, is with glucagon or diazoxide.

INSULIN

A. Physiology: Insulin is synthesized as a prohormone, **proinsulin,** an 86-amino-acid single-chain polypeptide. Cleavage of proinsulin and cross-linking result in the two-chain 51-peptide insulin molecule and a 31-amino-acid residual **C-peptide.** C-peptide (connecting peptide) is of clinical interest because it can be measured by immunoassay independently of insulin. Neither proinsulin nor C-peptide appears to have any physiologic actions.

B. Effects: Insulin has important effects in almost every tissue of the body. Its actions on liver, muscle, and adipose tissue are listed in Table 41–1. The insulin receptor, a transmembrane tyro-

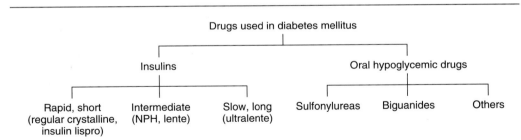

Figure 41–1. Subgroups of hypoglycemic drugs discussed in this chapter.

303

Table 41–1. Endocrine effects of insulin.*

Category of Effect	Result
Effects on liver	
Reversal of catabolic features of insulin deficiency	Inhibits glycogenolysis; inhibits conversion of fatty acids and amino acids to keto acids; inhibits conversion of amino acids to glucose
Anabolic action	Promotes glucose storage as glycogen (induces glucokinase and glycogen synthase; inhibits phosphorylase); increases triglyceride synthesis and very-low-density lipoprotein formation
Effects on muscle	
Increased protein synthesis	Increases amino acid transport; increases ribosomal protein synthesis
Increased glycogen synthesis	Increases glucose transport; induces glycogen synthase and inhibits phosphorylase
Effect on adipose tissue	
Increased triglyceride storage	Induces and activates lipoprotein lipase to hydrolyze triglycerides from lipoproteins; increases glucose transport into the cell to provide glycerol phosphate and permit esterification of fatty acids supplied by lipoprotein transport; inhibits intracellular lipase

*Modified and reproduced, with permission, from Katzung BG (editor): *Basic & Clinical Pharmacology*, 7th ed. Appleton & Lange, 1998.

sine kinase, phosphorylates itself and a variety of intracellular proteins when activated by the hormone. The major target organs for insulin action include the following:

1. **Liver:** Insulin increases the storage of glucose as glycogen in the liver. This involves insertion of additional GLUT 2 glucose transport molecules in cell walls, increased synthesis of the enzymes pyruvate kinase, phosphofructokinase, and glucokinase, and suppression of several other enzymes. Insulin also decreases protein catabolism.

2. **Muscle:** Insulin stimulates glycogen synthesis and protein synthesis. Glucose transport into muscle cells is facilitated by insertion of additional GLUT 4 transport molecules into cell walls.

3. **Adipose tissue:** Insulin facilitates triglyceride storage by activating plasma lipoprotein lipase, by increasing glucose transport into cells via GLUT 4 transporters, and by reducing intracellular lipolysis.

C. **Types of Insulin Available:** Two animal insulin preparations are available (from pork and beef). Human insulin is manufactured by bacterial recombinant DNA technology or by chemical modification of pork insulin. Because the insulin molecule has a half-life of only a few minutes in the circulation, many preparations for use in diabetes are formulated to release the hormone slowly into the circulation.

The insulin forms available provide four rates of onset and durations of effect: ultra-rapid onset, rapid onset with short action, intermediate onset and action, and slow onset with long action (Table 41–2). All insulin preparations contain zinc; it is the ratio of zinc (and other substances) to insulin that determines the rate of release of active hormone from the site of administration and the duration of action.

1. **Ultra-rapid onset and very short action:** **Insulin lispro,** a new recombinant human insulin, contains a transposition of two amino acids, lysine and proline. This transposition alters the physical properties of the peptide so that insulin lispro dissolves more rapidly at its site of administration and enters the circulation approximately twice as fast as regular crystalline insulin. It is considered ultra-rapid in onset and is suitable for use immediately before meals for closer ("tight") glycemic control than is possible with older preparations. Unlike other insulin preparations, increasing the dose of insulin lispro increases only the intensity of effect and not its duration.

2. **Rapid onset and short action:** **Crystalline zinc (regular) insulin,** a rapid-onset preparation, is used intravenously in emergencies or administered subcutaneously in ordinary maintenance regimens, alone or mixed with intermediate- or long-acting preparations. Before the development of insulin lispro, it was the primary rapid onset agent for use in tight control regimens but required administration an hour or more before each meal.

Table 41–2. Insulin: Types and activity.

Pharmacokinetic Type	Species Type	Activity (hours)	
		Peak	Duration
Ultra-rapid-acting Insulin lispro	Human, modified	0.25–0.5	3–4
Rapid-acting Insulin injection USP (regular, crystalline zinc)	Human, beef, pork	0.5–3	5–7
Intermediate-acting NPH insulin (isophane insulin suspension USP)	Human, pork, or beef-pork mixture	8–12	18–24
Lente insulin (insulin zinc suspension USP)	Human, pork, or beef-pork mixture	8–12	18–24
Long-acting Ultralente insulin (insulin zinc suspension extended USP)	Human	8–16	24–36

3. **Intermediate onset and action:** These preparations include isophane insulin suspension (NPH insulin) and lente zinc suspension. Both preparations are given by subcutaneous injection; they are not suitable for intravenous use.

4. **Slow onset and long action:** Ultralente insulin is a long-acting insulin. It is often given in the morning or in the morning and evening to provide maintenance or basal levels for 12–24 hours. This basal insulin level may be supplemented with individual injections of insulin lispro or regular insulin during the day to meet the requirements of carbohydrate intake. Protamine zinc insulin, another long-acting preparation, is no longer available in the USA. These agents cannot be given intravenously.

The time course of effect of these preparations is shown in Figure 41–2.

D. **Hazards of Insulin Use:** Diabetic patients who use insulin are subject to two types of complications; hypoglycemia, from excessive insulin effect; and immunologic toxic effects, from the development of antibodies. Hypoglycemia is very hazardous because brain damage may result. Prompt administration of glucose (sugar or candy by mouth, glucose by vein) or of glucagon (by intramuscular injection) is essential.

The most common and most important insulin-induced immunologic complication is the formation of insulin antibodies, which results in resistance to the action of the drug. Of the forms available, beef insulin is the most antigenic, human the least, and pork insulin intermediate. Lipodystrophy, a change in fatty tissue at the site of injection, was relatively common in the past. Use of more purified, less antigenic forms of insulin has almost eliminated this complication.

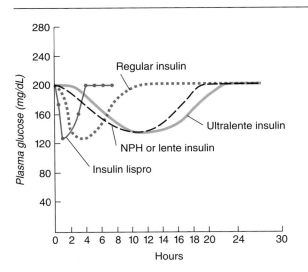

Figure 41–2. Extent and duration of action of various types of insulin (in a fasting diabetic). The durations of action shown are typical of average therapeutic doses; except for insulin lispro, duration increases when dosage is increased. (Reproduced, with permission, from Katzung BG [editor]: *Basic & Clinical Pharmacology,* 7th ed. Appleton & Lange, 1998.)

ORAL HYPOGLYCEMIC AGENTS

Two older groups of drugs are used for the oral treatment of diabetes: the sulfonylureas and the biguanides. Newer groups include the agents troglitazone and acarbose. Some members of these groups are listed in Table 41–3.

A. Sulfonylureas:
1. **Mechanism and effects:** The primary action of the sulfonylureas is to stimulate the release of endogenous insulin. These drugs close potassium channels in the B cell membrane; channel closure depolarizes the cell; and depolarization triggers insulin release. The sulfonylureas are not effective in patients with insulin-dependent diabetes or in adult diabetics who lack functioning islet cells. Furthermore, it has been proposed that these drugs may reduce glucagon release and that they may increase the number of functional insulin receptors in peripheral tissues. The "second-generation" sulfonylureas (**glyburide, glipizide, glimepiride**) are considerably more potent than the older agents (**tolbutamide, chlorpropamide, tolazamide,** others).
2. **Toxicities:** Adverse effects are relatively uncommon with the sulfonylureas: hypoglycemia due to overdosage, rash (occasionally), and sulfonamide allergy are reported. Chlorpropamide has a long duration of action, and liver or kidney disease may greatly increase the blood levels of the drug. Because of their great potency, hypoglycemia is somewhat more common with glyburide and glipizide.

B. Biguanides: The biguanides act by an unknown mechanism. They are effective in some patients who lack functional islet cells. Mechanisms that have been proposed include stimulation of glycolysis in peripheral tissues, reduced hepatic gluconeogenesis, reduction of glucose absorption from the gastrointestinal tract, and reduction of plasma glucagon levels. Several biguanides are in use overseas. **Metformin,** a newer biguanide, is the primary member of this group in the USA. It has a better safety record than **phenformin,** which was associated with an apparent increase in the incidence of lactic acidosis and no evidence of long-term benefit. Phenformin was withdrawn from the regular market but is available for use in special cases.

C. Newer Oral Hypoglycemic Agents:
1. **Thiazolidinediones:** **Troglitazone** is the first member of this group to be approved. Its mechanism of action is not fully understood, but the drug appears to reduce insulin resistance, a common problem in non-insulin-dependent diabetes. As a result, both fasting and postprandial hyperglycemia are reduced.
2. **Acarbose:** Acarbose is a carbohydrate analog that acts within the intestine to inhibit α-glucosidase, an enzyme necessary for the rapid absorption of most sugars. As a result of slowed absorption, postprandial hyperglycemia is reduced. The drug has no effect on fasting blood sugar.

Table 41–3. Representative oral antidiabetic drugs.

Drug	Dose	Duration of Action (hours)
Sulfonylureas		
Chlorpropamide	100–500 mg/d	Up to 60
Tolbutamide	500–2000 mg/d	6–12
Glimepiride	1–30 mg/d	12–24
Glipizide	5–20 mg/d	10–24
Glyburide	1.25–20 mg/d	10–24
Biguanides		
Metformin	1–3 g/d	10–12
Phenformin	25–150 mg/d	4–6
Others		
Troglitazone	400–600 mg/d	12–24
Acarbose	150–300 mg/d	3–4

TREATMENT OF DIABETES MELLITUS

Diabetes is diagnosed on the basis of more than one fasting blood sugar determination in excess of 140 mg/dL. Two major forms of the disease have been identified: **insulin-dependent diabetes mellitus (IDDM, type I)** and **non-insulin-dependent diabetes mellitus (NIDDM, type II).** The clinical history and the course of these two forms differ considerably, but treatment in both cases requires careful attention to diet and blood sugar levels.

Insulin-dependent diabetes (often called juvenile-onset diabetes) usually has its onset during childhood and results from destruction of the B cells in the pancreatic islets. IDDM is associated with a much higher incidence of ketoacidosis than NIDDM. Non-insulin-dependent diabetes usually has its onset in adulthood and is frequently associated with obesity and insulin resistance rather than insulin deficiency.

A. **Insulin-Dependent Diabetes:** Therapy of insulin-dependent diabetes involves dietary instruction, parenteral insulin (often a mixture of shorter- and longer-acting forms that mimic physiologic variations in insulin secretion and maintain a stable blood sugar during the day and night), and careful attention by the patient to things that change insulin requirements: exercise, infections, other forms of stress, and deviations from the regular diet. Recent large clinical studies indicate that close control of blood sugar—by frequent blood sugar testing and insulin injections—will reduce the incidence of vascular complications, including renal and retinal damage. The risk of hypoglycemic reactions is increased in close control regimens but not enough to negate the benefits of better control. A case of diabetes is presented in Case 10 (Appendix IV).

B. **Non-Insulin-Dependent Diabetes:** Therapy of non-insulin-dependent diabetes starts with attempts to eliminate obesity and to lower blood glucose by dietary means. If this is unsuccessful, oral hypoglycemic agents are begun. A sulfonylurea agent is given to maximum effect or to the onset of side effects. Insulin is added if both diet and oral hypoglycemic drugs are unsuccessful in controlling the blood sugar. The roles of troglitazone and acarbose have not yet been defined. Patients with marked hyperinsulinemia would appear to be reasonable candidates for treatment with troglitazone.

HYPERGLYCEMIC DRUGS: GLUCAGON & DIAZOXIDE

A. **Glucagon:**
1. **Chemistry, mechanism, and effects:** Glucagon is the product of the A cells of the endocrine pancreas. Like insulin, glucagon is a peptide; but unlike insulin, glucagon acts on G protein-coupled receptors. Activation of glucagon receptors located in heart, smooth muscle, and liver results in activation of adenylyl cyclase and increases intracellular cAMP. The effect is to stimulate heart rate and the force of contraction, to increase hepatic glycogenolysis and gluconeogenesis, and to relax smooth muscle. The smooth muscle effect is particularly marked in the gut.
2. **Clinical use:** Glucagon is used to treat severe hypoglycemia in diabetics, but its hyperglycemic action requires intact hepatic glycogen stores. The drug is given intramuscularly or intravenously. A nasal spray for self-administration is in clinical trials. Glucagon is also valuable for x-ray studies of the bowel or abdomen when temporary reduction of motility is necessary for optimal visualization. In the management of severe beta-blocker overdose, glucagon may be the most effective method for stimulating the depressed heart, since it increases cardiac cAMP without requiring access to beta adrenoceptors.

B. **Diazoxide:**
1. **Chemistry, mechanism, and effects:** Diazoxide, which is used primarily in the treatment of hypertensive emergencies (Chapter 11), also has hyperglycemic effects. By opening potassium channels (the opposite of sulfonylureas), diazoxide reduces insulin release from the pancreas and from insulin-secreting tumors. Severe hypoglycemia is thus prevented.
2. **Clinical use:** Diazoxide is used orally in the treatment of chronic hypoglycemic conditions, especially insulinomas that are not amenable to surgical cure.

DRUG LIST

The following drugs are important members of the groups discussed in this chapter. Prototypes should be learned in detail; the other significant agents should be recognized as belonging to a specific subclass.

Subclass	Prototype	Other Significant Agents
Insulins	Insulin lispro, regular, lente, NPH, ultralente	
Sulfonylureas	Chlorpropamide	Tolbutamide, tolazamide, glipizide, glimepiride, glyburide
Biguanides	Metformin	Phenformin
Other oral hypoglycemic drugs	Troglitazone, acarbose	
Drugs that increase blood sugar	Glucagon, diazoxide	

QUESTIONS

DIRECTIONS: Each of the numbered items or incomplete statements in this section is followed by answers or by completions of the statement. Select the ONE lettered answer or completion that is BEST in each case.

Items 1–2: A 13-year-old boy, reported to have had a viral infection 3 months earlier, is brought to the hospital complaining of dizziness. He has a recent history of weight loss, polyuria, and polydipsia. Laboratory findings include severe hyperglycemia, ketoacidosis, and a blood pH of 7.15.

1. In order to achieve rapid control of the severe ketoacidosis in this diabetic boy, the appropriate antidiabetic agent to use is
   (A) Crystalline zinc insulin
   (B) Isophane (NPH) insulin
   (C) Ultralente insulin
   (D) Tolbutamide
   (E) Glyburide

2. Possible complications of insulin therapy in this patient include
   (A) Dilutional hyponatremia
   (B) Hypoglycemia
   (C) Pancreatitis
   (D) Increased bleeding tendency
   (E) All of the above

3. A 24-year-old woman with insulin-dependent diabetes wishes to try close control of her diabetes to improve her long-term prognosis. Which of the following regimens is most appropriate?
   (A) Morning injections of mixed lente and ultralente insulins
   (B) Evening injections of mixed regular and lente insulins
   (C) Morning and evening injections of regular insulin, supplemented by small amounts of lente insulin at mealtimes
   (D) Morning injections of ultralente insulin, supplemented by small amounts of insulin lispro at mealtimes
   (E) Morning injection of semilente insulin and evening injection of lente insulin

4. All of the following drugs act by the same mechanism EXCEPT
   (A) Tolbutamide
   (B) Tolazamide
   (C) Chlorpropamide
   (D) Glipizide
   (E) Phenformin

5. Effects of insulin include all of the following EXCEPT
   (A) Increased glucose transport into cells
   (B) Induction of lipoprotein lipase
   (C) Decreased gluconeogenesis
   (D) Stimulation of glycogenolysis
   (E) Decreased conversion of amino acids into glucose

DIRECTIONS (Items 6–15): Each set of matching questions in this section consists of a list of three to twenty-six lettered options (some of which may be figures) followed by several numbered items. For each numbered item, select the ONE lettered option that is most closely associated with it. Each lettered option may be selected once, more than once, or not at all.

   (A) Human NPH insulin
   (B) Porcine regular crystalline zinc insulin
   (C) Human ultralente insulin
   (D) Pork lente insulin
   (E) Beef lente insulin
   (F) Insulin lispro
   (G) Glucagon
   (H) Glyburide
   (I) Metformin
   (J) Tolbutamide
   (K) Troglitazone

6. Longest-acting insulin preparation
7. Most antigenic insulin preparation
8. Less potent agent whose primary action is to release endogenous insulin
9. Oral agent that is not dependent on functioning pancreatic islet cells
10. Most potent oral hypoglycemic agent
11. Drug that acts on G protein-coupled receptors and increases cAMP
12. Parenteral drug with the fastest onset of hypoglycemic action
13. Human insulin with transposition of two amino acids
14. Produced in A cells of the pancreas
15. Oral agent that appears to sensitize tissue to insulin; no effect on insulin release

ANSWERS

1. Oral antidiabetic agents are inappropriate in this patient because he clearly has insulin-dependent diabetes (suggested by his age, history, and ketoacidosis). He needs a rapidly acting insulin preparation that can be given intravenously (Table 41–2). The answer is **(A)**.
2. Because of the risk of brain damage, the most important complication of insulin therapy is hypoglycemia. The other choices are not common effects of insulin. The answer is **(B)**.
3. Insulin regimens for close control usually take the form of establishing a basal level of insulin with a small amount of a long-acting preparation (ultralente) and supplementing the insulin levels, when called for by food intake, with short-acting insulin lispro. Less tight control may be achieved with two injections of intermediate-acting insulin per day. Because intake of glucose is mainly during the day, long-acting insulins are usually given in the morning, not at night. The answer is **(D)**.
4. Phenformin is a biguanide oral antidiabetic agent; the others are all sulfonylureas (Table 41–3). The answer is **(E)**.
5. Insulin stimulates the storage of glucose as glycogen (Table 41–1). The answer is **(D)**.
6. The longest-acting insulin is ultralente. The answer is **(C)**.
7. Pork insulin differs from the human hormone by only one amino acid. Beef insulin differs from human by three amino acids and is therefore the most antigenic. The answer is **(E)**.
8. The sulfonylureas are inactive in patients without functioning B cells, ie, these drugs cause the release of endogenous insulin. In contrast, the biguanides lower blood sugar in some patients with IDDM. Tolbutamide is much less potent than glyburide. The answer is **(J)**.
9. The biguanides lower blood sugar even in the absence of insulin. The answer is **(I)**, metformin.
10. The most potent oral hypoglycemic drugs are the second-generation sulfonylureas. The answer is glyburide, **(H)**.

11. Glucagon activates adenylyl cyclase and increases cAMP. The answer is **(G)**.
12. Insulin lispro is the insulin with the fastest onset of action. Like all insulins, it must be given parenterally. The answer is **(F)**.
13. The name "lispro" is derived from the lysine and proline amino acids that are transposed in this recombinant mutant human insulin. The answer is **(F)**.
14. Glucagon is produced in the A cells of the pancreas. The answer is **(G)**.
15. Troglitazone is a member of a new group of oral hypoglycemic drugs and appears to lower insulin resistance. The answer is **(K)**.

42 Drugs That Affect Bone Mineral Homeostasis

OBJECTIVES

You should be able to:

- List the agents useful in hypercalcemia.
- List the major and minor hormonal regulators of bone mineral homeostasis.
- Describe the major effects of parathyroid hormone on the intestine, the kidney, and bone.
- Describe the major effects of the vitamin D derivatives on the intestine, the kidney, and bone.
- Describe the therapeutic and toxic effects of bisphosphonates.
- Describe the therapeutic and toxic effects of fluoride ion.

CONCEPTS

Calcium and phosphorus are the two major elements of bone. They are also important in the metabolism of other cells in the body, and bone therefore functions as a storage reservoir. The two hormones of primary importance in the regulation of bone mineral homeostasis are parathyroid hormone (PTH) and vitamin D. Less important regulators include calcitonin, glucocorticoids, and estrogens. Exogenous agents of importance in the treatment of bone mineral disorders include the bisphosphonates and fluoride (Figure 42–1).

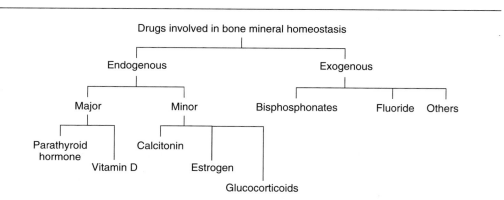

Figure 42–1. Subgroups of drugs discussed in this chapter.

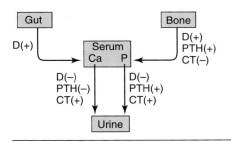

Figure 42–2. Some effects of vitamin D (D), parathyroid hormone (PTH), and calcitonin (CT) on calcium and phosphorus metabolism. Vitamin D increases absorption of calcium from both gut and bone, while PTH increases reabsorption from bone. Both vitamin D and parathyroid hormone reduce urinary excretion of calcium. (Reproduced, with permission, from Katzung BG [editor]: *Basic & Clinical Pharmacology,* 7th ed. Appleton & Lange, 1998.)

ENDOGENOUS SUBSTANCES

A. Parathyroid Hormone: Parathyroid hormone (PTH) is an 84-amino-acid peptide. The peptide acts on membrane G protein-coupled receptors to increase cAMP in cells. Increasing cAMP regulates calcium and phosphorus flux across cell membranes in bone and in the renal tubule. At high doses, the hormone increases blood calcium and decreases phosphorus by increasing net bone resorption (Figure 42–2). At low doses (physiologic levels), the agent may actually increase net bone formation (Table 42–1). A 34-amino-acid agent similar to PTH is under study for the treatment of osteoporosis.

B. Vitamin D: Vitamin D, a derivative of 7-dehydrocholesterol, is formed in the skin under the influence of ultraviolet light. Vitamin D is also found in some foods and is commonly used as a food supplement in milk. Several forms of the hormone occur (calcitriol, calciferol, and secalciferol), differing primarily in the number of hydroxyl groups on the molecule (Table 42–2). Some vitamin D is stored in adipose tissue; the rest is cleared by the liver.

Calcitriol is the best-studied of the active vitamin D metabolites, and specific receptors for this molecule have been identified. The actions of vitamin D include increased intestinal calcium and phosphorus absorption, decreased renal excretion of these substances, and a net increase in blood levels of both (Figure 42–2, Table 42–1). Bone formation may be increased by one of the isomers of the hormone (secalciferol; 24,25-dihydroxyvitamin D).

C. Calcitonin: Calcitonin, a peptide hormone secreted by the thyroid gland, decreases bone resorption and serum calcium and phosphate (Figure 42–2). Bone formation is not impaired initially, but ultimately it is reduced. Therefore, calcitonin is not useful in treating conditions in which bone mass is reduced, eg, osteoporosis. The hormone has been used in conditions in which an acute reduction of serum calcium is needed, eg, Paget's disease and hypercalcemia. No disease involving a primary abnormality of calcitonin secretion has been recognized. Although human calcitonin is available, salmon calcitonin is most often selected for clinical use because of its longer half-life and greater potency.

Table 42–1. Actions of PTH and vitamin D on intestine, kidney, and bone.*

Organ	PTH	Vitamin D
Intestine	Increased calcium and phosphate absorption (by increased 1,25[OH]$_2$D production)	Increased calcium and phosphate absorption (by 1,25[OH]$_2$D)
Kidney	Decreased calcium excretion, increased phosphate excretion	Calcium and phosphate excretion may be decreased by 25(OH)D and 1,25(OH)$_2$D
Bone	Calcium and phosphate resorption increased by high doses. Low doses may increase bone formation	Increased calcium and phosphate resorption by 1,25(OH)$_2$D. Bone formation may be increased by 24,25(OH)$_2$D
Net effect on serum levels	Serum calcium increased, serum phosphate decreased	Serum calcium and phosphate both increased

*Reproduced, with permission, from Katzung BG (editor): *Basic & Clinical Pharmacology,* 7th ed. Appleton & Lange, 1998.

Table 42–2. Vitamin D and its clinically available metabolites and analogs.*

Chemical Name	Abbreviation	Generic Name
Vitamin D$_3$	D$_3$	Cholecalciferol
Vitamin D$_2$	D$_2$	Ergocalciferol
25-Hydroxyvitamin D$_3$	25(OH)D$_3$	Calciferol
1,25-Dihydroxyvitamin D$_3$	1,25(OH)$_2$D$_3$	Calcitriol
24,25-Dihydroxyvitamin D$_3$	24,25(OH)$_2$D$_3$	Secalciferol
Dihydrotachysterol	DHT	Dihydrotachysterol

*Reproduced, with permission, from Katzung BG (editor): *Basic & Clinical Pharmacology,* 7th ed. Appleton & Lange, 1998.

D. **Estrogens:** Estrogens can prevent or delay bone loss in postmenopausal women (Chapter 40). Their action may involve the inhibition of parathyroid hormone-stimulated bone resorption. Because of estrogen's proved efficacy in slowing the progression of osteoporosis, many experts strongly recommend these drugs for general use (unless contraindicated) in postmenopausal women.

E. **Glucocorticoids:** The glucocorticoids have several effects already referred to (eg, protein catabolism; see Chapter 39) that inhibit bone mineral maintenance. As a result, chronic systemic use of these drugs may cause osteoporosis. However, these hormones are useful in the intermediate-term treatment of hypercalcemia.

EXOGENOUS AGENTS

A. **Bisphosphonates:** The bisphosphonates (**etidronate, pamidronate, alendronate**) are short-chain organic polyphosphate compounds that reduce both the resorption and the formation of bone by an action on the basic hydroxyapatite crystal structure. Recent studies suggest that chronic bisphosphonate therapy halts the progress of postmenopausal osteoporosis and reduces fractures, an extremely promising result. Because these drugs can be very irritating to the esophagus, the prescription of bisphosphonates requires that the patient be informed about taking large quantities of water with the tablets and avoiding situations (lying down) that permit esophageal reflux.

B. **Fluoride:** Appropriate concentrations of fluoride ion in drinking water (0.5–1 ppm) or as a dentifrice additive have a well-documented ability to reduce dental caries. Chronic exposure to the ion, especially in high concentrations, may increase new bone synthesis. It is not clear, however, whether this new bone is normal in strength. Acute toxicity of fluoride (usually caused by ingestion of rat poison) is manifested by gastrointestinal and neurologic symptoms. Chronic toxicity (fluorosis) includes ectopic bone formation and exostoses.

C. **Other Drugs With Effects on Calcium and Bone:** Plicamycin (**mithramycin**) is an antibiotic used to reduce serum calcium and bone resorption in Paget's disease and hypercalcemia. The **thiazide diuretics** (see Chapter 15) reduce the excretion of calcium by the kidney and have been used to decrease kidney stone formation. The loop diuretics, eg, **furosemide,** are often used (with saline infusion) to reduce serum calcium in acute hypercalcemia.

QUESTIONS

DIRECTIONS: Each of the numbered items or incomplete statements in this section is followed by answers or by completions of the statement. Select the ONE lettered answer or completion that is BEST in each case.

1. All of the following are useful in the therapy of hypercalcemia EXCEPT
   (A) Calcitonin
   (B) Glucocorticoids

      (C) Plicamycin
      (D) Parenteral infusion of phosphate
      (E) Thiazides
  2. Characteristics of vitamin D include which one of the following?
      (A) It is a prohormone produced in the liver
      (B) Active metabolites of vitamin D decrease serum calcium
      (C) Active metabolites of vitamin D increase serum phosphorus
      (D) Active metabolites of vitamin D increase cellular cAMP
      (E) All of the above
  3. Which one of the following conditions is an indication for the use of calcitonin?
      (A) Osteoporosis
      (B) Paget's disease
      (C) Rickets
      (D) Intestinal osteodystrophy
      (E) Hypoparathyroidism

DIRECTIONS (Items 4–10): Each set of matching questions in this section consists of a list of three to twenty-six lettered options (some of which may be figures) followed by several numbered items. For each numbered item, select the ONE lettered option that is most closely associated with it. Each lettered option may be selected once, more than once, or not at all.

      (A) Calcitonin
      (B) Estrogen
      (C) Fluoride
      (D) Furosemide
      (E) Alendronate
      (F) Parathyroid hormone
      (G) Prednisone
      (H) Vitamin D
  4. A hormone secreted by the human thyroid; the more commonly used preparation is obtained from salmon
  5. An inorganic ion that appears to facilitate new bone formation, especially if ingested in high concentrations
  6. Causes decreased renal calcium excretion and increased plasma phosphorus
  7. A diuretic used to rapidly lower serum calcium
  8. A drug that causes osteoporosis through inhibition of protein synthesis
  9. A synthetic phosphate derivative that shows promise in halting or reversing loss of bone density in osteoporosis
  10. Drug most commonly used to slow osteoporosis in postmenopausal women

ANSWERS

  1. Thiazides increase calcium reabsorption from the urine (see Chapter 15) and are never used in patients with hypercalcemia. The answer is **(E)**.
  2. Vitamin D is a prohormone produced in the skin whose metabolites increase serum phosphorus. They also increase serum calcium (Table 42–1). The active metabolites are produced in the skin, not the liver. Parathyroid hormone, not vitamin D, acts via cAMP. The answer is **(C)**.
  3. Rickets, hypoparathyroidism, and intestinal osteodystrophy are treated with vitamin D. Calcitonin is often used in Paget's disease to control hypercalcemia. The answer is **(B)**.
  4. The answer is **(A)**, calcitonin.
  5. The answer is **(C)**, fluoride.
  6. The answer is **(H)**, vitamin D (Table 42–1).
  7. Furosemide is used—with saline infusion to prevent hemoconcentration—to reduce serum calcium in the emergency management of hypercalcemia. The answer is **(D)**.
  8. Systemic glucocorticoids, eg, prednisone, cause significant osteoporosis when used chronically. The answer is **(G)**.
  9. The bisphosphonates are simple synthetic phosphate derivatives that slow or reverse osteoporosis. The answer is **(E)**.
  10. The answer is **(B)**, estrogen.

Part VIII: Chemotherapeutic Drugs

43 Beta-Lactam Antibiotics & Other Cell Wall Synthesis Inhibitors

OBJECTIVES

You should be able to:

- Describe the mechanism of antibacterial action of beta-lactam antibiotics.
- Describe the mechanisms underlying the resistance of bacteria to beta-lactam antibiotics.
- Identify the important drugs in each subclass of penicillins and describe their antibacterial activity and clinical uses.
- Identify the four subclasses of cephalosporins and describe their antibacterial activities and clinical uses.
- List the major adverse effects of the penicillins and the cephalosporins.
- Identify the important features of aztreonam and imipenem.
- Describe the clinical uses and toxicities of vancomycin, fosfomycin, and bacitracin.

Learn the definitions that follow.

Table 43–1. Definitions.

Term	Definition
Bactericidal	An antimicrobial drug that can eradicate an infection in the absence of host defense mechanisms; kills bacteria
Bacteriostatic	An antimicrobial drug that inhibits microbial growth but requires host defense mechanisms to eradicate the infection; does not kill bacteria
Beta-lactam antibiotics	Drugs with structures containing a beta-lactam ring; includes the penicillins and cephalosporins. This ring must be intact for antimicrobial action
Beta-lactamases	Bacterial enzymes (penicillinases, cephalosporinases) that hydrolyze the beta-lactam ring of certain penicillins and cephalosporins
Minimal inhibitory concentration (MIC)	Lowest concentration of antimicrobial drug capable of inhibiting growth of an organism in a defined growth medium
Penicillin-binding proteins (PBPs)	Bacterial cytoplasmic membrane proteins that act as the initial receptors for penicillins and other beta-lactam antibiotics
Peptidoglycan, murein	Polymeric chains of polysaccharides and polypeptides that are cross-linked to form the bacterial cell wall
Selective toxicity	More toxic to the invader than to the host; a property of useful antimicrobial drugs
Transpeptidases	Bacterial enzymes involved in the cross-linking of linear peptidoglycan chains, the final step in cell wall synthesis

CONCEPTS

Penicillins and cephalosporins are the major antibiotics that inhibit bacterial cell wall synthesis. They are called beta-lactams because of the unusual four-member ring that is common to all their members. These two large classes of beta-lactams include some of the most effective, widely used, and well-tolerated agents available for the treatment of microbial infections. Vancomycin, fosfomycin, and bacitracin also inhibit cell wall synthesis but for various reasons are not nearly as important as the beta-lactam drugs. The **selective toxicity** of the drugs discussed in this chapter is mainly due to specific actions on the synthesis of a cellular structure that is unique to the microorganism. Over 60 antibiotics that act as cell wall synthesis inhibitors are currently available, with individual spectrums of activity that afford a wide range of clinical applications.

The emergence of **microbial resistance** poses a constant challenge to the use of antimicrobial drugs. Mechanisms underlying microbial resistance to cell wall synthesis inhibitors include the production of antibiotic-inactivating enzymes, changes in the structure of target receptors, and decreases in the permeability to antibiotics of the cellular membranes of microbes. Strategies designed to combat microbial resistance include the use of adjunctive agents that can protect against antibiotic inactivation, the use of antibiotic combinations, the introduction of new (and often expensive) chemical derivatives of established antibiotics, and efforts to avoid the indiscriminate use or misuse of antibiotics.

PENICILLINS

A. Classification: All penicillins are derivatives of 6-aminopenicillanic acid and contain a beta-lactam ring structure that is essential for antibacterial activity. Penicillin subclasses have additional chemical substituents that confer differences in antimicrobial activity, susceptibility to acid and enzymatic hydrolysis, and biodisposition.

B. Pharmacokinetics: Penicillins vary in their resistance to gastric acid and therefore in their oral bioavailability. They are polar compounds and are not metabolized extensively. They are usually excreted unchanged in the urine via glomerular filtration and tubular secretion, the latter process being inhibited by probenecid. Ampicillin and nafcillin are excreted partly in the bile. The plasma half-lives of most penicillins vary from 0.5 to 1 hour. Procaine and benzathine forms of penicillin G are administered intramuscularly and have long plasma half-lives because the active drug is released very slowly into the bloodstream. Most penicillins cross the blood-brain barrier only when the meninges are inflamed.

C. Mechanisms of Action and Resistance: Beta-lactam antibiotics are **bactericidal** drugs. They act to inhibit cell wall synthesis by the following steps (see Figure 43–2): (1) binding of the drug to specific receptors **(penicillin-binding proteins; PBPs)** located in the bacterial cytoplasmic membrane; (2) inhibition of **transpeptidase** enzymes that act to cross-link linear peptidoglycan chains that form part of the cell wall; and (3) activation of autolytic enzymes that cause lesions in the bacterial cell wall.

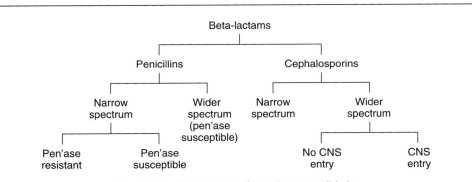

Figure 43–1. Subdivisions of beta-lactam antibiotics.

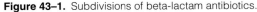

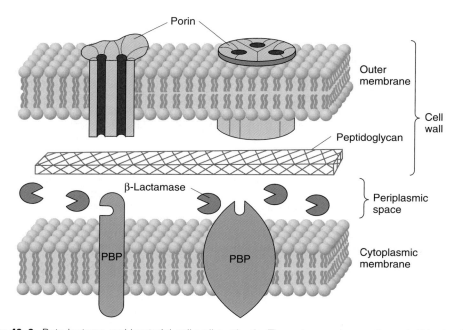

Figure 43–2. Beta-lactams and bacterial cell wall synthesis. The outer membrane shown in this simplified diagram is present only in gram-negative organisms. It is penetrated by proteins (porins) that are permeable to hydrophilic substances such as beta-lactam antibiotics. The peptidoglycan chains (mureins) are cross-linked by transpeptidases located in the cytoplasmic membrane, closely associated with penicillin-binding proteins (PBPs). Beta-lactam antibiotics bind to PBPs and inhibit transpeptidation, the final step in cell wall synthesis. They also activate autolytic enzymes that cause lesions in the cell wall. Beta-lactamases, which inactivate beta-lactam antibiotics, may be present in the periplasmic space or on the outer surface of the cytoplasmic membrane. (Reproduced, with permission, from Katzung BG [editor]: *Basic & Clinical Pharmacology,* 7th ed. Appleton & Lange, 1998.)

Enzymatic hydrolysis of the beta-lactam ring results in loss of antibacterial activity. The formation of **beta-lactamases (penicillinases)** by microorganisms is thus a major mechanism of bacterial resistance. Inhibitors of these bacterial enzymes (eg, **clavulanic acid, sulbactam, tazobactam**) are sometimes used in combination with penicillins to prevent their inactivation. Structural change in target PBPs is another mechanism of resistance and is responsible for methicillin resistance in staphylococci and for resistance to penicillin G in pneumococci. In gram-negative rods, changes in the porin structures in the outer membrane may contribute to resistance by impeding access of penicillins to PBPs.

D. **Clinical Uses:**
1. **Narrow-spectrum, penicillinase-susceptible agents:** **Penicillin G** is the prototype of a subclass of penicillins that have a limited spectrum of antibacterial activity and are susceptible to beta-lactamases. Clinical uses include therapy of infections caused by common streptococci, pneumococci, meningococci, gram-positive bacilli, and spirochetes. Most strains of *Staphylococcus aureus* and many strains of the gonococcus are resistant via production of beta-lactamases. Activity against enterococci is enhanced by aminoglycoside antibiotics. Penicillin V is an oral drug used mainly in oropharyngeal infections.
2. **Very narrow spectrum, penicillinase-resistant drugs:** This subclass of penicillins includes **methicillin** (the prototype), **nafcillin**, and **oxacillin.** The primary use of these agents is in the treatment of known or suspected staphylococcal infections. Methicillin-resistant staphylococci (MRSA) are resistant to members of this subgroup and may be resistant to multiple antimicrobial drugs.

3. **Wider-spectrum, penicillinase-susceptible drugs:**
   a. **Ampicillin and amoxicillin:** These drugs comprise a penicillin subgroup that has a wider spectrum of antibacterial activity than penicillin G but remains susceptible to penicillinases. Their clinical uses include indications similar to indications for penicillin G as well as infections due to enterococci, *Listeria monocytogenes, Escherichia coli, Proteus mirabilis,* and *Haemophilus influenzae,* though resistant strains occur. When used in combination with inhibitors of penicillinases (clavulanic acid, etc), their antibacterial activity is enhanced. In enterococcal and listerial infections, ampicillin is synergistic with aminoglycosides.
   b. **Piperacillin and ticarcillin:** These drugs have activity against several gram-negative rods, including *Pseudomonas* and *Enterobacter* species. Most drugs in this subgroup have synergistic actions when used with aminoglycosides against such organisms. Piperacillin and ticarcillin are susceptible to penicillinases and are often used in combination with penicillinase inhibitors to enhance their activity.

E. **Toxicity:**
   1. **Allergy:** Allergic reactions include urticaria, severe pruritus, fever, joint swelling, hemolytic anemia, nephritis, and anaphylaxis. About 5–10% of persons with a past history of penicillin reaction have an allergic response when given a penicillin again. Methicillin causes nephritis more often than do other penicillins, and nafcillin is associated with neutropenia. Antigenic determinants include degradation products of penicillins, such as penicilloic acid. Complete **cross-allergenicity** between different penicillins should be assumed. Ampicillin frequently causes a maculopapular skin rash that may not be an allergic reaction.
   2. **Gastrointestinal disturbances:** Nausea and diarrhea may occur with oral penicillins, especially with ampicillin. Gastrointestinal upsets may be caused by direct irritation or by overgrowth of gram-positive organisms or yeasts. Ampicillin has been implicated in pseudomembranous colitis.
   3. **Cation toxicity:** Toxic effects from Na^+ or K^+ may occur when high doses of penicillin salts are used in patients with cardiovascular or renal disease.

CEPHALOSPORINS

A. **Classification:** The cephalosporins are derivatives of 7-aminocephalosporanic acid and contain the beta-lactam ring structure. Many members of this group are in clinical use. They are classified on the basis of their antibacterial activity, but are designated first-, second-, third-, or fourth-generation drugs according to the time of their introduction into clinical use.

B. **Pharmacokinetics:** Several cephalosporins are available for oral use, but most are administered parenterally. Cephalosporins with side chains may undergo hepatic metabolism, but the major elimination mechanism for drugs in this class is renal excretion via active tubular secretion. Cefoperazone and ceftriaxone are excreted mainly in the bile. Most first- and second-generation cephalosporins do not enter the cerebrospinal fluid even when the meninges are inflamed.

C. **Mechanisms of Action and Resistance:** Cephalosporins bind to PBPs on bacterial cell membranes to inhibit bacterial cell wall synthesis by mechanisms similar to those described for the penicillins. Cephalosporins are bactericidal against susceptible organisms.
   Structural differences from penicillins render cephalosporins less susceptible to penicillinases produced by staphylococci, but many bacteria are resistant through the production of other beta-lactamases that can inactivate cephalosporins. Resistance can also result from decreases in membrane permeability to cephalosporins and by changes in PBPs. Methicillin-resistant staphylococci are also resistant to most cephalosporins.

D. **Clinical Uses:**
   1. **First-generation drugs:** **Cefazolin** (parenteral) and **cephalexin** (oral) are examples of this subgroup. They are active against gram-positive cocci, including staphylococci and

common streptococci. Many strains of *Enterobacter coli* and *Klebsiella pneumoniae* are also sensitive. Clinical uses include treatment of infections caused by these organisms and surgical prophylaxis in selected cases. These drugs have minimal activity against gram-negative cocci, enterococci, methicillin-resistant staphylococci, and most gram-negative rods.

2. **Second-generation drugs:** Drugs in this subgroup usually have less activity against gram-positive organisms than the first-generation drugs but have an extended gram-negative coverage. Marked differences in activity occur among the drugs in this subgroup. Examples of clinical uses include infections caused by *Bacteroides fragilis* (**cefotetan, cefoxitin**) and by *H influenzae* or *Branhamella catarrhalis* (**cefuroxime, cefaclor**).

3. **Third-generation drugs:** Characteristic features of third-generation drugs (eg, **cefoperazone, cefotaxime**) include increased activity against gram-negative organisms resistant to other beta-lactam drugs and ability to penetrate the blood-brain barrier (except cefoperazone and cefixime). Most are active against *Enterobacter, Providencia, Serratia marcescens,* and beta-lactamase-producing strains of *H influenzae* and *Neisseria*. Individual drugs also have activity against *Pseudomonas* (**ceftazidime**) and *B fragilis* (**ceftizoxime**). Drugs in this subclass should usually be reserved for treatment of serious infections, eg, bacterial meningitis. **Ceftriaxone** (parenteral) and **cefixime** (oral), currently the drugs of choice in gonorrhea, are exceptions. Likewise, in acute otitis media, a single injection of ceftriaxone is as effective as a 10-day course of treatment with amoxicillin or cefaclor.

4. **Fourth-generation drugs:** **Cefepime** is more resistant to beta-lactamases produced by gram-negative organisms, including *Enterobacter, Haemophilus,* and *Neisseria*.

E. **Toxicity:**
1. **Allergy:** Cephalosporin use is associated with a range of allergic reactions from skin rashes to anaphylactic shock. These reactions occur less frequently with cephalosporins than with penicillins. Complete cross-hypersensitivity between different cephalosporins should be assumed. Cross-reactivity between penicillins and cephalosporins is incomplete (5–10%), so patients allergic to penicillin are sometimes treated successfully with a cephalosporin. However, patients with a history of *anaphylaxis* to penicillins should not be treated with a cephalosporin.

2. **Other adverse effects:** Cephalosporins may cause pain at intramuscular injection sites and phlebitis after intravenous administration. They may increase the nephrotoxicity of aminoglycosides when the two are administered together. Drugs containing a methylthiotetrazole group (cefoperazone, cefotetan, moxalactam) cause hypoprothrombinemia and may cause disulfiram-like reactions with ethanol. Moxalactam also decreases platelet function and may cause severe bleeding.

OTHER BETA-LACTAM DRUGS

A. **Aztreonam:** Aztreonam is a **monobactam** that is resistant to beta-lactamases produced by certain gram-negative rods, including *Klebsiella, Pseudomonas,* and *Serratia.* The drug has no activity against gram-positive bacteria or anaerobes. It is an inhibitor of cell wall synthesis, preferentially binding to PBPs, and is synergistic with aminoglycosides.

Aztreonam is administered intravenously and is eliminated via renal tubular secretion. Its half-life is prolonged in renal failure. Adverse effects include gastrointestinal upset with possible superinfection, vertigo and headache, and (rarely) hepatotoxicity. Though skin rash may occur, there is no cross-allergenicity with penicillins.

B. **Imipenem:** Imipenem is a **carbapenem** (chemically different from penicillins but retaining the beta-lactam ring structure) with low susceptibility to beta-lactamases. The drug has wide activity against gram-positive cocci (including some penicillin-resistant pneumococci), gram-negative rods, and anaerobes. It is administered parenterally and is especially useful for infections caused by organisms resistant to other antibiotics. It is currently the drug of choice for infections due to *Enterobacter.*

Imipenem is rapidly inactivated by renal dehydropeptidase I and is administered in fixed combination with cilastatin, an inhibitor of this enzyme. Cilastatin increases the plasma half-life of imipenem and inhibits the formation of a potentially nephrotoxic metabolite.

Adverse effects of imipenem-cilastatin include gastrointestinal distress, skin rash, and, at very high plasma levels, CNS toxicity (confusion, encephalopathy, seizures). There is partial cross-allergenicity with the penicillins. **Meropenem** is similar to imipenem except that it is not metabolized by renal dehydropeptidases and is less likely to cause seizures.

C. **Beta-Lactamase Inhibitors:** **Clavulanic acid, sulbactam,** and **tazobactam** are used in fixed combinations with certain hydrolyzable penicillins. They are most active against plasmid-encoded beta-lactamases such as those produced by gonococci, streptococci, *E coli,* and *H influenzae.* They are not good inhibitors of inducible chromosomal beta-lactamases formed by *Enterobacter* and *Pseudomonas.*

OTHER INHIBITORS OF CELL WALL SYNTHESIS

A. **Vancomycin:** Vancomycin is a bactericidal glycoprotein that binds to the D-Ala-D-Ala terminal of the nascent peptidoglycan pentapeptide side chain and inhibits transglycosylation. This action prevents elongation of the peptidoglycan chain and interferes with cross-linking. Resistance involves a decreased affinity of vancomycin for the binding site due to the replacement of the terminal D-Ala by D-lactate. Vancomycin has a narrow spectrum of activity and is used for serious infections caused by drug-resistant gram-positive organisms, including methicillin-resistant staphylococci, penicillin-resistant pneumococci and *C difficile.*

Vancomycin-resistant enterococci have emerged recently, a serious clinical problem since such organisms usually exhibit multiple drug resistance. Vancomycin is not absorbed from the gastrointestinal tract and may be given orally for bacterial enterocolitis. When given parenterally, vancomycin penetrates most tissues and is eliminated unchanged in the urine. Dosage modification is mandatory in patients with renal impairment. Toxic effects of vancomycin include chills, fever, phlebitis, ototoxicity, and nephrotoxicity. Rapid intravenous infusion may cause diffuse flushing ("red man syndrome").

B. **Fosfomycin:** Fosfomycin is an antimetabolite inhibitor of cytosolic enolpyruvate transferase. This action prevents the formation of *N*-acetylmuramic acid, an essential precursor molecule for peptidoglycan chain formation. Resistance to fosfomycin occurs via decreased intracellular accumulation of the drug.

Fosfomycin is excreted by the kidney, with urinary levels exceeding the **minimal inhibitory concentrations (MICs)** for many urinary tract pathogens. In a single dose the drug is less effective than a 7-day course of treatment with fluoroquinolones. With multiple dosing, resistance emerges rapidly and diarrhea is common. Fosfomycin may be synergistic with beta-lactam and quinolone antibiotics in specific infections.

C. **Bacitracin:** Bacitracin is a peptide antibiotic that interferes with a late stage in cell wall synthesis in gram-positive organisms. Because of its marked nephrotoxicity, the drug is limited to topical use.

D. **Cycloserine:** Cycloserine is an antimetabolite that blocks the incorporation of D-Ala into the pentapeptide side chain of the peptidoglycan. Because of its potential neurotoxicity (tremors, seizures, psychosis) cycloserine is used only to treat tuberculosis caused by organisms resistant to first-line antituberculosis drugs.

DRUG LIST

The following drugs are important members of the group discussed in this chapter. Prototypes should be learned in detail; features of the major variants should be known well enough so that the variants can be distinguished from prototypes and from each other.

Subclass	Prototype	Major Variants
Penicillins		
Limited spectrum	Penicillin G	Penicillin V
Beta-lactamase-resistant	Methicillin	Nafcillin, oxacillin, cloxacillin
Wider spectrum	Ampicillin, carbenicillin	Amoxicillin, piperacillin, ticarcillin
Cephalosporins		
First-generation	Cefazolin	Cephalexin, cephradine, cephapirin
Second-generation	Cefamandole	Cefaclor, cefotetan, cefoxitin
Third-generation	Cefoperazone	Cefotaxime, ceftazidime, ceftriaxone
Carbapenem	Imipenem	Meropenem
Monobactam	Aztreonam	
Beta-lactamase inhibitors[1]	Clavulanic acid	Sulbactam, tazobactam
Miscellaneous	Vancomycin	Fosfomycin, bacitracin, cycloserine

[1]Negligible antimicrobial activity when given alone.

QUESTIONS

DIRECTIONS: Each of the numbered items or incomplete statements in this section is followed by answers or by completions of the statement. Select the ONE lettered answer or completion that is BEST in each case.

1. Which one of the following statements about the biodisposition of penicillins and cephalosporins is most accurate?
   (A) Oral bioavailability is affected by first-pass hepatic metabolism
   (B) Only third-generation cephalosporins cross the blood-brain barrier
   (C) Procaine penicillin G is the most commonly used intravenous form of the antibiotic
   (D) Renal tubular reabsorption of beta-lactams is inhibited by probenecid
   (E) Nafcillin and ceftriaxone are eliminated mainly via biliary secretion

2. The mechanism of antibacterial action of cephalosporins involves
   (A) Inhibition of the synthesis of precursors of peptidoglycans
   (B) Interference with the synthesis of ergosterol
   (C) Inhibition of transpeptidation reactions
   (D) Inhibition of beta-lactamases
   (E) Binding to cytoplasmic receptor proteins

Items 3–4: A 21-year-old man was seen in a clinic with a complaint of dysuria and urethral discharge of yellow pus. He had a painless clean-based ulcer on the penis and nontender enlargement of the regional lymph nodes. A Gram stain of the urethral exudate showed gram-negative diplococci within polymorphonuclear leukocytes. The patient informed the clinic staff that he was unemployed and had not eaten for 3 days.

3. The most appropriate treatment of gonorrhea in this patient is
   (A) Amoxicillin orally for 7 days
   (B) Ceftriaxone intramuscularly as a single dose
   (C) Procaine penicillin G intramuscularly as a single dose plus 1 gram of probenecid
   (D) Tetracycline orally for 7 days
   (E) Vancomycin intramuscularly as a single dose

4. Immunofluorescent microscopic examination of fluid expressed from the penile chancre of this patient revealed treponemes. Since he appears to be infected with *T pallidum*, the best course of action would be to
   (A) Treat with spectinomycin
   (B) Treat with oral tetracycline
   (C) Inject intramuscular benzathine penicillin G
   (D) Give a single oral dose of fosfomycin
   (E) Give no other antibiotics, since drug treatment of gonorrhea provides coverage for incubating syphilis

5. Which one of the following statements about imipenem is most accurate?
   (A) The drug has a narrow spectrum of antibacterial action
   (B) It is used in fixed combination with sulbactam
   (C) Imipenem is highly susceptible to beta-lactamases produced by *Enterobacter* species
   (D) In renal dysfunction, dosage reductions are necessary to avoid seizures
   (E) Imipenem is active against methicillin-resistant staphylococci

6. An elderly debilitated patient has a fever believed to be due to an infection. He has extensive skin lesions, scrapings of which reveal the presence of large numbers of gram-positive cocci. The most appropriate drug to use for treatment of this patient is
   (A) Amoxicillin
   (B) Aztreonam
   (C) Moxalactam
   (D) Nafcillin
   (E) Penicillin G

7. A 36-year-old woman recently treated for leukemia is admitted to hospital with malaise, chills, and high fever. Gram's stain of a blood smear reveals the presence of gram-negative bacilli. The initial diagnosis is bacteremia, and parenteral antibiotics are indicated. The patient's records reveal that she had a severe urticarial rash, hypotension, and respiratory difficulty following oral penicillin V about 6 months previously. The most appropriate drug regimen for empiric treatment is
   (A) Ampicillin plus sulbactam
   (B) Aztreonam
   (C) Cefazolin
   (D) Imipenem plus cilastatin
   (E) Ticarcillin plus clavulanic acid

Items 8–10:   A 52-year-old man (weight 70 kg) is brought to the hospital emergency room in a confused and delirious state. He has had an elevated temperature for over 24 hours, during which time he complained of a severe headache and had suffered from nausea and vomiting. Lumbar puncture reveals an elevated opening pressure, and CSF findings include elevated protein, decreased glucose, and increased neutrophils. You are informed that the patient has a long history of antibiotic treatment for sinusitis but is not currently taking any drugs other than ibuprofen. A Gram-stained smear of CSF reveals gram-positive diplococci and a preliminary diagnosis of purulent meningitis is made. The microbiology report informs you that for approximately 15% of *Streptococcus pneumoniae* isolates in the community, the minimal inhibitory concentration for penicillin G is greater than 2 μg/mL.

8. Treatment of this patient should be initiated immediately with
   (A) Ampicillin, 2 g IV every 6 hours
   (B) Cefoperazone, 2 g IV every 12 hours
   (C) Cefotaxime, 1.5 g IV every 6 hours
   (D) Nafcillin, 2 g IV every 4 hours
   (E) Penicillin G, 2 million units IV every 4 hours

9. The molecular basis for the resistance of pneumococci to penicillin G is
   (A) The production of beta-lactamases
   (B) Structural changes in penicillin-binding proteins
   (C) Decreased intracellular accumulation of penicillin G
   (D) Changes in the D-Ala-D-Ala building block of peptidoglycan precursor
   (E) Changes in porin structure

10. If this patient had been 82 years old and the Gram stain of the CSF smear had revealed gram-positive rods resembling diphtheroids, the antibiotic regimen for empiric treatment would include
    (A) Ampicillin
    (B) Cefazolin
    (C) Moxalactam
    (D) Ticarcillin
    (E) Vancomycin

DIRECTIONS (Items 11–15):   Each set of matching questions in this section consists of a list of three to twenty-six lettered options (some of which may be figures) followed by several numbered items. For each numbered item, select the ONE lettered option that is most closely associated with it. Each lettered option may be selected once, more than once, or not at all.

(A) Ampicillin
(B) Aztreonam
(C) Bacitracin
(D) Cefaclor
(E) Cefotetan
(F) Cefoxitin
(G) Dicloxacillin
(H) Fosfomycin
(I) Meropenem
(J) Nafcillin
(K) Penicillin VK
(L) Ticarcillin
(M) Vancomycin

11. This drug has activity against anaerobes and would be appropriate for prophylaxis in gynecologic surgery. Administration of a single dose of this antibiotic has led to disulfiram-like reactions following ingestion of alcoholic beverages

12. When used with gentamicin, this drug would be appropriate for treatment of enterococcal endocarditis in a patient who has experienced an anaphylactic reaction to penicillin G

13. This drug has activity against many strains of *Pseudomonas aeruginosa*. However, when it is used alone, resistance has emerged during the course of treatment. The drug should not be used in penicillin-allergic patients. Its activity against gram-negative rods is enhanced if it is given in combination with clavulanic acid

14. Of the drugs listed, this antibiotic is the most active against staphylococci, including strains resistant to methicillin

15. This antibiotic undergoes enterohepatic cycling and is partly eliminated in the feces. It may cause superinfections through disturbances of gastrointestinal and urogenital flora. When used in patients who have viral infections, the drug causes a high incidence of maculopapular rashes

ANSWERS

1. Stability in gastric acid is the main determinant of the oral bioavailability of beta-lactam antibiotics. Cefuroxime (a second-generation cephalosporin) and cefepime (fourth-generation) both cross the blood-brain barrier. Several third-generation cephalosporins (eg, cefoperazone) do not achieve CSF levels high enough to be useful in bacterial meningitis. Procaine penicillin G is given by intramuscular injection (not intravenously) and is rarely used now because of resistance on the part of gonococci and pneumococci. The elimination half-lives of many beta-lactam antibiotics are prolonged by probenecid, which inhibits their proximal tubular secretion. Biliary excretion is the major mode of elimination of nafcillin and ceftriaxone. The answer is **(E).**

2. The cephalosporins bind to PBPs present on the cytoplasmic membrane and act at the transpeptidation stage of cell wall synthesis (the final step) to inhibit peptidoglycan cross-linking. Like penicillins, they also activate autolysins that break down the bacterial cell wall. Vancomycin is an inhibitor of transglycosylation and, like fosfomycin, interferes with the synthesis of precursor molecules needed for peptidoglycan chain formation. The answer is **(C).**

3. Currently the treatment of choice for gonorrhea is a single dose of ceftriaxone (intramuscularly) or of cefixime (orally). Note that neither of these third-generation cephalosporins has activity against *Chlamydia* or other organisms responsible for nongonococcal urethritis. Because of the high incidence of beta-lactamase-producing gonococci, the use of penicillin G or amoxicillin is no longer appropriate for gonorrhea. Similarly, many strains of gonococci are resistant to tetracyclines. Back-up drugs (not listed) include spectinomycin and certain quinolone antibiotics. The answer is **(B).**

4. This patient with gonorrhea also has primary syphilis. The penile chancre, enlarged nontender lymph nodes, and the microscopic identification of treponemes in fluid expressed from the lesion are essential elements of the diagnosis. Serologic tests for syphilis (eg, VRDL) are likely to be positive. While a single dose of ceftriaxone may cure incubating syphilis, it cannot be relied upon for treating primary syphilis. The most appropriate course of action in this patient is

to administer a single intramuscular injection of 2.4 million units of benzathine penicillin G. For penicillin-allergic patients, oral doxycycline or tetracycline for 15 days is effective in most cases. However, lack of compliance may be a problem with oral therapy. Fosfomycin and spectinomycin have no significant activity against spirochetes. The answer is **(C)**.

5. Imipenem has a wide spectrum of activity that includes anaerobes and many beta-lactamase producing gram-negative rods, including *Enterobacter*. The drug is hydrolyzed by renal dehydropeptidases and is given in combination with cilastatin, an inhibitor of this enzyme. The chemical structure of imipenem is related to the beta-lactams, and the drug displays partial cross-allergenicity with the penicillins. Severe CNS toxicity, including seizures, will occur if the dose of imipenem is not reduced in patients with renal impairment. The answer is **(D)**.

6. Bacterial lesions of the skin are often caused by staphylococci or streptococci and may lead to systemic infections; they should be treated promptly. Virtually all strains of *S aureus* are penicillinase-producing, so amoxicillin and penicillin G would not be effective. Aztreonam is only active against gram-negative bacilli, and the third-generation cephalosporin (moxalactam) has limited activity against gram-positive organisms. In addition, moxalactam carries the risk of bleeding disorders in elderly debilitated patients. Nafcillin is resistant to penicillinases and has activity against most strains of *S aureus* and common streptococci. The answer is **(D)**.

7. Each of the drugs listed has activity against some gram-negative bacilli. All penicillins should be avoided in patients with a history of allergic reactions to any individual penicillin drug. Cephalosporins should also be avoided in patients who have had anaphylaxis or other severe hypersensitivity reactions following use of a penicillin. There is no cross-reactivity between the penicillins and aztreonam. The answer is **(B)**.

8. Pneumococcal isolates with a minimal inhibitory concentration for penicillin G of greater than 2 μg/mL are highly resistant. Such strains are not killed by the concentrations of penicillin G or ampicillin that can be achieved in the cerebrospinal fluid. Nafcillin would be of value in a purulent meningitis suspected to be due to staphylococci but has minimal activity against penicillin-resistant pneumococci. Cefotaxime and ceftriaxone (not listed) are the most active cephalosporins against penicillin-resistant pneumococci and the addition of vancomycin or rifampin is recommended in the case of highly resistant strains. Cefoperazone does not readily cross the blood-brain barrier and is of marginal value in bacterial meningitis with the possible exception of that caused by *Pseudomonas aeruginosa*. The answer is **(C)**.

9. Many gram-positive cocci, especially staphylococci, are resistant to penicillin G via the production of penicillinases. Beta-lactamase formation is also the mechanism of resistance of gonococci and many gram-negative rods. Pneumococcal resistance is due to changes in the chemical structures of penicillin-binding proteins located in the bacterial cytoplasmic membrane. A similar mechanism underlies the resistance of staphylococci to methicillin (MRSA strains). Changes in porin structure may play a role in penicillin resistance in gram-negative rods. Structural alterations in the D-Ala-D-Ala component of the pentapeptide side chains of peptidoglycans constitute a mechanism of resistance to vancomycin. The answer is **(B)**.

10. The presence of diphtheroid-like gram-positive rods in the cerebrospinal fluid smear of an 82-year-old patient is indicative of the presence of *Listeria monocytogenes*. In addition to the role of *Listeria* as a potential causative agent in neonatal meningitis, infections with this pathogen are more common in the elderly patient and in those who have received immunosuppressive therapy. Treatment consists of ampicillin with or without gentamicin. Resistant strains are rare. The answer is **(A)**.

11. Cephalosporins are commonly used in surgical prophylaxis, especially first-generation drugs such as cefazolin. Those with activity against anaerobes include cefotetan and cefoxitin, and the latter is an important component of antibiotic regimens for management of pelvic inflammatory disease. Cephalosporins containing the methylthiotetrazole ring (cefotetan, cefoperazone, moxalactam) may cause hypoprothrombinemia and disulfiram-like interactions with ethanol. The answer is **(E)**.

12. In patients who have had a severe reaction to a penicillin, it is inadvisable to administer a cephalosporin or a carbapenem such as meropenem. Aztreonam has no significant activity against gram-positive cocci, so the logical treatment in this case is vancomycin, usually with an aminoglycoside for synergistic activity against enterococci. The answer is **(M)**.

13. Several drugs listed have activity against strains of *Pseudomonas aeruginosa*, including aztreonam, imipenem and ticarcillin. When any of these drugs are used as sole agents in pseudomonal infections, resistance can emerge rapidly. However, aztreonam is quite safe in patients with established allergy to the penicillins. Ticarcillin (not imipenem) has greater activity

against beta-lactamase-producing gram-negative rods when used with clavulanic acid. The answer is **(L)**.

14. Vancomycin continues to have the greatest antistaphylococcal activity among the inhibitors of bacterial cell wall synthesis. While several of the other drugs listed are effective against beta-lactamase-producing staphylococci, only vancomycin has useful activity against strains of methicillin-resistant staphylococci. The answer is **(M)**.

15. Most antibiotics are capable of disturbing normal microflora, and in some cases this action can lead to opportunistic superinfections. Ampicillin causes yeast infections in the upper gastrointestinal and urogenital tracts and may cause colitis due to infection with staphylococcal or clostridial species. Maculopapular rashes occur quite frequently during use of ampicillin, especially if the drug is administered to patients with viral infections, including infectious mononucleosis. The answer is **(A)**.

44
Chloramphenicol, Tetracyclines, Macrolides, & Clindamycin

OBJECTIVES

You should be able to:

- Describe the mechanisms of action of these inhibitors of bacterial protein synthesis.
- Describe the mechanisms responsible for clinical bacterial resistance to these drugs.
- List the major clinical uses of these drugs.
- Describe the pharmacokinetic features of these agents that are most relevant to their clinical use.
- List the main toxic effects of these drugs.

CONCEPTS

The antimicrobial drugs reviewed in this chapter selectively inhibit bacterial protein synthesis (Figure 44–1). The mechanisms of protein synthesis in microorganisms are not identical to those of mammalian cells. Bacteria have 70 S ribosomes whereas mammalian cells have 80 S ribosomes. Differences exist in ribosomal subunits and in the chemical composition and functional specificities of component nucleic acids and proteins. Such differences form the basis for the selective toxicity of these drugs against microorganisms without major effects on protein synthesis in mammalian cells.

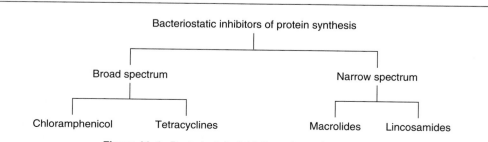

Figure 44–1. Bacteriostatic inhibitors of protein synthesis.

Chloramphenicol and the tetracyclines were among the first inhibitors of bacterial protein synthesis to be discovered. Because they had a broad spectrum of antibacterial activity and were thought to have low toxicities, they were overused. Many bacterial species once highly susceptible have become resistant and these drugs are now used for more selected targets. Erythromycin, a macrolide antibiotic, has a narrower spectrum of action but continues to be active against several important pathogens. Azithromycin and clarithromycin are semisynthetic macrolides with some distinctive properties compared to erythromycin.

MECHANISM OF ACTION

All of the antibiotics reviewed in this chapter are bacteriostatic inhibitors of protein synthesis acting at the ribosomal level (Figure 44–2). The binding sites for chloramphenicol, macrolides, and clindamycin are close to each other on the 50 S ribosomal subunit. Chloramphenicol indirectly inhibits transpeptidation (catalyzed by peptidyltransferase) by blocking the binding of the aminoacyl moiety of the charged tRNA molecule to the acceptor site on the ribosome-mRNA complex. Thus, the peptide at the donor site cannot be transferred to its amino acid acceptor. Macrolides and clindamycin block translocation of peptidyl tRNA from the acceptor site to the donor site. Incoming charged tRNA cannot access the occupied acceptor site, so the next amino acid cannot be added to the nascent peptide chain. Macrolides also block formation of the initiation complex. Tetracyclines bind to the 30 S ribosomal subunit at a site that blocks the binding of amino acid-charged tRNA to the acceptor site of the ribosome-mRNA complex.

Selective toxicity of these protein synthesis inhibitors against microorganisms may be explained by target differences. Chloramphenicol does not bind to the 80 S ribosomal RNA of mammalian cells, though it can inhibit the functions of *mitochondrial* ribosomes, which contain 70 S ribosomal RNA. Tetracyclines have little effect on mammalian protein synthesis because an active efflux mechanism prevents their intracellular accumulation.

CHLORAMPHENICOL

A. Classification and Pharmacokinetics: Chloramphenicol has a simple and distinctive structure, and no other antimicrobials have been discovered in this chemical class. It is effective orally as well as parenterally and is distributed throughout all tissues; it readily crosses the placental and blood-brain barriers. The drug undergoes enterohepatic cycling, and a small fraction of the dose is excreted in the urine unchanged. Most of the drug is inactivated by a hepatic glucuronosyltransferase.

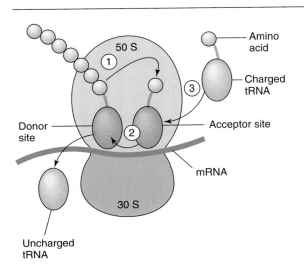

Figure 44–2. Steps in protein synthesis and sites of action of (1) chloramphenicol, (2) macrolides and clindamycin, and (3) tetracyclines. The 70 S ribosomal mRNA complex is shown with its 50 S and 30 S subunits. The peptidyl tRNA at the donor site donates the growing peptide chain to the aminoacyl tRNA at the acceptor site in a reaction catalyzed by peptidyl transferase. The tRNA, discharged of its peptide, is released from the donor site to make way for translocation of the newly formed peptidyl tRNA. The acceptor site is then free to be occupied by the next "charged" aminoacyl tRNA. See text for additional details. (Reproduced, with permission, from Katzung BG [editor]: *Basic & Clinical Pharmacology,* 7th ed. Appleton & Lange, 1998.)

B. **Antimicrobial Activity:**   Chloramphenicol has a wide spectrum of antimicrobial activity and is usually bacteriostatic. Some strains of *H influenzae, N meningitidis,* and *Bacteroides* are highly susceptible, and for these organisms chloramphenicol may be bactericidal. It is not active against *Chlamydia.* Resistance to chloramphenicol, which is plasmid-mediated, occurs through the formation of acetyltransferases that inactivate the drug.

C. **Clinical Uses:**   Because of its toxicity, chloramphenicol has very few uses as a systemic drug. It is a backup drug for severe infections caused by *Salmonella* and for the treatment of pneumococcal and meningococcal meningitis in beta-lactam-sensitive persons. Some *H influenzae* strains are resistant to chloramphenicol, and ceftriaxone or another third-generation cephalosporin is usually preferred. Chloramphenicol is sometimes used for rickettsial diseases and for infections caused by anaerobes such as *Bacteroides fragilis.* The drug is commonly used as a topical antimicrobial agent.

D. **Toxicity:**
   1. **Gastrointestinal disturbances:**   These may occur from direct irritation and from superinfections, especially candidiasis.
   2. **Bone marrow:**   Inhibition of red cell maturation leads to a decrease in circulating red cells. This action is dose-dependent and reversible.
   3. **Aplastic anemia:**   This is a rare (approximately one case in 25,000–40,000 patients treated) idiosyncratic reaction. It is usually irreversible and may be fatal.
   4. **Gray baby syndrome:**   This syndrome occurs in infants and is characterized by cyanosis and cardiovascular collapse. Neonates—especially premature neonates—are deficient in hepatic glucuronosyltransferase, the enzyme required for chloramphenicol elimination. They are therefore very sensitive to doses of the drug that would be tolerated in older infants.
   5. **Drug interactions:**   Chloramphenicol inhibits the metabolism of several drugs, including phenytoin, coumarins, and tolbutamide.

TETRACYCLINES

A. **Classification:**   Drugs in this class are structural congeners that have a broad range of antimicrobial activity and only minor differences in their activities against specific organisms.

B. **Pharmacokinetics:**   Oral absorption is variable, especially for the older drugs, and may be impaired by foods and multivalent cations (calcium, iron, aluminum). These drugs have a wide tissue distribution and cross mammalian cell membranes. They cross the placental barrier, but CNS penetration is limited. All of the tetracyclines undergo enterohepatic cycling. Doxycycline is excreted mainly in feces; the other drugs are eliminated primarily in the urine. The half-lives of doxycycline and minocycline are longer than those of other tetracyclines.

C. **Antibacterial Activity:**   Tetracyclines are broad-spectrum antibiotics with activity against gram-positive and gram-negative bacteria, rickettsiae, chlamydiae, mycoplasmas, and some protozoa. Susceptible organisms accumulate tetracyclines intracellularly via energy-dependent transport systems in their cell membranes.

   Plasmid-mediated resistance to tetracyclines is widespread. Tetracycline-resistant organisms show decreased intracellular accumulation of the drugs. Resistance mechanisms include decreased activity of the uptake systems and the development of mechanisms (efflux pumps) for active extrusion of tetracyclines. Plasmids that include genes involved in the production of efflux pumps for tetracyclines commonly include resistance genes for multiple antibiotics.

D. **Clinical Uses:**
   1. **Primary uses:**   Tetracyclines are the drugs of first choice in the treatment of infections caused by *Mycoplasma pneumoniae* (in adults), chlamydiae, rickettsiae, and vibrios.
   2. **Secondary uses:**   Tetracyclines are alternative drugs in the treatment of syphilis. They are also used in the treatment of respiratory infections caused by susceptible organisms, for prophylaxis against infection in chronic bronchitis, in the treatment of leptospirosis, and in the treatment of acne.

3. **Selective uses:** Specific tetracyclines are used in the treatment of gastrointestinal ulcers caused by *Helicobacter pylori* (tetracycline), in Lyme disease (doxycycline), and in the meningococcal carrier state (minocycline). Doxycycline is also used for the prevention of malaria and the treatment of amebiasis (Chapter 53). Demeclocycline inhibits the renal actions of ADH and is used in the management of patients with ADH-secreting tumors (Chapter 15).

E. **Toxicity:**
1. **Gastrointestinal disturbances:** Effects on the gastrointestinal system range from mild nausea and diarrhea to severe, possibly life-threatening colitis. Disturbances in the normal flora lead to candidiasis (oral and vaginal) and, more rarely, to bacterial superinfections with *Staphylococcus aureus* or *Clostridium difficile*.
2. **Bony structures and teeth:** Fetal exposure to tetracyclines may lead to tooth enamel dysplasia and irregularities in bone growth. Treatment of younger children may cause enamel dysplasia and crown deformations when permanent teeth appear.
3. **Hepatic toxicity:** High doses of tetracyclines, especially in pregnant patients or in patients with preexisting hepatic disease, may impair liver function and lead to hepatic necrosis.
4. **Renal toxicity:** One form of renal tubular acidosis, Fanconi's syndrome, has been attributed to use of outdated tetracyclines. Though not directly nephrotoxic, tetracyclines may exacerbate preexisting renal dysfunction.
5. **Photosensitivity:** Tetracyclines—especially demeclocycline—may cause enhanced skin sensitivity to ultraviolet light.
6. **Vestibular toxicity:** Dose-dependent, reversible dizziness, and vertigo have been noted with minocycline.

MACROLIDES

A. **Classification and Pharmacokinetics:** The macrolide antibiotics (**erythromycin, azithromycin,** and **clarithromycin**) are large cyclic lactone-ring structures with attached sugars. The drugs have good oral bioavailability, but azithromycin absorption is impeded by food. Macrolides distribute to most body tissues, but azithromycin is unique in that the levels achieved in tissues and in phagocytes are considerably higher (10- to 100-fold) than those in the plasma. The elimination of erythromycin (via biliary excretion) and clarithromycin (via hepatic metabolism and urinary excretion of intact drug) is fairly rapid (half-life 2–5 hours). Azithromycin is eliminated slowly (half-life 2–4 days), mainly in the urine as unchanged drug.

B. **Antibacterial Activity:** Erythromycin has activity against many species of *Campylobacter, Chlamydia, Mycoplasma, Legionella,* gram-positive cocci, and some gram-negative organisms. The spectrums of activity of azithromycin and clarithromycin are similar but include greater activity against *Chlamydia, Mycobacterium avium* complex, and *Toxoplasma.*

Resistance to the macrolides in gram-positive organisms involves production of a methylase that adds a methyl group to the ribosomal binding site. Resistance in gram-negative rods is the result of formation of drug-metabolizing esterases. Cross-resistance between the individual macrolides is complete.

C. **Clinical Uses:** Erythromycin is effective in the treatment of infections caused by *Mycoplasma pneumoniae, Corynebacterium, Chlamydia trachomatis, Legionella pneumophila, Ureaplasma urealyticum,* and *Bordetella pertussis.* The drug is also active against gram-positive cocci including pneumococci and beta-lactamase-producing staphylococci (but not methicillin-resistant strains).

Azithromycin has a similar spectrum of activity but is more active against *H influenzae, M catarrhalis,* and *Neisseria.* Because of its long half-life, a single dose of azithromycin is effective in the treatment of urogenital infections due to *C trachomatis,* and a 4-day course of treatment is effective in community-acquired pneumonia.

Clarithromycin is currently approved for prophylaxis against and treatment of *M avium* complex and as a component of drug regimens for ulcers due to *H pylori.*

D. **Toxicity:** Adverse effects include gastrointestinal irritation (common), skin rashes, and eosinophilia. A hypersensitivity-based acute cholestatic hepatitis may occur with erythromycin estolate, but this is rare in children. Erythromycin inhibits several forms of hepatic cytochrome P450 and can increase the plasma levels of anticoagulants, astemizole, carbamazepine, cisapride, digoxin, terfenadine, and theophylline. Cardiac arrhythmias have occurred when erythromycin is administered to patients taking astemizole or terfenadine. Similar drug interactions have also occurred with clarithromycin. The lactone ring structure of azithromycin is slightly different from that of other macrolides, and drug interactions are uncommon since azithromycin does not inhibit hepatic cytochrome P450.

CLINDAMYCIN

A. **Classification and Pharmacokinetics:** The lincosamides, **lincomycin** and **clindamycin,** inhibit bacterial protein synthesis via a mechanism similar to that of the macrolides, though they are not chemically related. Mechanisms of resistance include methylation of the binding site on the 50 S ribosomal subunit and enzymatic inactivation. Cross-resistance between lincosamides and macrolides is common. Good tissue penetration occurs after oral absorption. The lincosamides are eliminated partly by metabolism and partly by biliary and renal excretion.

B. **Clinical Use and Toxicity:** The main use of clindamycin is in the treatment of severe infections due to certain anaerobes such as *Bacteroides.* Clindamycin has been used as a backup drug against gram-positive cocci and is currently recommended for prophylaxis of endocarditis in patients with valvular disease patients who are penicillin-allergic. The drug is also active against *Pneumocystis carinii* and *Toxoplasma gondii.* The toxicity of clindamycin includes gastrointestinal irritation, skin rashes, neutropenia, hepatic dysfunction, and possible superinfections such as *C difficile* pseudomembranous colitis.

DRUG LIST

The following drugs are important members of the group discussed in this chapter. Prototypes should be learned in detail; features of the major variants should be known well enough so that the variants can be distinguished from prototypes and from each other; the other significant agents should be recognized as belonging to a specific subclass.

Subclass	Prototype	Major Variants	Other Significant Agents
Chloramphenicol	Chloramphenicol		
Tetracyclines	Tetracycline	Demeclocycline	Doxycycline, minocycline
Macrolides	Erythromycin	Azithromycin	Clarithromycin
Lincosamides	Lincomycin	Clindamycin	

QUESTIONS

DIRECTIONS: Each of the numbered items or incomplete statements in this section is followed by answers or by completions of the statement. Select the ONE lettered answer or completion that is BEST in each case.

1. A 2-year-old child is brought to the hospital after ingesting pills a parent had used for bacterial dysentery when traveling outside the United States. The child has been vomiting for over 24 hours and has had diarrhea with green stools. He is now lethargic, with an ashen skin color. Other signs and symptoms include hypothermia, hypotension, and abdominal distention. The drug most likely to be the cause of this problem is
   (A) Ampicillin
   (B) Chloramphenicol

    (C) Clindamycin

    (D) Doxycycline

    (E) Erythromycin

2. The mechanism of antibacterial action of tetracyclines involves

    (A) Binding to a component of the 50 S ribosomal subunit

    (B) Inhibition of translocase activity

    (C) Blockade of binding of aminoacyl-tRNA to bacterial ribosomes

    (D) Selective inhibition of ribosomal peptidyl transferases

    (E) Inhibition of DNA-dependent RNA polymerase

3. A 24-year-old woman has primary syphilis. She has a history of penicillin hypersensitivity, so tetracycline will be used to treat the infection. Which one of the following statements about the proposed drug treatment of this patient is LEAST accurate?

    (A) She will have to take the drug for 15 days

    (B) She should avoid the consumption of milk products at the same time as she takes the drug

    (C) She may experience anorexia and gastrointestinal distress

    (D) She should eat plenty of yogurt to prevent vaginal candidiasis

    (E) She should call her physician if she develops severe diarrhea

4. Clarithromycin and erythromycin have very similar spectrums of antimicrobial activity. The major advantage of clarithromycin is that it

    (A) Eradicates mycoplasmal infections in a single dose

    (B) Is active against strains of streptococci that are resistant to erythromycin

    (C) Is more active against *M avium* complex

    (D) Does not inhibit liver drug-metabolizing enzymes

    (E) Acts on methicillin-resistant strains of staphylococci

5. The primary mechanism underlying the resistance of gram-positive organisms to macrolide antibiotics is

    (A) Methylation of binding sites on the 50 S ribosomal subunit

    (B) Formation of esterases that hydrolyze the lactone ring

    (C) Increased activity of efflux mechanisms

    (D) Formation of drug-inactivating acetyltransferases

    (E) Decreased drug permeability of the cytoplasmic membrane

6. A 26-year-old woman allergic to beta-lactams was treated for gonorrhea at a neighborhood clinic. A single intramuscular injection of spectinomycin was administered, and she was given a prescription for oral doxycycline for 7 days. Two weeks later, she returns to the clinic with a mucopurulent cervicitis. On questioning, she admits that she did not have the prescription filled because she had no money. The best course of action at this point would be to

    (A) Give her the money for the prescription

    (B) Treat her with a single oral dose of cefixime

    (C) Write a prescription for oral erythromycin for 7 days

    (D) Treat her with a single oral dose of azithromycin

    (E) Delay drug treatment until the infecting organism is identified

7. A 55-year-old patient with a prosthetic heart valve is to undergo a periodontal procedure involving scaling and root planing. Several years ago, the patient had a severe allergic reaction when given procaine penicillin G. Regarding prophylaxis against bacterial endocarditis, which one of the following is most appropriate?

    (A) No prophylaxis is needed, since this patient is in the negligible risk category

    (B) Give 600 mg of clindamycin orally 1 hour before the procedure

    (C) Give 500 mg of erythromycin orally 1 hour before the procedure and at 4 hours after the procedure

    (D) Administer intravenous vancomycin prior to the procedure

    (E) Give 2 grams of amoxicillin orally 1 hour before the procedure

Items 8–10: A 24-year-old accountant comes to a clinic with complaints of a dry cough, headache, fever, and malaise which have lasted 3 or 4 days. The patient appears to have some respiratory difficulty, and chest examination reveals rales but no other obvious signs of pulmonary involvement. However, extensive patchy infiltrates are seen on a chest x-ray. A Gram-stained smear of expectorated sputum fails to reveal any bacterial pathogens. The patient informs the attending physician that her husband is not sick but that one of her colleagues at work has symptoms similar to those she is experiencing. The patient has no history of serious medical problems. She and her husband have no children and want to start a family when he finishes graduate school. The patient is taking loratadine for allergies, multivitamins, and supplementary iron tablets. She is an avid consumer of coffee and caffeinated beverages. The physician makes an initial diagnosis of community-acquired pneumonia.

8. Regarding the drug management of this patient, which one of the following statements is most accurate?
   (A) No antibiotics should be given since this patient has a viral pneumonia
   (B) A single oral dose of clindamycin is indicated
   (C) Amoxicillin should be given for 7 days
   (D) She should be treated with erythromycin for 14 days
   (E) A 7-day course of cefaclor is the best choice in this case

9. If this patient is treated with the macrolide, she should
   (A) Temporarily discontinue the antihistamine to prevent cardiotoxicity
   (B) Avoid exposure to sunlight
   (C) Cut down her consumption of caffeinated beverages
   (D) Avoid taking supplementary iron tablets
   (E) Have her BUN or plasma creatinine checked prior to treatment

10. This patient is not an ideal candidate for treatment with tetracycline hydrochloride because
    (A) It may cause vaginal candidiasis
    (B) Her pulmonary infection may be due to pneumococci
    (C) Tetracyclines inhibit hepatic cytochrome P450
    (D) Tetracycline has no activity against *M pneumoniae*
    (E) The drug causes a high incidence of vestibular dysfunction

DIRECTIONS (Items 11–15): Each set of matching questions in this section consists of a list of three to twenty-six lettered options (some of which may be figures) followed by several numbered items. For each numbered item, select the ONE lettered option that is most closely associated with it. Each lettered option may be selected once, more than once, or not at all.

   (A) Azithromycin
   (B) Chloramphenicol
   (C) Clarithromycin
   (D) Clindamycin
   (E) Demeclocycline
   (F) Doxycycline
   (G) Erythromycin
   (H) Minocycline
   (I) Streptomycin
   (J) Tetracycline
   (K) Ticarcillin

11. The appearance of markedly vacuolated, nucleated red cells in the marrow, anemia, and reticulocytopenia is a characteristic dose-dependent side effect of this drug

12. This antibiotic has been used as a backup drug to vancomycin in the treatment of infections caused by methicillin-resistant staphylococci

13. This drug is prophylactic against traveler's diarrhea and has been used in triple-drug regimens for treatment of gastrointestinal ulcers associated with *Helicobacter pylori*. Decreases in renal function have little effect on the rate of its elimination, and its long plasma half-life permits once-daily dosing

14. In addition to its antibacterial actions, this drug has ADH-inhibiting effects. It has caused photosensitivity

15. This inhibitor of bacterial protein synthesis has a narrow spectrum of antibacterial activity. It is useful in the management of abdominal abscess thought to be due to *Bacteroides fragilis*

ANSWERS

1. Although the gray baby syndrome was initially described in neonates, a similar syndrome has occurred with overdosage of chloramphenicol in older children and adults, especially those with hepatic dysfunction. The answer is **(B)**.

2. Tetracyclines inhibit bacterial protein synthesis by interfering with the binding of aminoacyl-tRNA molecules to bacterial ribosomes. Peptidyl transferase is inhibited by chloramphenicol. The answer is **(C)**.

3. The ingestion of foods containing multivalent cations (yogurt contains calcium and magnesium) can interfere with gastrointestinal absorption of tetracyclines and impair their clinical efficacy. The answer is **(D)**.

4. Clarithromycin can be administered less frequently than erythromycin, but it is not effective in single doses against susceptible organisms. Organisms resistant to erythromycin, including pneumococci and methicillin-resistant staphylococci, are also resistant to other macrolides. Drug interactions have occurred with clarithromycin through its ability to inhibit cytochrome P450. Clarithromycin is more active than erythromycin against *M avium* complex, *T gondii,* and *H pylori.* The answer is **(C)**.

5. Methylase production and methylation of the receptor site accounts for the resistance of gram-positive organisms to macrolide antibiotics. Such enzymes may be inducible by macrolides or constitutive; in the latter case, cross-resistance occurs between macrolides and clindamycin. Esterase formation is a mechanism of macrolide resistance seen in coliforms. Resistance to tetracyclines occurs either from increased activity of efflux mechanisms or changes in cell membrane permeability, leading to decreases in intracellular levels of such drugs. Resistance to chloramphenicol involves plasmid-mediated formation of a drug-inactivating acetyltransferase. The answer is **(A)**.

6. Cervicitis or urethritis that appears 2–3 weeks after treatment of gonorrhea is often caused by *C trachomatis.* Such infections may have been acquired at the same time as gonorrhea but develop more slowly owing to the long incubation period of chlamydial infection. Treatment with oral doxycycline for 7 days would have eradicated *C trachomatis* and most other organisms commonly associated with nongonococcal cervicitis or urethritis. Given the uncertain compliance of this patient, the best course of action would be the administration (in the clinic) of a single oral dose of azithromycin. In addition, she should encourage her sexual partner to come to the clinic for treatment. The answer is **(D)**.

7. This patient is in the high-risk category for bacterial endocarditis and should receive prophylactic antibiotics prior to many dental procedures, including root planing and extractions. The American Heart Association now recommends that clindamycin be used in patients allergic to penicillins. Oral erythromycin is not recommended, since it is no more effective than clindamycin and causes more gastrointestinal side effects. Intravenous vancomycin, sometimes with gentamicin, is recommended for prophylaxis in high-risk penicillin-allergic patients undergoing genitourinary and lower gastrointestinal surgical procedures. Complete cross-allergenicity must be assumed between individual penicillins. The answer is **(B)**.

8. It is often difficult to establish a definite microbial etiology of pneumonia. The most common pathogens involved in community-acquired pneumonia in otherwise healthy young adults are *Streptococcus pneumoniae, Mycoplasma pneumoniae,* respiratory viruses, and *Chlamydiae pneumoniae.* Empiric antibiotic therapy is initiated in most cases because the physical signs and a Gram-stained smear of sputum do not often indicate a specific etiologic agent. Gradual onset of the condition, with many extrapulmonary symptoms, may be indicative of atypical pneumonia but does not rule out bacterial pneumonia. Erythromycin would provide coverage for both pneumococcal and atypical pathogens (not viral) and should be given for 10–14 days. None of the other antibiotics listed are active against *Chlamydia* or *Mycoplasma.* The answer is **(D)**.

9. The inhibition of liver cytochrome P450 by erythromycin has led to serious drug interactions. Inhibition of the CYP3A4 isoform of the enzyme has resulted in cardiac arrhythmias with the nonsedating antihistamines astemizole and terfenadine but not with loratadine. However, erythromycin also inhibits the CYP1A2 form of cytochrome P450, which metabolizes methylxanthines. Consequently, cardiac and central nervous system toxicity may occur with excessive ingestion of caffeine. Unlike the tetracyclines, the oral absorption of erythromycin is not affected by cations and the drug does not cause photosensitivity. Since erythromycin undergoes biliary excretion there is little reason to assess renal function prior to treatment. The answer is **(C)**.

10. Tetracyclines have activity against both chlamydial and mycoplasmal pathogens involved in community-acquired pneumonia. However, their widespread use for minor infections has led to emergence of resistant strains of gram-positive cocci, including *Streptococcus pneumoniae.* Consequently, tetracycline does not provide antibacterial coverage equivalent to that of erythromycin when used empirically in pneumonia. Alterations in normal flora caused by tetracy-

clines may lead to oral or vaginal candidiasis, but this is not the primary reason why erythromycin is the treatment of choice. The tetracyclines do not inhibit liver drug-metabolizing enzymes. Minocycline causes vestibular dysfunction. Loss of balance, dizziness, nausea, and tinnitus may occur in up to 70% of patients receiving this drug for meningococcal prophylaxis. The answer is **(B)**.

11. Reversible, dose-dependent bone marrow maturation arrest occurs with chloramphenicol. Serum iron concentration increases and blood levels of phenylalanine decrease. These actions are unrelated to the rare occurrence of aplastic anemia. The answer is **(B)**.

12. Minocycline is the only inhibitor of bacterial protein synthesis with significant activity against methicillin-resistant *S aureus.* The answer is **(H)**.

13. Doxycycline offers a number of pharmacologic advantages over conventional tetracyclines. It has good bioavailability, effective tissue penetration, and a long half-life. Doxycycline is also more effective against pathogens associated with acute exacerbations of chronic bronchitis (pneumococci, *H influenzae, M catarrhalis*) and has better activity in Lyme disease than other tetracyclines. The answer is **(F)**.

14. Photosensitivity reactions can occur with any tetracycline but appear to be more common with demeclocycline. Photosensitivity has also been reported for azithromycin. The answer is **(E)**.

15. Of the drugs listed, only chloramphenicol, clindamycin, and ticarcillin (with clavulanic acid) are reliably active against *B fragilis.* Chloramphenicol is a broad-spectrum antibiotic, and ticarcillin inhibits bacterial cell wall synthesis. The answer is **(D)**.

45

Aminoglycosides

OBJECTIVES

You should be able to:

- Describe the mechanisms of action of aminoglycoside antibiotics and the mechanisms by which bacterial resistance to this class of drugs occurs.
- List the major clinical applications of aminoglycosides and describe their main toxic effects.
- Describe the pharmacokinetics of this drug class, with special reference to the importance of renal clearance and its relationship to toxicity.
- Understand the concepts of time-dependent and concentration-dependent killing actions of antibiotics and know what is meant by postantibiotic effect (PAE).

CONCEPTS

A. Modes of Antibacterial Action: In the treatment of microbial infections with antibiotics, multiple daily dosage regimens traditionally have been designed to maintain serum concentrations above the minimal inhibitory concentration (MIC) for as long as possible. However, the in vivo effectiveness of some antibiotics, including aminoglycosides, results from a **concentration-dependent** killing action. As the plasma level is increased above the MIC, aminoglycosides kill an increasing proportion of bacteria and do so at a more rapid rate. Other antibiotics, including penicillins and cephalosporins, cause **time-dependent** killing of microorganisms, wherein their in vivo efficacy is directly related to time of exposure above MIC and becomes independent of concentration once the MIC has been reached.

Aminoglycosides are also capable of exerting a **postantibiotic effect (PAE)** such that their killing action continues when their plasma levels have declined below measurable levels. Consequently, aminoglycosides have greater efficacy when administered as a few large daily doses than when given as multiple smaller doses. The toxicity of aminoglycosides (in contrast to their antibacterial efficacy) depends both on a critical plasma concentration and on the time during which such a level is exceeded. The time above such a threshold will be shorter with administration of a single large dose of an aminoglycoside than when multiple smaller doses are given. These concepts form the basis for the recently introduced **once-daily dosing protocol** for aminoglycosides, which can be more effective and less toxic than traditional dosing regimens.

B. Classification: The drugs in this class are structurally related amino sugars attached by glycosidic linkages. The main differences among the individual drugs lie in their activities against specific organisms, particularly gram-negative rods.

C. Pharmacokinetics: Aminoglycosides are polar compounds and are not absorbed after oral administration. They must be given parenterally for systemic effect and have limited tissue penetration. Aminoglycosides are not significantly metabolized by the patient (but bacteria may inactivate them). Glomerular filtration is the major mode of excretion, and plasma levels of these drugs are greatly affected by changes in renal function. Excretion of aminoglycosides is directly proportionate to creatinine clearance. Dosage adjustments must be made in renal insufficiency to avoid toxic accumulation of aminoglycosides. Monitoring of plasma levels of aminoglycosides is an important requirement for safe and effective dosage selection and adjustment. For traditional dosing regimens (two or three times daily), peak serum levels are measured 30–60 minutes after administration and trough levels just before the next dose. Note, however, that once-daily dosing is now recommended for many infections (see above).

D. Mechanism of Action: Aminoglycosides are bactericidal inhibitors of protein synthesis. Their penetration through the bacterial cell envelope is partly a function of oxygen-dependent active transport, and they have little activity against strict anaerobes. Aminoglycoside transport can be enhanced by cell wall synthesis inhibitors, which may be the basis of antimicrobial synergism. Inside the cell, streptomycin (the best-studied aminoglycoside) binds to the 30 S ribosomal subunit and interferes with protein synthesis in three ways: (1) it blocks formation of the initiation complex, which prevents the latter's transition to a chain-elongating functional ribosomal complex; (2) it causes misreading of the code on the mRNA template, which causes miscoding of amino acids in the peptide; and (3) it disrupts polysomes (mRNA with multiple ribosomes on it), resulting in nonfunctional monosomes (Figure 45–1). Other aminoglycosides have a similar but not identical mechanism of action.

E. Mechanism of Resistance: The primary mechanism of resistance to aminoglycosides at the clinical level involves the plasmid-mediated formation of inactivating enzymes. These enzymes are **group transferases** that catalyze the acetylation of amine functions and the transfer of phosphoryl or adenylyl groups to the oxygen atoms of hydroxyl groups on the aminoglycoside. Individual aminoglycosides have varying susceptibilities to such enzymes. Currently, **netilmicin** is susceptible to only a few such enzymes, and this drug may be active against more strains of organisms than other aminoglycosides.

F. Clinical Uses:
   1. **Primary uses:** Three aminoglycosides (gentamicin, tobramycin, amikacin) are important drugs for the treatment of serious infections caused by aerobic gram-negative bacteria, including *E coli* as well as *Enterobacter, Klebsiella, Proteus, Pseudomonas,* and *Serratia* species (Table 45–1). Drug choice depends on susceptibility patterns. Antibacterial synergy may occur when aminoglycosides are used in combination with beta-lactam antibiotics. Examples include their combined use in the treatment of serious pseudomonal and enterococcal infections.
   2. **Other indications:**
      a. **Streptomycin:** Streptomycin is used in the treatment of tuberculosis, plague, and tularemia. Because of the risk of ototoxicity, streptomycin should not be used when other drugs will serve.
      b. **Neomycin:** Owing to its toxic potential, neomycin is only used topically or locally, eg, in the gastrointestinal tract.
      c. **Netilmicin:** Netilmycin is usually reserved for treatment of serious infections caused by organisms resistant to the other aminoglycosides.
      d. **Spectinomycin:** Spectinomycin is an aminocyclitol related to the aminoglycosides. It is a backup drug for the treatment of gonorrhea.

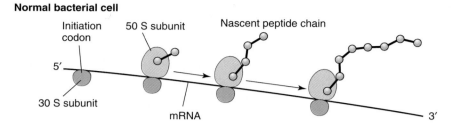

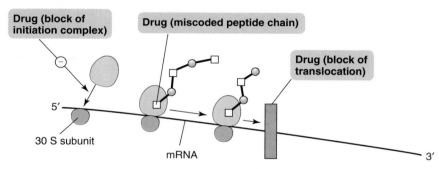

Figure 45–1. Putative mechanisms of action of the aminoglycosides. Normal protein synthesis is shown in the top panel. At least three different aminoglycoside effects have been described as shown in the bottom panel: block of formation of the initiation complex; miscoding of amino acids in the emerging peptide chain due to misreading of the mRNA; and block of translocation on mRNA. Block of movement of the ribosome may occur after the formation of a single initiation complex, resulting in an mRNA chain with only a single ribosome on it, a so-called monosome.

G. **Toxicity:**
   1. **Ototoxicity:** Auditory or vestibular nerve damage (or both) may occur with any amino-glycoside and may be irreversible. Ototoxicity risk is proportionate to the plasma levels and thus is especially high if dosage is not appropriately modified in a patient with renal dysfunction. Ototoxicity may be increased by the use of loop diuretics.
   2. **Nephrotoxicity:** Renal toxicity usually takes the form of acute tubular necrosis. This adverse effect, which is often reversible, is more common in elderly patients and in those concurrently receiving amphotericin B, cephalosporins, or vancomycin.
   3. **Neuromuscular blockade:** Though rare, a curare-like block may occur at high doses of aminoglycosides and may result in respiratory paralysis. It is usually reversible by treatment with calcium and neostigmine, but ventilatory support may be required.
   4. **Skin reactions:** Allergic skin reactions may occur in patients, and contact dermatitis may occur in personnel handling the drug. Of the aminoglycosides, neomycin is the most likely to cause this adverse effect.

Table 45–1. Clinical applications of the aminoglycosides.

Drug	Application
Gentamicin, amikacin, tobramycin, netilmicin	Serious infections with aerobic gram-negative bacteria, including *E coli*, *Enterobacter*, *Klebsiella*, *Proteus*, *Pseudomonas*, and *Serratia*
Streptomycin	Tuberculosis; rarely plague, brucellosis, tularemia, and infective endocarditis
Neomycin, kanamycin	Bowel sterilization, skin infections
Spectinomycin	Gonorrhea

DRUG LIST

The following drugs are important members of the group discussed in this chapter. Prototypes should be learned in detail; features of the major variants should be known well enough so that the variants can be distinguished from prototypes and from each other; the other significant agents should be recognized as belonging to a specific subclass.

Subclass	Prototype	Major Variants	Other Significant Agents
Aminoglycosides Systemic	Gentamicin	Tobramycin	Amikacin, netilmicin, streptomycin
Local	Neomycin		Gentamicin, kanamycin
Aminocyclitols	Spectinomycin		

QUESTIONS

DIRECTIONS: Each of the numbered items or incomplete statements in this section is followed by answers or by completions of the statement. Select the ONE lettered answer or completion that is BEST in each case.

1. Which one of the following statements about the mechanism of action of aminoglycosides is LEAST accurate?
   (A) They induce misreading of the code on the mRNA template
   (B) They promote polysome instability
   (C) They inhibit peptidyl transferase
   (D) They block the formation of the initiation complex
   (E) They are bactericidal inhibitors of protein synthesis

2. A 70-kg patient with creatinine clearance of over 90 mL/min has a gram-negative infection. Amikacin is administered intramuscularly at a dosage of 5 mg/kg every 8 hours, and the patient begins to respond. After 2 days, creatinine clearance declines to 30 mL/min. Assuming that no information is available about amikacin plasma levels, what would be the most reasonable approach to management of the patient at this point?
   (A) Decrease daily dose to a total of 100 mg
   (B) Decrease the dosage to 120 mg every 8 hours
   (C) Maintain the patient on the present dosage and test auditory function
   (D) Administer 5 mg/kg every 12 hours
   (E) Discontinue amikacin and switch to gentamicin

3. Which one of the following statements about the clinical uses of the aminoglycosides is LEAST accurate?
   (A) Owing to their polar nature, aminoglycosides are not absorbed following oral administration
   (B) Aminoglycosides are often used in combination with cephalosporins in the empiric treatment of life-threatening bacterial infections
   (C) Netilmycin is more likely than streptomycin to be effective in the treatment of a hospital-acquired infection caused by *Serratia marcescens*
   (D) The spectrum of antimicrobial activity of aminoglycosides includes *Bacteroides fragilis*
   (E) Gentamicin is used with ampicillin for synergistic effects in the treatment of enterococcal endocarditis

4. Which one of the following statements about bacterial resistance to aminoglycosides is most accurate?
   (A) Resistance is due to the production of peptidyltransferases
   (B) Bacteria resistant to aminoglycosides have characteristic alterations in the pathway of folic acid synthesis
   (C) Emergence of resistance during the course of drug treatment is common
   (D) Clinical resistance occurs mainly through plasmid-mediated formation of group transferase enzymes
   (E) Methicillin-resistant staphylococci are usually sensitive to aminoglycosides

5. Which one of the following antibiotics is likely to be the most effective agent in the treatment of an infection due to enterococci if used in conjunction with penicillin G?
   (A) Amikacin
   (B) Gentamicin
   (C) Netilmicin
   (D) Streptomycin
   (E) Tobramycin

6. Regarding the antibacterial action of gentamicin, which one of the following statements is most accurate?
   (A) Efficacy is directly proportionate to the time the plasma level of the drug is greater than the minimal inhibitory concentration
   (B) The antibacterial action of gentamicin is not concentration-dependent
   (C) Gentamicin continues to exert antibacterial effects even after plasma levels decrease below detectable levels
   (D) Antibacterial activity is often reduced by the presence of an inhibitor of cell wall synthesis
   (E) The antibacterial action of gentamicin is time-dependent

7. An adult patient (weight 70 kg) has bacteremia suspected to be due to a gram-negative rod. Tobramycin is to be administered using a once-daily dosing regimen, and the loading dose must be calculated to achieve a peak plasma level of 20 mg/L. Assume the patient has normal renal function. Pharmacokinetic parameters of tobramycin in this patient are: $V_d = 20$ L; $t_{1/2} = 3$h; and CL = 80 mL/min. What loading dose should be given?
   (A) 100 mg
   (B) 200 mg
   (C) 300 mg
   (D) 400 mg
   (E) 800 mg

8. Which one of the following drugs is most likely to be effective against multidrug-resistant strains of *M tuberculosis,* including those resistant to streptomycin?
   (A) Amikacin
   (B) Clarithromycin
   (C) Gentamicin
   (D) Meropenem
   (E) Spectinomycin

9. A 57-year-old man is seen in a hospital emergency room complaining of pain in and behind the right ear. Physical examination shows edema of the external otic canal with purulent exudate and weakness of the muscles on the right side of the face. There are no obvious signs of systemic infection. The patient informs the physician that he is a diabetic, taking glipizide daily but no insulin. He is also taking a "baby" aspirin daily but no other drugs. A Gram-stained smear of the exudate from the ear shows many polymorphonucleocytes and gram-negative rods. Samples of the exudate are sent to the microbiology laboratory for culture and drug susceptibility testing. A preliminary diagnosis is made of external otitis. At this point, which of the following is most appropriate?
   (A) Analgesics should be prescribed for pain, but antibiotics should be withheld pending the results of lab cultures
   (B) The patient should be sent home with a prescription for oral cefaclor
   (C) The patient should be hospitalized and treatment with gentamicin plus ticarcillin started
   (D) The patient should be hospitalized and treatment started with intravenous imipenem-cilastatin
   (E) The patient should be hospitalized and treatment started with spectinomycin

10. Regarding the toxicity of gentamicin, which one of the following statements is most accurate?
    (A) Ototoxicity is reduced if loop diuretics are used to facilitate gentamicin excretion
    (B) Systemic neomycin is usually safer than gentamicin
    (C) Gentamicin is more likely to cause ototoxic effects than renal damage
    (D) With traditional dosage regimens, the earliest sign of nephrotoxicity is a reduced creatinine clearance
    (E) Ototoxicity due to gentamicin is usually irreversible and manifests itself as vestibular dysfunction

DIRECTIONS (Items 11–15): Each set of matching questions in this section consists of a list of three to twenty-six lettered options (some of which may be figures) followed by several numbered items. For each numbered item, select the ONE lettered option that is most closely associated with it. Each lettered option may be selected once, more than once, or not at all.

(A) Amikacin
(B) Ampicillin
(C) Gentamicin
(D) Neomycin
(E) Netilmicin
(F) Penicillin G
(G) Spectinomycin
(H) Streptomycin
(I) Ticarcillin
(J) Tobramycin
(K) Vancomycin

11. The systemic use of this drug has been largely abandoned due to its toxicity. It is still used topically and for its local effects in the gastrointestinal tract

12. This drug is used in the treatment of bubonic plague and tularemia. When administered in combination with other agents in tuberculosis, this drug delays the emergence of resistant mycobacteria

13. This drug has a spectrum of activity and pharmacokinetic properties almost identical to those of gentamicin. However, the drug in question shows poor activity in combination with penicillin against enterococci

14. This drug is the LEAST susceptible of the aminoglycosides to degradation by enzymes produced by resistant bacteria

15. In the empiric treatment of severe bacterial infections of unidentified cause, this drug may be used with an aminoglycoside to provide coverage against resistant staphylococci

ANSWERS

1. Aminoglycosides are bactericidal inhibitors of protein synthesis binding to specific components of the 30 S ribosomal subunit. Their actions include block of the formation of the initiation complex, miscoding, and polysomal breakup. Peptidyl transferase is inhibited by chloramphenicol, not aminoglycosides. The answer is (C).

2. Monitoring plasma drug levels is important when aminoglycosides are used. In this case the patient seems to be improving, so a decrease of the amikacin dose in proportion to decreased creatinine clearance is most appropriate. Since creatinine clearance is only one-third of the starting value, a dose reduction should be made to one-third of that given initially. The answer is (B).

3. The intracellular accumulation of aminoglycoside by bacteria is oxygen-dependent. Anaerobic bacteria are inherently resistant. The answer is (D).

4. Clinical resistance to aminoglycosides results from the formation of drug-metabolizing transferases. The emergence of resistance during drug treatment is rare. Aminoglycosides are not active against staphylococci resistant to methicillin. The answer is (D).

5. When used in combination with penicillin G, streptomycin continues to be a useful agent for treating enterococcal infections. About 15% of enterococcal isolates that are resistant to gentamicin and the other systemic aminoglycosides remain susceptible to streptomycin. The answer is (D).

6. The antibacterial action of aminoglycosides is concentration-dependent rather than time-dependent. The activity of the drug continues to increase as its plasma level rises above the minimal inhibitory concentration (MIC). When the plasma level of gentamicin falls below the MIC, the drug continues to exert antibacterial effects for several hours (postantibiotic effect). Inhibitors of bacterial cell wall synthesis often exert synergistic effects with aminoglycosides, possibly by increasing the intracellular accumulation of the aminoglycoside. The answer is (C).

7. The loading dose of any drug is calculated by multiplying the desired plasma concentration (mg/L) by the volume of distribution (L). The answer is (D).

8. Strains of multidrug-resistant *M tuberculosis* resistant to streptomycin are usually susceptible to amikacin. None of the other drugs listed (including gentamicin) have significant antituberculosis activity. In the treatment of tuberculosis, amikacin and streptomycin are backup drugs and if used are always included in combination regimens with other antituberculosis agents. The answer is (A).

9. The diabetic patient with external otitis is at special risk because of the danger of spread to the middle ear and possibly the meninges, so hospitalization is advisable. Based on the results of the Gram stain, the likely pathogens include *E coli* and *Pseudomonas aeruginosa,* and coverage must be provided for these and perhaps other gram-negative rods. The combination of an aminoglycoside plus a wider spectrum penicillin is most suitable in this case and is synergistic against many *Pseudomonas* strains. Imipenem-cilastatin is also a possible choice, but resistant strains of *Pseudomonas aeruginosa* have emerged during treatment. Cefaclor is used for otitis media in ambulatory patients, but it lacks anti-pseudomonal activity. The answer is (C).

10. The incidence of nephrotoxic effects with gentamicin is two to three times greater than the incidence of ototoxicity. With traditional dosage regimens, the first indication of potential nephrotoxicity is an increase in trough serum levels of aminoglycosides, followed by an increase in blood creatinine. While ototoxicity due to gentamicin usually involves irreversible effects on vestibular function, hearing loss can also occur. Ototoxicity is enhanced by loop diuretics. Neomycin is not used systemically because it is *more* toxic than other aminoglycosides. The answer is (E).

11. When used parenterally, neomycin causes renal damage and ototoxicity. It is used topically and for local actions, including gastrointestinal tract infections, for sterilization prior to bowel surgery, and to reduce ammonia intoxication in hepatic coma. The answer is (D).

12. Streptomycin is not commonly used to treat infections caused by gram-negative rods, since many organisms are resistant. The drug does have special clinical uses, including the treatment of plague, tularemia, and tuberculosis. The answer is (H).

13. Tobramycin is almost identical to gentamicin in both its pharmacodynamic and pharmacokinetic properties. However, it is much less active than either gentamicin or streptomycin when used in combination with a penicillin in the treatment of enterococcal endocarditis. The answer is (J).

14. Chemical substitutions on the ring structure of netilmicin sterically protect the molecule from enzymatic degradation. Thus, netilmicin is not inactivated by as many group transferase enzymes produced by bacteria as other aminoglycosides such as gentamicin and tobramycin. The answer is (E).

15. In most cases involving the empiric use of aminoglycosides, coverage for possible staphylococcal infection would involve combined use with nafcillin or a cephalosporin (neither type of drug is listed). In cases of suspected drug-resistant staphylococci, vancomycin can be used in combination with an aminoglycoside. However, such combinations confer a higher risk of oto- and nephrotoxicity. The answer is (K).

46

Sulfonamides, Trimethoprim, & Fluoroquinolones

OBJECTIVES

You should be able to:

- Describe the mechanisms of antibacterial action of sulfonamides and trimethoprim on bacterial folic acid synthesis and the mechanisms involved in bacterial resistance to the antifolate drugs.
- List the major clinical uses of sulfonamides and trimethoprim, singly and in combination; describe their pharmacokinetic properties and toxic effects.

- Describe the mechanisms of action of the fluoroquinolone antibiotics and the mechanisms involved in bacterial resistance to these agents.
- List the major clinical uses of fluoroquinolones and describe their pharmacokinetic properties and toxic effects.

Learn the definitions that follow.

Table 46–1. Definitions.

Term	Definition
Antimetabolite	A drug that through chemical similarity is able to interfere with the role of an endogenous compound in cellular metabolism. The category includes antibacterial agents that inhibit bacterial folic acid metabolism
Sequential blockade	The combined action of two drugs that inhibit sequential steps in a pathway of bacterial metabolism

CONCEPTS

Sulfonamides and trimethoprim are examples of drugs that act as **antimetabolites.** Having a chemical structure close to that of naturally occurring compounds, they are able to interfere with folic acid synthesis, which is critical to many microorganisms. Sulfonamides (structural congeners of para-aminobenzoic acid) inhibit dihydropteroic acid synthase, an early step in folic acid synthesis. Trimethoprim (an analog of dihydrofolic acid) inhibits the enzyme dihydrofolate reductase, which converts dihydrofolic acid to an active form, tetrahydrofolic acid. The combination of a sulfonamide and trimethoprim causes a sequential blockade of folic acid synthesis, resulting in a bactericidal and synergistic action.

The development of fluoroquinolones in the mid 1980s represented an important advance, since these drugs have a broad spectrum of antimicrobial activity that includes strains of many common pathogens resistant to older antibiotics. Fluoroquinolones have good oral bioavailability and cause few side effects, characteristics that have contributed to their widespread use in the past decade. Unfortunately, the emergence of resistant strains of formerly susceptible organisms is starting to reduce the clinical value of these drugs. Increasing numbers of fluoroquinolone-resistant strains of pneumococci and streptococci now limit the effectiveness of these drugs in infections caused by such common pathogens.

ANTIFOLATE DRUGS

A. Classification and Pharmacokinetics:

1. **Sulfonamides:** The sulfonamides are weakly acidic compounds that have a common chemical nucleus resembling *p*-aminobenzoic acid (PABA). Members of this group differ mainly in their pharmacokinetic properties and clinical uses. Pharmacokinetic features include modest tissue penetration, hepatic metabolism, and excretion of both intact drug and acetylated metabolites in the urine. Solubility may be decreased in acidic urine, resulting in precipitation of the drug or its metabolites. Because of the solubility limitation, a combination of three separate sulfonamides (triple sulfas) has been used to reduce the likelihood that any one drug will precipitate. The sulfonamides may be classified as short-acting (eg, sulfisoxazole), intermediate-acting (eg, sulfamethoxazole), and long-acting (eg, sulfadoxine). Sulfonamides bind to plasma proteins at sites shared by bilirubin and by other drugs.

2. **Trimethoprim:** This drug is structurally similar to folic acid. It is a weak base and is trapped in acidic environments, reaching high concentrations in prostatic and vaginal fluids. (The trapping of a congener, pyrimethamine, is illustrated in Figure 1–1.) A large fraction of trimethoprim is excreted unchanged in the urine. The half-life of this drug is similar to that of sulfamethoxazole (10–12 hours).

B. Mechanisms of Action:
   1. **Sulfonamides:** The sulfonamide drugs are bacteriostatic inhibitors of folic acid synthesis. As antimetabolites of PABA, they are competitive inhibitors of dihydropteroate synthase (Figure 46–1). They can also act as substrates for this enzyme, resulting in the synthesis of nonfunctional forms of folic acid. The selective toxicity of sulfonamides results from the inability of mammalian cells to synthesize folic acid; they must use preformed folic acid that is present in the diet.
   2. **Trimethoprim:** Trimethoprim is a selective inhibitor of bacterial dihydrofolate reductase that prevents the formation of the active tetrahydro form of folic acid (Figure 46–1). Bacterial dihydrofolate reductase is four to five orders of magnitude more sensitive than the mammalian enzyme to inhibition by trimethoprim.
   3. **Trimethoprim plus sulfamethoxazole:** When the two drugs are used in combination, antimicrobial synergy results from the **sequential blockade** of folate synthesis (Figure 46–1). The drug combination is bactericidal against susceptible organisms.

C. Resistance: Bacterial resistance to sulfonamides is common and may be plasmid-mediated. It can result from decreased intracellular accumulation of the drugs, increased production of PABA by bacteria, or a decrease in the sensitivity of dihydropteroate synthase to the sulfonamides. Clinical resistance to trimethoprim most commonly results from the production of dihydrofolate reductase that has a reduced affinity for the drug.

D. Clinical Uses:
   1. **Sulfonamides:** The sulfonamides are active against a wide range of gram-positive and gram-negative organisms, *Chlamydia,* and *Nocardia.* Specific members of the sulfonamide group are used by the following routes for the conditions indicated:
      a. **Simple urinary tract infections:** Oral (eg, triple sulfas, sulfisoxazole).
      b. **Ocular infections:** Topical (eg, sulfacetamide).
      c. **Burn infections:** Topical (eg, mafenide, silver sulfadiazine).
      d. **Ulcerative colitis:** Oral (eg, sulfasalazine).
   2. **Trimethoprim and sulfamethoxazole (TMP-SMZ):** This important drug combination is currently accepted treatment for complicated urinary tract infections and for respiratory, ear, and sinus infections due to *H influenzae* and *Moraxella catarrhalis.* In the immunocompromised patient, TMP-SMZ is used for infections due to *Aeromonas hydrophila* and in *Pneumocystis carinii* pneumonia. TMP-SMZ is the agent of choice for typhoid fever; it is also active against *Shigella* and *Serratia* and is a backup drug for treatment of infections due to methicillin-resistant staphylococci and *Listeria monocytogenes.*

E. Toxicity of Sulfonamides:
   1. **Hypersensitivity:** Allergic reactions, including skin rashes and fever, occur commonly. Cross-allergenicity between the individual drugs, including other sulfonamide families (di-

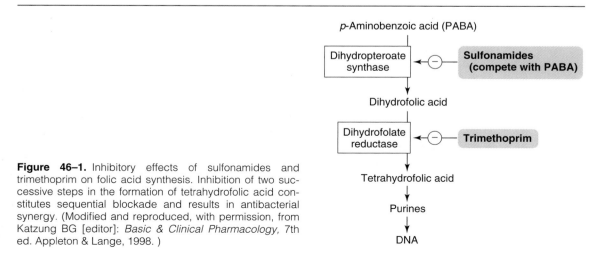

Figure 46–1. Inhibitory effects of sulfonamides and trimethoprim on folic acid synthesis. Inhibition of two successive steps in the formation of tetrahydrofolic acid constitutes sequential blockade and results in antibacterial synergy. (Modified and reproduced, with permission, from Katzung BG [editor]: *Basic & Clinical Pharmacology,* 7th ed. Appleton & Lange, 1998.)

uretics, oral hypoglycemics, etc), should be assumed. Exfoliative dermatitis, polyarteritis nodosa, and Stevens-Johnson syndrome have also occurred, though rarely.

2. **Gastrointestinal:** Nausea, vomiting, and diarrhea occur commonly. Mild hepatic dysfunction can occur, but hepatitis is uncommon.

3. **Hematotoxicity:** Though such effects are rare, sulfonamides can cause granulocytopenia, thrombocytopenia, and aplastic anemia. Acute hemolysis may occur in persons with glucose-6-phosphate dehydrogenase deficiency.

4. **Nephrotoxicity:** Sulfonamides may precipitate in the urine at acidic pH, causing crystalluria and hematuria.

5. **Drug interactions:** Competition with warfarin and methotrexate for plasma protein binding transiently increases the plasma levels of these drugs. Sulfonamides can displace bilirubin from plasma proteins, with the risk of kernicterus in the neonate.

F. **Toxicity of Trimethoprim:** Trimethoprim may cause the predictable adverse effects of an antifolate drug, including megaloblastic anemia, leukopenia, and granulocytopenia. These effects are usually ameliorated by supplementary folinic acid. The combination of trimethoprim plus sulfamethoxazole may cause any of the adverse effects associated with the sulfonamides. AIDS patients given TMP-SMZ have a high incidence of adverse effects, including fever, rashes, leukopenia, and diarrhea.

FLUOROQUINOLONES

A. **Classification and Pharmacokinetics:** The original fluoroquinolone is **norfloxacin;** others in the group include **ciprofloxacin, ofloxacin, levofloxacin, lomefloxacin,** and **sparfloxacin.** All of the drugs have good oral bioavailability, and most penetrate body tissues, with the exception of the CNS. However, norfloxacin does not achieve adequate plasma levels for use in most systemic infections. Elimination of fluoroquinolones is partly by metabolism but mainly through the kidneys via active tubular secretion (which can be blocked by probenecid). Half-lives are usually in the range of 3–8 hours, but sparfloxacin has a half-life of 24 hours. Dosage reductions of the fluoroquinolones are needed in renal dysfunction.

B. **Mechanism of Action:** The fluoroquinolones interfere with bacterial DNA synthesis by inhibiting topoisomerase II (DNA gyrase) and topoisomerase IV. They block the relaxation of supercoiled DNA that is catalyzed by DNA gyrase—a step required for normal transcription and duplication. Inhibition of topoisomerase IV by fluoroquinolones interferes with the separation of replicated chromosomal DNA during cell division. Fluoroquinolones are usually bactericidal against susceptible organisms.

C. **Resistance:** Fluoroquinolone resistance occurs during treatment with a frequency of about one in 10^8 organisms, especially staphylococci, *Pseudomonas,* and *Serratia.* Mechanisms of resistance include decreased intracellular accumulation of the drug and changes in the sensitivity of target enzymes via point mutations in the fluoroquinolone binding regions. In coliforms, changes in DNA gyrase sensitivity are most important, while in gram-positive cocci, resistance is mainly due to changes in the sensitivity of topoisomerase IV.

D. **Clinical Use:** Fluoroquinolones are effective in the treatment of infections of the urogenital and gastrointestinal tracts caused by gram-negative organisms including gonococci, *E coli, Klebsiella pneumoniae, Campylobacter jejuni, Enterobacter, Pseudomonas aeruginosa, Salmonella,* and *Shigella.* They have been used widely for respiratory tract, skin, and soft tissue infections, but their effectiveness is now variable because of the emergence of resistant strains of pneumococci and staphylococci. Fluoroquinolones have also been used in the meningococcal carrier state, the treatment of tuberculosis, and in prophylactic treatment of neutropenic patients. Ofloxacin is effective in chlamydial infections of the urogenital system. Sparfloxacin has activity against penicillin-resistant pneumococci.

E. **Toxicity:** Gastrointestinal distress is the most common side effect. The fluoroquinolones may cause skin rashes, headache, dizziness, insomnia, abnormal liver function tests, phototoxicity, and tendonitis. Superinfections due to *C albicans* and streptococci have occurred. The fluoroquinolones are not recommended for use in persons less than 18 years of age or in pregnancy because these drugs have caused cartilage erosion in young animals. Ciprofloxacin increases the plasma levels of theophylline and other methylxanthines, enhancing their toxicity. Sparfloxacin prolongs the QT interval and may increase the risk of cardiac arrhythmias. Severe photosensitivity due to sparfloxacin occurs in up to 10% of patients.

DRUG LIST

The following drugs are important members of the group discussed in this chapter. Prototypes should be learned in detail; features of the major variants should be known well enough so that the variants can be distinguished from prototypes and from each other; the other significant agents should be recognized as belonging to a specific subclass.

Subclass	Prototype	Major Variants	Other Significant Agents
Sulfonamides Oral agents	Sulfisoxazole	Triple sulfas, sulfamethoxazole	Sulfadiazine
Local agents, drugs for special applications	Sulfacetamide, sulfasalazine, mafenide		
Combination	Trimethoprim-sulfamethoxazole		Pyrimethamine-sulfadoxine
Folate reductase inhibitors	Trimethoprim		Pyrimethamine
Fluoroquinolones	Norfloxacin	Ciprofloxacin, sparfloxacin	Ofloxacin, levofloxacin

QUESTIONS

DIRECTIONS: Each of the numbered items or incomplete statements in this section is followed by answers or by completions of the statement. Select the ONE lettered answer or completion that is BEST in each case.

1. Which one of the following statements about sulfonamides is LEAST accurate?
   (A) Sulfonamides inhibit bacterial dihydrofolate reductase
   (B) Dysfunction of the basal ganglia may occur in the newborn if sulfonamides are administered late in pregnancy
   (C) Cross-allergenicity may occur between sulfonamides and thiazides
   (D) Sulfonamide crystalluria is most likely to occur at low urinary pH
   (E) Sulfonamides are antimetabolites of PABA

2. The combination of trimethoprim and sulfamethoxazole is effective against which one of the following opportunistic infections in the AIDS patient?
   (A) Disseminated herpes simplex
   (B) Cryptococcal meningitis
   (C) Toxoplasmosis
   (D) Oral candidiasis
   (E) Tuberculosis

3. A 24-year-old woman has returned from a vacation abroad suffering from traveler's diarrhea, and her problem has not responded to antidiarrheal drugs. A pathogenic gram-negative bacillus is suspected. Which one of the following drugs is most likely to be effective in the treatment of this patient?
   (A) Ampicillin
   (B) Ciprofloxacin
   (C) Sulfacetamide
   (D) Trimethoprim
   (E) Vancomycin

4. Which one of the following statements about the clinical use of sulfonamides is LEAST accurate?
   (A) Resistant bacterial strains may have decreased intracellular accumulation of sulfonamides

    (B) Sulfonamides have activity against *C trachomatis* and can be used topically for the treatment of chlamydial infections of the eye

    (C) Sulfonamides are effective in Rocky Mountain spotted fever in patients allergic to tetracyclines

    (D) A sulfonamide is unlikely to be effective as the sole antibacterial agent in the treatment of chronic prostatitis

    (E) Some strains of bacteria become resistant to sulfonamides by an increased production of PABA

5. A 31-year-old man has gonorrhea. He has no drug allergies, but he remembers that a few years ago while in Africa he had acute hemolysis following use of an antimalarial drug. The physician is concerned that the patient has an accompanying urethritis due to *C trachomatis* infection, though no culture or enzyme tests have been conducted. Which of the following drugs is most likely to be effective against gonococci and also eradicate *C trachomatis* in this patient?

    (A) Cefixime

    (B) Ciprofloxacin

    (C) Ofloxacin

    (D) Spectinomycin

    (E) Sulfamethoxazole

6. Which of the following statements about the fluoroquinolones is LEAST accurate?

    (A) Antacids may decrease the oral bioavailability of fluoroquinolones

    (B) Pneumococcal resistance to fluoroquinolones may involve changes in topoisomerase IV

    (C) Modification of fluoroquinolone dosage is required in patients if creatinine clearance is less than 50 mL/min

    (D) A fluoroquinolone is the drug of choice for treatment of an uncomplicated urinary tract infection in a 10-year-old girl

    (E) Fluoroquinolones inhibit relaxation of positively supercoiled DNA

Items 7–8: A 55-year-old man complains of periodic bouts of diarrhea with lower abdominal cramping and intermittent rectal bleeding. He appears well-nourished, with a blood pressure in the normal range. Examination reveals moderate abdominal pain and tenderness. His current medications are limited to ibuprofen for tennis elbow and over-the-counter loperamide for his diarrhea. The patient has no other significant medical history. Sigmoidoscopy reveals mucosal edema, friability, and some pus. Laboratory findings include mild anemia and decreased serum albumin. Stool cultures and mucosal biopsies do not reveal any evidence for bacterial, amebic, or cytomegalovirus involvement. A preliminary diagnosis is made of mild to moderate ulcerative colitis.

7. The most appropriate drug to use in this patient is

    (A) Ciprofloxacin

    (B) Ganciclovir

    (C) Metronidazole

    (D) Sulfasalazine

    (E) Trimethoprim-sulfamethoxazole

8. The mechanism by which sulfasalazine exerts its primary action in ulcerative colitis is inhibition of

    (A) Dihydrofolate reductase

    (B) Cyclooxygenase

    (C) Phospholipase A_2

    (D) Proton pump activity

    (E) The formation of interleukins

9. Which one of the following statements about the combination of trimethoprim plus sulfamethoxazole is LEAST accurate?

    (A) This combination is effective in the treatment of pneumonia due to *Pneumocystis carinii*

    (B) The drugs produce a sequential blockade of folic acid synthesis

    (C) Fever and pancytopenia occur frequently when these drugs are used in AIDS patients

    (D) The combination is appropriate for the treatment of streptococcal pharyngitis

    (E) The combination is effective in the management of acute exacerbations of chronic bronchitis

10. All of the following adverse effects may occur with sulfonamide therapy EXCEPT

    (A) Neurologic effects, including headache, dizziness, and lethargy

    (B) Hematuria

(C) Fanconi's aminoaciduria syndrome
(D) Kernicterus in the newborn
(E) Urticaria

DIRECTIONS (Items 11–15): Each set of matching questions in this section consists of a list of three to twenty-six lettered options (some of which may be figures) followed by several numbered items. For each numbered item, select the ONE lettered option that is most closely associated with it. Each lettered option may be selected once, more than once, or not at all.

(A) Ciprofloxacin
(B) Ofloxacin
(C) Mafenide
(D) Nalidixic acid
(E) Sparfloxacin
(F) Sulfadiazine
(G) Sulfasalazine
(H) Sulfisoxazole
(I) Trimethoprim
(J) Vancomycin

11. This drug is the preferred agent for treatment of nocardiosis and, in combination with pyrimethamine, is prophylactic against *Pneumocystis carinii* infections in AIDS patients

12. This drug is frequently active against amoxicillin-resistant strains of *H influenzae;* in combination with erythromycin, it can be used to treat otitis media caused by such strains

13. Supplementary folinic acid may prevent anemia in folate-deficient persons who use this drug; it is a weak base and achieves tissue levels similar to those in plasma

14. This drug is used topically in burn patients; systemic absorption can lead to metabolic acidosis

15. When used orally, this drug does not achieve systemic concentrations adequate for treatment of infections other than those in the urinary tract. It is the prototype of the quinolone-fluoroquinolone class of antibiotic agents

ANSWERS

1. Make sure that you know the specific enzymes in bacterial folic acid synthesis that are inhibited by sulfonamides and trimethoprim: sulfonamides inhibit dihydropteroate synthase; dihydrofolate reductase is inhibited by trimethoprim. The answer is **(A).**

2. Trimethoprim-sulfamethoxazole is not effective in the treatment of infections due to viruses, fungi, or mycobacteria. However, the drug combination is active against certain protozoans, including *Toxoplasma,* and can be used both for prophylaxis against and treatment of toxoplasmosis in the AIDS patient. The answer is **(C).**

3. The fluoroquinolones are very effective in diarrhea caused by bacterial pathogens, including *E coli, Shigella,* and *Salmonella.* None of the other drugs listed would be appropriate. Many coliforms are now resistant to ampicillin. Sulfacetamide is a topical agent used for bacterial conjunctivitis. While trimethoprim is available as a single drug, resistance may emerge during treatment unless it is used for urinary tract infections, where high concentrations are achieved. Vancomycin has no activity against gram-negative bacilli. The answer is **(B).**

4. Sulfonamides have minimal therapeutic actions in rickettsial infections. Chloramphenicol may be used for Rocky Mountain spotted fever in patients with established allergy or other contraindications to tetracyclines. The answer is **(C).**

5. While cefixime in a single oral dose is effective in gonorrhea, it has no activity against organisms causing nongonococcal urethritis. Both ciprofloxacin and spectinomycin are active against gonococci, but neither drug will eradicate a urogenital chlamydial infection. However, another fluoroquinolone, ofloxacin, is effective in both gonorrhea and chlamydial urethritis. In practice, this patient would best be treated by single oral doses of cefixime and azithromycin (not listed). Sulfamethoxazole would not be useful and may cause an acute hemolytic episode in this patient. The answer is **(C).**

6. The fluoroquinolones should not be used to treat uncomplicated first-time urinary tract infections. In this child, the infection is almost certainly due to a strain of *E coli* that is sensitive to many other drugs, including beta-lactam antibiotics. In addition, because of possible effects on

cartilage, fluoroquinolones are not recommended for use in patients under the age of 18 years. The answer is **(D)**.

7. Oral antimicrobial agents sometimes have beneficial effects in inflammatory bowel disease. However, in the absence of any evidence pointing toward a definite microbial cause of the colitis in this patient, a drug that decreases inflammation is indicated. Sulfasalazine has significant anti-inflammatory action, and its oral use results in symptomatic improvement in 50–75% of patients. The answer is **(D)**.

8. Sulfasalazine is degraded by intestinal flora to sulfapyridine and 5-aminosalicylate. Release of high concentrations of salicylate in the colon exerts anti-inflammatory action, the major benefit of the use of sulfasalazine in ulcerative colitis. 5-Aminosalicylic acid is an effective inhibitor of cyclooxygenases and decreases formation of inflammatory mediators such as prostaglandins. The answer is **(B)**.

9. The combination of trimethoprim and sulfamethoxazole is often effective in respiratory infections due to susceptible *S pneumoniae* and *H influenzae*. However, in streptococcal pharyngitis, the organisms are not eradicated. The answer is **(D)**.

10. Renal dysfunction, including crystalluria, hematuria, nephrosis, and allergic nephritis, occurs with sulfonamides. However, Fanconi's syndrome, characterized by low back pain, aminoaciduria, polydipsia, and polyuria, is associated with the use of outdated tetracyclines. The answer is **(C)**.

11. Sulfadiazine is the preferred drug in nocardiosis. In combination with pyrimethamine (an effective dihydrofolate reductase inhibitor in protozoans), sulfadiazine is effective in toxoplasmosis and is prophylactic against PCP in the AIDS patient. The answer is **(F)**.

12. Sulfisoxazole is very soluble in the urine and is commonly used for the treatment of acute, uncomplicated urinary tract infections. The drug is also active against some common causative agents of otitis media, including *H influenzae* and pneumococci. For the treatment of otitis media, sulfisoxazole is usually given in a fixed-ratio combination with erythromycin. The answer is **(H)**.

13. Trimethoprim is the only weak base listed. Its high lipid solubility at blood pH allows penetration of the drug into prostatic and vaginal fluid to reach levels similar to those in plasma. Leukopenia and thrombocytopenia may occur in folate deficiency when the drug is used alone or in combination with sulfamethoxazole. The answer is **(I)**.

14. Mafenide is a sulfonamide used solely as a topical agent to prevent bacterial colonization and infection of burn wounds. Topical application of mafenide is painful and may lead to fungal superinfections. Systemic absorption from burn sites may result in metabolic acidosis through inhibition of carbonic anhydrase. The answer is **(C)**.

15. Fluoroquinolones are fluorinated analogs of nalidixic acid, a quinolone that is excreted too rapidly to have systemic antibacterial effects. Nalidixic acid can be used as a urinary antiseptic, but it has been largely replaced by the more effective fluoroquinolones. The answer is **(D)**.

Antimycobacterial Drugs

47

OBJECTIVES

You should be able to:

- Describe the special problems associated with chemotherapy of mycobacterial infections.
- Describe the pharmacodynamic and pharmacokinetic properties of the first-line drugs used in tuberculosis (isoniazid, ethambutol, pyrazinamide, rifampin, and streptomycin).
- Identify the second-line drugs used in tuberculosis and list their limitations.
- Identify the drugs used in leprosy and in atypical mycobacterial diseases and describe their major toxic effects.

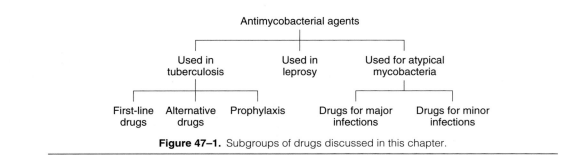

Figure 47–1. Subgroups of drugs discussed in this chapter.

CONCEPTS

The chemotherapy of infections caused by *M tuberculosis, M leprae,* and *M avium-intracellulare* is complicated by numerous factors, including (1) limited information about the mechanisms of antimycobacterial drug actions; (2) the development of resistance; (3) the intracellular location of mycobacteria; and (4) the chronic nature of mycobacterial disease, which requires protracted drug treatment and is associated with drug toxicities. Chemotherapy of mycobacterial infections almost always involves the use of **drug combinations** to delay the emergence of resistance and to enhance antimycobacterial efficacy. The major drugs used in tuberculosis are **isoniazid (INH), rifampin, ethambutol, pyrazinamide,** and **streptomycin.** Suppression of *M avium-intracellulare—M avium* complex (MAC)—in the immunocompromised patient also requires multidrug treatment. The primary drug for leprosy is **dapsone,** commonly given with either **rifampin** or **clofazimine.** The subgroups of drugs used in these conditions are shown in Figure 47–1.

DRUGS FOR TUBERCULOSIS

A. Isoniazid:
1. **Mechanisms:** Isoniazid (INH) is a structural congener of pyridoxine. Its mechanism of action involves inhibition of enzymes required for the synthesis of mycolic acids and mycobacterial cell walls. Resistance can emerge rapidly if the drug is used alone. In some cases, resistance may be associated with deletion of a gene *(katG)* that codes for catalase and peroxidase enzymes in mycobacteria.
2. **Pharmacokinetics:** INH is well absorbed orally and penetrates cells to act on intracellular mycobacteria. The liver metabolism of INH is by acetylation and is under genetic control. Patients may be fast (half-life 1 hour) or slow (half-life 3 hours) inactivators of the drug. The proportion of fast acetylators is higher among people of Asian origin (including Native Americans) than those of European or African origin. Fast acetylators often require higher dosage than slow acetylators for equivalent therapeutic effects.
3. **Clinical use:** INH is the single most important drug used in tuberculosis, and it is a component of most drug combination regimens. In the prophylaxis of skin test converters—and in close contacts of patients with active disease—INH is given as the sole drug.
4. **Toxicity and interactions:** Neurotoxic effects are common and include peripheral neuritis, restlessness, muscle twitching, and insomnia. These effects can be alleviated (without blocking the antibacterial effect) by administration of pyridoxine. INH is hepatotoxic and may cause abnormal liver function tests, jaundice, and hepatitis. Fortunately, hepatotoxicity is rare in children. INH may inhibit the hepatic metabolism of drugs, eg, phenytoin. Hemolysis has occurred in patients with glucose-6-phosphate dehydrogenase deficiency. Drug-induced systemic lupus erythematosus has been reported.

B. Rifampin:
1. **Mechanisms:** Rifampin, a derivative of rifamycin, is bactericidal to *M tuberculosis.* The drug inhibits DNA-dependent RNA polymerase in *M tuberculosis* and many other microorganisms. Resistance, via changes in drug sensitivity of the polymerase, emerges rapidly if the drug is used alone.
2. **Pharmacokinetics:** When given orally, rifampin is well absorbed and is distributed to most body tissues, including the CNS. The drug undergoes enterohepatic cycling and is

partially metabolized in the liver. Both free drug and metabolites (which are orange-colored) are eliminated mainly in the feces.

3. **Clinical uses:**   In tuberculosis, rifampin is usually used in combination with other drugs. In leprosy, rifampin given monthly delays the emergence of resistance to dapsone. Rifampin can be used as the sole drug in prophylaxis against tuberculosis in INH-intolerant patients or close contacts of patients with INH-resistant strains of the organism. Other uses of rifampin include the meningococcal and staphylococcal carrier states.

4. **Toxicity and interactions:**   Rifampin commonly causes light chain proteinuria and may impair antibody responses. Occasional side effects include skin rashes, thrombocytopenia, nephritis, and liver dysfunction. If given less often than twice weekly, rifampin may cause a flu-like syndrome and anemia. Rifampin strongly induces liver drug-metabolizing enzymes and enhances the elimination rate of many drugs, including anticonvulsants, contraceptive steroids, cyclosporine, ketoconazole, methadone, and warfarin.

C. **Ethambutol:**
   1. **Mechanisms:**   Ethambutol inhibits the synthesis of arabinogalactan, a component of mycobacterial cell walls. Resistance occurs rapidly if the drug is used alone.
   2. **Pharmacokinetics:**   The drug is well absorbed orally and distributed to most tissues including the CNS. A large fraction of drug is eliminated unchanged in the urine. Dose reduction is necessary in renal failure.
   3. **Clinical use:**   The only use of ethambutol is in tuberculosis, and it is always given in combination with other drugs.
   4. **Toxicity:**   The most common adverse effects are dose-dependent visual disturbances, including decreased visual acuity, optic neuritis, and possible retinal damage (with prolonged use at high doses). Most of these effects regress when the drug is stopped. Other neurotoxic effects include headache, confusion, and peripheral neuritis.

D. **Pyrazinamide:**
   1. **Mechanisms:**   The mechanism of action of pyrazinamide is not known; however, its bacteriostatic action appears to require metabolic conversion via pyrazinamidases present in *M tuberculosis.* Resistant mycobacteria lack these enzymes, and resistance develops rapidly if the drug is used alone. There is minimal cross-resistance with other antimycobacterial drugs.
   2. **Pharmacokinetics:**   Pyrazinamide is well absorbed orally and penetrates most body tissues including the CNS. It is partly metabolized to pyrazinoic acid, and both parent molecule and metabolite are excreted in the urine. The plasma half-life of pyrazinamide is increased in hepatic or renal failure.
   3. **Clinical use:**   The combined use of pyrazinamide with other antituberculosis drugs is an important factor in the success of "short-course" (6-month) treatment regimens.
   4. **Toxicity:**   Approximately 40% of patients develop nongouty polyarthralgia. Hyperuricemia occurs commonly but is usually asymptomatic. Other adverse effects include myalgia, gastrointestinal irritation, maculopapular rash, hepatic dysfunction, porphyria, and photosensitivity reactions.

E. **Streptomycin:**   This aminoglycoside is now used more frequently than hitherto because of the growing prevalence of drug-resistant strains of *M tuberculosis.* Streptomycin is used principally in drug combinations for the treatment of life-threatening disease, including tuberculous meningitis, miliary dissemination, and severe organ tuberculosis. The pharmacodynamic and pharmacokinetic properties of streptomycin are similar to those of other aminoglycosides (see Chapter 45).

F. **Alternative Drugs:**   The second-line antimycobacterial drugs are used in cases resistant to first-line agents; they are considered second-line drugs because they are no more effective and their toxicities are often more serious than those of the major drugs.
   1. **Amikacin** is indicated for treatment of tuberculosis suspected to be caused by streptomycin-resistant or multidrug-resistant mycobacterial strains. To avoid emergence of resistance, amikacin should always be used in combination drug regimens.
   2. **Ciprofloxacin** and **ofloxacin** are often active against strains of *M tuberculosis* resistant to first-line agents. The fluoroquinolones must always be used in combination with two or more other active agents.
   3. **Ethionamide** is a congener of INH, but cross-resistance does not occur. The major disadvantage of ethionamide is severe gastrointestinal irritation and adverse neurologic effects at doses needed for effective plasma levels.

4. **p-Aminosalicylic acid (PAS)** is now rarely used because primary resistance is common. In addition, its toxicity includes gastrointestinal irritation, peptic ulceration, hypersensitivity reactions, and effects on kidney, liver, and thyroid function.

5. Other drugs of limited use because of their toxicity include **capreomycin** (ototoxicity, renal dysfunction) and **cycloserine** (peripheral neuropathy, CNS dysfunction).

DRUGS FOR LEPROSY

A. Sulfones: **Dapsone** (diaminodiphenylsulfone) remains the most active drug against *M leprae*. The mechanism of action of sulfones may involve inhibition of folic acid synthesis. Resistance can develop, especially if low doses are given. Dapsone can be given orally, penetrates tissues well, undergoes enterohepatic cycling, and is eliminated in the urine, partly as acetylated metabolites. Common adverse effects include gastrointestinal irritation, fever, skin rashes, and methemoglobinemia. Hemolysis may occur, especially in patients with glucose-6-phosphate dehydrogenase deficiency.

    Acedapsone is a repository form of dapsone that provides inhibitory plasma concentrations for several months. In addition to its use in leprosy, dapsone is an alternative drug for the treatment of *Pneumocystis carinii* pneumonia in AIDS patients.

B. Other Agents: Alternative drugs for leprosy include rifampin (see above) and **clofazimine.** Clofazimine is given in cases of dapsone resistance or intolerance. The drug causes gastrointestinal irritation and marked skin discoloration.

DRUGS FOR ATYPICAL MYCOBACTERIAL INFECTIONS

Infections due to atypical mycobacteria (eg, *M marinum, M avium-intracellulare, M ulcerans*), though sometimes asymptomatic, may be treated with the described antimycobacterial drugs (eg, ethambutol, rifampin) or with other antibiotics (eg, erythromycin, amikacin).

    M avium complex (MAC) is a frequent cause of disseminated infections in AIDS patients. Currently, clarithromycin or azithromycin is recommended for prophylaxis in patients with CD4 counts less than 100/μL. Treatment of MAC infections requires a combination of drugs, one favored regimen consisting of azithromycin or clarithromycin plus ethambutol and sometimes rifabutin, a congener of rifampin. Most of the conventional antimycobacterial drugs have also been used in combinations for MAC infections. Clofazimine should not be used in such regimens since it may increase morbidity in the AIDS patient.

DRUG LIST

The following drugs are important members of the group discussed in this chapter. Prototypes should be learned in detail; other significant agents should be recognized as belonging to a specific subclass.

Subclass	Prototype	Other Significant Agents
Drugs for tuberculosis Pyridines	Isoniazid	Ethionamide, pyrazinamide
Rifamycins	Rifampin	Rifabutin
Diamines	Ethambutol	
Aminoglycosides	Streptomycin	Amikacin
Others		Ciprofloxacin, ofloxacin, aminosalicylic acid, capreomycin, cycloserine, viomycin
Drugs for leprosy Sulfones	Dapsone	Acedapsone
Phenazines	Clofazimine	
Drugs for *M avium* complex		A combination of azithromycin or clarithromycin with ethambutol, with or without rifabutin, is favored

QUESTIONS

DIRECTIONS: Each of the numbered items or incomplete statements in this section is followed by answers or by completions of the statement. Select the ONE lettered answer or completion that is BEST in each case.

1. The primary reason for the use of drug combinations in the treatment of tuberculosis is to
   (A) Ensure patient compliance with the drug regimen
   (B) Lower the incidence of adverse effects
   (C) Enhance activity against metabolically inactive mycobacteria
   (D) Delay or prevent the emergence of resistance
   (E) Provide prophylaxis against other bacterial infections

Items 2–5: A 21-year-old woman from Thailand has been staying with family members in California for the past 3 months and looking after her sister's preschool children during the day. Since she has difficulty with the English language, her sister escorts her to the emergency room of a local hospital. She tells the staff that the patient has been feeling very tired for the past month, has a poor appetite, and has lost weight. Two weeks ago she had symptoms of the "flu," with fever and night sweats. The patient has been feeling better lately except for a cough that produces a greenish sputum, sometimes specked with blood. With the exception of rales in the left upper lobe, the physical exam of the patient is unremarkable and she does not seem to be acutely ill. Lab values show a white count of 12,000/μL and a hematocrit of 33%. Chest x-ray reveals an infiltrate in the left upper lobe with a possible cavity. A Gram-stained smear of the sputum shows mixed flora with no dominance. An acid-fast stain reveals many thin rods of pinkish hue. A preliminary diagnosis is made of pulmonary tuberculosis. Sputum is sent to the laboratory for culture.

2. At this point, the most appropriate course of action is to
   (A) Send the patient home to await the culture results
   (B) Prescribe isoniazid for prophylaxis and send the patient home to await culture results
   (C) Start outpatient treatment with isoniazid and rifampin
   (D) Hospitalize the patient and start treatment with four antimycobacterial drugs
   (E) Hospitalize the patient and start treatment with isoniazid, rifampin, and ethambutol

3. When treatment is started, which one of the following drug regimens should be initiated in this patient?
   (A) Amikacin, isoniazid, pyrazinamide, streptomycin
   (B) Ciprofloxacin, cycloserine, isoniazid, PAS
   (C) Ethambutol, isoniazid, rifabutin, streptomycin
   (D) Ethambutol, pyrazinamide, rifampin, streptomycin
   (E) Isoniazid, rifampin, pyrazinamide, ethambutol

4. Which of the following statements concerning the possible use of isoniazid (INH) in this patient is LEAST accurate?
   (A) She may experience flushing, palpitations, sweating, and dyspnea after ingestion of tyramine-containing foods
   (B) Persons from Southeast Asia require lower maintenance doses of INH than most other persons in the USA
   (C) She should take 10 mg of pyridoxine daily
   (D) Symptoms of peripheral neuritis may occur during treatment
   (E) Her risk of developing hepatitis due to INH is less than 0.5%

5. On her release from the hospital, the patient is advised not to rely solely on oral contraceptives to avoid pregnancy, since they may be less effective while she is being maintained on antimycobacterial drugs. The agent most likely to interfere with the action of oral contraceptives is
   (A) Ethambutol
   (B) Isoniazid
   (C) Pyrazinamide
   (D) Rifampin
   (E) Streptomycin

6. The mechanism of high-level INH resistance of *M tuberculosis* is
   (A) Formation of drug-inactivating *N*-acetyltransferase
   (B) Reduced expression of the *katG* gene
   (C) Decreased intracellular accumulation of INH

     (D) Mutation in the *inhA* gene

     (E) Change in the pathway of mycolic acid synthesis

7. Which one of the following statements concerning drugs used in leprosy is LEAST accurate?

     (A) The mechanism of action of dapsone probably involves inhibition of folic acid synthesis

     (B) Single intramuscular injections of acedapsone maintain inhibitory levels of dapsone in tissues for up to 3 months

     (C) Monthly doses of rifampin delay the emergence of resistance to dapsone

     (D) Clofazimine should not be given to patients who are intolerant of dapsone or who fail to improve during treatment with dapsone

     (E) Clofazimine may cause skin discoloration

8. A patient with AIDS and a CD4 cell count of 100/μL has persistent fever and weight loss associated with invasive pulmonary disease that is due to *M avium* complex. The optimal management of this patient is to

     (A) Treat with rifabutin since it prevents the development of MAC bacteremia

     (B) Select an antibiotic regimen based on drug susceptibility of the cultured organism

     (C) Start treatment with INH and pyrazinamide

     (D) Treat the patient with clarithromycin, ethambutol, and rifabutin

     (E) Treat with trimethoprim-sulfamethoxazole

9. A patient with pulmonary tuberculosis due to an INH-susceptible strain of *M tuberculosis* has been treated with INH, rifampin, and pyrazinamide for a total of 2 months. If the pyrazinamide is stopped at this time, treatment should be continued with INH and rifampin for a further minimum time period of at least

     (A) 2 months

     (B) 4 months

     (C) 6 months

     (D) 12 months

     (E) 18 months

10. A 10-year-old boy has uncomplicated pulmonary tuberculosis. After initial hospitalization, he is now being treated at home with isoniazid, rifampin, and ethambutol. Which one of the following statements about this case is LEAST accurate?

     (A) Caregivers should not worry about orange-colored tears if he cries

     (B) Periodic tests of liver function should be considered

     (C) Pyridoxine should be administered in an amount equivalent to the dose of INH

     (D) His mother (who takes care of him) should receive INH prophylaxis, but this is inadvisable for his younger siblings

     (E) The boy may develop symptoms similar to those of influenza

DIRECTIONS (Items 11–15): Each set of matching questions in this section consists of a list of three to twenty-six lettered options (some of which may be figures) followed by several numbered items. For each numbered item, select the ONE lettered option that is most closely associated with it. Each lettered option may be selected once, more than once, or not at all.

     (A) Azithromycin

     (B) Clofazimine

     (C) Dapsone

     (D) Ethambutol

     (E) Isoniazid

     (F) *p*-Aminosalicylic acid (PAS)

     (G) Pyrazinamide

     (H) Rifabutin

     (I) Rifampin

     (J) Streptomycin

11. This drug eliminates a majority of meningococci from carriers, but highly resistant strains may be selected out during treatment

12. Patients taking this drug might be advised to test their vision by reading the small print in the newspaper from time to time

13. Once weekly administration of this antibiotic has prophylactic activity against bacteremia due to *M avium* complex in AIDS patients

14. Provocation of an attack of acute gouty arthritis is possible with this drug

15. Of the drugs listed, this agent is most likely to cause loss of equilibrium and auditory damage

ANSWERS

1. While it is sometimes possible to achieve synergistic effects against mycobacteria with drug combinations, the primary reason for their use is to delay the emergence of resistance. The answer is **(D)**.

2. Despite the fact that this patient does not appear to be acutely ill, she should be treated with four drugs that have activity against *M tuberculosis*. This is because organisms infecting patients from Southeast Asia are commonly INH-resistant and coverage must be provided with three other antituberculosis drugs in addition to isoniazid. This patient should be hospitalized for several reasons, including potential difficulties with compliance regarding the drug regimen and the fact that young children are in the home where she is living. The answer is **(D)**.

3. Sputum cultures will not be available for several weeks, and no information is available regarding drug susceptibility of the organism at this stage. For optimal coverage, the initial regimen should include INH, rifampin, pyrazinamide, and ethambutol. INH-resistant organisms are usually sensitive to both rifampin and pyrazinamide. Streptomycin is usually reserved for use in severe forms of tuberculosis or for infections known to be resistant to first-line drugs. Likewise, amikacin and ciprofloxacin are possible agents for treatment of multidrug-resistant strains of *M tuberculosis*. Cycloserine, PAS, and rifabutin are alternative second-line drugs that may be used in cases of failed response to more conventional agents. The answer is **(E)**.

4. Peripheral neuropathy caused by INH is due to pyridoxine deficiency. It is more common in the diabetic, malnourished, or AIDS patient and can be prevented by a daily dose of 10 mg of pyridoxine. INH can inhibit monoamine oxidase type A and has caused tyramine reactions. Hepatotoxicity is age-dependent, with an incidence of 0.3% in patients aged 21–35 and greater than 2% in patients over the age of 50 years. Patients from Pacific Rim countries do not require lower doses of INH. Fast acetylators, including Native Americans, may require higher doses of the drug than others. The answer is **(B)**.

5. Rifampin induces the formation of several microsomal drug-metabolizing enzymes, including cytochrome P450 isoforms. This action increases the rate of elimination of a number of drugs, including anticoagulants, ketoconazole, methadone, and oral contraceptives. The pharmacologic activity of these drugs can be reduced in patients taking rifampin. The answer is **(D)**.

6. Mutations in the *katG* gene result in the underproduction of mycobacterial catalase, an enzyme that facilitates the interaction of isoniazid with its target protein. The result is high-level resistance to isoniazid but without cross-resistance to pyrazinamide. Mutations in the *inhA* gene result in low-level resistance, with cross-resistance to pyrazinamide. The answer is **(B)**.

7. Clofazimine is not related chemically to dapsone, and there is little cross-resistance. The drug is used in sulfone-resistant leprosy and for patients unable to tolerate dapsone. The answer is **(D)**.

8. Combinations of antibiotics are essential for suppression of disease caused by *M avium* complex in the AIDS patient, and treatment should be started before culture results are available. While rifabutin is prophylactic against MAC bacteremia, when used as sole therapy in active disease, resistant strains of the organism emerge rapidly. MAC is much less susceptible than *M tuberculosis* to conventional antimycobacterial drugs. Both isoniazid and pyrazinamide have minimal activity against MAC. Currently, the optimal regimen consists of clarithromycin (or azithromycin) with ethambutol and rifabutin. The answer is **(D)**.

9. The duration of antimycobacterial drug therapy depends on the severity and location of the infection, the drug susceptibility characteristics of the infecting organism, and the effectiveness of the individual drugs used in the combination regimens. In pulmonary tuberculosis, treatment with INH, rifampin, and pyrazinamide should be continued for a total of 6 months, with pyrazinamide included for the first 2 months only. If pyrazinamide is not used during the first 2 months, INH and rifampin must be given for a total of 9 months. The answer is **(B)**.

10. Hepatic dysfunction due to INH is rare in patients under 20 years of age. However, periodic tests of liver function may be advisable in younger patients who are also receiving rifampin, especially if higher doses of these drugs are used. Prophylaxis with INH is advisable for all household members and very close contacts of patients with active tuberculosis, *especially* children. A flu-like syndrome has occurred following intermittent high dose administration of rifampin. The answer is **(D)**.

11. Resistance emerges rapidly when rifampin is used as a single agent in the treatment of bacterial infections. When it is used to treat the meningococcal carrier state, up to 10% of treated carriers may harbor rifampin-resistant organisms. The answer is **(I)**.

12. Decreased visual acuity, optic neuritis, and possible retinal damage are characteristic adverse effects of ethambutol. Ocular toxicity is dose-dependent and is usually reversible when ethambutol is discontinued. Periodic testing of visual acuity is advisable during treatment. The answer is (**D**).

13. Owing to its long elimination half-life (3–4 days), weekly administration of azithromycin has proved to be equivalent to daily administration of clarithromycin when used for prophylaxis against *M avium* complex in AIDS patients. The answer is (**A**).

14. The major adverse effect of pyrazinamide is hepatotoxicity. However, the drug uniformly causes hyperuricemia and may provoke acute gouty arthritis. The answer is (**G**).

15. Ototoxicity is characteristic of the aminoglycoside antibiotics. While disturbances of equilibrium may occur with overdosage, PAS does not cause hearing loss. The answer is (**J**).

48

Antifungal Agents

OBJECTIVES

You should be able to:

- Describe the mechanisms of action of the major drugs used for fungal infections.
- Describe the clinical uses and pharmacokinetics of amphotericin B, flucytosine, fluconazole, itraconazole, ketoconazole, griseofulvin, and terbinafine.
- Indicate the major toxic effects of the antifungal drugs listed above.
- Identify the major antifungal agents for topical use.

CONCEPTS

Fungal infections are difficult to treat, particularly in the immunocompromised or neutropenic patient. Most fungi are resistant to conventional antimicrobial agents, and only a few drugs are available for the treatment of systemic fungal diseases. Amphotericin B and the azoles (fluconazole, itraconazole, and ketoconazole) are useful in systemic infections and are selectively toxic to fungi because they interact with ergosterol or inhibit its synthesis. Ergosterol is a sterol that is unique to the fungal cell membrane.

DRUGS FOR SYSTEMIC FUNGAL INFECTIONS

A. Amphotericin B:
1. Classification and pharmacokinetics: Amphotericin B is a polyene antibiotic related to nystatin. Amphotericin is poorly absorbed from the gastrointestinal tract and is usually ad-

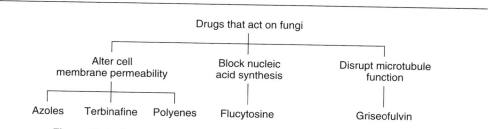

Figure 48–1. Subgroups of the antifungal drugs discussed in this chapter.

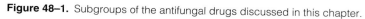

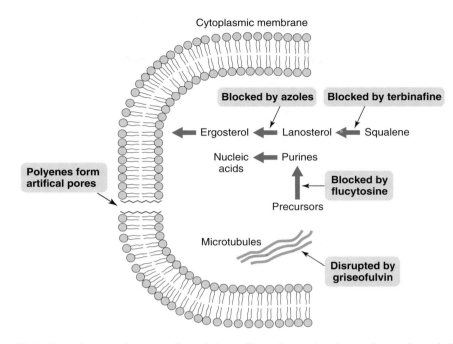

Figure 48–2. Sites of action of some antifungal drugs. The cell cytoplasmic membrane shown is that of a typical fungus. Because ergosterol is not a component of mammalian membranes, significant selective toxicity is achieved with the azole drugs.

ministered intravenously as a colloidal suspension. The drug is widely distributed to all tissues except the CNS. Elimination is mainly via slow hepatic metabolism; the half-life is approximately 2 weeks. A small fraction of the drug is excreted in the urine; dosage modification is necessary only in extreme renal dysfunction. Amphotericin B is not dialyzable.

2. **Mechanism of action:** The fungicidal action of amphotericin B is due to its effects on the permeability and transport properties of fungal membranes. Polyenes are molecules with both hydrophilic and lipophilic characteristics, ie, they are amphipathic. They bind to **ergosterol,** a sterol specific to fungal cell membranes, and cause the formation of artificial pores (Figure 48–2). Resistance can occur via a decreased level of—or a structural change in—membrane ergosterol.

3. **Clinical uses:** Amphotericin B is the most important drug for the treatment of systemic mycoses and is often used for initial induction regimens prior to follow-up treatment with an azole. It has the widest antifungal spectrum of any agent and remains the drug of choice for most systemic infections caused by *Aspergillus, Candida albicans, Cryptococcus, Histoplasma,* and *Mucor.* Amphotericin B is usually given by slow intravenous infusion, but in fungal meningitis intrathecal administration may be necessary.

4. **Toxicity:** Adverse effects related to intravenous infusion commonly include fever, chills, muscle spasms, vomiting, and a shock-like fall in blood pressure. These effects may be attenuated by a slow infusion rate and by premedication with antihistamines, antipyretics, or glucocorticoids. Amphotericin B decreases glomerular filtration rate and causes renal tubular acidosis with magnesium and potassium wasting. Anemia may result from decreases in the renal formation of erythropoietin. While concomitant saline infusion may reduce renal damage, the nephrotoxic effects of the drug are dose-limiting. Dose reduction (with lowered toxicity) is possible in some infections when amphotericin B is used with flucytosine. Liposomal preparations of amphotericin B have reduced nephrotoxic effects, possibly due to decreased binding of the drug to renal cells. Intrathecal administration of the drug may cause seizures and neurologic damage.

B. Flucytosine (5-Fluorocytosine, 5-FC):

1. **Classification and pharmacokinetics:** 5-FC is a pyrimidine antimetabolite related to the anticancer drug 5-fluorouracil (5-FU). 5-FC is effective orally and is distributed to most body tissues, including the CNS. The drug is eliminated intact in the urine, and the dose must be reduced in patients with renal impairment.

2. **Mechanism of action:** Flucytosine is accumulated in fungal cells by the action of a membrane permease and converted by cytosine deaminase to 5-FU, an inhibitor of thymidylate synthase (Figure 48–2). Selective toxicity occurs because mammalian cells have low levels of permease and deaminase. Resistance can occur rapidly and involves decreased activity of the fungal permeases or deaminases. When 5-FC is given with amphotericin B, emergence of resistance is decreased and synergistic antifungal effects may occur.

3. **Clinical uses:** The antifungal spectrum of 5-FC is narrow; its clinical use is limited to the treatment, in combination with amphotericin B, of infections due to *Cryptococcus* and *C albicans.*

4. **Toxicity:** Prolonged high plasma levels of flucytosine cause reversible bone marrow depression, alopecia, and liver dysfunction. The hematotoxic effects can be reduced by administration of uracil.

C. Azole Antifungal Agents:

1. **Classification and pharmacokinetics:** The azoles used for systemic mycoses include **ketoconazole, fluconazole,** and **itraconazole.** Oral bioavailability is variable (normal gastric acidity is required), and the drugs are distributed to most body tissues. With the exception of fluconazole, drug levels achieved in the CNS are low. Liver metabolism is responsible for the elimination of ketoconazole and itraconazole. Fluconazole is more reliably absorbed via the oral route than the other azoles. This drug is distributed widely and readily enters the CNS. Fluconazole is eliminated by the kidneys, largely in unchanged form.

2. **Mechanism of action:** The azoles interfere with fungal cell membrane permeability by inhibiting the synthesis of ergosterol. These drugs act at the step of 14α-demethylation of lanosterol, which is catalyzed by a cytochrome P450 isozyme. With increasing use of azole antifungals, especially long-term prophylaxis in immunocompromised and neutropenic patients, resistance is appearing, possibly via changes in the sensitivity of the target enzymes.

3. **Clinical uses:**

   a. **Ketoconazole:** This drug has a narrow antifungal spectrum and is considered to be a backup drug for systemic infections caused by certain strains of *Blastomyces, Coccidioides,* and *Histoplasma.* Ketoconazole has been used commonly for chronic mucocutaneous candidiasis, and when given orally it is also effective against dermatophytes.

   b. **Fluconazole:** Fluconazole has a wide spectrum of antifungal activity, but in systemic mycoses it is usually an alternative agent to amphotericin B. Fluconazole is currently the drug of choice in esophageal and oropharyngeal candidiasis and for most infections due to *Coccidioides.* Since it readily penetrates into the CSF, fluconazole can suppress cryptococcal meningitis in immunodeficient patients.

   c. **Itraconazole:** This azole is currently the drug of choice for systemic infections due to *Blastomyces* and *Sporothrix* and for subcutaneous chromoblastomycosis. Itraconazole is an alternative agent in the treatment of infections caused by *Aspergillus, Coccidioides, Cryptococcus,* and *Histoplasma.* In esophageal candidiasis, the drug is active against some strains resistant to fluconazole. Itraconazole is also active in dermatophytoses.

4. **Toxicity:** Adverse effects of the azoles include vomiting, diarrhea, rash, and sometimes hepatotoxicity (especially in patients with preexisting liver dysfunction). Ketoconazole inhibits hepatic cytochrome P450 isozymes and may increase the plasma levels of other drugs including anticoagulants, oral hypoglycemics, and phenytoin. The same inhibition of drug metabolism is responsible for life-threatening cardiotoxicity when astemizole or terfenadine is given concomitantly with ketoconazole. Inhibition of cytochrome P450 isoforms by ketoconazole interferes with the synthesis of adrenal and gonadal steroids and may lead to gynecomastia, menstrual irregularities, and infertility. The newer azoles appear to be more selective inhibitors of fungal cytochrome P450 and are much less likely than ketoconazole to cause drug interactions or endocrine dysfunction.

SYSTEMIC DRUGS FOR SUPERFICIAL FUNGAL INFECTIONS

    A. Griseofulvin:
        1. Pharmacokinetics: Oral absorption of griseofulvin depends on the physical state of the drug (ultramicrosize formulations, which have finer crystals or particles, are more effectively absorbed) and is aided by high-fat foods. The drug is distributed to the stratum corneum, where it binds to keratin. Biliary excretion is responsible for its elimination.
        2. Mechanism of action: Griseofulvin interferes with microtubule function (Figure 48–2) and may also inhibit the synthesis and polymerization of nucleic acids. Sensitive fungi take up the drug by an energy-dependent mechanism, and resistance can occur via decrease in this transport. Griseofulvin is fungistatic.
        3. Clinical uses and toxicity: Activity of griseofulvin is restricted to dermatophytes. The drug is indicated for severe dermatophytoses of the skin, hair, and nails. Adverse effects include headaches, mental confusion, gastrointestinal irritation, photosensitivity, and changes in liver function. A drug interaction may enhance coumarin metabolism, resulting in decreased anticoagulant effect.

    B. Terbinafine:
        1. Mechanism of action: Terbinafine inhibits a fungal enzyme, squalene epoxidase. It causes accumulation of toxic levels of squalene, which can interfere with ergosterol synthesis. Terbinafine is fungicidal.
        2. Clinical use and toxicity: Like griseofulvin, terbinafine accumulates in keratin, but it is much more effective in onychomycosis. Adverse effects include gastrointestinal upsets, rash, headache, and taste disturbances. Terbinafine does not inhibit cytochrome P450.

    C. Azoles:
        1. Pulse dosing: All three of the azoles used for systemic antifungal infections have activity against dermatophytes. Pulse or intermittent dosing with itraconazole is as effective in onychomycoses as continuous dosing because the drug persists in the nails for several months. Typically, treatment for 1 week is followed by 3 weeks without drug. Advantages of pulse dosing include a lower incidence of side effects and major cost savings. Similar dosing regimens may be applicable to fluconazole and terbinafine.

TOPICAL DRUGS FOR SUPERFICIAL INFECTIONS

A number of antifungal drugs are used topically for superficial infections caused by *C albicans* and dermatophytes. **Nystatin** is a polyene antibiotic (related to amphotericin) that disrupts fungal membranes by binding to ergosterol. Nystatin is commonly used topically to suppress local *Candida* infections and has been used orally to eradicate gastrointestinal fungi in patients with impaired defense mechanisms. Other topical antifungal agents include the azole compounds **miconazole** and **clotrimazole** and the nonazoles **haloprogin, tolnaftate,** and **undecylenic acid.**

DRUG LIST

The following drugs are important members of the group discussed in this chapter. Prototypes should be learned in detail; the other significant agents should be recognized as belonging to a specific subclass.

Subclass	Prototype	Other Significant Agents
Drugs for systemic mycoses		
Polyenes	Amphotericin B	
Azoles	Ketoconazole	Fluconazole, itraconazole
Pyrimidine	Flucytosine	
Systemic drugs for superficial infections	Griseofulvin	Terbinafine, ketoconazole, fluconazole, itraconazole
Drugs for topical or local use	Nystatin	Miconazole, clotrimazole, tolnaftate

QUESTIONS

DIRECTIONS: Each of the numbered items or incomplete statements in this section is followed by answers or by completions of the statement. Select the ONE lettered answer or completion that is BEST in each case.

1. Chemical interactions between this drug and cell membrane components can result in the formation of pores lined by hydrophilic groups present in the drug molecule.
   (A) Dactinomycin
   (B) Griseofulvin
   (C) Fluconazole
   (D) Nystatin
   (E) Terbinafine

2. Which one of the following statements about fluconazole is most accurate?
   (A) It is highly effective in treatment of aspergillosis
   (B) It does not penetrate the blood-brain barrier
   (C) Its oral bioavailability is less than that of ketoconazole
   (D) It inhibits demethylation of lanosterol
   (E) It is a potent inhibitor of hepatic drug-metabolizing enzymes

Items 3–6: A 20-year-old woman with leukemia was undergoing chemotherapy with intravenous antineoplastic drugs. During treatment, she developed a fever and other symptoms suggesting that she had developed a systemic infection due to an opportunistic pathogen. There was no erythema or edema at the catheter insertion site. A white vaginal discharge was observed. After appropriate specimens for culture were obtained, empiric antibiotic therapy was started with gentamicin, nafcillin, and ticarcillin intravenously. This regimen was maintained for 72 hours, during which time the patient's condition did not improve significantly. Her throat was sore, and white plaques had appeared in her pharynx. On day 4, none of the cultures had shown any bacterial growth, but both the blood and urine cultures grew out *Candida albicans*.

3. At this point, the best course of action is to
   (A) Continue current antibiotics and start flucytosine
   (B) Stop current antibiotics and start ketoconazole
   (C) Continue current antibiotics and start amphotericin B
   (D) Continue current antibiotics and start fluconazole
   (E) Stop current antibiotics and start amphotericin B

4. If given amphotericin B, the patient should be premedicated with
   (A) Diphenhydramine
   (B) Ibuprofen
   (C) Prednisone
   (D) Any or all of the above
   (E) None of the above

5. The dose-limiting toxicity of amphotericin B is
   (A) Myelosuppression
   (B) Infusion-related adverse effects
   (C) Renal tubular acidosis
   (D) Hypotension
   (E) Hepatitis

6. The opportunistic candidal infection in this patient could have been prevented by prophylaxis with
   (A) Fluconazole
   (B) Itraconazole
   (C) Ketoconazole
   (D) Nystatin
   (E) None of the above

Items 7–8: An African-American man living on the East Coast was transferred by his employer to California for 6 months. On his return he complains of having influenza-like symptoms with fever and a cough. He also has red, tender nodules on his shins. His physician suspects that these symptoms are due to coccidioidomycosis, contracted during his stay in California.

7. This patient should be treated immediately with
   (A) None of the following drugs
   (B) Amphotericin B
   (C) Griseofulvin
   (D) Itraconazole
   (E) Ketoconazole

8. Which one of the following drugs is LEAST likely to be useful if this patient is suffering from persistent lung lesions or disseminated disease due to *Coccidioides immitis*?
   (A) Amphotericin B
   (B) Fluconazole
   (C) Ketoconazole
   (D) Itraconazole
   (E) Terbinafine

9. Which one of the following drugs is LEAST likely to be effective in the treatment of esophageal candidiasis if it is used by the oral route?
   (A) Amphotericin B
   (B) Clotrimazole
   (C) Fluconazole
   (D) Griseofulvin
   (E) Ketoconazole

DIRECTIONS (Items 10–14): Each set of matching questions in this section consists of a list of three to twenty-six lettered options (some of which may be figures) followed by several numbered items. For each numbered item, select the ONE lettered option that is most closely associated with it. Each lettered option may be selected once, more than once, or not at all.

   (A) Amphotericin B
   (B) Clotrimazole
   (C) Fluconazole
   (D) Flucytosine
   (E) Griseofulvin
   (F) Itraconazole
   (G) Ketoconazole
   (H) Miconazole
   (I) Nystatin
   (J) Terbinafine

10. After oral administration of this antimetabolite, the cerebrospinal fluid levels achieved are almost as high as plasma levels. Resistance may emerge during the treatment of systemic mycoses if the drug is used as the sole antifungal agent

11. The oral absorption of this drug is impaired by antacids and by histamine H_2 receptor-blocking agents. Cardiac arrhythmias have occurred during concomitant administration of astemizole

12. This drug is fungicidal via inhibition of squalene epoxidase

13. This azole is not a substrate for hepatic drug-metabolizing enzymes; it is eliminated in unchanged form via the kidney

14. Of the drugs listed, this is the most likely to cause anemia due to reduced erythropoietin

ANSWERS

1. The polyene antifungal drugs are amphipathic molecules that can interact with ergosterol in fungal cell membranes to form artificial pores. In these structures, the lipophilic groups on the drug molecule are arranged on the outside of the pore and the hydrophilic regions are located on the inside. The fungicidal action of amphotericin B and nystatin derives from this interaction, which results in leakage of intracellular constituents. The answer is **(D)**.

2. The only azole with activity against *Aspergillus* is itraconazole. Fluconazole is the best-absorbed of the azoles by the oral route and is the only azole that readily penetrates into cerebrospinal fluid. Fluconazole has minimal effects on hepatic cytochrome P450. The answer is **(D)**.

3. The antibiotic regimen should be stopped on the grounds that the condition of the patient had not improved over 3 days of such treatment, the cultures were negative for bacteria, the clinical picture suggested that the patient had a *Candida* infection, and the blood culture results confirmed a fungal infection. Intravenous amphotericin B should be started as soon as possible. The answer is **(E)**.

4. Infusion-related adverse effects of amphotericin B include chills and fevers (the "shake and bake" syndrome), muscle spasms, nausea, headache, and hypotension. Antipyretics, antihistamines, and glucocorticoids have all been shown to be helpful. The administration of a 1 mg test dose of amphotericin B is sometimes useful in predicting the severity of infusion-related toxicity. The answer is **(D)**.

5. Renal toxicity is dose-limiting with amphotericin B. Azotemia is commonplace and sometimes is severe enough to warrant dialysis. Decreases in glomerular filtration rate may be reversible, but irreversible damage can occur, presenting as renal tubular acidosis with hypokalemia and hypomagnesemia. The answer is **(C)**.

6. Infection is a leading cause of death in patients with neutropenia. In the case of opportunistic candidal infections in the immunocompromised patient, no prophylactic drugs have been shown to be effective. Prophylaxis against other fungi may be effective in some instances, including suppression of cryptococcal meningitis in AIDS patients with fluconazole. However, prophylactic use of azoles may be contributory to the development of fungal resistance. The answer is **(E)**.

7. A travel history can be important in the diagnosis of fungal disease. If this patient has a fungal infection of the lungs, it is likely to be due to *C immitis,* which is endemic in dry regions of the western United States. Pulmonary symptoms of coccidioidomycosis are usually self-limiting, and drug therapy is not commonly required. The presence of red, tender nodules on extensor surfaces is a sign of a good prognosis. Erythema nodosum is a delayed hypersensitivity response to fungal antigens. No organisms are present in the lesions, and it is not a sign of disseminated disease. The answer is **(A)**.

8. In progressive or disseminated forms of coccidioidomycosis, systemic antifungal drug treatment is needed. Until recently, amphotericin B was the recommended therapy, but fluconazole may be more suitable in pulmonary disease or in meningitis. The antifungal activity of terbinafine is restricted to dermatophytes. Note that the risk of dissemination is much greater in African-Americans (10% incidence) and in pregnant women during the third trimester. The answer is **(E)**.

9. Griseofulvin has no activity against *Candida albicans* and is not effective in the treatment of systemic or superficial infections caused by such organisms. "Swish and swallow" formulations of clotrimazole and nystatin have been used commonly, and a similar formulation of amphotericin B is now available for use in resistant candidiasis. Most of the azoles are effective in esophageal candidiasis. The answer is **(D)**.

10. Flucytosine is converted to the antimetabolite 5-fluorouracil, which causes inhibition of thymidylate synthase. Flucytosine is usually used in combination with amphotericin B. The answer is **(D)**.

11. An acidic environment is required for the dissolution of ketoconazole. Cardiotoxicity has occurred when ketoconazole was combined with astemizole (or terfenadine), due to the ability of ketoconazole to inhibit hepatic drug-metabolizing enzymes. The answer is **(G)**.

12. Terbinafine has a unique action to interfere with ergosterol synthesis in dermatophytes by causing the intracellular accumulation of squalene to toxic levels. The answer is **(J)**.

13. The pharmacokinetic properties of fluconazole are different from those of other azoles used in systemic fungal infections. It is the azole most reliably absorbed orally; it achieves effective cerebrospinal fluid levels after oral administration; and it is not eliminated by hepatic metabolism. The answer is **(C)**.

14. Damage to renal tubular cells during treatment with amphotericin B can lead to a decreased production of erythropoietin. Hematotoxicity is also an adverse effect of flucytosine due to its myelosuppressant actions. The answer is **(A)**.

Antiviral Chemotherapy & Prophylaxis   **49**

OBJECTIVES

You should be able to:

- Identify the main steps in viral replication.
- Describe the mechanisms of action and of resistance for the major antiherpes drugs.
- Describe the pharmacokinetic properties, the clinical uses, and the toxic effects of the antiherpes drugs.
- Describe the mechanisms of action and of resistance for the major antiretroviral drugs.
- Describe the pharmacokinetic properties, the clinical uses, and the toxic effects of the antiretroviral drugs.
- Identify the significant antiviral properties of amantadine, interferons, and ribavirin.

CONCEPTS

Most clinically useful antiviral agents exert their actions on viral replication, either at the stage of nucleic acid synthesis or at the stage of late protein synthesis and processing (Figure 49–1). With the exception of foscarnet, all of the drugs active against herpesviruses and against the human immunodeficiency virus (HIV) are antimetabolites, structurally similar to naturally occurring compounds. In order to interfere with viral nucleic acid synthesis or the late synthesis of viral proteins, they must first undergo conversion to active forms, usually triphosphate derivatives. For example, drugs such as **zidovudine (AZT)** undergo phosphorylation by host cell kinases to form nucleotide analogs that may

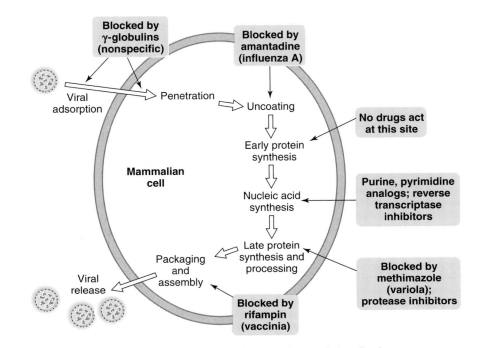

Figure 49–1. The major sites of drug action on viral replication.

359

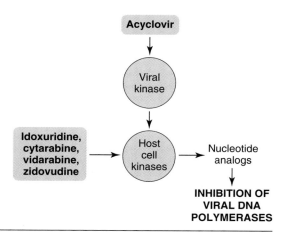

Figure 49–2. Antiviral actions of purine and pyrimidine analogs. Acyclovir (top) is metabolized first by viral kinase to an intermediate. This intermediate and the drugs shown on the left are then metabolized by host cell kinases to nucleotide analogs that inhibit viral replication.

inhibit viral DNA polymerases (Figure 49–2). Selective toxicity results because viral DNA polymerases are more sensitive to inhibition by these antimetabolites than are mammalian polymerases.

Acyclovir is more selectively toxic than the drugs that require phosphorylation only by host cell enzymes. This increased selectivity is partly a result of initial phosphorylation of acyclovir by a *viral* thymidine kinase that is absent in uninfected cells (Figure 49–2, top).

One of the most important recent trends in antiviral chemotherapy has been combination therapy. The strategy is similar to that of cancer chemotherapy where treatment with combinations of drugs can result in greater effectiveness and prevent or delay the emergence of resistance. The limited success of monotherapy in treatment of HIV disease has been the major stimulus to combination antiviral chemotherapy. The current approach to treatment of infection with HIV is the initiation of treatment with two or three drugs, if possible before symptoms appear. When three drugs are used, the combination usually includes two inhibitors of reverse transcriptase plus an inhibitor of HIV protease. Such drug combinations can slow or reverse the increases in viral RNA titers that normally accompany progression of disease. They may also delay the emergence of resistant strains of HIV and provide a survival advantage over traditional monotherapy.

ANTIHERPES DRUGS

A. **Acyclovir (Acycloguanosine):**
1. **Mechanisms:** Acyclovir is a guanosine analog active against herpes simplex virus (HSV) and varicella-zoster virus (VZV). The drug is activated to form acyclovir triphosphate, a competitive substrate for DNA polymerase, leading to chain termination following its incorporation into viral DNA (Figure 49–2). Resistance of herpes can involve changes in viral DNA polymerase. However, many resistant strains of HSV (TK⁻ strains) lack thymidine kinase, the enzyme involved in the initial *virus-specific* phosphorylation of acyclovir. Such strains are cross-resistant to famciclovir, ganciclovir, and valacyclovir.
2. **Pharmacokinetics:** Acyclovir can be administered by the topical, oral, and intravenous routes. Renal excretion is the major route of elimination of acyclovir and dosage should be reduced in patients with renal impairment.
3. **Clinical uses and toxicity:** Oral acyclovir is used for treatment of mucocutaneous and genital herpes lesions and for prophylaxis in AIDS and in other immunocompromised patients (eg, those undergoing organ transplantation). The oral drug is well tolerated but may cause gastrointestinal distress and headache. Intravenous administration is used for severe herpes disease (including encephalitis) and for neonatal HSV infection. Toxic effects with parenteral administration include delirium, tremor, seizures, hypotension, and nephrotoxicity. Acyclovir has no significant toxicity on the bone marrow.
4. **Acyclovir congeners:** Several new antiviral agents have characteristics similar to acyclovir. **Famciclovir** is a prodrug converted to penciclovir by first-pass metabolism in the liver. Used orally in genital herpes and for herpes zoster, famciclovir is well tolerated and

is similar to acyclovir in its pharmacokinetic properties. **Penciclovir** also undergoes activation by viral thymidine kinase, and the triphosphate form inhibits DNA polymerase but does not cause chain termination. **Valacyclovir** is converted to acyclovir by hepatic metabolism after oral administration and reaches plasma levels three to five times greater than those achieved by acyclovir. Valacyclovir has a longer duration of action than acyclovir but is otherwise identical.

B. Foscarnet:
    1. Mechanisms: Foscarnet is a phosphonoformate derivative that does not require phosphorylation for antiviral activity. Though not an antimetabolite, foscarnet inhibits viral RNA polymerase, DNA polymerase, and HIV reverse transcriptase. A known mechanism of resistance involves point mutations in the DNA polymerase gene.
    2. Pharmacokinetics: Foscarnet is given intravenously and penetrates well into tissues, including the CNS. Up to a third of a dose may be deposited in bone. The drug undergoes renal elimination in direct proportion to creatinine clearance.
    3. Clinical uses and toxicity: The drug is used for prophylaxis and treatment of cytomegalovirus (CMV) infections (including CMV retinitis) and has activity against ganciclovir-resistant strains of this virus (Table 49–1). Foscarnet inhibits herpes DNA polymerase in acyclovir-resistant strains that are thymidine kinase-deficient and may suppress such resistant herpetic infections in patients with AIDS. Adverse effects include nephrotoxicity with disturbances in electrolyte balance (especially calcium and phosphate), genitourinary ulceration, and central nervous system symptoms (headache, hallucinations, seizures).

C. Ganciclovir:
    1. Mechanisms: Ganciclovir, a guanine derivative, is triphosphorylated to form a nucleotide that inhibits DNA polymerases of CMV and HSV but does not cause chain termination. The first phosphorylation step is catalyzed by virus-specific enzymes in both CMV- and HSV-infected cells. CMV resistance mechanisms include changes in DNA polymerase and mutations in the gene that codes for the activating viral phosphotransferase. Thymidine kinase-deficient HSV strains are resistant to ganciclovir.
    2. Pharmacokinetics: Ganciclovir is usually given intravenously and penetrates well into tissues, including the eye and the CNS. The drug undergoes renal elimination in direct proportion to creatinine clearance. Although oral bioavailability is less than 10%, an oral formulation is available for maintenance therapy.
    3. Clinical uses and toxicity: Ganciclovir is used for the prophylaxis and treatment of CMV retinitis and other CMV infections in immunocompromised patients. Systemic toxic effects include leukopenia, thrombocytopenia, mucositis, hepatic dysfunction, and seizures. The drug may cause severe neutropenia when used with zidovudine or other myelosuppressive agents.

D. Cidofovir:
    1. Mechanisms and pharmacokinetics: Cidofovir is activated exclusively by host cell kinases and inhibits DNA polymerases of HSV, CMV, adenovirus, and papillomavirus. Resistance is due to mutations in the DNA polymerase gene. The drug has been used by intravenous and topical administration and by intravitreal injection. Cidofovir undergoes renal elimination in proportion to creatinine clearance.

Table 49–1. Major clinical uses of antiviral drugs.

Virus	Drug of Choice	Alternative Drugs
Cytomegalovirus	Ganciclovir	Foscarnet, cidofovir
Hepatitis viruses B and C	Interferon α-2b	Lamivudine
Herpes simplex virus	Acyclovir	Foscarnet, ganciclovir, cidofovir, vidarabine
HIV	Zidovudine, indinavir	Didanosine, lamivudine, zalcitabine
Influenza A	Amantadine	Rimantadine
Respiratory syncytial virus	Ribavirin	
Varicella-zoster virus	Acyclovir	Foscarnet

   2. **Clinical uses and toxicity:**   Cidofovir is effective in CMV retinitis. It may also be valu-
      able in mucocutaneous HSV infections, including those resistant to acyclovir, and in genital
      warts. Nephrotoxicity is the major dose-limiting toxicity.

  E. **Other Antiherpes Drugs:**
   1. **Vidarabine:**   Vidarabine is an adenine analog and has activity against HSV, VZV, and
      CMV. Its use for systemic infections is limited by rapid metabolic inactivation and by
      marked toxic potential. However, it has been used intravenously for severe HSV infections,
      including those resistant to acyclovir, and it also prevents the dissemination of varicella-
      zoster virus in immunocompromised patients. Vidarabine is used topically for herpes kerati-
      tis, but it has no effect on genital lesions. Toxic effects with systemic use include gastroin-
      testinal irritation, paresthesias, tremor, convulsions, and hepatic dysfunction. Vidarabine is
      teratogenic in animals.
   2. **Sorivudine:**   Sorivudine is a pyrimidine analog with activity against HSV-1, VZV, and
      Epstein-Barr virus (EBV). This investigational drug is approximately 1000 times more po-
      tent than acyclovir against HSV strains. However, thymidine-deficient strains of HSV are
      resistant to sorivudine.
   3. **Idoxuridine and trifluridine:**   These pyrimidine analogs are used topically in herpes ker-
      atitis. They are too toxic for systemic use.

ANTI-HIV AGENTS: REVERSE TRANSCRIPTASE INHIBITORS

  A. **Zidovudine (ZDV, AZT):**
   1. **Mechanisms:**   Formerly called azidothymidine, zidovudine is an antimetabolite that re-
      quires triphosphorylation by host cell kinases to form a nucleotide analog that both inhibits
      reverse transcriptase of HIV-1 and HIV-2 and causes chain termination in viral DNA. Re-
      sistance, common in patients with advanced HIV infection, is due to mutations at several
      sites on the *pol* gene, which encodes for several proteins including reverse transcriptase.
   2. **Pharmacokinetics:**   Zidovudine is active orally (with 60% bioavailability) and is dis-
      tributed to most tissues, including the CNS. Elimination of the drug involves both hepatic
      metabolism to glucuronides and renal excretion. Dosage reduction is necessary in uremic
      patients and those with cirrhosis. The half-life of zidovudine is 1–3 hours.
   3. **Clinical uses:**   Zidovudine temporarily reduces mortality and morbidity in patients with
      AIDS and AIDS-related complex. In asymptomatic HIV-positive individuals, zidovudine
      slows the rate of progression to AIDS. Monotherapy is not recommended because of rapid
      emergence of resistance, but zidovudine continues to be the most frequently used reverse
      transcriptase inhibitor in combination drug therapy regimens. Zidovudine is also of value in
      prophylaxis against HIV infection through accidental needle sticks and against vertical
      transmission from mother to neonate.
   4. **Toxicity:**   The primary toxicity is bone marrow suppression leading to anemia and neu-
      tropenia, which may require transfusions. Bone marrow toxicity is additive with other
      myelosuppressants. Gastrointestinal distress, thrombocytopenia, headaches, myalgia, acute
      cholestatic hepatitis, agitation, and insomnia may also occur.
   5. **Drug interactions:**   Drugs that undergo hepatic glucuronidation, including acetaminophen,
      benzodiazepines, cimetidine, and sulfonamides, may increase plasma levels of zidovudine.
      Metabolism of zidovudine may also be inhibited by azole antifungals and by protease in-
      hibitors. Rifampin increases the clearance of zidovudine.

  B. **Didanosine (ddI):**
   1. **Mechanisms:**   Didanosine, an analog of deoxyadenosine, is activated by host cell kinases
      to a triphosphate form that inhibits reverse transcriptase and causes chain termination. Re-
      sistant strains are associated with point mutations of the *pol* gene, and there is complete
      cross-resistance with zalcitabine (ddC) but only partial cross-resistance with zidovudine.
      High-level resistance has not been noted to date.
   2. **Pharmacokinetics and clinical use:**   Oral bioavailability of ddI is reduced by food and
      by chelating agents. The drug is eliminated by glomerular filtration and active tubular se-
      cretion, and the dose must be reduced in patients with renal dysfunction. While the drug
      may slow the progression of AIDS when used as sole anti-HIV therapy, ddI is usually used

in combination regimens with zidovudine, other reverse transcriptase inhibitors, and protease inhibitors.

   3. Toxicity: Pancreatitis is dose-limiting and occurs more frequently in alcoholic patients and those with hypertriglyceridemia. Other adverse effects include peripheral neuropathy, diarrhea, hepatic dysfunction, hyperuricemia, and central nervous system effects.

C. Zalcitabine (ddC):

   1. Mechanisms: Zalcitabine is a pyrimidine nucleoside, and the mechanisms of its inhibition of reverse transcriptase and of resistance development are similar to those of zidovudine and didanosine. Depending on specific sites of mutation on the *pol* gene, resistance may emerge to ddC alone, or cross-resistance between other RT inhibitors may occur. High-level resistance has not been noted to date.

   2. Pharmacokinetics and clinical use: Zalcitabine's bioavailability is high following oral use. Dosage adjustment is needed in patients with renal insufficiency. Zalcitabine is almost always used in combination with other anti-HIV drugs.

   3. Toxicity: Dose-dependent peripheral neuropathy is the major adverse effect of ddC. Pancreatitis, esophageal ulceration, stomatitis, and arthralgias may also occur.

D. Lamivudine (3TC):

   1. Mechanisms: Like other reverse transcriptase inhibitors, lamivudine requires activation by host cell kinases, and the drug is active against HIV-1, including strains resistant to zidovudine. If the drug is used alone, high-level resistance emerges rapidly via mutations on the gene encoding for reverse transcriptase. Lamivudine is also effective in hepatitis B, and HBV nucleic acid is undetectable after treatment for 12 weeks.

   2. Pharmacokinetics and clinical uses: Lamivudine is used orally in combination regimens with zidovudine. Dosage adjustment is needed in patients with renal insufficiency.

   3. Toxicity: Adverse effects of lamivudine are usually mild and include gastrointestinal distress, headache, insomnia, and fatigue.

E. Stavudine (d4T):

   1. Mechanisms: Stavudine is a thymidine analog; its mechanisms of inhibition of reverse transcriptase and of resistance development are similar to those of other reverse transcriptase inhibitors. Depending on specific sites of mutation on the reverse transcriptase gene, resistance may emerge to stavudine alone, or cross-resistance between other reverse transcriptase inhibitors may occur.

   2. Pharmacokinetics and clinical uses: Stavudine is almost always used in combination with zidovudine and other anti-HIV drugs. The drug has good oral bioavailability and penetrates most tissues, including the CNS. Dosage adjustment is needed in renal insufficiency.

   3. Toxicity: Peripheral neuropathy is dose-limiting.

F. Nonnucleosides: Several nonnucleoside inhibitors of reverse transcriptase have been introduced for treatment of HIV infections. These include **delaviridine** and **nevirapine.** Neither drug can be used as monotherapy because of rapid emergence of resistance. In addition, nevirapine has caused a life-threatening rash in AIDS patients. These drugs may have a niche in combination regimens by increasing the efficacy of the nucleoside reverse transcriptase inhibitors.

ANTI-HIV AGENTS: PROTEASE INHIBITORS

A. Indinavir:

   1. Mechanisms: Indinavir inhibits HIV-1 protease, an enzyme that cleaves viral precursor proteins and is critical to the production of mature infectious virions. The protease is encoded by the *pol* gene, and resistance to indinavir is mediated by multiple point mutations. Up to 70% of indinavir-resistant strains are cross-resistant with ritonavir and saquinavir.

   2. Pharmacokinetics and clinical use: Oral bioavailability is good except in the presence of food. Clearance is mainly via the liver, with about 10% renal excretion. Indinavir is recommended for use in conjunction with zidovudine with or without other reverse transcriptase inhibitors.

   3. Toxicity: Nausea, diarrhea, thrombocytopenia, hyperbilirubinemia, and nephrolithiasis occur. To reduce renal damage, it is important to maintain good hydration. Indinavir is a substrate for and inhibitor of the cytochrome P450 isoform CYP3A4 and is implicated in drug interactions. Serum levels of indinavir are increased by azole antifungals and decreased by rifamycins. Indinavir increases the serum levels of antihistamines, benzodiazepines, and rifampin.

B. Ritonavir:

    1. Mechanisms: Mechanisms of action and resistance are quite similar to those of indinavir. Cross-resistance occurs between the two drugs.

    2. Pharmacokinetics and clinical use: Oral bioavailability is good, and the drug should be taken with meals. Clearance is mainly via the liver and dosage reduction is necessary in patients with hepatic impairment. Ritonavir is recommended for use in combination regimens with zidovudine and other reverse transcriptase inhibitors.

    3. Toxicity: The most common adverse effects of the drug are gastrointestinal irritation and a bitter taste. Paresthesias and elevations of hepatic aminotransferases and triglycerides in the plasma also occur. Drug interactions are of major concern. Drugs that increase the activity of the cytochrome P450 isoform CYP3A4 (anticonvulsants, rifamycins) lower serum levels of ritonavir, and drugs that inhibit this enzyme (azole antifungals, cimetidine, erythromycin) elevate serum levels of the antiviral drug. Ritonavir inhibits the metabolism of a wide range of drugs, including dronabinol, erythromycin, ketoconazole, prednisone, rifampin, and saquinavir.

C. Saquinavir:

    1. Mechanisms: The mechanism of action and resistance of saquinavir are similar to those of the other protease inhibitors. Cross-resistance is not common, and saquinavir-resistant strains usually retain susceptibility to indinavir.

    2. Pharmacokinetics and clinical use: Saquinavir must be taken with meals to avoid gastrointestinal distress and has only 4% oral bioavailability. The drug has additive or synergistic effects against HIV-1 when used in combination with reverse transcriptase inhibitors.

    3. Toxicity: In addition to marked gastrointestinal effects, saquinavir may cause headache and neutropenia. Serum levels of the drug are increased by ingestion of ketoconazole, ritonavir, or grapefruit juice.

D. Nelfinavir: This recently introduced protease inhibitor causes significant reductions in HIV blood titer when used in combination with zidovudine. It may prove to be of value when other protease inhibitors are ineffective or contraindicated.

MISCELLANEOUS ANTIVIRAL AGENTS

A. Amantadine and Rimantidine:

    1. Mechanisms: Amantadine and rimantidine inhibit the first steps in the replication of the influenza A and rubella viruses (Figure 49–1). These steps involve viral adsorption to the host cell membrane, penetration into the cell via endocytosis, and virus particle uncoating. The inhibitory action of these drugs may be due to their alkaline reaction, which raises the endosomal pH. At low concentrations, amantadine also binds to a specific protein in the surface coat of the influenza virus to prevent fusion. Drug-resistant influenza A virus mutants can emerge and infect contacts of patients in treatment.

    2. Clinical uses and toxicity: These drugs are prophylactic with 80% efficacy against influenza A virus infection. They can reduce the duration of symptoms if given within 48 hours after contact. Toxic effects include gastrointestinal irritation, dizziness, ataxia, and slurred speech. Rimantadine has activity equal to that of amantadine, but it has a longer half-life and requires no dosage adjustment in renal failure.

B. Interferons:

    1. Mechanisms: Interferons are glycoproteins produced in human leukocytes (IFN-α), fibroblasts (IFN-β), and immune cells (IFN-γ). They exert multiple actions that affect viral RNA and DNA synthesis. Interferons induce the formation of enzymes, including a protein kinase that phosphorylates a factor that blocks peptide chain initiation, a phosphodiesterase that degrades terminal nucleotides of tRNA, and enzymes that activate RNase.

2. **Clinical use and toxicity:** Interferon-α is approved for use in chronic hepatitis A and B infections, Kaposi's sarcoma, papillomatosis, and topically for genital warts. Another possible use of interferons is to prevent herpes zoster virus dissemination in cancer patients. Toxic effects include dose-limiting neutropenia, gastrointestinal irritation, fatigue, myalgia, mental confusion, and a reversible cardiomyopathy.

C. **Ribavirin:**
1. **Mechanisms:** Although the precise antiviral mechanism of ribavirin is not known, the drug inhibits guanosine triphosphate formation, prevents capping of viral mRNA, and can block RNA-dependent RNA polymerases.
2. **Clinical use and toxicity:** Ribavirin is used in aerosol form for respiratory syncytial virus infections and may shorten the symptoms of influenza A and B infections. Early intravenous administration decreases mortality in Lassa fever and other viral hemorrhagic fevers. Aerosol ribavirin may cause conjunctival or bronchial irritation. Systemic use results in dose-dependent myelosuppression.

D. **Topical Antiviral Drugs:** Several antiviral agents with marked systemic toxicity (bone marrow, hepatic, renal) are used mainly as topical drugs for herpes simplex eye infections, including corneal keratitis. These drugs include three antimetabolites: **idoxuridine, cytarabine,** and **trifluridine.**

DRUG LIST

The following drugs are important members of the group discussed in this chapter. Prototypes should be learned in detail; features of the other significant agents should be known well enough to distinguish them from the prototypes and from each other.

Subclass	Prototype	Other Significant Agents
Antiherpes drugs Topical	Idoxuridine	Trifluridine
Systemic (HSV, VZV)	Acyclovir	Famciclovir, valacyclovir
Systemic (CMV)	Ganciclovir	Foscarnet, cidofovir
Anti-HIV drugs Reverse transcriptase inhibitors	Zidovudine	Didanosine, lamivudine, stavudine, zalcitabine
Protease inhibitors	Indinavir	Ritonavir, saquinavir
Miscellaneous drugs	Amantadine, interferons, ribavirin	Rimantadine

QUESTIONS

DIRECTIONS: Each of the numbered items or incomplete statements in this section is followed by answers or by completions of the statement. Select the ONE lettered answer or completion that is BEST in each case.

1. Which one of the following statements about the mechanisms of action of antiviral drugs is LEAST accurate?
(A) The initial step in activation of famciclovir in HSV-infected cells is its phosphorylation by viral thymidine kinase
(B) The reverse transcriptase of HIV is 30–50 times more sensitive to inhibition by indinavir than host cell DNA polymerases
(C) Ganciclovir inhibits viral DNA polymerase but does not cause chain termination
(D) Increased activity of host cell phosphodiesterases that degrade tRNA is one of the antiviral actions of interferons
(E) Foscarnet has no requirement for activation by phosphorylation

Items 2–3: A 30-year-old male patient who is HIV-positive has a CD4 count of 500/μL and a viral RNA concentration of 5000 copies/mL. His treatment involves a three-drug antiviral regimen consisting of zidovudine, didanosine, and saquinavir. Because of weight loss, he is taking dronabinol. Nystatin had been used for oral candidiasis, but for the past week the patient has been taking ketoconazole. He now complains of anorexia, nausea and vomiting, and abdominal pain. His abdomen is tender in the epigastric area. Lab results reveal an amylase activity of 220 units/L and a preliminary diagnosis is made of acute pancreatitis.

2. If this patient has acute pancreatitis, the drug most likely to be responsible is
    (A) Didanosine
    (B) Dronabinol
    (C) Ketoconazole
    (D) Saquinavir
    (E) Zidovudine

3. In the further treatment of this patient, the drug causing the pancreatitis should be terminated and replaced by
    (A) Acyclovir
    (B) Ganciclovir
    (C) Indinavir
    (D) Lamivudine
    (E) Trifluridine

4. Which one of the following statements about antiviral agents is LEAST accurate?
    (A) Interferons may prevent dissemination of herpes zoster in cancer patients and reduce CMV shedding after renal transplantation
    (B) The oral absorption of acyclovir is slow and incomplete, but this process is not affected by foods
    (C) Dosage modification of amantadine is required in renal insufficiency
    (D) Peripheral neuropathy is the major dose-limiting toxic effect of ganciclovir
    (E) Topical use of vidarabine requires caution during pregnancy because systemic absorption occurs, and the drug is potentially mutagenic and teratogenic

5. In an accidental needle stick, an unknown quantity of blood from an AIDS patient is injected into a nurse. The most recent lab data on the AIDS patient shows a CD4 count of 20/μL and a viral RNA concentration of $> 10^7$ copies/mL. The most appropriate course of action regarding treatment of the nurse is to
    (A) Monitor the nurse's blood to see if HIV transmission has occurred
    (B) Treat him with full doses of zidovudine for 2 weeks
    (C) Treat him with full doses of zidovudine for 4 weeks
    (D) Add acyclovir to the 4-week zidovudine regimen
    (E) Administer zidovudine with lamivudine for 4 weeks

Items 6–7: A patient with AIDS has a CD4 count of 45/μL. He is being maintained on a three-drug regimen of indinavir, zalcitabine, and zidovudine. For prophylaxis against opportunistic infections he is also receiving cidofovir, fluconazole, rifabutin, and trimethoprim-sulfamethoxazole.

6. The drug most likely to be suppress herpetic infections in this patient and provide prophylaxis against CMV retinitis is
    (A) Cidofovir
    (B) Fluconazole
    (C) Indinavir
    (D) Rifabutin
    (E) Zalcitabine

7. The plasma levels of indinavir in this patient will be considerably lower than those achieved if indinavir is given as the sole drug. The reason for this is that
    (A) Cidofovir increases the renal clearance of other drugs
    (B) Indinavir must be taken with meals
    (C) Rifabutin increases liver drug-metabolizing enzymes
    (D) Sulfamethoxazole displaces indinavir from plasma proteins
    (E) Zidovudine slows gastric emptying

8. Which of the following drugs is most likely to cause additive anemia and neutropenia if administered to an AIDS patient taking zidovudine?
    (A) Acyclovir

    (B) Amantadine
    (C) Ganciclovir
    (D) Pentamidine
    (E) Stavudine

Items 9–10: A 27-year-old nursing mother is diagnosed as suffering from herpes simplex genitalis. She has a prior history of this viral infection. Previously, she responded to a drug used topically. Apart from her current problem, she is in good health.

  9. Which of the following drugs is most likely to be prescribed at this time?
    (A) Acyclovir
    (B) Amantadine
    (C) Foscarnet
    (D) Ritonavir
    (E) Trifluridine

 10. Which one of the following statements about the drug management of herpes simplex genitalis in this patient is LEAST accurate?
    (A) Topical administration of the antiviral drug will provide minimal clinical benefit
    (B) Oral use of the antiviral drug will reduce pain and shorten the duration of disease manifestations
    (C) It is probably advisable to terminate use of the antiviral drug if she becomes pregnant
    (D) Prompt intravenous treatment with the antiviral drug will prevent recurrent disease
    (E) She should not breast-feed the infant while taking the antiviral drug

DIRECTIONS (Items 11–15): Each set of matching questions in this section consists of a list of three to twenty-six lettered options (some of which may be figures) followed by several numbered items. For each numbered item, select the ONE lettered option that is most closely associated with it. Each lettered option may be selected once, more than once, or not at all.

    (A) Acyclovir
    (B) Amantadine
    (C) Foscarnet
    (D) Ganciclovir
    (E) Indinavir
    (F) Interferon alfa
    (G) Ribavirin
    (H) Ritonavir
    (I) Stavudine
    (J) Zalcitabine
    (K) Zidovudine

 11. The antiviral actions of this drug include inhibition of both RNA and DNA synthesis. The drug is used for the treatment of severe respiratory syncytial virus infections in neonates
 12. At the initiation of therapy with this drug, most patients experience a flu-like syndrome. Its clinical uses include the treatment of Kaposi's sarcoma, hairy cell leukemias, and genital warts
 13. Over 90% of this drug is excreted in the urine in intact form. Because its urinary solubility is low, patients should be well hydrated to prevent nephrotoxicity
 14. In prophylaxis against influenza A, this drug has efficacy equivalent to that of vaccines
 15. This thymidine analog has excellent oral bioavailability. Its major dose-limiting toxicity is peripheral sensory neuropathy

ANSWERS

   1. Indinavir is an inhibitor of HIV protease and has no significant effect on reverse transcriptase. Note that initial monophosphorylation by viral thymidine kinase is a characteristic of the activation not only of acyclovir but also of its congeners famciclovir and valacyclovir. The answer is **(B).**
   2. Gastrointestinal problems occur with most antiviral drugs used in the HIV-positive patient, and acute pancreatitis has been reported for several reverse transcriptase inhibitors. However, didanosine is the drug most likely to be responsible, since its most characteristic adverse effect is a dose-limiting acute pancreatitis. Other risk factors that are relative contraindications to didanosine are advanced AIDS, hypertriglyceridemia, and alcoholism. The answer is **(A).**

3. Acyclovir and ganciclovir have minimal activity against retroviruses and would not be useful components of a three-drug anti-HIV regimen. Use of a second protease inhibitor (indinavir) has not yet been shown to be as effective as regimens that include two reverse transcriptase inhibitors and will greatly increase the possibility of drug interactions. Trifluridine is a topical antiherpes drug. Lamivudine (3TC) is known to have additive effects with zidovudine and would be the best choice for replacement in this case. The answer is **(D)**.

4. The adverse effects of ganciclovir are similar to those caused by radiation therapy. The major dose-limiting adverse effects—myelosuppression, gastrointestinal distress, and mucositis—occur commonly. The toxic effects of ganciclovir are enhanced by concomitant administration of other drugs that suppress bone marrow. The answer is **(D)**.

5. The viral RNA concentration in the blood from the AIDS patient in this case is very high, and needle stick must be regarded as a high-risk event. While giving full doses of zidovudine for 4 weeks has been shown to have prophylactic value, combination regimens are favored in high-risk situations. Optimal prophylaxis in this case might best be provided by the combination of zidovudine with lamivudine, and some experts would advise adding a protease inhibitor. The answer is **(E)**.

6. Foscarnet and ganciclovir have been the most commonly used drugs for prevention and treatment of CMV infections in the immunocompromised patient. Foscarnet has activity also against thymidine kinase-deficient strains of HSV. Cidofovir is very effective in CMV retinitis and has good activity against many strains of herpesviruses, including those resistant to acyclovir. The answer is **(A)**.

7. Drug interactions can be severe in the immunocompromised patient, since many of the drugs administered can influence the pharmacokinetic properties of other drugs. Rifabutin, like rifampin, acts as an inducer of several isoforms of hepatic cytochrome P450. This action can result in increased clearance of other drugs, including indinavir, decreasing their usefulness. Cidofovir is more likely to decrease the renal clearance of other drugs since nephrotoxicity is dose-limiting. The answer is **(C)**.

8. Like zidovudine, ganciclovir is myelosuppressant, and over 40% of patients treated with ganciclovir as a single agent develop granulocytopenia or thrombocytopenia. When the two drugs are coadministered, there is a much higher incidence of anemia and neutropenia. Colony stimulating factors may be needed if the two drugs must be given together. None of the other drugs listed have significant hematotoxicity. The answer is **(C)**.

9. Three of the drugs listed (acyclovir, foscarnet, trifluridine) are active against strains of herpes simplex virus. Foscarnet is not used in genital infections (HSV-2) because clinical efficacy has not been established and the drug causes many toxic effects. Trifluridine is used topically but only for herpetic keratoconjunctivitis (HSV-1). The answer is **(A)**.

10. First episodes of genital HSV usually respond to topical acyclovir, but oral or parenteral administration is necessary to treat recurrent disease. Acyclovir treatment, by any mode of administration, does not eradicate latent herpes and will not prevent recurrence of the disease. Note that the drug is secreted in breast milk and, while there are no reports of human teratogenicity, acyclovir is a potential mutagen. The answer is **(D)**.

11. The antiviral actions of ribavirin include inhibition of RNA polymerases, inhibition of DNA and RNA synthesis, and interference with viral coating. Ribavirin is used by aerosol inhalation for respiratory syncytial virus infections in premature infants and children with cardiopulmonary disease. The answer is **(G)**.

12. Headache, fever, chills, and muscle aches are common side effects of treatment with interferons. Patients are advised to take acetaminophen, since aspirin aggravates gastrointestinal irritation and may promote bleeding. Interferons may also cause neurotoxicity, cardiovascular dysfunction, and bone marrow depression. The answer is **(F)**.

13. Acyclovir is eliminated in the urine by glomerular filtration and by active tubular secretion, which is inhibited by probenecid. Nephrotoxic effects, including hematuria and crystalluria, are enhanced in patients who are dehydrated or who have preexisting renal dysfunction. The answer is **(A)**.

14. In high-risk persons oral amantadine reduces the risk of influenza A infection by 70–90%. This is in the same range of effectiveness as that of influenza vaccines. The answer is **(B)**.

15. Stavudine (d4T) is a thymidine analog with activity against the reverse transcriptase of HIV-1. While it has only minor hematotoxic potential, the drug is markedly neurotoxic. Peripheral neuropathy may also occur with other reverse transcriptase inhibitors, including didanosine and zidovudine, but such toxicity is not dose-limiting in the case of these drugs. The answer is **(I)**.

Miscellaneous Antimicrobial Agents & Urinary Antiseptics

50

OBJECTIVES

You should be able to:

- Describe the antibacterial actions, clinical uses, and toxicities of metronidazole, mupirocin, and polymyxins.
- Identify nitrofurantoin, methenamine, and nalidixic acid as urinary antiseptics and describe their toxic effects.
- List the compounds used as antiseptics and disinfectants and describe their advantages and disadvantages.

Learn the definitions that follow.

Table 50–1. Definitions.

Term	Definition
Antiseptic	An agent used to inhibit bacterial growth in vitro and in vivo
Disinfectant	An agent used to kill microorganisms in an inanimate environment
Sterilization	Procedures that kill microorganisms on instruments and dressings; methods include autoclaving, dry heat, and exposure to ethylene oxide
Chlorine demand	The amount of chlorine bound to organic matter in water and thus unavailable for antimicrobial activity

MISCELLANEOUS ANTIMICROBIAL AGENTS

A. **Metronidazole:**
  1. **Mechanisms and pharmacokinetics:** Metronidazole is an imidazole derivative with activity against protozoa and bacteria. The drug undergoes a reductive bioactivation of its nitro group by ferredoxin (present in anaerobic parasites) to form reactive cytotoxic products that interfere with nucleic acid synthesis.
  2. **Pharmacokinetics:** Metronidazole is effective orally and is distributed widely to tissues, achieving CSF levels similar to those in the blood. The drug can also be given intravenously. Elimination of metronidazole requires hepatic metabolism, and dosage reduction may be needed in patients with liver dysfunction.
  3. **Clinical use:** As an antibacterial agent, metronidazole has greatest activity against *Bacteroides* and *Clostridium*. Metronidazole is the drug of choice for treatment of pseudomembranous colitis due to *C difficile* and is effective in anaerobic or mixed intra-abdominal infections and in brain abscess. Metronidazole is the antiprotozoal drug of choice in trichomoniasis and is important in the treatment of intestinal amebiasis and amebic hepatic abscess.
  4. **Toxicity:** Adverse effects include gastrointestinal irritation, headache, and discoloration of urine. More serious toxicity includes leukopenia, dizziness, and ataxia. Drug interactions with metronidazole include a disulfiram-like reaction with ethanol and potentiation of coumarin anticoagulant effects. Although it is not contraindicated in pregnancy, the drug should be used with caution because of teratogenic effects of high doses in rodents.

B. **Mupirocin:**
  1. **Mechanisms:** Mupirocin is a fermentation product of *Pseudomonas fluorescens* and is unrelated to any other antimicrobial drug. It acts on gram-positive cocci and inhibits protein

369

synthesis by specifically binding to isoleucyl-tRNA synthetase. Low level resistance involves point mutations on a noninducible gene for this enzyme, and high-level resistance results from increased expression of a second, plasmid-encoded gene.

2. **Pharmacokinetics and clinical use:** Mupirocin is used topically and is not absorbed. This drug is indicated for impetigo caused by staphylococci (including methicillin-resistant strains), beta-hemolytic streptococci, and *Streptococcus pyogenes.* It is also used intranasally to eliminate staphylococcal carriage by patients and medical personnel.

3. **Toxicity:** Local itching and burning sensations are common. Mupirocin may also cause rash, erythema, and contact dermatitis.

C. Polymyxins:

1. **Mechanisms:** The polymyxins are fatty acid-containing basic polypeptides that are bactericidal against gram-negative bacteria. These drugs interact with a specific lipopolysaccharide component of the outer cell membrane that is also a binding site for calcium. Membrane lipid structure is distorted, with an increase in permeability to polar molecules, resulting in marked changes in cell metabolism.

2. **Clinical uses:** Because of their toxicity, the clinical applications of the polymyxins are limited to topical therapy of resistant gram-negative infections, including those caused by *Enterobacter* and *Pseudomonas.* These drugs are occasionally administered into infected cavities, eg, the joints and the pleural and peritoneal cavities.

3. **Toxicity:** If the polymyxins are absorbed into the systemic circulation, adverse effects include neurotoxicity (paresthesias, dizziness, ataxia) and acute renal tubular necrosis (hematuria, proteinuria, nitrogen retention).

URINARY ANTISEPTICS

Urinary antiseptics are oral drugs that are rapidly excreted into the urine and act there to suppress bacteriuria. The drugs lack systemic antibacterial effects but may be toxic. Urinary antiseptics are often administered with acidifying agents, because low pH is an independent inhibitor of bacterial growth in urine.

A. Nitrofurantoin: This drug is active against many urinary tract pathogens (but not *Proteus* or *Pseudomonas*), and resistance emerges slowly. Single daily doses of the drug can prevent recurrent urinary tract infections. The drug is active orally and is excreted in the urine via filtration and secretion; toxic levels may occur in the blood of patients with renal dysfunction. Adverse effects of nitrofurantoin include gastrointestinal irritation, skin rashes, neuropathies, and hemolysis in patients with glucose-6-phosphate dehydrogenase deficiency.

B. Nalidixic Acid: This quinolone drug acts against many gram-negative organisms (but not *Proteus* or *Pseudomonas*) by mechanisms that may involve acidification or inhibition of DNA gyrase. Resistance emerges rapidly. The drug is active orally and is excreted in the urine partly unchanged and partly as the inactive glucuronide. Toxic effects include gastrointestinal irritation, glycosuria, skin rashes, photosensitization, visual disturbances, and CNS stimulation.

C. Methenamine: Methenamine mandelate and methenamine hippurate combine urine acidification with the release of the antibacterial compound formaldehyde at pH levels below 5.5. These drugs are not usually active against *Proteus* because those organisms alkalinize the urine. Insoluble complexes form between formaldehyde and sulfonamides, and the drugs should not be used together.

DISINFECTANTS & ANTISEPTICS

Although the terms are often used interchangeably, a **disinfectant** is a compound that is used to kill microorganisms in an inanimate environment, whereas an **antiseptic** is one that is used to inhibit bacterial growth both in vitro and upon contact with the surfaces of living tissues. Disinfectants and antiseptics do not have selective toxicity, and their clinical use is therefore limited. Most antiseptics delay wound healing.

A. **Alcohols, Aldehydes, and Acids:** **Ethanol** (70%) and **isopropanol** (70–90%) are effective skin antiseptics because they denature microbial proteins. **Formaldehyde,** which also denatures proteins, is too irritating for topical use but is a disinfectant for instruments. **Acetic acid** (1%) is used in surgical dressings and has activity against gram-negative bacteria, including *Pseudomonas,* when used as a urinary irrigant and in the external ear. **Salicylic acid** and **undecylenic acid** are useful in the treatment of dermatophyte infections.

B. **Halogens:** **Iodine tincture** is an effective antiseptic for intact skin and, though it can cause dermatitis, is commonly used in preparing the skin before taking blood samples. Iodine complexed with povidone **(povidone-iodine)** is widely used, particularly as a preoperative skin antiseptic, but solutions can become contaminated with aerobic gram-negative bacteria.

 Hypochlorous acid, formed when **chlorine** dissolves in water, is antimicrobial. This is the basis for the use of chlorine and **halazone** in water purification. Organic matter binds chlorine, thus preventing antimicrobial actions. In a given water sample, this process is referred to as the **"chlorine demand,"** since the chlorine-binding capacity of the organic material must be exceeded before bacterial killing is accomplished. Many preparations of chlorine for water purification do not eradicate all bacteria or *Entamoeba* cysts.

 Sodium hypochlorite is the active component in household bleach, a 1:10 dilution of which is recommended by the CDC for the disinfection of blood spills that may contain HIV or hepatitis B virus (HBV).

C. **Oxidizing Agents:** **Hydrogen peroxide** exerts a short-lived antimicrobial action through the release of molecular oxygen. The agent is used as a mouthwash, for cleansing wounds, and for disinfection of contact lenses. **Potassium permanganate** is an effective bactericidal agent but has the disadvantage of causing persistent brown stains on skin and clothing.

D. **Heavy Metals:** **Mercury** and **silver** precipitate proteins and inactivate sulfhydryl groups of enzymes, but because of their toxicity they are rarely used. Organic mercurials such as **nitromersol** and **thimerosal** frequently cause hypersensitivity reactions, but they continue to be used as preservatives for vaccines, antitoxins, and immune sera. **Merbromin** is a weak antiseptic and stains tissues a bright red color. **Silver nitrate** was commonly used at one time for prevention of neonatal gonococcal ophthalmia, but it has been largely replaced by topical antibiotics. **Silver sulfadiazine** (a sulfonamide) is used to decrease bacterial colonization in burns.

E. **Chlorinated Phenols:** Because of its toxicity, **phenol** itself is used only as a disinfectant of inanimate objects. Mixtures of phenolic derivatives are used in antiseptics but can cause skin irritation. **Hexachlorophene** has been widely used in surgical scrub routines and in deodorant soaps, where it forms antibacterial deposits on the skin, decreasing the population of resident bacteria. Repeated use on the skin in infants can lead to absorption of the drug, resulting in CNS white matter degeneration. Antiseptic soaps may also contain other chlorinated phenols such as **triclocarban** and **chlorhexidine.** Chlorhexidine is mainly active against gram-positive cocci and is commonly used in hospital scrub routines to cleanse skin sites. All antiseptic soaps may cause allergies or photosensitization.

 Lindane (gamma benzene hexachloride) is used to treat infestations with mites or lice and as an agricultural insecticide. The agent can be absorbed through the skin; if excessive amounts are applied, toxic effects, including blood dyscrasias and convulsions, may occur.

F. **Cationic Surfactants:** **Benzalkonium chloride** and **cetylpyridinium chloride** are used as disinfectants of surgical instruments and surfaces such as floors and bench-tops. Since they are effective against most bacteria and fungi and are not irritating, they are also used as antiseptics. However, when they are used on the skin, the antimicrobial action of these agents is antagonized by soaps and multivalent cations. Recently, the CDC recommended that benzalkonium chloride and similar quaternary compounds *not* be used as antiseptics because outbreaks of infection have occurred as a result of growth of gram-negative bacteria (eg, *Pseudomonas*) in such antiseptic solutions.

DRUG LIST

The following drugs are important members of the group discussed in this chapter. Prototypes should be learned in detail; features of the major variants should be known well enough so that the variants can be distinguished from prototypes and from each other.

Subclass	Prototype	Major Variants
Miscellaneous antimicrobials		
Nitroimidazoles	Metronidazole	
Pseudomonic acid	Mupirocin	
Basic peptides	Polymyxin B	Polymyxin E
Urinary tract antiseptics		
Quinolones	Nalidixic acid	Cinoxacin
Methenamine salts	Methenamine mandelate	Methenamine hippurate
Nitrofurans	Nitrofurantoin	
Disinfectants and antiseptics		
Alcohols, aldehydes, and acids	Ethanol, formaldehyde, acetic acid	Isopropanol, glutaraldehyde, salicylic acid
Halogens	Iodine, chlorine	Povidone-iodide, halazone, sodium hypochlorite (household bleach)
Heavy metals	Silver nitrate, mercury bichloride	Silver sulfadiazine, nitromersol, thimerosal
Chlorinated phenols	Hexachlorophene	Triclocarban, chlorhexidine
Cationic surfactants	Benzalkonium chloride	Cetylpyridinium chloride

QUESTIONS

DIRECTIONS: Each of the numbered items or incomplete statements in this section is followed by answers or by completions of the statement. Select the ONE lettered answer or completion that is BEST in each case.

1. Infections due to gram-negative bacilli have occurred when this agent has been used as a skin antiseptic.
   (A) Acetic acid
   (B) Benzalkonium chloride
   (C) Hexachlorophene
   (D) Merbromin
   (E) Thimerosal

Items 2–3: A young woman with no past medical problems is brought to a hospital emergency room with intense abdominal pain of 2 days' duration. The pain has spread to the right lower quadrant and is accompanied by nausea, vomiting, and fever. In the ER, her blood pressure is 85/45 mm Hg, pulse 120/min, and temperature 40 °C. Her abdomen has a board-like rigidity with diffuse pain to palpation. Lab values include WBC 20,000/μL and creatinine 1.5 mg/dL. Following abdominal x-rays, a preliminary diagnosis is made of abdominal sepsis, possibly due to bowel perforation. After appropriate samples are sent to the lab for culture, the patient is hospitalized and antimicrobial therapy is started with intravenous ampicillin and gentamicin.

2. Regarding the treatment of this patient, which one of the following statements is most accurate?
   (A) Cultures are pointless, since this is probably a mixed infection
   (B) A Gram-stained smear of blood would provide positive identification of the specific organism involved in this infection
   (C) Metronidazole should be included in the antibiotic regimen
   (D) Empiric antimicrobial therapy of abdominal sepsis should always include a third-generation cephalosporin
   (E) The combination of ampicillin and gentamicin provides good coverage for all likely pathogens

3. If the antibiotic regimen in this patient is modified to include metronidazole,
   (A) The patient should be monitored for candidiasis
   (B) Gentamicin should be excluded from the regimen
   (C) Metronidazole should not be used intravenously
   (D) Ampicillin should be excluded from the regimen
   (E) Coverage will be extended to methicillin-resistant staphylococci

4. Which one of the following compounds is used topically to treat scabies and pediculosis?
   (A) Lindane
   (B) Mupirocin
   (C) Nitrofurazone
   (D) Polymyxin B
   (E) Silver sulfadiazine

5. Methenamine salts are used as urinary antiseptics. The reason why they lack systemic antibacterial action is that they are
   (A) Not absorbed into the systemic circulation following oral ingestion
   (B) Rapidly metabolized by liver drug-metabolizing enzymes
   (C) Converted to formaldehyde only at low urinary pH
   (D) Substrates for active tubular secretion
   (E) Over 98% bound to plasma proteins

6. Which one of the following statements about the actions of antimicrobial agents is LEAST accurate?
   (A) Polymyxins act as cationic detergents to disrupt bacterial cell membranes
   (B) Resistance to nitrofurantoin emerges rapidly, and there is cross-resistance with sulfonamides
   (C) Salicylic acid has useful antidermatophyte activity when applied topically
   (D) Neonatal gonococcal ophthalmia can be prevented by silver nitrate
   (E) Isoleucyl-tRNA synthetase is inhibited by mupirocin

7. Which one of the following antiseptics *promotes* wound healing?
   (A) Cetylpyridinium chloride
   (B) Chlorhexidine
   (C) Hexachlorophene
   (D) Iodine
   (E) None of the above

8. A 22-year-old man with gonorrhea is to be treated with cefixime and will need another drug to provide coverage for possible urethritis due to *C trachomatis*. Which one of the following drugs is LEAST likely to be effective in nongonococcal urethritis?
   (A) Azithromycin
   (B) Ciprofloxacin
   (C) Erythromycin
   (D) Nitrofurantoin
   (E) Tetracycline

9. A patient with AIDS has an extremely high viral RNA load. While blood is being drawn from this patient, the syringe is accidentally dropped, contaminating the floor, which is made of porous material. The best way to deal with this is to
   (A) Completely replace the contaminated part of the floor
   (B) Clean the floor with soap and water
   (C) Seal the room and decontaminate with ethylene oxide
   (D) Clean the floor with a 10% solution of household bleach
   (E) Neutralize the spill with a solution of potassium permanganate

DIRECTIONS (Items 10–16):   Each set of matching questions in this section consists of a list of three to twenty-six lettered options (some of which may be figures) followed by several numbered items. For each numbered item, select the ONE lettered option that is most closely associated with it. Each lettered option may be selected once, more than once, or not at all.
   (A) Benzalkonium chloride
   (B) Chlorhexidine

    (C) Formaldehyde
    (D) Halazone
    (E) Hexachlorophene
    (F) Methenamine
    (G) Metronidazole
    (H) Nalidixic acid
    (I) Nitrofurantoin
    (J) Polymyxin B
    (K) Salicylic acid

10. This compound is used in tablet form to purify drinking water. If a large quantity of organic material is present, cysts of *Entamoeba histolytica* may not be eradicated

11. This agent has activity against gram-negative bacteria in urinary tract infections, but resistance may develop during the course of treatment. There is cross-resistance with cinoxacin. The drug has no useful systemic antibacterial effects

12. Daily use of this substituted phenol results in a bacteriostatic deposit on the skin. The compound may be absorbed and has caused neurotoxic effects in neonates when used as an antistaphylococcal agent

13. Neuropathies are more likely to occur with this agent when it is used in patients with renal dysfunction. The drug may cause acute hemolysis in patients with G6PD deficiency

14. This agent is commonly incorporated into soaps used for skin antisepsis and surgical scrub procedures. The compound has minimal activity against *Pseudomonas* and *Serratia*

15. A urinary antiseptic, this agent is not effective in the treatment of urinary tract infections caused by *Proteus*. Mutual antagonism may occur if this drug is used concomitantly with sulfonamides

16. Consumption of ethanol together with this drug will cause nausea, vomiting, abdominal cramps, flushing, and headache in some patients

ANSWERS

1. *Pseudomonas* and other gram-negative bacteria have caused infections following the use of cationic surfactants, partly because they form a film on the skin under which microorganisms can survive. In addition, some gram-negative bacilli are able to grow in solutions containing benzalkonium salts. Bacterial growth may also occur in solutions of povidone-iodine. The answer is **(B)**.

2. Abdominal sepsis is commonly a mixed infection, with the most likely pathogens being *Bacteroides fragilis,* Enterobacteriaceae, and *Enterococcus faecalis.* An antibiotic regimen that includes only ampicillin and gentamicin will not control *B fragilis.* Empiric treatment in this case should include a drug active against this pathogen—eg, metronidazole, cefoxitin, cefotetan, clindamycin, or imipenem. The answer is **(C)**.

3. Fungal superinfections, especially from *Candida albicans,* occur quite frequently during treatment with metronidazole. In most cases of abdominal sepsis, metronidazole would be given by slow intravenous infusion. Both ampicillin and gentamicin should be maintained until the infection is controlled, at which point surgery is indicated. Metronidazole has no activity against aerobes. The combination of ampicillin, gentamicin, and metronidazole does not provide coverage for methicillin-resistant staphylococci. The answer is **(A)**.

4. Of the agents listed, only lindane is an effective scabicide and pediculicide. There is some concern about the systemic absorption of topically applied lindane, which may cause neurotoxicity. Accidental ingestion has caused seizures in children. The answer is **(A)**.

5. Below pH 5.5 methenamine releases formaldehyde, which is antibacterial. This pH is achieved in the urine but nowhere else in the body. Ascorbic acid is sometimes given with methenamine salts when they are used in urinary tract infections to ensure a low urinary pH. The answer is **(C)**.

6. Clinical drug resistance emerges very slowly when nitrofurantoin is used as a urinary antiseptic. There is no cross-resistance between this drug and other drugs used in the treatment of bacterial infections of the urinary tract. The answer is **(B)**.

7. No antiseptic in current use is able to promote wound healing, and most agents do the opposite. In general, cleansing of abrasions and superficial wounds with soap and water is just as effective as and less damaging than the application of topical antiseptics. The answer is **(E)**.

8. Urinary tract infections due to *C trachomatis* are likely to respond to all of the drugs listed except nitrofurantoin. However, nitrofurantoin is effective against many bacterial urinary tract pathogens with the exception of *Pseudomonas aeruginosa* and strains of *Proteus*. The answer is **(D)**.

9. Household bleach contains sodium hypochlorite. A 1:10 dilution of bleach is effective for disinfection of a direct blood spill on a porous surface. In addition to inactivating HIV, sodium hypochlorite solutions also have disinfectant activity against other viruses, including hepatitis B virus. The answer is **(D)**.

10. The addition of 4–8 mg of halazone per liter will sterilize most water samples in about 30 minutes but will not kill cysts of *Entamoeba histolytica*. The answer is **(D)**.

11. Nalidixic acid, a quinolone, is structurally related to cinoxacin. Both drugs are used in the treatment of urinary tract infections, and cross-resistance may occur. Quinolone derivatives may lower the seizure threshold in susceptible individuals. The answer is **(H)**.

12. Repeated bathing of newborns with hexachlorophene to prevent staphylococcal colonization may permit systemic absorption, which leads to neurotoxic effects (eg, spongiform degeneration of white matter). The answer is **(E)**.

13. Acute hemolytic reactions in G6PD deficiency occur with drugs that are oxidizing agents, including antimalarials, nalidixic acid, sulfonamides, and the nitrofurans. Severe polyneuropathies, with both motor and sensory nerve degeneration, may occur with nitrofurantoin. These reactions are more likely to occur in patients with renal dysfunction. The answer is **(I)**.

14. Chlorhexidine is a biguanide that disrupts bacterial cytoplasmic membranes, especially of gram-positive organisms. The agent is less effective against *Pseudomonas* and *Serratia*. Hospital uses include hand-washing, wound cleansing, and preparation of skin sites for operative procedures. The answer is **(B)**.

15. The activity of methenamine as a urinary antiseptic is mainly due to the release of formaldehyde at acidic pH. Sulfonamides may form insoluble complexes with formaldehyde, resulting in mutual antagonism. *Proteus* organisms alkalinize the urine, preventing the release of formaldehyde. The answer is **(F)**.

16. Metronidazole inhibits aldehyde dehydrogenase and may cause a disulfiram-like reaction in patients who consume alcoholic beverages while taking the drug. The answer is **(G)**.

Clinical Use of Antimicrobials   51

OBJECTIVES

You should be able to:

- List the steps that should be taken prior to the initiation of empiric antimicrobial therapy.
- Describe the importance of susceptibility testing and analyses of serum drug levels or bactericidal titers in antimicrobial chemotherapy.
- Identify the antimicrobial drugs that require major modifications of dosage when renal or hepatic function changes or when dialysis is used.
- List the reasons for use of antimicrobial drugs in combination and the probable mechanisms involved in drug synergy.
- Describe the principles underlying valid antimicrobial chemoprophylaxis and give examples of surgical and nonsurgical prophylaxis.

Learn the definitions that follow.

Table 51–1. Definitions.

Term	Definition
Antimicrobial prophylaxis	The use of antimicrobial drugs to decrease the risk of infection
Combination antimicrobial drug therapy	The use of two or more drugs together to achieve efficacy greater than can be achieved with a single agent
Empiric (presumptive) antimicrobial therapy	Initiation of drug treatment prior to identification of a specific pathogen
Minimal inhibitory concentration (MIC)	An estimate of the drug sensitivity of pathogens for comparison with anticipated levels in blood or tissues
Postantibiotic effect (PAE)	Antibacterial effect that persists after drug concentration falls below the minimum inhibitory concentration
Susceptibility testing	Laboratory methods to determine the sensitivity of the isolated pathogen to antimicrobial drugs

CONCEPTS

A. Guidelines for Antimicrobial Therapy: Empiric antimicrobial therapy is antimicrobial therapy that is begun before a specific pathogen has been identified and is based on the presumption of an infection that requires immediate drug treatment. Prior to initiation of such therapy, accepted practice involves making a clinical diagnosis of microbial infection, obtaining specimens for laboratory analyses, making a microbiologic diagnosis, deciding whether treatment should precede the results of laboratory tests, and, finally, selecting the optimal drug or drugs. A variety of publications provide annually updated lists of antimicrobial drugs of choice for specific pathogens. Such lists can provide a useful guide to empiric therapy based on presumptive microbiologic diagnosis. Table 51–2 sets forth the current drugs of choice and alternative agents for various common pathogens.

B. Principles of Antimicrobial Therapy: Antimicrobial therapy in established infections is guided by the following principles:

1. **Susceptibility testing:** The results of susceptibility testing establish the drug sensitivity of the organism. These results usually predict the **minimal inhibitory concentrations (MICs)** of a drug for comparison with anticipated blood or tissue levels. The two most common methods of susceptibility testing are disk diffusion (Kirby-Bauer) and broth dilution. For some bacteria (eg, gonococci, enterococci, *H influenzae*), a direct test for beta-lactamase can be substituted, since susceptibility patterns are identical for all strains except for the production of beta-lactamase.

2. **Drug concentration in blood:** The measurement of drug concentration in the blood may be appropriate when using agents with a low therapeutic index (eg, aminoglycosides, vancomycin) and when investigating poor clinical response to a drug treatment regimen.

3. **Serum bactericidal titers:** In certain infections in which host defenses may contribute minimally to cure, the estimation of serum bactericidal titers can confirm the appropriateness of choice of drug and dosage. Serial dilutions of serum are incubated with standardized quantities of the pathogen isolated from the patient; killing at a dilution of 1:8 is generally considered satisfactory.

4. **Route of administration:** Parenteral therapy is preferred in most cases of serious microbial infections. Chloramphenicol, the fluoroquinolones, and trimethoprim-sulfamethoxazole (TMP-SMZ) may be effective orally.

5. **Monitoring of therapeutic response:** Therapeutic responses to drug therapy should be monitored clinically and microbiologically to detect the development of resistance or superinfections. The duration of drug therapy required depends on the pathogen (eg, longer courses of therapy are required for infections due to fungi or mycobacteria), the site of infection (eg, endocarditis and osteomyelitis require longer duration of treatment), and the immunocompetence of the patient.

6. **Clinical failure of antimicrobial therapy:** Inadequate clinical or microbiologic response to antimicrobial therapy can result from laboratory testing errors, problems with the drug (eg, incorrect choice, poor tissue penetration, inadequate dose), the patient (poor host defenses, undrained abscesses), or the pathogen (resistance, superinfection).

Table 51–2. Examples of empiric antimicrobial therapy based on microbiologic etiology.

Pathogen	Drugs of First Choice	Alternative Drugs
Gram-positive cocci		
Pneumococcus	Penicillin G, ampicillin	Erythromycin, cephalosporin, vancomycin
Streptococcus (common)	Penicillin G	Erythromycin, cephalosporin
Staphylococcus (penicillinase-producing)	Penicillinase-resistant penicillin	Cephalosporin, vancomycin, macrolide
Staphylococcus (methicillin-resistant)	Vancomycin	TMP-SMZ, minocycline
Enterococcus	Penicillin G plus gentamicin	Vancomycin plus gentamicin
Gram-negative cocci		
Gonococcus	Ceftriaxone, cefixime	Fluoroquinolone, spectinomycin
Meningococcus	Penicillin G, ampicillin	Cefotaxime, cefuroxime, chloramphenicol
Gram-negative rods		
E coli, Proteus, Klebsiella	First- or second-generation cephalosporin, TMP-SMZ	Aminoglycoside, fluoroquinolone, extended-spectrum penicillin
Shigella	Fluoroquinolone	TMP-SMZ, ampicillin
Enterobacter, Citrobacter, Serratia	Imipenem, TMP-SMZ, fluoroquinolone	Extended-spectrum penicillin, amino-glycoside
Haemophilus	Cefuroxime or third-generation cephalosporin	TMP-SMZ, ampicillin, chloramphenicol
Pseudomonas aeruginosa	Aminoglycoside plus extended-spectrum penicillin	Ceftazidime, aztreonam, imipenem
Bacteroides fragilis	Metronidazole, clindamycin	Imipenem, chloramphenicol, ampicillin with sulbactam
Miscellaneous		
Mycoplasma pneumoniae	Erythromycin, tetracycline	Fluoroquinolones
Treponema pallidum	Penicillin G	Erythromycin, tetracycline

C. Factors Influencing Antimicrobial Drug Use:

   1. Bactericidal versus bacteriostatic actions: Antibiotics classified as bacteriostatic include clindamycin, macrolides, sulfonamides, and tetracyclines. For bacteriostatic drugs, the concentrations that inhibit growth are much lower than those that kill bacteria. Antibiotics classified as bactericidal include the aminoglycosides, beta-lactams, fluoroquinolones, metronidazole, most antimycobacterial agents, and vancomycin. For such drugs there is little difference between the concentrations that inhibit growth and those that kill bacteria. Bactericidal drugs are preferred for the treatment of infections in patients with impaired defense mechanisms, especially immunocompromised patients.

   Some bactericidal agents (aminoglycosides, quinolones) cause **concentration-dependent** killing. Maximizing peak blood levels of such drugs increases the rate and the extent of their bactericidal effects. This is one of the factors responsible for the clinical effectiveness of high-dose, once-daily administration of aminoglycosides. Other bactericidal agents (beta-lactams, vancomycin) cause **time-dependent** killing. Their killing action is independent of drug concentration and continues only when blood levels are maintained above the minimal bactericidal concentration (MBC).

   Inhibition of bacterial growth that continues after antibiotic blood concentrations have fallen to low levels is called the **postantibiotic effect (PAE).** The mechanisms of PAE are unclear but may reflect the lag time required by bacteria to synthesize new enzymes and cellular components, the possible persistence of antibiotic at the target site, or an enhanced susceptibility of bacteria to phagocytic and other defense mechanisms. PAE may be another factor contributing to the clinical effectiveness of high-dose, once-daily administration of aminoglycosides.

   2. Drug elimination mechanisms: Changes in hepatic and renal function—and the use of dialysis—can influence the pharmacokinetics of antimicrobials and may necessitate dosage modifications. The major mechanisms of elimination of commonly used antimicrobial drugs are shown in Table 51–3. In anuria (creatinine clearance < 5 mL/min), the elimination half-life of drugs that are eliminated by the kidney is markedly increased, usually necessitating major reductions in drug dosage. Erythromycin, clindamycin, chloramphenicol, rifampin, and ketoconazole are notable exceptions, requiring no change in dosage in renal failure. In patients with biliary dysfunction or cirrhosis, reductions in dosage may be required for drugs that undergo hepatic elimination. Dialysis, especially hemodialysis, may markedly decrease the plasma levels of many antimicrobials; supplementary doses of such drugs may be required to reestablish effective plasma levels following these procedures. Drugs that are *not* removed from the blood by hemodialysis include amphotericin B, cefonicid, cefoperazone, ceftriaxone, erythromycin, nafcillin, tetracyclines, and vancomycin.

3. **Pregnancy and the neonate:** Antimicrobial therapy during pregnancy and the neonatal period requires special consideration. Tetracyclines cause tooth enamel dysplasia and inhibition of bone growth. Sulfonamides, by displacing bilirubin from serum albumin, may cause kernicterus in the neonate. Chloramphenicol may cause the gray baby syndrome. Other drugs that should be used with extreme caution during pregnancy include most antiviral and antifungal agents. The fluoroquinolones are not recommended for use in pregnancy or in children because of possible effects on growing cartilage.

4. **Drug interactions:** Interactions sometimes occur between antimicrobials and other drugs (see also Chapter 61). Interactions include enhanced nephrotoxicity or ototoxicity when aminoglycosides are given with loop diuretics, vancomycin, or cisplatin. Several drug interactions with sulfonamides are based on competition for plasma protein binding; these include excessive hypoglycemia with sulfonylureas and increased hypoprothrombinemia with warfarin. Disulfiram-like reactions to ethanol occur with metronidazole and with several newer cephalosporins (see Chapter 43). Erythromycin inhibits the hepatic metabolism of a number of drugs, including phenytoin, terfenadine, theophylline, and warfarin. Rifampin, a strong inducer of hepatic drug-metabolizing enzymes, decreases the effects of digoxin, ketoconazole, oral contraceptives, propranolol, quinidine, and warfarin.

D. Antimicrobial Drug Combinations: Therapy with multiple antimicrobials may be indicated in the following clinical situations:

1. **Emergency situations:** In severe infections (eg, sepsis, meningitis), combinations of antimicrobial drugs are used empirically to suppress all of the most likely pathogens.

2. **To delay resistance:** The combined use of drugs is valid in situations where the rapid emergence of resistance impairs the chances for cure. For this reason, combined drug therapy is especially important in the treatment of tuberculosis.

3. **Mixed infections:** Multiple organisms may be involved in some infections. For example, peritoneal infections may be caused by several pathogens (eg, anaerobes and coliforms); a combination of drugs may be required to achieve coverage. Skin infections are often due to mixed bacterial, fungal, or viral pathogens.

4. **To achieve synergistic effects:** The use of a drug combination against a specific pathogen may result in an effect greater than that achieved with a single drug. Examples include the use of penicillins with gentamicin in enterococcal endocarditis, the use of an

Table 51–3. Elimination of commonly used antimicrobial agents.

Mode of Elimination	Drugs or Drug Groups
Renal	Acyclovir, aminoglycosides, amphotericin B, most cephalosporins, imipenem, most penicillins, most quinolones, sulfonamides, tetracyclines (except doxycycline), TMP-SMZ, vancomycin
Hepatic	Amphotericin B, ampicillin, cefoperazone, chloramphenicol, clindamycin, erythromycin, isoniazid, ketoconazole, nafcillin, rifampin
Hemodialysis	Acyclovir (and most other antiviral agents), aminoglycosides, cephalosporins (not cefonicid, cefoperazone, ceftriaxone), penicillins (not nafcillin), sulfonamides

extended-spectrum penicillin plus an aminoglycoside in *Pseudomonas aeruginosa* infections, and the combined use of amphotericin B and flucytosine in cryptococcal meningitis.

In terms of bactericidal actions, the outcome of the combined use of two antimicrobials may be indifference, synergism, potentiation, or antagonism (see Chapter 61). Such actions are more readily demonstrated in vitro than at the clinical level. Some mechanisms that may account for synergism follow.

   a. Sequential blockade: The combined use of drugs may cause inhibition of two or more steps in a metabolic pathway. For example, trimethoprim and sulfamethoxazole block different steps in the formation of tetrahydrofolic acid.

   b. Blockade of drug-inactivating enzymes: Clavulanic acid, sulbactam, and tazobactam inhibit penicillinases and are often combined with penicillinase-sensitive beta-lactam drugs.

   c. Enhanced drug uptake: Increased permeability to aminoglycosides after exposure of certain bacteria to cell wall-inhibiting antimicrobials (eg, beta-lactams) is thought to underlie some synergistic effects.

E. Antimicrobial Chemoprophylaxis: The general principles of antimicrobial chemoprophylaxis can be summarized as follows: (1) Prophylaxis should always be directed toward a **specific pathogen;** (2) **no resistance** should develop during the period of drug use; (3) prophylactic drug use should be of **limited duration;** (4) conventional **therapeutic doses** should be employed; and (5) prophylaxis should be employed only in situations of documented **drug efficacy.**

Examples of clinical situations in which nonsurgical antimicrobial prophylaxis is highly effective are given in Table 51–4. These include contacts of patients with meningococcal infections, gonorrhea, syphilis, and tuberculosis as well as prophylaxis against streptococcal infections in patients with rheumatic fever. Though somewhat less effective, antimicrobial prophylaxis is also commonly used for animal or human bite wounds, influenza A, recurrent otitis media, and chronic bronchitis. Severely leukopenic patients are often given prophylactic antibiotics.

Prophylaxis against postsurgical infections should be limited to procedures that are associated with infection in more than 5% of untreated cases under optimal conditions. Prophylaxis should embody the principles listed above, with drug selection based on the most likely infecting organism and treatment initiated just prior to surgery and continued throughout the procedure. Ideally, the agent should be nontoxic and not essential for treatment of severe microbial infections. Situations in which surgical prophylaxis is of benefit (or commonly used) include gastrointestinal procedures, vaginal hysterectomy, cesarean section, joint replacement, open fracture surgery, and dental procedures in patients with valvular disease or prostheses.

Table 51–4. Examples of nonsurgical antimicrobial prophylaxis with established efficacy.

Disease Prevented	Subjects for Prophylaxis	Drugs	Comments
Group A streptococcal infection	Prior rheumatic fever or rheumatic heart disease	Penicillin G, sulfadiazine	Does not prevent endocarditis
Meningococcal infection	Close contacts of index case	Rifampin, minocycline	
Gonorrhea	Contacts of index case	As for patient with gonorrhea	
	Newborn	Silver nitrate	
Syphilis	Contacts of index case	Benzathine penicillin G	
Urinary tract infections	History of recurrent UTI	TMP-SMZ	Alternatively, treat each episode
Pneumocystis carinii pneumonia	Immunosuppressed	TMP-SMZ	Aerosolized pentamidine is an alternative

QUESTIONS

DIRECTIONS: Each of the numbered items or incomplete statements in this section is followed by answers or by completions of the statement. Select the ONE lettered answer or completion that is BEST in each case.

Items 1–3: A hospitalized AIDS patient is receiving zidovudine but no antimicrobial prophylaxis. He develops sepsis with fever, suspected to be caused by a gram-negative bacillus. Treatment will include antibiotics, and the drugs under consideration include aminoglycosides, cephalosporins, fluoroquinolones, and imipenem.

1. Antimicrobial treatment of this severely immunodepressed patient should not be initiated before
   (A) The pathogen has been identified by the microbiology laboratory
   (B) Specimens have been taken for laboratory tests and examinations
   (C) The results of a Gram stain are available
   (D) Antipyretic drugs have been given to reduce body temperature
   (E) The results of antibacterial drug susceptibility tests are available

2. If gentamicin is used systemically in the treatment of this patient, monitoring of the serum drug level may be advised because
   (A) If administered orally, the drug is unstable in gastric acid
   (B) The drug's antibacterial action will be antagonized by cephalosporins
   (C) Gentamicin is hematotoxic
   (D) The drug will not readily penetrate into the cerebrospinal fluid
   (E) Gentamicin has a narrow therapeutic window

3. A combination of drugs might be given to this patient to provide coverage of multiple organisms or to obtain a synergistic action. Examples of antimicrobial drug synergism established at the clinical level include all of the following EXCEPT
   (A) Amphotericin B and flucytosine in cryptococcal meningitis
   (B) Carbenicillin and gentamicin in pseudomonal infections
   (C) Penicillin and tetracycline in bacterial meningitis
   (D) Penicillin and vancomycin in enterococcal infections
   (E) Trimethoprim and sulfamethoxazole in coliform infections

Items 4–5: A 27-year-old pregnant patient with a past history of pyelonephritis has developed a severe upper respiratory tract infection that appears to be due to a bacterial pathogen. The woman is hospitalized and an antibacterial agent is to be selected for treatment.

4. Assuming that the physician is concerned about the effects of renal impairment on drug dosage in this patient, which one of the following drugs is LEAST likely to require dosage reduction even if creatinine clearance is less than 10 mL/min?
   (A) Ampicillin
   (B) Cefazolin
   (C) Clindamycin
   (D) Tetracycline
   (E) Trimethoprim-sulfamethoxazole

5. Which one of the following antibacterial agents appears to be quite safe for the treatment of infections in the pregnant patient?
   (A) Ciprofloxacin
   (B) Erythromycin
   (C) Metronidazole
   (D) Sulfadiazine
   (E) Tetracycline

6. A common drug interaction that occurs with the use of antimicrobial drugs—particularly drugs that have a wide antibacterial spectrum of activity—is
   (A) Disulfiram-like reactions when ethanol is ingested
   (B) Increased ototoxicity if administered to a patient taking furosemide
   (C) Enhancement of the anticoagulant effects of warfarin
   (D) Increased adverse effects if acetaminophen is administered as an antipyretic
   (E) Hypertension with ingestion of red wine and cheese

7. There is no evidence that antimicrobial prophylaxis is of established benefit in
   (A) Contacts of the index case in mycoplasmal pneumonia
   (B) Traveler's diarrhea
   (C) Contacts of the index case in gonorrhea
   (D) Recurrent urinary tract infection
   (E) Tuberculin converters

8. Which one of the following is NOT an established mechanism of antimicrobial drug synergy?
   (A) Drugs A and B block successive steps in a bacterial metabolic pathway
   (B) Drug A promotes the accumulation of drug B within the bacterium
   (C) Drug A induces enzymes that convert drug B to a more polar form
   (D) Drug A inhibits an enzyme that inactivates drug B

Items 9–10: A 48-year-old patient is scheduled for a vaginal hysterectomy. An antimicrobial drug will be used for prophylaxis against postoperative infection. It is proposed that cefazolin, a first-generation cephalosporin, be given intravenously at the normal therapeutic dose immediately prior to surgery and continued until the patient is released from the hospital.

9. Which one of the following statements about the proposed drug management of this patient is LEAST accurate?
   (A) Without prophylaxis, the infection rate following this procedure exceeds 5% under optimal conditions
   (B) This drug will not be effective against *Bacteroides*
   (C) Probable pathogens do not become rapidly resistant to this drug
   (D) Nosocomial (hospital-acquired) infection will be prevented by treatment throughout the period of hospitalization
   (E) Prophylaxis has documented efficacy in this type of surgical procedure

10. If the above patient had been scheduled for elective colonic surgery, optimal prophylaxis against infection would be achieved by mechanical bowel preparation and the use of
    (A) Intravenous cefotetan
    (B) Oral ampicillin
    (C) Oral neomycin and erythromycin
    (D) An intravenous third-generation cephalosporin
    (E) Oral fluoroquinolone

11. Which one of the following antimicrobial drugs is LEAST likely to affect the hepatic metabolism of other drugs or endogenous compounds?
    (A) Ampicillin
    (B) Chloramphenicol
    (C) Erythromycin
    (D) Ketoconazole
    (E) Rifampin

12. Which one of the following antimicrobial drugs does NOT require supplementation of dosage during hemodialysis?
    (A) Ampicillin
    (B) Cefazolin
    (C) Ganciclovir
    (D) Tobramycin
    (E) Vancomycin

13. The persistent suppression of bacterial growth that may occur following limited exposure to some antimicrobial drugs is called
    (A) Time-dependent killing
    (B) The postantibiotic effect
    (C) Clinical synergy
    (D) Concentration-dependent killing
    (E) Sequential blockade

14. If ampicillin and piperacillin are used in combination in the treatment of infections due to *Pseudomonas aeruginosa,* antagonism may occur. The most likely explanation is
    (A) The two drugs form an insoluble complex
    (B) Piperacillin blocks the attachment of ampicillin to penicillin-binding proteins
    (C) Ampicillin induces beta-lactamase production

(D) Autolytic enzymes are inhibited by piperacillin
(E) Ampicillin is bacteriostatic

ANSWERS

1. To delay therapy until laboratory results are available is inappropriate in serious bacterial infections, but specimens for possible microbial identification must be obtained before drugs are administered. The answer is **(B)**.

2. Monitoring plasma aminoglycoside levels is important because these drugs have a low therapeutic index; toxicity occurs when plasma levels are only three to four times higher than their minimal inhibitory concentrations. Decreases in renal function may elevate the plasma levels of aminoglycosides to toxic levels within a few hours. The answer is **(E)**.

3. Combinations of antimicrobial drugs are not always synergistic. In the treatment of bacterial meningitis, two drugs may *not* be better than one. For example, the combination of penicillin and a tetracycline cures fewer patients with pneumococcal meningitis than the same dose of penicillin used alone. The answer is **(C)**.

4. Antimicrobial drugs that are eliminated via hepatic metabolism or biliary excretion include erythromycin, cefoperazone, clindamycin, doxycycline, isoniazid, ketoconazole, and nafcillin. The answer is **(C)**.

5. Several groups of antimicrobial drugs are relatively safe in pregnancy, including penicillins, cephalosporins, the macrolides, and the lincosamides. The answer is **(B)**.

6. Disturbance of the gut microbial flora often leads to decreased availability of vitamin K, with enhancement of the anticoagulant effects of coumarins. The answer is **(C)**. Can you name the drugs in the other drug interactions listed?

7. Tetracycline has been administered to subjects exposed to mycoplasmal pneumonia, but the effectiveness of such treatment has not been documented. The answer is **(A)**.

8. Increased activity of enzymes that make drugs more polar is likely to inactivate an antimicrobial drug and will not lead to increased antibacterial activity. Specific examples of mechanisms that *do* result in synergy include choice **(A)**, the combination of trimethoprim and sulfamethoxazole; choice **(B)**, the combination of a penicillin and an aminoglycoside; and choice **(D)**, the combination of clavulanic acid and amoxicillin. The answer is **(C)**.

9. With few exceptions, the prophylactic use of antibiotics in surgery should not extend beyond the duration of the procedure. After routine surgical procedures, the risk of superinfection (from disturbances in microbial flora) *increases* in a hospitalized patient if prophylaxis is prolonged; there is also more likelihood of drug toxicity. The answer is **(D)**.

10. Second-generation cephalosporins, including cefoxitin and cefotetan, are more active than cefazolin against bowel anaerobes such as *B fragilis* and are sometimes used for prophylaxis in "dirty" surgical procedures. However, for elective bowel surgery, most authorities favor the oral use of neomycin together with a poorly absorbed formulation of erythromycin. In cases of bowel perforation, the use of a second- or third-generation cephalosporin is more appropriate. The answer is **(C)**.

11. Chloramphenicol, ketoconazole, and erythromycin can inhibit the hepatic metabolism of various drugs. Rifampin is an inducer of liver microsomal drug-metabolizing enzymes. The answer is **(A)**.

12. Vancomycin is not removed from the blood during hemodialysis, and no change in dosage is required. The answer is **(E)**.

13. Many antibiotics continue to exert effects on the growth of bacteria when blood levels are lower than those normally thought of as the minimal inhibitory concentration. This is called the postantibiotic effect (PAE). The PAE may contribute to the clinical effectiveness of antibiotics, especially in the case of bactericidal agents such as aminoglycosides and fluoroquinolones, which exert concentration-dependent killing. For example, once-daily dosing with an aminoglycoside is as effective as conventional dosage regimens and is less likely to cause toxicity. The answer is **(B)**.

14. Gram-negative rods such as *Enterobacter* and *Pseudomonas aeruginosa* have inducible beta-lactamases. Several beta-lactam antibiotics, including ampicillin, cefoxitin, and imipenem, are potent inducers of beta-lactamase production. When such inducers are used in combination with a hydrolyzable penicillin (eg, piperacillin), antagonism may result. The answer is **(C)**.

Principles of Antiparasitic Chemotherapy

52

OBJECTIVES

You should be able to:

- Describe the mechanisms of drugs whose targets are enzymes unique to parasites, ie, not found in host cells.
- Describe the mechanisms of drugs whose targets are enzymes indispensable to parasites but not to their hosts.
- Describe the mechanisms of drugs whose targets are biochemical functions common to host and parasite cells.

Learn the definitions that follow.

Table 52–1. Definitions.	
Term	**Definition**
Glycosome	A membrane-bounded intracellular organelle in trypanosomes that contains glycolytic enzymes
Hydrogenosome	A membrane-bounded intracellular organelle in certain anaerobic protozoans that contains hydrogenase
Salvage enzymes	Nucleoside phosphotransferases involved in the salvage of purines and pyrimidines in protozoans
Sequential blockade	Actions of two or more drugs that interfere with sequential steps in a metabolic pathway
Suicide substrate	A chemical that forms a stable complex with an enzyme leading to its irreversible inhibition; suicide compounds are chemically related to natural enzyme substrates

CONCEPTS

Rational approaches to antiparasite chemotherapy utilize the principle of **selective toxicity,** which exploits biochemical and physiologic differences between parasite and host cells. Many antiparasitic agents target enzymes that are unique to—or indispensable to—parasites; other drugs affect cellular functions common to both host and parasite cells (Table 52–2).

A. **Mechanisms Involving Enzymes Unique to Parasites:** These enzymes are not found in the host's cells.

1. **Dihydropteroate synthase:** Sporozoans (eg, *Plasmodium, Toxoplasma,* and *Eimeria* species) lack the ability to utilize exogenous folate and therefore possess enzymes for its synthesis; these enzymes can be inhibited by drugs. **Sulfonamides,** which are antimetabolites of PABA, inhibit dihydropteroate synthase. **Sequential blockade** can be achieved with a sulfonamide and an inhibitor of dihydrofolate reductase (eg, pyrimethamine); such drug combinations are effective in malaria and toxoplasmosis.

2. **Pyruvate-ferredoxin oxidoreductase:** Certain anaerobic protozoans *(Trichomonas, Entamoeba)* lack mitochondria and possess a pyruvate-ferredoxin oxidoreductase of low redox potential that generates acetyl-CoA via electron transport. In trichomonal flagellates, this enzyme is coupled to a hydrogenase located in hydrogenosomes. Under anaerobic conditions, electron transport results in formation of hydrogen. The system also transfers electrons from pyruvate to the nitro groups of nitroimidazoles (eg, **metronidazole**), forming cytotoxic products that inhibit growth by binding to the parasite's proteins and DNA.

Table 52–2. Identified targets and mechanisms of action of some antiparasitic drugs.

Mechanism	Parasites	Examples of Drugs
Act on enzyme specific to parasites		
Dihydropteroate synthase	Sporozoa	Sulfonamides, sulfones
Pyruvate-ferredoxin oxidoreductase	Anaerobic protozoa	Nitroimidazoles
Nucleoside phosphotransferase	Flagellated protozoa	Allopurinol riboside
Trypanothione reductase	Kinetoplastida	Nifurtimox, melarsoprol
Act on enzymes indispensable to parasites		
Purine phosphoribosyl transferase	Protozoa	Allopurinol
Ornithine decarboxylase	Protozoa	α-Difluoromethylornithine
Glycolytic enzymes	Kinetoplastida	Glycerol plus salicylhydroxamic acid and suramin
Act on functions common to both host and parasites[1]		
Thiamin transporter	Coccidia	Amprolium
Mitochondrial electron transporter	Coccidia	4-Hydroxyquinolines
Microtubules	Helminths	Benzimidazoles
Neurotransmission, muscle contraction	Helminths and ectoparasites	Levamisole, piperazines, avermectins, milbemycins

[1]Differences in the structures of regulatory macromolecules among parasites and host cells and differences in drug access may account for the selective toxicities of drugs in this subgroup.

3. **Nucleoside phosphotransferases:** Protozoan parasites depend critically on purine salvage pathways because these organisms are unable to synthesize purine nucleotides de novo. In *Leishmania,* purine nucleoside phosphotransferase (a **salvage enzyme** that transfers phosphate groups to the 5′ position of purine nucleosides) also phosphorylates purine nucleoside analogs such as **allopurinol riboside, formycin B,** and **thiopurinol riboside.** The triphosphate derivatives of these drugs may be incorporated into nucleic acids or may inhibit enzymes in purine metabolism. Toxicity is low because mammalian cells lack this salvage enzyme.

Trichomonads need to salvage pyrimidines (as well as purines), since these organisms lack dihydrofolate reductase and thymidylate synthase. Conversion of exogenous thymidine to thymidine 5′-phosphate can only be carried out in these parasites by the action of a thymidine phosphotransferase. This enzyme can be selectively inhibited by antimetabolites (eg, **guanosine**).

4. **Trypanothione reductase:** In the protozoans known as kinetoplastidans, glutathione exists largely in the form of trypanothione, a unique conjugate with spermidine. Trypanothione, via the action of a specific trypanothione reductase, plays a central role in maintaining the reduced state of intracellular thiols and is essential for the survival of such parasites. **Nifurtimox** and certain trivalent arsenicals used as antitrypanosomal agents inhibit trypanothione reductase.

B. **Mechanisms Involving Enzymes Indispensable to Parasites:** These enzymes are present in the host as well as the parasite, but they are essential only to the parasite or they differ in their substrate specificities.

1. **Purine phosphoribosyl transferases:** Hypoxanthine-guanine phosphoribosyltransferase (HGPRTase) is a key enzyme in purine synthesis in many parasites, including *Leishmania, Schistosoma,* and *Trypanosoma* species. **Allopurinol** is a good substrate for this enzyme in certain parasites (but not for the mammalian enzyme); the drug is metabolized to the ribotide, which is incorporated after phosphorylation into RNA forms that interfere with normal growth. Purine salvage in *Giardia* depends critically on adenine phosphoribosyltransferase and guanine phosphoribosyltransferase. Unlike mammalian forms of these enzymes, the parasite enzymes do not utilize hypoxanthine, xanthine, or adenine as substrates and are thus amenable to inhibition by a designed inhibitor.

2. **Ornithine decarboxylase:** This enzyme controls the formation of putrescine (a polyamine) and appears to be more critical for the growth of certain parasites than for the growth of mammalian cells. **Alpha-difluoromethylornithine (DFMO)** is a **suicide substrate** of ornithine decarboxylase and has antiparasitic activity against *Trypanosoma, Plasmodium,* and *Giardia* species. In *T brucei,* DFMO transforms the organism into a nondividing form that can be eliminated by the host immune system.

3. **Glycolytic enzymes:** The bloodstream form of the African trypanosome *T brucei* is entirely dependent on glycolysis for generation of ATP. The enzymes involved are arranged in close proximity to each other in glycosomes. Glycerol-3-phosphate oxidase is a key enzyme that can be inhibited by **salicylhydroxamic acid (SHAM),** bringing the parasite into an anaerobic state. The addition of glycerol inhibits the reversed glycerol kinase reaction, stops glycolysis, and results in the death of the parasite. Biogenesis of glycosomes may also be a target for antiparasitic drugs. Suramin, a very large, polar molecule, binds to glycolytic enzymes and may prevent the incorporation of the enzymes into the glycosome.

C. **Mechanisms Involving Biochemical Functions Common to Host and Parasite:** Several processes that occur in both parasites and hosts are nevertheless more susceptible to inhibition in the parasite.

1. **Thiamin transporter:** Carbohydrate metabolism is the primary energy source in coccidia. Inhibition of the cellular transport of thiamin by the structurally similar agent **amprolium** leads to a deficiency of this cofactor in coccidia.

2. **Mitochondrial electron transporter:** **4-Hydroxyquinoline** drugs with anticoccidial effects interact with components of the respiratory chain that are specific to *Eimeria* species and inhibit electron transport in the mitochondria of these organisms. Mitochondrial respiration in other parasites and in mammals is not inhibited by these drugs.

3. **Microtubules:** The microtubules of the cytoskeleton and mitotic spindle consist of tubulin polymers. These tubulins are heterogeneous among species. Structural features of alpha-tubulins in helminths may account for the selective toxicity of benzimidazole drugs (eg, **mebendazole**). These agents bind to microtubules in helminths to block transport processes.

4. **Neurotransmission and muscle contraction:** The antiparasitic effect of nicotinic agonist drugs (eg, **levamisole, pyrantel pamoate**) in nematodes is caused by stimulation of neuromuscular transmission, which leads to muscle contraction. **Piperazine** acts as a GABA receptor agonist in nematodes, causing flaccid paralysis; facilitation of the actions of GABA appears to underlie the actions of **milbemycins** and **avermectins.** These natural products do not cross the blood-brain barrier in mammalian hosts and are relatively nontoxic. **Praziquantel,** an antischistosomal and antitapeworm agent, stimulates Ca^{2+} entry into muscles of these parasites and causes unphysiologic contraction.

QUESTIONS

DIRECTIONS: Each of the numbered items or incomplete statements in this section is followed by answers or by completions of the statement. Select the ONE lettered answer or completion that is BEST in each case.

1. Certain anaerobic protozoan parasites lack mitochondria and generate energy-rich compounds, such as acetyl-CoA, by means of enzymes present in organelles called hydrogenosomes. An important enzyme involved in this process is
   (A) Cytochrome P450
   (B) Glycerol-3-phosphate oxidase
   (C) Hypoxanthine-guanine phosphoribosyltransferase
   (D) Pyruvate-ferredoxin oxidoreductase
   (E) Thymidylate synthase

2. Which of the following compounds is a good substrate for hypoxanthine-guanine phosphoribosyltransferase in trypanosomes (but not mammals) and is eventually converted into metabolites that are incorporated into RNA?
   (A) Allopurinol
   (B) Alpha-difluoromethylornithine

    (C)   Glycerol
    (D)   Mebendazole
    (E)   Salicylhydroxamic acid

3.   One chemotherapeutic strategy used to eradicate the bloodstream form of African try-panosomes is based on the absolute dependence of the organism on
    (A)   Cytochrome-dependent electron transfer
    (B)   Dihydropteroate synthesis
    (C)   Glycolysis
    (D)   Lactate dehydrogenase
    (E)   Mitochondrial respiration

4.   Which of the following drugs enhances GABA actions on the neuromuscular junctions of nematodes and arthropods?
    (A)   Glutamic acid
    (B)   Ivermectin
    (C)   Picrotoxin
    (D)   Pyrantel pamoate
    (E)   Thiamine

5.   Which of the following drugs is an antimetabolite that inhibits a trypanosomal enzyme involved in putrescine synthesis?
    (A)   Alpha-difluoromethylornithine
    (B)   Alpha-fluorodeoxyuridine
    (C)   Metronidazole
    (D)   Polymyxin
    (E)   Thiopurinol riboside

6.   All of the following statements about the mechanisms of action of antiparasitic drugs are accurate EXCEPT
    (A)   4-Hydroxyquinolines inhibit phospholipase C
    (B)   Mebendazole binds to tubulins to alter the transport functions of microtubules
    (C)   Metronidazole is activated in the parasite to a cytotoxic product
    (D)   Salicylhydroxamic acid is an inhibitor of glycerol-3-phosphate oxidase
    (E)   Sulfonamides inhibit the activity of 7,8-dihydropteroate synthase

7.   Which one of the following enzymes is NOT unique to parasites?
    (A)   Dihydropteridine pyrophosphokinase
    (B)   Hypoxanthine-guanine phosphoribosyltransferase
    (C)   Lanosterol demethylase
    (D)   Purine nucleoside phosphotransferase
    (E)   Trypanothione reductase

8.   Which one of the following statements about specific antiparasitic drugs is LEAST accurate?
    (A)   Amprolium is an inhibitor of thiamin transport in *Eimeria* species
    (B)   Allopurinol riboside is a potent inhibitor of mitochondrial electron transfer
    (C)   Sulfadoxine is an inhibitor of dihydropteroate synthase in the malaria parasite
    (D)   Suramin binds to glycolytic enzymes and prevents their incorporation into glycosomes
    (E)   The mechanism of action of diloxanide furoate in amebiasis is unknown

ANSWERS

1.   In *T vaginalis,* conversion of pyruvate to acetyl-CoA takes place via the actions of pyruvate-ferredoxin oxidoreductase. The answer is **(D).**

2.   Allopurinol is a good substrate for HGPRTase in trypanosomes but not in mammals. Recall that allopurinol is also an inhibitor of xanthine oxidase and is used in gout and cancer chemotherapy. The answer is **(A).**

3.   Glycolytic enzyme inhibitors (such as SHAM) that inhibit glycerol-3-phosphate oxidase may be selectively toxic to African trypanosomes. The answer is **(C).**

4.   Several antiparasitic drugs enhance GABA neurotransmission in nematodes and arthropods and cause muscle paralysis. These drugs include piperazine, milbemycins, and avermectins (eg, ivermectin). The answer is **(B).**

5.   DFMO is a suicide inhibitor of ornithine decarboxylase. Although it also inhibits mammalian ornithine decarboxylase, DMFO is less toxic to the host because of more rapid turnover and replacement of the irreversibly inhibited enzyme in the host than in parasites. The answer is **(A).**

6. The anticoccidial 4-aminoquinolines inhibit mitochondrial respiration in *Eimeria* species, probably through interaction with a component between NADH oxidase and cytochrome b in the electron transport chain. The answer is **(A)**.

7. HGPRTase, an enzyme involved in purine salvage, is present in both parasites and mammals. Note that in *Leishmania* and *T cruzi* ergosterol is an essential component of the plasma membrane. In such species the antifungal azoles inhibit a cytochrome P450 isoform that converts lanosterol to ergosterol via demethylation. The answer is **(B)**.

8. *Leishmania* species possess the unique salvage enzyme purine nucleoside phosphotransferase. This enzyme phosphorylates allopurinol riboside to form the corresponding nucleotide, which interferes with purine and nucleic acid metabolism. The answer is **(B)**.

Antiprotozoal Drugs

53

OBJECTIVES

You should be able to:

- List the major groups of antiprotozoal drugs.
- Describe the pharmacodynamic and pharmacokinetic properties of the major antimalarial drugs (chloroquine, quinine, primaquine, and the antifolate agents).
- Describe the pharmacodynamic and pharmacokinetic properties of the major amebicides (diloxanide, emetine, iodoquinol, and metronidazole). List other clinical applications of metronidazole.
- Identify the drugs useful for prophylaxis and treatment of pneumocystosis and toxoplasmosis and know their toxic effects.
- Identify the major drugs used for trypanosomiasis and leishmaniasis and know their toxic effects.

CONCEPTS

DRUGS FOR MALARIA

Malaria parasites have a complex life cycle that permits drug action at several points. *Plasmodium* species that infect humans *(P falciparum, P malariae, P ovale, P vivax)* are spread by the female *Anopheles* mosquito and, after inoculation into the human host, undergo a primary developmental stage in the liver (primary tissue phase). They then enter the blood and parasitize erythrocytes (erythrocytic phase). *P falciparum* and *P malariae* have only one cycle of liver cell invasion; thereafter, multiplication is confined to erythrocytes. The other species have a dormant hepatic stage (in which they become **hypnozoites**) that is responsible for recurrent infections and relapses after apparent recovery of the host from the initial infection.

Primary **tissue schizonticides** (eg, primaquine) kill schizonts in the liver soon after infection, whereas **blood schizonticides** (eg, chloroquine, quinine) kill these parasitic forms only in the erythrocyte. Antimalarial drugs may exert multiple actions. Primaquine is **gametocidal,** since it kills gametes in the blood; the drug also destroys the secondary exoerythrocytic (liver) schizonts that cause the relapsing fevers of malaria. **Sporonticides** (proguanil, pyrimethamine) prevent sporogony and multiplication in the mosquito (Table 53–1).

A. **Chloroquine:**
1. **Classification and pharmacokinetics:** Chloroquine is a 4-aminoquinoline derivative. The drug is rapidly absorbed when given orally, is widely distributed to tissues, and has an extremely large volume of distribution. Chloroquine is excreted largely unchanged in the urine.

Table 53–1. Drugs used in malaria.

Drug	Use in Acute Attacks?	Use for Eradication of Liver Stages?	Use for Prophylaxis?
Chloroquine	Yes	No	Yes, except in regions where *P falciparum* is resistant
Quinine, mefloquine	Yes, in resistant *P falciparum*	No	Yes, mefloquine is used in regions with chloroquine-resistant *P falciparum*
Primaquine	No	Yes *(P vivax, P ovale)*	Yes, but only if exposed to *P vivax* or *P ovale*
Antifols	Yes, but only in resistant *P falciparum*	No	Not usually advised

2. **Mechanism of action:** Chloroquine forms a complex with hemin that has deleterious effects on cellular membranes. Chloroquine is a weak base and may buffer intracellular pH, thereby inhibiting cellular invasion by parasitic organisms. The selective toxicity of the drug is due to an energy-dependent carrier mechanism in parasitized cells. Chloroquine-resistant parasites are able to expel the drug via a membrane P-glycoprotein pump (see Chapter 55).

3. **Clinical use:** Chloroquine is used for acute attacks of malaria and for prophylaxis except in regions where *P falciparum* is resistant. The drug is solely a blood schizonticide and will not eradicate secondary tissue schizonts. Chloroquine is also used in amebic liver disease and in autoimmune disorders.

4. **Toxicity:** At low doses, chloroquine causes gastrointestinal irritation, skin rash, and headaches. High doses may cause severe skin lesions, peripheral neuropathies, myocardial depression, retinal damage, auditory impairment, and toxic psychosis. Chloroquine may also precipitate attacks of porphyria.

B. Quinine and Mefloquine:

1. **Classification and pharmacokinetics:** Quinine is the principal alkaloid derived from the bark of the cinchona tree. Quinine is rapidly absorbed orally and is metabolized before renal excretion. Intravenous administration of quinine is possible in severe infections.

   Mefloquine is a synthetic 4-quinoline derivative chemically related to quinine. Because of local irritation, mefloquine can only be given orally, though it is subject to variable absorption. Mefloquine binds to plasma and tissue proteins and has a long plasma half-life (> 6 days).

2. **Mechanism of action:** Quinine complexes with double-stranded DNA to prevent strand separation, resulting in block of DNA replication and transcription to RNA. The mechanism of action of mefloquine is unknown but does not appear to involve binding to DNA. Quinine and mefloquine are blood schizonticides and have no effect on liver stages of the malaria parasite.

3. **Clinical use:** The main use of these drugs is in *P falciparum* infections resistant to chloroquine. To delay emergence of resistance, the drugs should not be used routinely for prophylaxis.

4. **Toxicity:** Quinine commonly causes **cinchonism,** whose symptoms include gastrointestinal distress, headache, vertigo, blurred vision, and tinnitus. Severe overdose results in disturbances in cardiac conduction that resemble quinidine toxicity. Hematotoxic effects occur, including hemolysis in G6PD-deficient patients. **Blackwater fever** (intravascular hemolysis) is a rare and sometimes fatal complication in quinine-sensitized persons.

   Mefloquine is less toxic than quinine; its adverse effects include gastrointestinal distress, skin rash, headache, and dizziness. At high doses, mefloquine may cause neurologic symptoms and seizures.

C. Primaquine:

1. **Classification and pharmacokinetics:** Primaquine is a synthetic 8-aminoquinoline. Absorption is complete after oral administration and is followed by extensive metabolism.

2. **Mechanism of action:** Primaquine forms quinoline-quinone metabolites, which are electron-transferring redox compounds that act as cellular oxidants. The drug is a tissue schizonticide and also limits malaria transmission by acting as a gametocide.

3. **Clinical use:** Primaquine is used to eradicate liver stages of *P vivax* and *P ovale* and should be used in conjunction with a blood schizonticide. Though not active alone in acute attacks of vivax and ovale malaria, a 14-day course of primaquine is standard following initial treatment with chloroquine.

4. **Toxicity:** Primaquine is usually well tolerated but may cause gastrointestinal distress, pruritus, headaches, and methemoglobinemia. More serious toxicity involves hemolysis in G6PD-deficient patients; this is thought to be a result of the formation of redox intermediates.

D. **Antifolate Drugs:**
1. **Classification and pharmacokinetics:** The antifolate group includes pyrimethamine, proguanil, sulfadoxine, and dapsone. All of these drugs are absorbed orally and are excreted in the urine, partly in unchanged form. Proguanil has a shorter half-life (12–16 hours) than other drugs in this subclass (half-life > 100 hours).

2. **Mechanisms of action:** Sulfonamides act as antimetabolites of PABA and block folic acid synthesis in certain protozoans by inhibiting dihydropteroate synthase. Proguanil (chloroguanide) is bioactivated to cycloguanil. Pyrimethamine and cycloguanil are selective inhibitors of protozoal dihydrofolate reductases, preventing formation of tetrahydrofolate. The combination of pyrimethamine with sulfadoxine has synergistic antimalarial effects through the **sequential blockade** of two steps in folic acid synthesis.

3. **Clinical use:** The antifols are blood schizonticides that act mainly against *P falciparum.* Pyrimethamine with sulfadoxine in fixed combination (Fansidar) is used in the treatment of chloroquine-resistant forms of this species, though the onset of activity is slow. Many strains of *P falciparum* are now resistant to antifols, and the drugs are not commonly used for prophylaxis because of their toxicities. However, pyrimethamine with sulfadiazine is the treatment of choice in toxoplasmosis.

4. **Toxicity:** The toxic effects of sulfonamides include skin rashes, gastrointestinal distress, hemolysis, kidney damage, and drug interactions caused by competition for plasma protein binding sites. Pyrimethamine may cause folic acid deficiency when used in high doses.

DRUGS FOR AMEBIASIS

Tissue amebicides (**chloroquine, emetines, metronidazole**) act on organisms in the bowel wall and in the liver; luminal amebicides (**diloxanide furoate, iodoquinol, paromomycin**) act only in the lumen of the bowel. The choice of drug depends on the form of amebiasis. For asymptomatic disease, diloxanide furoate is the choice. For mild to severe intestinal infection, metronidazole is used with diloxanide furoate or iodoquinol. The latter regimen, plus chloroquine, is recommended in amebic liver abscess (see Table 53–2). The mechanisms of amebicidal action of most drugs in this class are unknown.

A. **Diloxanide Furoate:** This drug is commonly used as the sole agent for the treatment of asymptomatic amebiasis and is useful also in mild intestinal disease. Diloxanide furoate is converted in the gut to the diloxanide free-base form, which is the active amebicide. Toxic effects are mild and are usually restricted to gastrointestinal symptoms.

Table 53–2. Drugs used in the treatment of amebiasis.*

Disease Form	Drugs of Choice	Alternative Drugs
Asymptomatic intestinal	Diloxanide furoate	Iodoquinol, paromomycin
Mild to severe intestinal	Metronidazole plus diloxanide or iodoquinol	Diloxanide (plus doxycycline), chloroquine, paromomycin
Hepatic abscess	Metronidazole plus diloxanide, followed by chloroquine	Emetines, followed by chloroquine plus diloxanide

*Adapted, with permission, from Katzung BG (editor): *Basic & Clinical Pharmacology,* 7th ed. Appleton & Lange, 1998.

B. Emetines: Emetine and dehydroemetine inhibit protein synthesis by blocking ribosomal movement along messenger RNA. These alkaloids are used as backup drugs for treatment of severe intestinal or hepatic amebiasis in hospitalized patients. Emetines are given parenterally, are widely distributed to tissues, and are excreted slowly by the kidney. The drugs may cause severe toxicity, including gastrointestinal distress, muscle weakness, and cardiovascular dysfunction (arrhythmias and congestive heart failure).

C. Iodoquinol: Iodoquinol is a halogenated hydroxyquinoline with an unknown mechanism of action. The drug is an orally active luminal amebicide used as an alternative drug for mild to severe intestinal infections. Adverse gastrointestinal effects are common but usually mild. Systemic absorption after high doses may lead to thyroid enlargement and neurotoxic effects, including peripheral neuropathy and visual dysfunction.

D. Metronidazole:
1. **Pharmacokinetics:** Metronidazole is effective orally and distributed widely to tissues. Elimination of the drug requires hepatic metabolism.
2. **Mechanism of action:** Metronidazole undergoes a reductive bioactivation of its nitro group by ferredoxin (present in anaerobic parasites) to form reactive cytotoxic products.
3. **Clinical use:** Metronidazole is the drug of choice in severe intestinal wall disease and in hepatic abscess and other extraintestinal amebic disease. Metronidazole is commonly used with a luminal amebicide. Other important clinical uses of metronidazole include treatment of trichomoniasis, giardiasis, and infections caused by *Gardnerella vaginalis* and anaerobic bacteria *(B fragilis, C difficile).*
4. **Toxicity:** Adverse effects of metronidazole include gastrointestinal irritation, headache, and discoloration of urine. More serious toxicity includes leukopenia, dizziness, and ataxia. Drug interactions with metronidazole include a disulfiram-like reaction with ethanol and potentiation of coumarin anticoagulant effects. Safety of metronidazole in pregnancy and in nursing mothers has not been established.

E. Paromomycin: This drug is an aminoglycoside antibiotic used as a second-line luminal amebicide. It may also have some efficacy against cryptosporidiosis in the AIDS patient. Adverse gastrointestinal effects are common, and systemic absorption may lead to headaches, dizziness, rashes, and arthralgia. Tetracyclines (eg, doxycycline) are sometimes used with a luminal amebicide in mild intestinal disease.

DRUGS FOR PNEUMOCYSTOSIS & TOXOPLASMOSIS

A. Pentamidine:
1. **Classification and pharmacokinetics:** Pentamidine is an aromatic diamidine. For systemic effect, the drug is administered parenterally. Pentamidine is strongly bound to tissues, has a long half-life (2–4 weeks), and is excreted unchanged in the urine. The drug may be used as an aerosol for prophylaxis of *Pneumocystis carinii* pneumonia.
2. **Mechanism of action:** Pentamidine's mechanism of action is unknown, but may involve inhibition of glycolysis or interference with nucleic acid metabolism of protozoans. Preferential accumulation of the drug by susceptible parasites may account for its selective toxicity.
3. **Clinical use:** Aerosol pentamidine (once monthly) can be used in primary and secondary prophylaxis, although oral TMP-SMZ is usually preferred. Daily intravenous or intramuscular administration of the drug for 21 days is needed in the treatment of active pneumocystosis in the HIV-infected patient. Pentamidine is also used in trypanosomiasis (see below).
4. **Toxicity:** Adverse effects following parenteral use include respiratory stimulation followed by depression, hypotension due to peripheral vasodilation, hypoglycemia, anemia, neutropenia, hepatitis, and pancreatitis. Systemic toxicity is minimal when pentamidine is used by inhalation.

B. Trimethoprim-Sulfamethoxazole (TMP-SMZ):
1. **Clinical use:** TMP-SMZ is usually considered to be the medication of first choice in prophylaxis and treatment of pneumocystis pneumonia (PCP). Clinical manifestations of pneumocystis infection in the AIDS patient do not usually occur until the CD4 count is less than

250 cells/μL. Prophylaxis is recommended when the CD4 count drops below 200 cells/μL. Oral treatment with the double-strength formulation three times weekly is usually effective in prophylaxis and for prevention of recurrences. The same regimen of TMP-SMZ is prophylactic against toxoplasmosis and infections due to *Isospora belli*. For treatment of active PCP, daily oral or intravenous administration of TMP-SMZ is required.

2. **Toxicity:** Adverse effects due to TMP-SMZ occur in up to 50% of AIDS patients. Toxicity includes gastrointestinal distress, rash, fever, neutropenia, and thrombocytopenia. These effects may be serious enough to warrant discontinuance of TMP-SMZ and its replacement by alternative drugs. (See Chapter 46 for additional information on TMP-SMZ.)

C. **Antifols: Pyrimethamine and Sulfonamides:**
1. **Clinical use:** The combination of pyrimethamine with sulfadiazine has synergistic activity against *Toxoplasma gondii* through the **sequential blockade** of two steps in folic acid synthesis. Pyrimethamine plus sulfadiazine is the regimen of choice for prophylaxis against toxoplasmosis and is an alternative to TMP-SMZ or pentamidine in prophylaxis against pneumocystis pneumonia in the AIDS patient. For treatment of active toxoplasmosis, the drug combination is given daily for 3–4 weeks, with leucovorin to offset hematologic toxicity.

For patients allergic to sulfonamides, clindamycin can be used in combination with pyrimethamine. For toxoplasma encephalitis in AIDS, high-dose treatment with pyrimethamine plus sulfadiazine (or clindamycin) must be maintained for at least 6 weeks.

2. **Toxicity:** High doses of pyrimethamine plus sulfadiazine are associated with gastric irritation, glossitis, neurologic symptoms (headache, insomnia, tremors, seizures), and hematotoxicity (megaloblastic anemia, thrombocytopenia). Antibiotic-associated colitis may occur during treatment with clindamycin.

D. **Atovaquone:**
1. **Mechanism and pharmacokinetics:** Atovaquone inhibits mitochondrial electron transport and probably folate metabolism. Used orally, it is poorly absorbed and should be given with food to maximize bioavailability. Most of the drug is eliminated in feces in unchanged form.
2. **Clinical use and toxicity:** Atovaquone is approved for use in mild to moderate pneumocystis pneumonia. It is less effective than TMP-SMZ or pentamidine but is better tolerated. Adverse effects include rash, cough, nausea, vomiting, diarrhea, fever, and abnormal liver function tests.

Atovaquone may also be effective in toxoplasmosis, and in falciparum malaria when combined with proguanil.

E. **Miscellaneous Agents:** Other alternative drug regimens for the treatment of pneumocystis pneumonia include trimethoprim plus dapsone, primaquine plus clindamycin, and trimetrexate plus leucovorin.

DRUGS FOR TRYPANOSOMIASIS

A. **Pentamidine:** Pentamidine is commonly used in the hemolymphatic stages of disease caused by *Trypanosoma gambiense* and *T rhodesiense*. Because it does not cross the blood-brain barrier, pentamidine is not used in later stages of trypanosomiasis. Other clinical uses include the prophylaxis and therapy of pneumocystis infections (see above) and treatment of the kala azar form of leishmaniasis (Table 53–3).

B. **Melarsoprol (Mel B):** This drug is an organic arsenical that inhibits enzyme sulfhydryl groups. Because it enters the CNS, melarsoprol is the drug of choice in African sleeping sickness. Melarsoprol is given parenterally because it causes gastrointestinal irritation; it may also cause a reactive encephalopathy that can be fatal.

C. **Nifurtimox:** This drug is a nitrofurazone derivative that inhibits the parasite-unique enzyme trypanothione reductase. Nifurtimox is the drug of choice in American trypanosomiasis and has also been effective in mucocutaneous leishmaniasis. The drug causes severe toxicity, including allergies, gastrointestinal irritation, and CNS effects.

Table 53–3. Drugs used in the treatment of other protozoal infections.

Drug	Primary Indications
Melarsoprol	Drug of choice in African sleeping sickness (late, CNS stage of trypanosomiasis); also used in mucocutaneous forms of the disease
Nifurtimox	Trypanosomiasis due to *T cruzi*
Pentamidine	Hemolymphatic stage of trypanosomiasis; also used in *Pneumocystis carinii* pneumonia
Pyrimethamine plus sulfadiazine	Drug combination of choice in toxoplasmosis
Sodium stibogluconate	Drug of choice for leishmaniasis (all species)
Suramin	Drug of choice for hemolymphatic stage of trypanosomiasis *(T brucei gambiense, T rhodesiense)*
Trimethoprim-sulfamethoxazole	Drug combination of choice in *Pneumocystis carinii* infections

D. Suramin: This polyanionic compound is a drug of choice for the early hemolymphatic stages of African trypanosomiasis (before CNS involvement). It is also an alternative to ivermectin in the treatment of onchocerciasis (see Chapter 54). Suramin is used parenterally and causes skin rashes, gastrointestinal distress, and neurologic complications.

DRUGS FOR LEISHMANIASIS

Leishmaniae—parasitic protozoa transmitted by flesh-eating flies—cause various diseases ranging from cutaneous or mucocutaneous lesions to splenic and hepatic enlargement with fever. **Sodium stibogluconate** (pentavalent antimony), the primary drug in all forms of the disease, appears to kill the parasite by inhibition of glycolysis or effects on nucleic acid metabolism. Alternative agents include pentamidine (for visceral leishmaniasis), metronidazole (for cutaneous lesions), and amphotericin B (for mucocutaneous leishmaniasis).

DRUG LIST

See drugs in Tables 53–1, 53–2, and 53–3.

QUESTIONS

DIRECTIONS: Each of the numbered items or incomplete statements in this section is followed by answers or by completions of the statement. Select the ONE lettered answer or completion that is BEST in each case.

1. Which one of the following statements about antiprotozoal drugs is LEAST accurate?
   - **(A)** A combination of primaquine and clindamycin is an alternative drug regimen for pneumocystis pneumonia
   - **(B)** Chloroquine is a blood schizonticide but does not affect secondary tissue schizonts
   - **(C)** Mefloquine destroys secondary exoerythrocytic schizonts
   - **(D)** Primaquine acts primarily on exoerythrocytic stages of the *Plasmodium* life cycle
   - **(E)** Proguanil is converted to a reactive metabolite that is sporonticidal
2. Which of the following antimalarial drugs causes a dose-dependent toxic state that includes flushed and sweaty skin, dizziness, nausea, diarrhea, tinnitus, blurred vision, and impaired hearing?
   - **(A)** Amodiaquine
   - **(B)** Primaquine
   - **(C)** Pyrimethamine
   - **(D)** Quinine
   - **(E)** Sulfadoxine

3. Plasmodial resistance to chloroquine is due to
   (A) Change in receptor structure
   (B) Decreased carrier-mediated drug transport
   (C) Increase in the activity of DNA repair mechanisms
   (D) Induction of inactivating enzymes
   (E) Inhibition of dihydrofolate reductase

Items 4–6: A photographer traveled in a jungle region where chloroquine-resistant *P falciparum* is endemic. She took a drug for prophylaxis but nevertheless developed a severe attack of *P vivax* malaria.

4. The drug she took for prophylaxis was probably
   (A) Chloroquine
   (B) Mefloquine
   (C) Primaquine
   (D) Proguanil
   (E) Pyrimethamine

5. Which of the following drugs should be used for oral treatment of the photographer's acute attack of *P vivax* malaria?
   (A) Chloroquine
   (B) Mefloquine
   (C) Primaquine
   (D) Pyrimethamine-sulfadoxine
   (E) Quinine

6. Which of the following drugs should be given later in order to eradicate schizonts and latent hypnozoites in the patient's liver?
   (A) Chloroquine
   (B) Mefloquine
   (C) Primaquine
   (D) Proguanil
   (E) Quinine

7. Which one of the following statements about amebicides is LEAST accurate?
   (A) Diloxanide furoate is a luminal amebicide
   (B) Emetine is contraindicated in pregnancy and in patients with cardiac disease
   (C) Metronidazole has little activity in the gut lumen
   (D) Paromomycin is effective in extraintestinal amebiasis
   (E) Systemic use of iodoquinol may cause thyroid enlargement and peripheral neuropathy

Items 8–9: A male patient presents with lower abdominal discomfort, flatulence, and occasional diarrhea. A diagnosis is made of intestinal amebiasis, and *Entamoeba histolytica* is identified in his diarrheal stools. An oral drug is prescribed and reduces the intestinal symptoms. Later he presents with severe dysentery, right upper quadrant pain, weight loss, fever, and an enlarged liver. Amebic liver abscess is diagnosed, and the patient is hospitalized. He has a past history of drug treatment for a tachyarrhythmia but is not taking antiarrhythmic drugs at present.

8. The preferred treatment that he *should* have received for the initial symptoms (which were indicative of mild to moderate intestinal infection) is
   (A) Diloxanide furoate
   (B) Emetine
   (C) Metronidazole
   (D) Metronidazole plus diloxanide furoate
   (E) Tetracycline

9. The drug regimen most likely to be effective in treating the hepatic abscess in this patient and in eradicating intestinal infection is
   (A) Chloroquine alone
   (B) Diloxanide furoate plus iodoquinol
   (C) Emetine plus diloxanide furoate plus chloroquine
   (D) Metronidazole plus chloroquine plus iodoquinol
   (E) Paromomycin plus mefloquine

10. Which one of the following statements about antiprotozoal drugs is LEAST accurate?
   (A) Blackwater fever occurs in patients sensitized to chloroquine

(B) Intravenous injection of pentamidine produces a sharp fall in blood pressure that is only partially blocked by atropine

(C) Metronidazole is the drug of choice for trichomoniasis

(D) Nifurtimox is selectively toxic to some protozoans because it inhibits trypanothione reductase

(E) Pyrimethamine is synergistic with sulfadoxine against malarial parasites (sequential blockade)

DIRECTIONS (Items 11–15): Each set of matching questions in this section consists of a list of three to twenty-six lettered options (some of which may be figures) followed by several numbered items. For each numbered item, select the ONE lettered option that is most closely associated with it. Each lettered option may be selected once, more than once, or not at all.

(A) Diloxanide furoate
(B) Emetine
(C) Melarsoprol
(D) Metronidazole
(E) Nifurtimox
(F) Paromomycin
(G) Pentamidine
(H) Primaquine
(I) Quinine
(J) Sodium stibogluconate

11. This drug is the antimalarial agent most commonly associated with causing an acute hemolytic reaction in patients with G6PD deficiency

12. This agent is used as an alternative drug in severe intestinal or hepatic amebiasis; atrial and ventricular arrhythmias have occurred during its use

13. This drug can clear trypanosomes from the blood and lymph nodes and is active in the late central nervous system stages of African sleeping sickness

14. The clinical uses of this drug include the treatment of amebiasis, giardiasis, and infections caused by anaerobic bacteria

15. This drug is recommended for oral treatment of an acute attack of malaria due to chloroquine-resistant *P falciparum* strains

ANSWERS

1. Mefloquine has many properties similar to those of quinine. Both drugs are effective blood schizonticides, and both have minimal effects on the secondary exoerythrocytic (liver) schizonts that cause the relapsing fevers of malaria. The answer is **(C).**

2. These dose-related symptoms are characteristic adverse effects of cinchona alkaloids (quinine, quinidine) and are termed cinchonism. The answer is **(D).**

3. Resistance occurs through decreases in the activity of a carrier-mediated transport system. The answer is **(B).**

4. Mefloquine is the preferred drug for prophylaxis in regions where chloroquine-resistant *P falciparum* is prevalent. One dose of mefloquine weekly, starting before travel and continuing until 4 weeks after leaving the region, is the preferred regimen. Doxycycline is an alternative drug for this indication. Another alternative for prophylaxis is chloroquine plus proguanil. The answer is **(B).**

5. Chloroquine is the drug of choice for the oral treatment of an acute attack of malaria due to *P vivax* but will not eradicate exoerythrocytic forms of the parasite. Quinine is used for the parenteral treatment of acute attacks. The answer is **(A).**

6. Primaquine is the only antimalarial drug that reliably acts on tissue schizonts in liver cells. Starting about day 4 following an acute attack, primaquine should be given daily for 2 weeks. The answer is **(C).**

7. Paromomycin is an aminoglycoside antibiotic used as a backup drug in the treatment of amebiasis. The drug acts only on organisms in the lumen of the bowel because the aminoglycosides are not absorbed when given orally. The answer is **(D).**

8. Metronidazole plus a luminal amebicide is the treatment of choice in mild to moderate amebic colitis. Diloxanide furoate is commonly used as the sole agent in asymptomatic intestinal infection. The answer is **(D)**.
9. Metronidazole given for 10 days is effective as monotherapy in many cases of hepatic abscess and has the dual advantage of being both amebicidal and active against anaerobic bacteria. However, treatment failures can occur, and follow-up therapy with chloroquine is highly recommended. Luminal amebicides should also be given to eradicate intestinal infection. Treatment with emetine is contraindicated in patients with a history of cardiac disease. The answer is **(D)**.
10. Massive intravascular hemolysis (blackwater fever) is now a rare complication of the treatment of malaria with quinine. Blackwater fever does not occur in the few patients who may be sensitive to chloroquine. The answer is **(A)**.
11. Primaquine is the prototypical drug that induces hemolysis in persons deficient in glucose-6-phosphate dehydrogenase. It may also occur (less frequently) during treatment with chloroquine or quinine. The answer is **(H)**.
12. Emetine causes severe side effects that include congestive heart failure, hypertension, and cardiac arrhythmias. The answer is **(B)**.
13. In African sleeping sickness, melarsoprol is the drug of choice because, unlike pentamidine, it effectively enters the CNS. The answer is **(C)**.
14. Of the drugs listed, only metronidazole has both antiprotozoal activity and clinically useful activity in bacterial infections. The answer is **(D)**.
15. Quinine sulfate is the standard drug for both oral and parenteral treatment of acute attacks of malaria due to chloroquine-resistant *P falciparum*. It should be used in combination with one or more other antimalarial drugs such as doxycycline, clindamycin, or pyrimethamine plus sulfadiazine. The answer is **(I)**.

Anthelmintic Drugs 54

OBJECTIVES

You should be able to:

- Identify the drugs of choice for treatment of common infections caused by nematodes, trematodes, and cestodes.
- Describe the mechanisms of action (if known), important pharmacokinetic features, and the major toxic effects of these drugs.
- Describe the main features of important backup anthelmintics.

CONCEPTS

Anthelmintic drugs have diverse chemical structures, mechanisms of action, and properties. Most were discovered by empiric screening methods; many act against specific parasites, and few are devoid of significant toxicity to host cells. In addition to the direct toxicity of the drugs, reactions to dead and dying parasites may cause serious toxicity in patients. In the text that follows, the drugs are divided into three groups on the basis of the type of helminth primarily affected (nematodes, trematodes, and cestodes). The drugs of choice and alternative agents for selected important helminthic infections are listed in Table 54–1.

Table 54–1. Major helminthic infections and the drugs used to treat them.

Infecting Organism	Drugs of Choice	Alternative Drugs
Nematodes		
Ascaris lumbricoides (roundworm)	Pyrantel pamoate, mebendazole	Albendazole, levamisole, piperazine
Necator americanus, Ancylostoma duodenale	Pyrantel pamoate, mebendazole	Albendazole, levamisole
Trichuris trichiura (whipworm)	Mebendazole	Albendazole, pyrantel pamoate
Strongyloides stercoralis (threadworm)	Ivermectin	Thiabendazole, albendazole
Enterobius vermicularis (pinworm)	Mebendazole, pyrantel pamoate	Albendazole
Larva migrans	Thiabendazole	Albendazole, diethylcarbamazine
Wuchereria bancrofti, Brugia malayi	Diethylcarbamazine	Ivermectin
Onchocerca volvulus	Ivermectin	Suramin
Trematodes (flukes)		
Schistosoma haematobium	Praziquantel	Metrifonate
Schistosoma mansoni	Praziquantel	Oxamniquine
Schistosoma japonicum	Praziquantel	None
Paragonimus westermani	Praziquantel	Bithionol
Fasciola hepatica	Bithionol	Praziquantel, emetine, dehydroemetine
Cestodes (tapeworms)		
Taenia saginata	Niclosamide, praziquantel	Mebendazole
Taenia solium	Niclosamide, praziquantel	
Cysticercosis (*T solium*, cysts)	Albendazole	Praziquantel
Diphyllobothrium latum	Niclosamide, praziquantel	
Echinococcus granulosus (hydatid disease)	Albendazole	Mebendazole

DRUGS THAT ACT AGAINST NEMATODES

The medically important intestinal nematodes responsive to drug therapy include *Enterobius vermicularis* (pinworm), *Trichuris trichiura* (whipworm), *Ascaris lumbricoides* (roundworm), *Ancylostoma* and *Necator* species (hookworms), and *Strongyloides stercoralis* (threadworm). Over 1 billion persons worldwide are estimated to harbor intestinal nematodes. Pinworm infections are common throughout the United States, while the hookworm and threadworm are endemic in the southern United States.

Tissue nematodes responsive to drug therapy include *Ancylostoma* species, which cause cutaneous larva migrans, seen primarily in southern USA. Species of *Dracunculus, Onchocerca, Toxocara,* and *Wuchereria bancrofti* (a cause of filariasis) are all responsive to drug treatment. The number of persons worldwide estimated to be infected by tissue nematodes exceeds 0.5 billion.

A. **Albendazole:**
   1. **Mechanisms:** The mechanism of action of albendazole is unclear. The drug blocks glucose uptake in both larval and adult parasites, which leads to decreased formation of ATP and subsequent parasite immobilization. The actions of albendazole may also include inhibition of microtubule assembly, as has been described for the other benzimidazoles, mebendazole and thiabendazole.
   2. **Clinical use:** Albendazole has a wide anthelmintic spectrum. It is a first-choice drug for larva migrans and an important alternative drug for ascariasis and for infections caused by roundworms, whipworms, hookworms, pinworms, and threadworms. Albendazole is also active against the pork tapeworm in the larval stage.

3. **Toxicity:** Albendazole has few toxic effects during short courses of therapy. Reversible leukopenia, alopecia, and changes in liver enzymes may occur with prolonged use. Long-term animal toxicity studies report bone marrow suppression and fetal toxicity.

B. **Diethylcarbamazine:**
1. **Mechanisms:** Diethylcarbamazine immobilizes microfilariae by an unknown mechanism, increasing their susceptibility to host defense mechanisms.
2. **Clinical use:** Diethylcarbamazine is the drug of choice for filariasis and an alternative drug, in combination with suramin, for onchocerciasis. Microfilariae are killed more readily than adult worms. The drug is rapidly absorbed from the gut and excreted in the urine.
3. **Toxicity:** Adverse effects include headache, malaise, weakness, and anorexia. Reactions to proteins released by dying filariae include fever, rashes, ocular damage, joint and muscle pain, and lymphangitis. In onchocerciasis, the **Mazzotti reaction** includes most of these symptoms as well as hypotension, pyrexia, respiratory distress, and prostration.

C. **Ivermectin:**
1. **Mechanisms:** Ivermectin intensifies GABA-mediated neurotransmission in nematodes and causes immobilization of parasites, facilitating their removal by the reticuloendothelial system. Selective toxicity results because in humans GABA is a neurotransmitter only in the CNS, and ivermectin does not cross the blood-brain barrier.
2. **Clinical use:** Ivermectin is the drug of choice for onchocerciasis; it acts more slowly than diethylcarbamazine but causes fewer systemic and ocular reactions. Ivermectin is also the drug of first choice for strongyloidiasis and an alternative agent in filariasis.
3. **Toxicity:** Single-dose oral treatment in onchocerciasis results in multiple reactions that include fever, headache, dizziness, rashes, pruritus, tachycardia, hypotension, and pain in joints, muscles, and lymph nodes. These symptoms are usually of short duration, and most can be controlled with antihistamines and nonsteroidal anti-inflammatory drugs.

D. **Mebendazole:**
1. **Mechanism:** Mebendazole acts by selectively inhibiting microtubule synthesis and glucose uptake in nematodes.
2. **Clinical use:** Mebendazole is the drug of choice for pinworm and whipworm infections. It is one of two drugs of choice (with pyrantel pamoate) for roundworm and for combined infections with ascarids and hookworm. Mebendazole can also be used as a backup drug in certain cestode and trematode infections. Less than 10% of the drug is absorbed systemically after oral use, and this portion is metabolized rapidly.
3. **Toxicity:** Mebendazole has a high therapeutic index, and its toxic effects are limited to gastrointestinal irritation. Mebendazole is contraindicated in pregnancy because of possible embryotoxicity.

E. **Piperazine:**
1. **Mechanism:** Piperazine paralyzes *Ascaris* by acting as an agonist at GABA receptors. The paralyzed roundworms are expelled live by normal peristalsis.
2. **Clinical use:** Piperazine is an alternative drug for ascariasis.
3. **Toxicity:** Mild gastrointestinal irritation is the most common side effect. Piperazine should not be used in patients with seizure disorders.

F. **Pyrantel Pamoate:**
1. **Mechanism:** Pyrantel pamoate and its congener, **oxantel pamoate,** stimulate nicotinic receptors present at neuromuscular junctions of nematodes. Contraction of muscles occurs followed by a depolarization-induced paralysis.
2. **Clinical use:** Pyrantel pamoate is one of two drugs of choice (with mebendazole) for infections due to hookworm, *Ascaris,* and *Trichostrongylus.* The drug is poorly absorbed when given orally.
3. **Toxicity:** Adverse effects are minor but include gastrointestinal distress, headache, and weakness.

G. **Thiabendazole:**
1. **Mechanism:** Thiabendazole is a structural congener of mebendazole and has a similar action on microtubules.

2. **Clinical use:** Thiabendazole is a drug of choice (the other is mebendazole) for visceral forms of larva migrans and is an effective drug for treatment of strongyloidiasis, cutaneous larva migrans, and threadworm infections. Thiabendazole is rapidly absorbed from the gut and metabolized by liver enzymes. The drug has anti-inflammatory and immunorestorative actions in the host.

3. **Toxicity:** Thiabendazole's toxic effects include gastrointestinal irritation, headache, dizziness, drowsiness, leukopenia, hematuria, and allergic reactions, including intrahepatic cholestasis. Reactions caused by dying parasites include fever, chills, lymphadenopathy, and skin rash.

DRUGS THAT ACT AGAINST TREMATODES

The medically important trematodes include *Schistosoma* species (blood flukes, estimated to affect over 150 million persons worldwide), *Clonorchis sinensis* (liver fluke, endemic in Southeast Asia), and *Paragonimus westermani* (lung fluke, endemic to both the Orient and India). With few exceptions, fluke infections respond well to praziquantel.

A. **Praziquantel:**
1. **Mechanism:** Praziquantel increases membrane permeability to calcium, causing marked contraction initially and then paralysis of trematode muscles; this is followed by vacuolization and parasite death.

2. **Clinical use:** Praziquantel has a wide anthelmintic spectrum that includes activity in both trematode and cestode infections. It is the drug of choice in schistosomiasis (all species), clonorchiasis, and paragonimiasis and for infections caused by small and large intestinal flukes. The drug is active against immature and adult schistosomal forms. Praziquantel is also one of two drugs of choice (with niclosamide) for infections due to cestodes (all common tapeworms) and in the treatment of cysticercosis.

3. **Pharmacokinetics:** Absorption from the gut is rapid, and the drug is metabolized by the liver to inactive products.

4. **Toxicity:** Common adverse effects include headache, dizziness, malaise, and, less frequently, gastrointestinal irritation, skin rash, and fever. Increased rates of abortion with praziquantel preclude its use in pregnancy.

B. **Bithionol:**
1. **Clinical use:** Bithionol is the drug of choice for treatment of fascioliasis (sheep liver fluke) and an alternative agent in paragonimiasis. The mechanism of action is unknown. Bithionol is orally effective and is eliminated in the urine.

2. **Toxicity:** Common adverse effects include nausea and vomiting, diarrhea and abdominal cramps, dizziness, and headache. Less frequently, pyrexia, tinnitus, proteinuria, and leukopenia may occur.

C. **Metrifonate:** Metrifonate is an organophosphate prodrug that is converted in the body to the cholinesterase inhibitor, dichlorvos. The active metabolite acts solely against *Schistosoma haematobium* (the cause of bilharziasis). Toxic effects occur from excess cholinergic stimulation.

D. **Oxamniquine:** Oxamniquine is effective solely in *Schistosoma mansoni* infections, acting on male immature forms and adult schistosomal forms. Dizziness is a common adverse effect; headache, gastrointestinal irritation, and pruritus may also occur. Reactions to dying parasites include eosinophilia, urticaria, and pulmonary infiltrates. It is not advisable to use the drug in pregnancy or in patients with a past history of seizure disorders.

DRUGS THAT ACT AGAINST CESTODES (TAPEWORMS)

The four medically important cestodes are *Taenia saginata* (beef tapeworm), *Taenia solium* (pork tapeworm, which can cause cysticerci in the brain and the eyes), *Diphyllobothrium latum* (fish tapeworm), and *Echinococcus granulosus* (dog tapeworm, which can cause hydatid cysts in the liver, lungs, and brain). The primary drugs for treatment of cestode infections are praziquantel (see above) and niclosamide.

A. **Niclosamide:**
1. **Mechanism:** Niclosamide may act by uncoupling oxidative phosphorylation or by activating ATPases.
2. **Clinical use:** Niclosamide is one of two drugs of choice (with praziquantel) for infections caused by beef, pork, and fish tapeworm infections. However, it is not effective in cysticercosis (for which praziquantel is used) or hydatid disease caused by *Echinococcus granulosus* (for which albendazole is used). Scoleces and cestode segments are killed, but ova are not. Niclosamide is effective in treatment of infections due to small and large intestinal flukes.
3. **Toxicity:** Toxic effects are usually mild but include gastrointestinal distress, headache, rash, and fever. Some of these effects may result from systemic absorption of antigens from disintegrating parasites.

DRUG LIST

See Table 54–1.

QUESTIONS

DIRECTIONS: Each of the numbered items or incomplete statements in this section is followed by answers or by completions of the statement. Select the ONE lettered answer or completion that is BEST in each case.

1. All of the following drugs are active against nematodes. Which one causes muscle paralysis by activating receptors for the inhibitory transmitter GABA?
   (A) Albendazole
   (B) Diethylcarbamazine
   (C) Mebendazole
   (D) Piperazine
   (E) Pyrantel pamoate
2. A patient with a tapeworm infection is to be treated with niclosamide. Which one of the following statements concerning the use of niclosamide is LEAST accurate?
   (A) A single dose achieves a cure rate of over 85% in the treatment of common tapeworm infections
   (B) Niclosamide is active against *Taenia* species and *Diphyllobothrium latum*
   (C) The patient probably became infected by eating raw or undercooked meat or fish
   (D) Niclosamide is only effective against intestinal worms
   (E) The drug will kill ova of the parasite
3. A missionary from Chicago is sent to work in a region of a Central American country where *Onchocerca volvulus* is endemic. Infections due to this tissue nematode (onchocerciasis) are a major cause of "river blindness," since microfilariae migrate through subcutaneous tissues and concentrate in the eyes. Which one of the following drugs can be used prophylactically to prevent onchocerciasis?
   (A) Bithionol
   (B) Ivermectin
   (C) Niclosamide
   (D) Oxamniquine
   (E) Suramin
4. A nonnative individual who contracts onchocerciasis in an endemic region would normally be treated with ivermectin and is likely to experience the Mazotti reaction. Which one of the following statements concerning this reaction is LEAST accurate?
   (A) The Mazotti reaction is more intense in nonnative adults than indigenous adults
   (B) Symptoms usually include headache, weakness, rash, muscle aches, hypotension, and peripheral edema
   (C) The reaction is due to drug toxicity
   (D) NSAIDs and steroids relieve symptoms of the reaction
   (E) The reaction is due to killing of microfilariae

5. Which one of the following statements about pyrantel pamoate is LEAST accurate?
   (A) It is highly effective in pinworm infections
   (B) Its action at the neuromuscular junction is similar to that of succinylcholine
   (C) Toxicity mainly concerns the gastrointestinal tract because only a small proportion of an oral dose is absorbed
   (D) The drug is equivalent in efficacy to niclosamide in the treatment of tapeworm infections
   (E) The drug kills adult worms in the colon but not the eggs

6. A medical student at a Caribbean university develops fever, chills, and diarrhea due to *S mansoni* infection, and oxamniquine is prescribed. Which one of the following statements about the proposed therapy is accurate?
   (A) It is not effective in late stages of the disease
   (B) If the patient has a history of seizure disorders, hospitalization is recommended during treatment
   (C) The drug is effective in other forms of schistosomiasis
   (D) Oxamniquine is safe for use in pregnancy
   (E) The drug blocks GABA receptors in trematodes

7. A 22-year-old Korean man has recently moved to Minnesota. He has symptoms of clonorchiasis (anorexia, upper abdominal pain, eosinophilia), presumably contracted in his homeland, where the Oriental liver fluke is endemic. He also has symptoms of diphyllobothriasis (abdominal discomfort, diarrhea, megaloblastic anemia), probably due to consuming raw fish from lakes near the Canadian border. Which one of the following drugs is most likely to be effective in the treatment of both clonorchiasis and diphyllobothriasis in this patient?
   (A) Albendazole
   (B) Ivermectin
   (C) Levamisole
   (D) Niclosamide
   (E) Praziquantel

8. Which one of the following infections due to helminths is LEAST likely to respond to treatment with praziquantel?
   (A) Hydatid disease
   (B) Opisthorchiasis
   (C) Paragonimiasis
   (D) Pork tapeworm infection
   (E) Schistosomiasis

Items 9–10: A sheepherder who lives most of the year in the mountains of eastern Nevada is hospitalized with liver cysts (hydatid disease) attributed to infection with *Echinococcus granulosus,* the dog tapeworm. He refuses to undergo surgery for removal of the cysts.

9. Which one of the following drugs is most likely to be of some help in this situation?
   (A) Albendazole
   (B) Ivermectin
   (C) Niclosamide
   (D) Oxamniquine
   (E) Suramin

10. Since the patient will have to undergo drug treatment for many months, he should be monitored for toxicity to the
    (A) Gonads
    (B) Kidney
    (C) Liver
    (D) Peripheral nerves
    (E) Retina

11. Which one of the following adverse effects occurs with the use of mebendazole during intestinal nematode therapy?
    (A) Cholestatic jaundice
    (B) Corneal opacities
    (C) Mazzotti reaction
    (D) Peripheral neuropathy
    (E) None of the above

12. A malnourished 12-year-old child who lives in a rural area of the southern United States presents with weakness, fever, cough, abdominal pain, and eosinophilia. His mother tells you that she has seen long, thin worms in the child's stools, sometimes with blood. A presumptive diagnosis of ascariasis is confirmed by the presence of the ova of *A lumbricoides* in the stools. However, microscopy also reveals that the stools contain the eggs of *Necator americanus*. The drug most likely to be effective in the treatment of this child is
    (A) Diethylcarbamazine
    (B) Ivermectin
    (C) Mebendazole
    (D) Niclosamide
    (E) Praziquantel

ANSWERS

1. Piperazine and ivermectin (not listed in the question) both cause muscle paralysis in nematodes by acting through GABA receptors. Pyrantel pamoate relaxes muscles by blocking nicotinic receptors. Diethylcarbamazine also causes muscle relaxation, but the mechanism is unknown. The benzimidazoles (albendazole, mebendazole) bind to alpha-tubulins in helminths to block transport processes. The answer is **(D)**.

2. Niclosamide is often used to treat tapeworm infections since it is usually effective in a single dose. It is minimally absorbed from the gastrointestinal tract and causes few side effects. The drug kills scoleces and cestode segments, but ova are not affected. The answer is **(E)**.

3. Ivermectin prevents onchocerciasis and is the drug of choice in the individual and mass treatment of the disease. The only other drugs effective against *Onchocerca volvulus* are suramin and diethylcarbamazine (not listed in the question). The World Health Organization no longer recommends diethylcarbamazine for onchocerciasis, since it is less effective and more toxic than ivermectin. Suramin is toxic to the kidney, liver, and nervous system and would not be used prophylactically in this case. The answer is **(B)**.

4. The Mazzotti reaction is due to the killing action of ivermectin on microfilariae, and its intensity correlates with the skin microfilaria load. It occurs more frequently and with greater severity in travelers and visitors than in the indigenous inhabitants of endemic areas. The reaction will occur with any drug capable of killing microfilariae, and it is not a drug toxicity. The answer is **(C)**.

5. Pyrantel pamoate is equivalent to mebendazole in the treatment of pinworm infections, but it is not effective in the treatment of infections caused by cestodes. The answer is **(D)**.

6. Oxamniquine may cause seizures, especially in persons with a history of convulsive disorders. Such persons should be hospitalized or treated with praziquantel. Oxamniquine is effective in all stages of disease caused by *S mansoni,* including advanced hepatosplenomegaly. It has been used extensively for mass treatment. The drug is not effective in other schistosomal diseases, and it is contraindicated in pregnancy. The answer is **(B)**.

7. Praziquantel is the drug of first choice for infections caused by the Oriental liver fluke and by the fish tapeworm. Both types of infection are acquired mainly from the consumption of raw fish. Niclosamide is one of two drugs of choice (with praziquantel) for fish tapeworm infections, but it is not active against *Clonorchis sinensis*. Albendazole is not effective in fish tapeworm infections but is useful in the pork tapeworm larval stage (cysticercosis). The answer is **(E)**.

8. Praziquantel has a wide spectrum of activity that includes many cestodes and trematodes. However, in hydatid disease, the drug has marginal efficacy because it does not affect the inner germinal membrane of *Echinococcus granulosus* present in hydatid cysts. The answer is **(A)**.

9. The optimal treatment of hydatid cysts is their surgical removal. Albendazole has been used—in high doses for 3 months or longer—for liver hydatid cysts. However, the cure rate, judged by shrinkage or disappearance of cysts, is less than 40%. The answer is **(A)**.

10. Elevations of aminotransferase occur most frequently (15–20% incidence) during long-term therapy with mebendazole. Jaundice has been reported in a few patients. With the exception of liver function, none of the other organ systems listed require periodic monitoring. The answer is **(C)**.

11. Mebendazole in the doses required for intestinal nematode therapy is almost free of adverse effects, even in the malnourished or debilitated patient. Gastrointestinal distress together with slight headache or dizziness may occur in children with ascariasis who are heavily parasitized. The answer is **(E)**.

12. Mebendazole and pyrantel pamoate (not listed in this question) are drugs of choice for the treatment of combined infections due to hookworm and roundworm. If this patient is also infected with *Trichuris trichiura* (whipworm), mebendazole would be more effective than pyrantel pamoate. The answer is **(C)**.

55   Cancer Chemotherapy

OBJECTIVES

You should be able to:

- Describe the relevance of cell cycle kinetics to the modes of action and clinical uses of anticancer drugs.
- Identify the major subclasses of anticancer drugs, describe the mechanisms of action of the main drugs in each subclass, and describe the mechanisms by which tumor cells develop drug resistance.
- Identify the drugs of choice for the more important neoplastic diseases and describe their pharmacokinetics and toxic effects.
- Understand the rationale underlying the strategies of combination drug chemotherapy and rescue therapies.

Learn the definitions that follow.

Table 55–1. Definitions.

Term	Definition
Cell cycle-specific (CCS) drug	An anticancer agent that acts selectively on tumor stem cells when they are traversing the cell cycle and not when they are in the G_0, or resting, phase
Cell cycle-nonspecific (CCNS) drug	An anticancer agent that acts on tumor stem cells when they are traversing the cell cycle and when they are in the resting phase
Log kill hypothesis	The concept developed to account for the observation that anticancer drugs kill a fixed proportion of a tumor cell population, not a fixed number of tumor cells. For example, a 1-log kill will decrease a tumor cell population by one order of magnitude, ie, 90% of the cells will be eradicated
Growth fraction	The proportion of cells in a tumor population that are actively dividing
Rescue therapy	The administration of endogenous metabolites to counteract the effects of anticancer drugs on normal (nonneoplastic) cells

CONCEPTS

The treatment of cancer requires a variety of different types of drugs, acting on several different targets (Figure 55–1).

CANCER CELL CYCLE KINETICS

A. Cell Cycle Kinetics: Cancer cell population kinetics and the cancer cell cycle are important determinants of the actions and clinical uses of anticancer drugs. Some anticancer drugs act specifically on tumor cells undergoing cycling (cell cycle-specific [CCS] drugs), and others

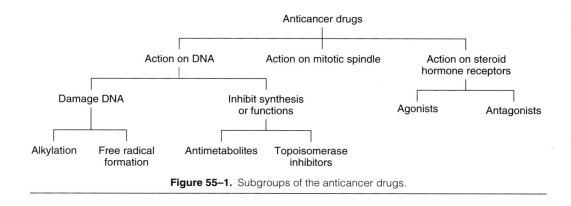

Figure 55–1. Subgroups of the anticancer drugs.

(cell cycle-nonspecific [CCNS] drugs) kill tumor cells in both cycling and resting phases of the cell cycle. CCS drugs are usually most active in a specific phase of the cell cycle (Figure 55–2). In general, CCS drugs are particularly effective when a large proportion of the tumor cells are proliferating (ie, when the growth fraction is high).

B.   The Log Kill Hypothesis: Cytotoxic drugs act with first-order kinetics, a given dose killing a constant *proportion* of a cell population rather than a constant *number* of cells. The log kill hypothesis proposes that the magnitude of tumor cell kill by anticancer drugs is a logarithmic function. For example, a 3-log kill dose of an effective drug will reduce a cancer cell population of 10^{12} cells to 10^{9} (a total kill of $10^{12} - 10^{9}$ or 999×10^{9} cells); the same dose would reduce a starting population of 10^{6} cells to 10^{3} cells (a kill of 999×10^{3} cells). In both cases, the dose reduces the numbers of cells by three orders of magnitude, or "3 logs."

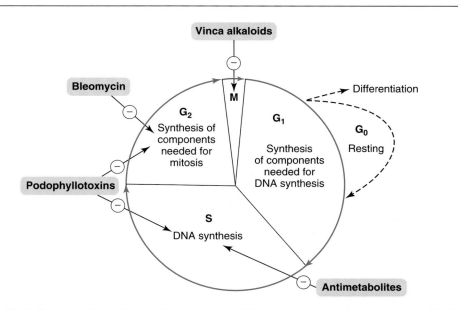

Figure 55–2. Phases of the cell cycle that are susceptible to the actions of cell cycle-specific (CCS) drugs. All cells—normal and neoplastic—must traverse these cell cycle phases before and during cell division. CCS drug actions may not be restricted to a specific phase, but tumor cells are usually most responsive to specific drugs (or drug groups) in the phases indicated. Cell cycle-nonspecific (CCNS) drugs act on tumor cells while they are actively cycling and while they are in the resting phase (G_0). (Adapted, with permission, from Katzung BG [editor]: *Basic & Clinical Pharmacology,* 7th ed. Appleton & Lange, 1998.)

C. **Resistance to Anticancer Drugs:** Drug resistance is a major problem in cancer chemotherapy. In many cases, the resistance mechanisms involve changes in gene expression in neoplastic cells that result in resistance either to an individual drug or to multiple anticancer drugs. Mechanisms of resistance include:

1. **Increased DNA repair:** An increased rate of DNA repair in tumor cells is responsible for resistance to several groups of anticancer drugs and is particularly important in the case of most alkylating agents and cisplatin.

2. **Formation of trapping agents:** Some tumor cells increase their production of thiol trapping agents (eg, glutathione), which interact with anticancer drugs that form reactive electrophilic species. This mechanism of resistance is seen with the alkylating agents as well as with bleomycin, cisplatin, and the anthracyclines.

3. **Changes in target enzymes:** Changes in the drug sensitivity of a target enzyme, dihydrofolate reductase, and increased synthesis of the enzyme are mechanisms of resistance of tumor cells to methotrexate. Resistance to the *Vinca* alkaloids can involve changes in the structure of their target, the tubulin proteins.

4. **Decreased activation of prodrugs:** Resistance to the purine antimetabolites (mercaptopurine, thioguanine) and the pyrimidine antimetabolites (cytarabine, fluorouracil) can result from a decrease in the activity of the tumor cell enzymes needed to convert these prodrugs to their cytotoxic metabolites.

5. **Inactivation of anticancer drugs:** Increased activity of enzymes capable of inactivating anticancer drugs is a mechanism of tumor cell resistance to most of the purine and pyrimidine antimetabolites.

6. **Decreased drug accumulation:** This form of multidrug resistance often involves the increased expression of a normal gene (the *MDR1* gene) for a cell surface glycoprotein (P-glycoprotein). This transport molecule is involved in the accelerated efflux of many anticancer drugs in resistant cells.

ALKYLATING AGENTS

The alkylating agents include nitrogen mustards (**chlorambucil, cyclophosphamide, mechlorethamine**), nitrosoureas (**carmustine [BCNU], lomustine [CCNU]**), and alkylsulfonates (**busulfan**). Other drugs that act in part as alkylating agents include **cisplatin, dacarbazine,** and **procarbazine.**

The alkylating agents are CCNS drugs. They form reactive molecular species that alkylate nucleophilic groups on DNA bases, particularly the N-7 position of guanine. This leads to cross-linking of bases, abnormal base pairing, and DNA strand breakage. Tumor cell resistance to the drugs occurs through increased DNA repair, decreased drug permeability, or the production of trapping agents such as thiols. Cross-resistance occurs commonly between the alkylating agents, except for the nitrosoureas.

A. **Cyclophosphamide:**

1. **Pharmacokinetics:** Hepatic cytochrome P450-mediated biotransformation of cyclophosphamide is needed for antitumor activity.

2. **Clinical use:** Cyclophosphamide is used in non-Hodgkin's lymphoma, breast and ovarian cancers, and neuroblastoma.

3. **Toxicity:** Gastrointestinal distress, myelosuppression, and alopecia are expected adverse effects. Hemorrhagic cystitis due to the formation of acrolein may be decreased by vigorous hydration and possibly by use of **mesna** (mercaptoethanesulfonate).

B. **Mechlorethamine:**

1. **Mechanism and pharmacokinetics:** Mechlorethamine is spontaneously converted in the body to a reactive cytotoxic product.

2. **Clinical use:** Mechlorethamine is best known for use in the MOPP regimen (see below) for Hodgkin's disease.

3. **Toxicity:** Gastrointestinal distress, myelosuppression, and alopecia are common. Mechlorethamine has marked vesicant actions.

C. **Carmustine (BCNU) and Lomustine (CCNU):**

1. **Pharmacokinetics:** BCNU and CCNU are nitrosoureas with high lipophilicity that facilitates CNS entry.

2. **Clinical use:** BCNU and CCNU are used as adjuncts in the treatment of brain tumors.
3. **Toxicity:** Adverse effects include gastrointestinal distress, myelosuppression, and CNS dysfunction.

D. Busulfan:
1. **Pharmacokinetics:** Busulfan is well absorbed orally and has a short duration of action owing to hepatic metabolism.
2. **Clinical use:** Busulfan is used as a component of most regimens for chronic myelogenous leukemia.
3. **Toxicity:** In addition to myelosuppression, busulfan causes hyperpigmentation, adrenal suppression, and pulmonary fibrosis.

E. Cisplatin and Carboplatin:
1. **Pharmacokinetics:** Cisplatin is used intravenously; the drug is distributed to most tissues and is cleared in unchanged form by the kidney. Carboplatin is similar.
2. **Clinical use:** Cisplatin is commonly used as a component of regimens for testicular carcinoma and for cancers of the bladder, lung, and ovary. Carboplatin has similar uses.
3. **Toxicity:** Cisplatin causes gastrointestinal distress and mild hematotoxicity and is neurotoxic (peripheral neuritis and acoustic nerve damage) and nephrotoxic. Renal damage may be reduced by the use of mannitol with forced hydration. Carboplatin is less nephrotoxic than cisplatin and is less likely to cause tinnitus and hearing loss, but it has greater myelosuppressant actions.

F. Procarbazine:
1. **Mechanisms:** Procarbazine is a reactive agent that forms hydrogen peroxide, which generates free radicals that cause DNA strand scission. Several of procarbazine's metabolites are cytotoxic, and one is an MAO inhibitor.
2. **Pharmacokinetics:** Procarbazine is orally active and penetrates into most tissues, including the CSF. It is eliminated via hepatic metabolism.
3. **Clinical use:** The primary use of the drug is as a component of the MOPP regimen for Hodgkin's disease.
4. **Toxicity:** Procarbazine is myelosuppressant and causes gastrointestinal irritation. The drug may also cause CNS dysfunction, peripheral neuropathy, and skin reactions. Procarbazine inhibits many enzymes, including those involved in hepatic drug metabolism. Disulfiram-like reactions have occurred with ethanol. The drug is leukemogenic.

G. Dacarbazine:
1. **Mechanisms:** Dacarbazine is activated by liver enzymes to form methylcarbonium species that act as alkylating agents and interfere with nucleic acid metabolism.
2. **Pharmacokinetics:** Dacarbazine is given intravenously; the drug is eliminated via hepatic metabolism.
3. **Clinical use:** Dacarbazine is used in Hodgkin's disease as part of the ABVD regimen (see below).
4. **Toxicity:** Gastrointestinal distress, myelosuppression, and alopecia are observed.

ANTIMETABOLITES

The antimetabolites are structurally similar to endogenous compounds and are antagonists of folic acid **(methotrexate)**, purines **(mercaptopurine, thioguanine)**, or pyrimidines **(fluorouracil, cytarabine)**. Antimetabolites are CCS drugs acting primarily in the S phase of the cell cycle. Their sites of action on DNA synthetic pathways are shown in Figure 55–3. In addition to their cytotoxic effects on neoplastic cells, the antimetabolites also have immunosuppressant actions. Some of the uses of the antimetabolites in neoplastic disease are listed in Table 55–2.

A. Methotrexate (MTX):
1. **Mechanisms of action and resistance:** Methotrexate is a substrate for (and inhibitor of) dihydrofolate reductase. This action leads to a decrease in the synthesis of thymidylate, purine nucleotides, and amino acids and thus interferes with nucleic acid and protein

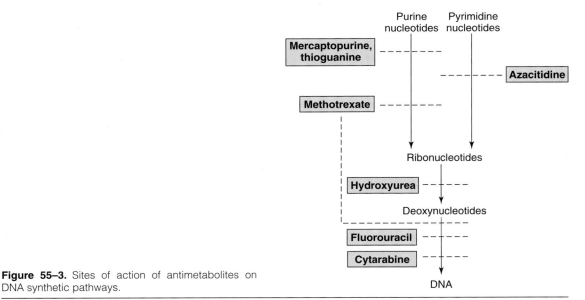

Figure 55–3. Sites of action of antimetabolites on DNA synthetic pathways.

metabolism. The formation of polyglutamate derivatives of methotrexate appears to be important for cytotoxic actions. Tumor cell resistance mechanisms include decreased drug accumulation, changes in the drug sensitivity or activity of dihydrofolate reductase, and decreased formation of polyglutamates.

2. **Pharmacokinetics:** Oral and intravenous administration of methotrexate affords good tissue distribution except to the CNS. Methotrexate is not metabolized, and its clearance is dependent on renal function.

3. **Clinical use:** Methotrexate is effective in choriocarcinoma and is also used for acute leukemias, non-Hodgkin's and cutaneous T cell lymphomas, and breast cancer. Methotrexate is also used in rheumatoid arthritis and psoriasis and is an abortifacient.

Table 55–2. Selected examples of effective cancer chemotherapy.*[1]

Diagnosis	Current Drug Therapy of Choice
Acute lymphocytic leukemia	Induction: Vincristine plus prednisone. Maintenance: Mercaptopurine, methotrexate, and cyclophosphamide in various combinations
Acute myelogenous leukemia	Induction: Cytarabine plus mitoxantrone or daunorubicin. Maintenance: Cytarabine plus etoposide or daunorubicin
Breast carcinoma (early stage)	Cyclophosphamide plus methotrexate and fluorouracil; tamoxifen if hormone receptor-positive
Burkitt's lymphoma	Cyclophosphamide plus methotrexate and vincristine
Ewing's sarcoma	Cyclophosphamide plus doxorubicin and vincristine
Hodgkin's disease	See text: examples of combination chemotherapy
Non-Hodgkin's lymphoma	Cyclophosphamide plus doxorubicin, vincristine, and prednisone
Small cell lung carcinoma	Multiple combinations that include cyclophosphamide, cisplatin, doxorubicin, etoposide, and vincristine
Trophoblastic (gestational) neoplasms	Methotrexate alone, or cisplatin plus etoposide
Testicular carcinoma	See text: examples of combination chemotherapy
Wilms' tumor	Dactinomycin plus vincristine (plus other agents for tumors with unfavorable histology)

*Modified and reproduced, with permission, from Katzung BG (editor): *Basic & Clinical Pharmacology,* 7th ed. Appleton & Lange, 1998.
[1]Cancers that respond to chemotherapy with prolonged patient survival and some cures.

4. **Toxicity:** Common adverse effects include bone marrow suppression and toxic effects on the skin and gastrointestinal mucosa (mucositis). The toxic effects of methotrexate on normal cells may be reduced by administration of folinic acid (leucovorin); this strategy is called **"leucovorin rescue."** Long-term use of methotrexate has led to hepatotoxicity. Salicylates, NSAIDs, sulfonamides, and sulfonylureas enhance the toxicity of methotrexate.

B. **Mercaptopurine (6-MP) and Thioguanine (6-TG):**
  1. **Mechanisms of action and resistance:** Mercaptopurine and thioguanine are purine antimetabolites. Both drugs are activated by hypoxanthine-guanine phosphoribosyltransferases (HGPRTases) to toxic nucleotides that inhibit several enzymes involved in purine metabolism. Resistant tumor cells have a decreased activity of HGPRTase, or they may increase their production of alkaline phosphatases that inactivate the toxic nucleotides.
  2. **Pharmacokinetics:** Mercaptopurine and thioguanine have low oral bioavailability as a result of first-pass metabolism by hepatic enzymes. Neither drug penetrates significantly into CSF. The metabolism of 6-MP by xanthine oxidase is inhibited by allopurinol.
  3. **Clinical use:** These purine antimetabolites are used mainly in the acute leukemias and chronic myelocytic leukemia.
  4. **Toxicity:** Bone marrow suppression is dose-limiting, but purine antimetabolites may also cause dose-dependent hepatic dysfunction (cholestasis, jaundice, necrosis).

C. **Cytarabine (Ara-C):**
  1. **Mechanisms of action and resistance:** Cytarabine (cytosine arabinoside) is a pyrimidine antimetabolite. The drug is activated by kinases to AraCTP, an inhibitor of DNA polymerases. Of all the antimetabolites, cytarabine is the most specific for the S phase of the tumor cell cycle. Resistance to cytarabine can occur through decreased uptake of Ara-C or a decreased conversion to AraCTP.
  2. **Pharmacokinetics:** The drug is used parenterally, and with slow IV infusion may reach appreciable levels in the CSF. Ara-C is eliminated via hepatic metabolism.
  3. **Clinical use:** Cytarabine is an important component in regimens for the treatment of acute leukemias.
  4. **Toxicity:** Ara-C causes gastrointestinal irritation and myelosuppression. High doses have led to neurotoxicity (cerebellar dysfunction and peripheral neuritis).

D. **Fluorouracil (5-FU):**
  1. **Mechanisms:** Fluorouracil is biotransformed to 5-fluoro-2′-deoxyuridine-5′-monophosphate (5-FdUMP), which inhibits thymidylate synthase and leads to "thymineless death" of cells. Tumor cell resistance mechanisms include decreased metabolism of 5-FU, increased thymidylate synthase activity, and reduced drug sensitivity of this enzyme.
  2. **Pharmacokinetics:** When given intravenously, fluorouracil is widely distributed, including into the CSF. Elimination is mainly by metabolism.
  3. **Clinical use:** Fluorouracil is used in bladder, breast, colon, head and neck, liver, and ovarian cancers. The drug can be used topically for keratoses and superficial basal cell carcinoma.
  4. **Toxicity:** Gastrointestinal distress, myelosuppression, and alopecia are common.

PLANT ALKALOIDS

The plant alkaloids are CCS drugs. The most important of these natural products are the *Vinca* alkaloids **(vinblastine, vincristine),** the podophyllotoxins **(etoposide, teniposide),** and the taxanes **(paclitaxel, docetaxel).**

A. **Vinblastine and Vincristine:**
  1. **Mechanisms:** Vinblastine and vincristine are **spindle poisons** that, by preventing the assembly of tubulin dimers into microtubules, block the formation of the mitotic spindle. They act primarily in the M phase of the cancer cell cycle. Resistance may occur from increased efflux of the drugs from tumor cells via the membrane drug transporter.
  2. **Pharmacokinetics:** Both drugs must be given parenterally. They penetrate most tissues except the CSF. Both drugs are cleared mainly via biliary excretion.

3. **Clinical use:** Vincristine is a component of the MOPP and COP combination drug regimens and is used in acute leukemias, lymphomas, Wilms' tumor, and choriocarcinoma. Vinblastine is a component of the ABVD regimen for Hodgkin's disease and is used for other lymphomas, neuroblastoma, testicular carcinoma, and Kaposi's sarcoma.

4. **Toxicity:** Vinblastine causes gastrointestinal distress, alopecia, and bone marrow suppression. Vincristine does not cause serious myelosuppression but has neurotoxic actions and may cause areflexia, peripheral neuritis, and paralytic ileus.

B. **Etoposide and Teniposide:**

1. **Mechanisms:** Etoposide increases degradation of DNA, possibly via interaction with topoisomerase II, and inhibits mitochondrial electron transport. The drug is most active in the late S and early G_2 phases of the cell cycle. Teniposide is an analog with very similar pharmacologic characteristics.

2. **Pharmacokinetics:** Etoposide is well absorbed after oral administration and distributed to most body tissues. Elimination of etoposide is mainly via the kidneys, and dose reductions should be made in patients with renal impairment.

3. **Clinical use:** These agents are used in combination drug regimens for therapy of lung (small cell), prostate, and testicular carcinoma.

4. **Toxicity:** Etoposide and teniposide are gastrointestinal irritants and cause alopecia and bone marrow suppression.

C. **Paclitaxel and Docetaxel:**

1. **Mechanisms:** Paclitaxel and docetaxel are spindle poisons and act differently from *Vinca* alkaloids: they prevent microtubule *disassembly* into tubulin monomers.

2. **Pharmacokinetics:** Paclitaxel and docetaxel are given intravenously.

3. **Clinical use:** Paclitaxel is approved for use in ovarian cancer and advanced breast cancer. Docetaxel is approved for use in advanced breast cancer.

4. **Toxicity:** Paclitaxel causes neutropenia, thrombocytopenia, a high incidence of peripheral neuropathy, and possible hypersensitivity reactions during infusion. Docetaxel causes neurotoxicity and bone marrow depression.

ANTIBIOTICS

This category of antineoplastic drugs is made up of several structurally dissimilar agents, including **doxorubicin, daunorubicin, bleomycin, dactinomycin, mitomycin,** and **mithramycin.**

A. **Doxorubicin and Daunorubicin:**

1. **Mechanisms:** These anthracyclines can intercalate between base pairs, interact with topoisomerase II, and generate free radicals. They block the synthesis of RNA and DNA and cause DNA strand scission. Membrane disruption also occurs. Anthracyclines are CCNS drugs.

2. **Pharmacokinetics:** Doxorubicin and daunorubicin must be given intravenously. They are metabolized in the liver, and the products are excreted in the bile.

3. **Clinical uses:** Doxorubicin is a component of the ABVD regimen used in Hodgkin's disease and is used in treatment of myelomas, sarcomas, and breast, endometrial, lung, ovarian, and thyroid cancers. The main use of daunorubicin is in the treatment of acute leukemias. **Idarubicin,** a new anthracycline, is approved for use in acute myelogenous leukemia.

4. **Toxicity:** Both drugs cause bone marrow suppression, gastrointestinal distress, and severe alopecia. Their most distinctive adverse effect is cardiotoxicity, which includes initial ECG abnormalities (with the possibility of arrhythmias) and slowly developing cardiomyopathy and congestive heart failure. **Dexrazoxane,** a free radical scavenger, may protect against cardiotoxicity.

B. **Bleomycin:**

1. **Mechanisms:** Bleomycin is a mixture of glycopeptides that generates free radicals that bind to DNA, cause strand breaks, and inhibit DNA synthesis. Bleomycin is a CCS drug active in the G_2 phase of the tumor cell cycle.

2. **Pharmacokinetics:** Bleomycin must be given parenterally. It is inactivated by tissue aminopeptidases, but some renal clearance of intact drug also occurs.
3. **Clinical use:** Bleomycin is a component of combination drug regimens for Hodgkin's disease and testicular cancer. It is also used for treatment of lymphomas and for squamous cell carcinomas.
4. **Toxicity:** The toxicity profile of bleomycin is unusual. Pulmonary toxicity (pneumonitis, fibrosis) develops slowly and is dose-limiting. Hypersensitivity reactions (chills, fever, anaphylaxis) are common, as are mucocutaneous reactions (alopecia, blister formation, hyperkeratosis).

C. **Dactinomycin:**
  1. **Mechanisms:** Dactinomycin is a CCNS drug that binds to double-stranded DNA and inhibits DNA-dependent RNA synthesis.
  2. **Pharmacokinetics:** Dactinomycin must be given parenterally, and both intact drug and metabolites are excreted in the bile.
  3. **Clinical use:** Dactinomycin is used in melanomas and Wilms' tumor.
  4. **Toxicity:** This drug causes bone marrow suppression, skin reactions, and gastrointestinal irritation.

D. **Mitomycin:**
  1. **Mechanisms:** Mitomycin is a CCNS drug that is metabolized by liver enzymes to form an alkylating agent which cross-links DNA.
  2. **Pharmacokinetics:** Mitomycin is given intravenously and rapidly cleared via hepatic metabolism.
  3. **Clinical use:** Mitomycin acts against hypoxic tumor cells and is used in combination regimens for adenocarcinomas of the cervix, stomach, pancreas, and lung.
  4. **Toxicity:** Mitomycin causes severe myelosuppression and can be nephrotoxic. A form of interstitial pneumonia can occur.

HORMONAL & MISCELLANEOUS ANTICANCER AGENTS

A. **Hormones and Hormone Antagonists:**
  1. **Glucocorticoids: Prednisone** is the most commonly used glucocorticoid in cancer chemotherapy. The steroid has applications in drug regimens for chronic lymphocytic leukemia, Hodgkin's disease (MOPP regimen), and other lymphomas.
  2. **Sex hormones:** The estrogens, progestins, and androgens are used in some hormone-dependent cancers to change the hormone balance.
  3. **Sex hormone antagonists: Tamoxifen,** an estrogen receptor partial agonist, blocks the binding of estrogen to receptors of estrogen-sensitive cancer cells. It is extremely useful in the therapy of breast cancer and also acts against progestin-resistant endometrial carcinoma. A large clinical trial is currently under way to determine whether it can *prevent* breast cancer in women at high risk. **Flutamide** is an androgen receptor antagonist used in prostatic carcinoma.
  4. **Gonadotropin-releasing hormone analogs: Leuprolide, goserelin,** and **nafarelin** are GnRH agonists. When administered in constant doses so as to maintain stable blood levels, they *inhibit* release of pituitary LH and FSH. These agents are as effective as diethylstilbestrol in prostatic carcinoma and cause fewer adverse effects.
  5. **Aromatase inhibitors: Anastrozole** and **aminoglutethimide** inhibit aromatase, the enzyme that catalyzes the conversion of androstenedione (an androgenic precursor) to estrone (an estrogenic hormone). Both drugs are used in advanced breast cancer in postmenopausal women. Aminoglutethimide also inhibits the conversion of cholesterol to pregnenolone, with major effects on the synthesis of adrenal steroids.

B. **Miscellaneous Anticancer Agents:**
  1. **Asparaginase:** Asparaginase is an enzyme that depletes serum asparagine; it is used in the treatment of T cell auxotrophic cancers (leukemia and lymphomas) that require exogenous asparagine for growth. Asparagine is given intravenously and may cause severe hypersensitivity reactions, acute pancreatitis, and bleeding.

2. **Mitoxantrone:** This anthracene compound probably acts via the alkylation of DNA bases. Mitoxantrone is used in combination regimens for refractory acute leukemia. Myelosuppression, gastrointestinal effects, and cardiac arrhythmias are toxic effects of the drug.

3. **Interferons:** The interferons are endogenous glycoproteins with antineoplastic, immunosuppressive, and antiviral actions. Alpha-interferons (see Chapter 56) are effective against a number of neoplasms, including hairy cell leukemia, the early stage of chronic myelogenous leukemia, and T cell lymphomas. Toxic effects of the interferons include myelosuppression and neurologic dysfunction.

STRATEGIES IN CANCER CHEMOTHERAPY

A. **Principles of Combination Therapy:**   Chemotherapy with combinations of anticancer drugs usually increases log kill markedly, and, in some cases, synergistic effects are achieved. Combinations are often cytotoxic to a heterogeneous population of cancer cells and may prevent development of resistant clones. Drug combinations using CCS and CCNS drugs may be cytotoxic to both dividing and resting cancer cells. The following principles are important for selecting appropriate drugs to use in combination chemotherapy:

(1) Each drug should be active when used alone against the particular cancer.
(2) The drugs should have different mechanisms of action.
(3) Cross-resistance between drugs should be minimal.
(4) The drugs should have different toxic effects.

B. **Examples of Combination Chemotherapy:**
1. **Hodgkin's disease:**
    a. **MOPP regimen:**   Mechlorethamine, Oncovin (vincristine), procarbazine, and prednisone. This regimen is effective and was the mainstay of drug treatment of stages III and IV of the disease for many years. It has now been replaced—for initial therapy—by the ABVD regimen.
    b. **ABVD regimen:**   Adriamycin (doxorubicin), bleomycin, vinblastine, and dacarbazine. The ABVD regimen is equally effective and appears to be less likely to cause sterility and secondary malignancies (leukemia) than the MOPP regimen. If the neoplasm becomes resistant, the MOPP regimen may be alternated with the ABVD regimen.
2. **Non-Hodgkin's lymphoma:**   The COP regimen, which includes cyclophosphamide, Oncovin (vincristine), and prednisone, is commonly used with or without doxorubicin (COP-D).
3. **Testicular carcinoma:**   The PVB regimen, which includes Platinol (cisplatin), vinblastine, and bleomycin, is the standard treatment and is very effective. A more recently introduced regimen, in which cisplatin is replaced by etoposide, appears to be equally effective.
4. **Breast carcinoma:**   Postoperative chemotherapy commonly involves use of the CMF regimen (cyclophosphamide, methotrexate, and fluorouracil) with or without tamoxifen.

C. **Additional Strategies for Cancer Chemotherapy:**
1. **Pulse therapy:**   Pulse therapy involves intermittent treatment with very high doses of an anticancer drug—doses that are too toxic to be used continuously. Intensive drug treatment every 3–4 weeks allows for maximum effects on neoplastic cells, with hematologic and immunologic recovery between courses. This type of regimen is used successfully in therapy of acute leukemias, testicular carcinomas, and Wilms' tumor.
2. **Recruitment and synchrony:**   The strategy of **recruitment** involves initial use of a CCNS drug to achieve a significant log kill, which results in the recruitment into cell division of previously resting cells in the G_0 phase of the cell cycle. With subsequent administration of a CCS drug active against dividing cells, maximal cell kill may be achieved. A similar approach involves **synchrony,** one example being the use of *Vinca* alkaloids to hold cancer cells in the M phase. Subsequent treatment with another CCS drug, such as the S phase-specific agent cytarabine, may result in a greater killing effect on the neoplastic cell population.
3. **Rescue therapy:**   Toxic effects of anticancer drugs can sometimes be alleviated by rescue strategy. For example, high doses of methotrexate may be given for 36–48 hours and terminated before severe toxicity occurs to cells of the gastrointestinal tract and bone marrow.

Leucovorin (folinic acid), which is accumulated more readily by normal than by neoplastic cells, is then administered. This results in rescue of the normal cells, since leucovorin bypasses the dihydrofolate reductase step in folic acid synthesis.

DRUG LIST

The following drugs are important members of the group discussed in this chapter. Prototypes should be learned in detail; features of the major variants should be known well enough so that the variants can be distinguished from prototypes and from each other; the other significant agents should be recognized as belonging to a specific subclass.

Subclass	Prototype	Major Variants	Other Significant Agents
Alkylating agents Nitrogen mustards	Mechlorethamine		Cyclophosphamide, chlorambucil
Nitrosoureas	Carmustine	Lomustine	Semustine
Alkylsulfonates	Busulfan		
Platinum complex	Cisplatin	Carboplatin	
Triazenes	Dacarbazine		
Hydrazines	Procarbazine		
Antimetabolites Folate analogs	Methotrexate		
Purine analogs	Mercaptopurine		Thioguanine
Pyrimidine analogs	Fluorouracil		Cytarabine
Plant alkaloids Vinca alkaloids	Vinblastine	Vincristine	
Podophyllotoxins	Etoposide	Teniposide	
Other	Paclitaxel		Docetaxel
Antibiotics Anthracyclines	Doxorubicin	Daunorubicin	
Bleomycins	Bleomycin		
Actinomycins	Dactinomycin		
Mitomycins	Mitomycin		
Hormones Adrenocorticoids	Prednisone	Hydrocortisone	
Androgens	Testosterone	Fluoxymesterone	
Estrogens	Diethylstilbestrol	Ethinyl estradiol	
Progestins	Hydroxyprogesterone	Medroxyprogesterone	
Antiestrogens	Tamoxifen	Anastrozole	
Antiandrogens	Flutamide		
Gonadotropin-releasing hormone agonists	Leuprolide	Goserelin, naferelin	

QUESTIONS

DIRECTIONS: Each of the numbered items or incomplete statements in this section is followed by answers or by completions of the statement. Select the ONE lettered answer or completion that is BEST in each case.

Items 1–3: A 32-year-old woman underwent segmental mastectomy for a breast tumor of 3 cm diameter. Lymph node sampling revealed two involved nodes. Since chemotherapy is of established value in her situation, she underwent postoperative treatment with antineoplastic drugs. The FAC-V regimen was employed, which consisted of a drug combination of fluorouracil, doxorubicin (Adriamycin), and cyclophosphamide plus vincristine. Six cycles of this chemotherapy regimen were planned, each 1 month apart. Adjunctive drugs used included tamoxifen, since the tumor cells were hormone receptor-positive.

1. Regarding the mechanisms of action and resistance of the antineoplastic drugs used in this case, which one of the following statements is most accurate?
    (A) Resistance to fluorouracil occurs via decreased activity of hypoxanthine-guanine phosphoribosyl transferase (HGPRT)
    (B) Cyclophosphamide is an irreversible inhibitor of dihydrofolic acid reductase
    (C) Resistance to doxorubicin occurs through the formation of enzymes that can degrade the drug
    (D) Vincristine causes DNA strand scission through effects on topoisomerase II
    (E) A metabolite of fluorouracil is cytotoxic because it causes "thymineless death" of cells

2. The chemotherapy undertaken by this patient caused considerable gastrointestinal and hematologic toxicity. Which one of the following statements concerning these and other adverse effects of the drugs she was taking is LEAST accurate?
    (A) The administration of doxorubicin probably caused local tissue necrosis
    (B) The patient should have been advised to maintain a high fluid intake to decrease the risk of dysuria and hematuria
    (C) The nausea and vomiting that she experienced was mainly due to tamoxifen
    (D) Granulocyte and platelet counts should be determined immediately prior to each cycle of drug treatment
    (E) Of the cytotoxic drugs used, vincristine was the least likely to contribute to myelosuppression

3. Between drug cycles 3 and 4, the patient was found to have a high resting pulse rate. A noninvasive radionuclide scan revealed evidence of cardiotoxicity, and a change in the drug regimen was suggested for the next cycle of treatment. Which one of the following changes is best?
    (A) Dosage of doxorubicin was reduced by 20%
    (B) Mesna (mercaptoethanesulfonate) was added to the drug regimen
    (C) Mitoxantrone was added and doxorubicin discontinued
    (D) Methotrexate replaced doxorubicin
    (E) Vincristine was discontinued

4. In a patient with diffuse lymphoma, the oncologist suggests a treatment strategy that involves the initial administration of doxorubicin to obtain a significant log kill, followed by the cell cycle-specific drugs cytarabine and vincristine. This therapeutic strategy is called
    (A) Pulse therapy
    (B) Recruitment
    (C) Rescue therapy
    (D) Sequential blockade
    (E) Synchrony

5. Which one of the following statements about the mechanisms of action of drugs used in cancer chemotherapy is LEAST accurate?
    (A) Alkylating agents commonly attack the nucleophilic N-7 position in guanine
    (B) Anthracyclines intercalate with base pairs to block nucleic acid synthesis
    (C) In steady doses, leuprolide inhibits the release of pituitary gonadotropins
    (D) Mercaptopurine is an irreversible inhibitor of HGPRTase
    (E) Paclitaxel acts mainly in the M phase of the cell cycle

Items 6–7: A patient with metastatic choriocarcinoma is to be treated with methotrexate (MTX) in a pulse dosage regimen, with the first drug course to continue for no more than 72 hours. Serum creatinine levels will be monitored, and rescue treatment with leucovorin is planned. Prior to drug treatment, glucose and bicarbonate will be given over 8–12 hours. Urine pH will be maintained above pH 6.5.

6. It is important to monitor serum MTX levels during the initial course of drug treatment because
    (A) High MTX levels in the blood require additional leucovorin rescue
    (B) Levels of MTX in the blood are predictive of gastrointestinal mucositis
    (C) MTX readily penetrates into the CSF
    (D) Renal toxicity due to MTX is likely to occur
    (E) Resistance to MTX occurs within a few days

7. Maintenance of a high urinary pH is important during methotrexate treatment in this patient because
   (A) Bladder irritation is reduced
   (B) It decreases renal tubular secretion of methotrexate
   (C) Leucovorin toxicity is increased in a dehydrated patient
   (D) Methotrexate is a weak acid
   (E) Reabsorption of purine metabolites occurs at high urinary pH

8. An adult patient is being treated for acute leukemia with a combination of anticancer drugs that includes cyclophosphamide, mercaptopurine, methotrexate, vincristine, and prednisone. He is also using dronabinol for emesis, a chlorhexidine mouthwash to reduce mucositis, and laxatives. The patient complains of "pins and needles" sensations in the extremities and muscle weakness. He is not able to execute a deep knee bend or get up out of a chair without using his arm muscles. He is also very constipated. If these problems are related to the chemotherapy, the most likely causative agent is
   (A) Chlorhexidine
   (B) Cyclophosphamide
   (C) Mercaptopurine
   (D) Prednisone
   (E) Vincristine

9. Which of the following agents is used in drug combination regimens to treat testicular carcinoma? (Adequate hydration of the patient and the use of an osmotic diuretic decrease the toxicity of the drug.)
   (A) Bleomycin
   (B) Cisplatin
   (C) Etoposide
   (D) Leuprolide
   (E) Vinblastine

10. Which one of the following is LEAST likely to be a mechanism of cancer cell resistance to antineoplastic drugs?
    (A) Change in properties of a target enzyme
    (B) Decreased activity of activating enzymes
    (C) Increase in drug-metabolizing cytochrome P450
    (D) Increase in DNA repair
    (E) Increase in production of drug-trapping molecules, eg, glutathione

Items 11–12: A 23-year-old man with Hodgkin's disease was treated unsuccessfully with the MOPP regimen. He subsequently underwent a successful course of therapy with the ABVD regimen.

11. Which one of the following classes of anticancer drugs used in the treatment of this patient is cell cycle-specific (CCS) and used in both the MOPP and ABVD regimens?
    (A) Alkylating agents
    (B) Antibiotics
    (C) Antimetabolites
    (D) Glucocorticoids
    (E) Plant alkaloids

12. During the second course of drug treatment (ABVD regimen), this patient developed dyspnea, a nonproductive cough, and intermittent fever. Chest x-ray revealed pulmonary infiltration. If these problems are due to the anticancer drugs that he has been exposed to, the most likely causative agent is
    (A) Bleomycin
    (B) Dacarbazine
    (C) Doxorubicin
    (D) Prednisone
    (E) Vinblastine

DIRECTIONS (Items 13–16): Each set of matching questions in this section consists of a list of three to twenty-six lettered options (some of which may be figures) followed by several numbered items. For each numbered item, select the ONE lettered option that is most closely associated with it. Each lettered option may be selected once, more than once, or not at all.

    (A) Busulfan
    (B) Cytarabine
    (C) Dacarbazine
    (D) Diethylstilbestrol
    (E) Doxorubicin
    (F) Etoposide
    (G) Flutamide
    (H) Leuprolide
    (I) Mechlorethamine
    (J) Mercaptopurine
    (K) Methotrexate
    (L) Paclitaxel
    (M) Procarbazine
    (N) Tamoxifen
    (O) Vincristine

13. This alkylating agent is the treatment of choice for palliation of chronic myelogenous leukemia. Its toxicity includes severe myelosuppression, hyperpigmentation, and a diffuse interstitial pulmonary fibrosis

14. If allopurinol is used adjunctively in cancer chemotherapy to offset hyperuricemia, the dosage of this drug should be reduced to 25% of normal

15. This drug is used in combination therapy for testicular carcinoma. It is a cell cycle-specific (CCS) drug that acts in the late S and early G_0 phases of the tumor cell cycle via interactions with topoisomerase II

16. This agent inhibits DNA polymerase and is one of the most active drugs in leukemias. Although myelosuppression is dose-limiting, the drug may also cause ataxia, dysarthria, and dysdiadochokinesia

ANSWERS

1. Fluorouracil (5-FU) undergoes metabolism to form 5-fluoro-2′-deoxyuridine 5′-phosphate (5dUMP). This metabolite forms a covalently bound ternary complex with thymidylate synthase and its coenzyme *N*-methylenetetrahydrofolate. The synthesis of thymine nucleotides is blocked and a "thymineless death" of cells results. The answer is **(E)**.

2. Cytotoxic anticancer drugs are much more likely to be the cause of nausea and vomiting than the estrogen receptor antagonist tamoxifen. Metoclopramide, ondansetron, dronabinol, dexamethasone, and phenothiazines are effective antiemetics used in cancer chemotherapy. The vesicant properties of doxorubicin may cause local tissue necrosis at injection sites; adequate hydration reduces the risk of hemorrhagic cystitis due to cyclophosphamide; vincristine is relatively sparing of the bone marrow. Blood counts are essential immediately before each cycle of pulse therapy since the drug dosages to be used depend on the extent of hematologic recovery. The answer is **(C)**.

3. A high resting pulse rate is one of the first signs of cardiotoxicity due to anthracyclines, which can include arrhythmias, cardiomyopathies, and congestive heart failure. The risk of cardiotoxicity depends on cumulative dosage, so doxorubicin should be discontinued and replaced by another agent with activity against breast tumors. The most logical drug for replacement is methotrexate, since the CMF regimen (cyclophosphamide, methotrexate, fluorouracil) has been commonly used in the postoperative chemotherapy of breast cancers. The answer is **(D)**.

4. Recruitment strategy in cancer chemotherapy involves the initial use of a CCNS drug (eg, doxorubicin) to achieve a significant log kill. This results in the recruitment into cell division of resting cells in the G_0 phase of the cell cycle. Subsequently, the administration of CCS drugs (eg, cytarabine, vincristine) active against dividing cells will achieve a maximal cell kill. The answer is **(B)**.

5. To exert anticancer activity, mercaptopurine (and thioguanine) must first be activated to nucleotides by HGPRTase. If mercaptopurine were an irreversible inhibitor of this enzyme, this activation process could not occur. The answer is **(D)**.

6. Resistance to methotrexate does not occur within a few days—a longer time period is required. Serum methotrexate levels are not predictive of mucositis but are related to potential myelosuppressive toxicity of the drug. Renal toxicity is unlikely to occur in this patient with the pro-

posed protocol. Intrathecal administration of methotrexate is required for central nervous system leukemia. The answer is **(A)**.

7. Nephrotoxicity can be a problem with high doses of methotrexate but is less likely to occur than myelosuppression, especially if the patient is well hydrated and the urine is alkalinized. MTX is a weak acid and is more water-soluble at alkaline pH; it is thus eliminated more rapidly in alkaline urine. The answer is **(D)**.

8. Neuropathy is a toxic side effect of vincristine. In its mildest form, paresthesias occur, but it progresses to significant muscle weakness—initially in the quadriceps muscle group. Constipation is the most common symptom of autonomic neuropathy. The answer is **(E)**.

9. The characteristic nephrotoxicity of cisplatin may be reduced by slow intravenous infusion, the maintenance of good hydration, and the administration of mannitol (to maximize urine flow). Bear in mind that cisplatin also has dose-dependent neurotoxic effects. The answer is **(B)**.

10. Increases in the activity of cytochrome P450 have not been reported as a mechanism of resistance to anticancer drugs. In fact, one might predict *enhanced* cytotoxic effects of drugs that are activated by this enzyme system, eg, cyclophosphamide. Increased drug inactivation through increased production of alkaline phosphatases is a mechanism of resistance to purine antimetabolites. The answer is **(C)**.

11. The cell cycle-specific drugs used in standard treatment protocols for Hodgkin's disease are bleomycin and the *Vinca* alkaloids. Vinblastine is used in the ABVD regimen, and vincristine (Oncovin) is used in the MOPP regimen. The answer is **(E)**.

12. The anticancer drugs most commonly associated with pulmonary toxicity include bleomycin, busulfan, and procarbazine. In the case of bleomycin, if pulmonary dysfunction with infiltration developed, the drug would be discontinued. High-dose steroids and empiric antibiotic therapy would also be indicated. Note that procarbazine (not listed), used in the MOPP regimen for Hodgkin's lymphoma, may also cause cough and pleural effusions. The answer is **(A)**.

13. For the palliative treatment of chronic myelogenous leukemia, busulfan is the treatment of choice. The drug has also been used to ablate the host's bone marrow prior to bone marrow transplantation. In addition to hematotoxicity, the drug may cause hyperpigmentation ("busulfan tan") and pulmonary fibrosis ("busulfan lung"). The answer is **(A)**.

14. Allopurinol, a xanthine oxidase inhibitor, is given to control the hyperuricemia that occurs as a result of large cell kills in the successful drug therapy of malignant diseases. The antimetabolite 6-mercaptopurine is metabolized by xanthine oxidase, and, in the presence of an inhibitor of this enzyme (eg, allopurinol), toxic levels of the drug may be reached rapidly. The answer is **(J)**.

15. Bleomycin, etoposide, and vinblastine are all CCS drugs used for the treatment of testicular carcinoma. Bleomycin is an antibiotic, not a plant alkaloid. Vinblastine is a spindle poison acting in the M phase of the cell cycle. The answer is **(F)**.

16. The pyrimidine antimetabolite cytarabine (Ara-C) is commonly used in drug regimens for the acute leukemias. Cytarabine, like most antimetabolites, is dose-limited by hematotoxicity. Cerebellar dysfunction may also occur with Ara-C, especially if the drug is used at high doses. The answer is **(B)**.

Immunopharmacology 56

OBJECTIVES

You should be able to:

- Describe cellular and serologic immunity.
- Identify the therapeutic similarities and differences between immunosuppressant and anticancer drugs.

- Describe the mechanisms of action, clinical uses, and toxicities of glucocorticoids, cyclosporine, azathioprine, and cyclophosphamide in immunopharmacology.
- Describe the mechanisms of action, clinical uses, and toxicities of antibodies used as immunosuppressants.
- Identify the major cytokines and other immunomodulating agents and know their clinical applications.
- Describe the different types of allergic reactions to drugs.

Learn the definitions that follow.

Table 56–1. Definitions.

Term	Definition
B cells	Lymphoid cells derived from the bone marrow that mediate serologic immunity through the formation of antibodies
T cells	Lymphoid cells derived from the thymus that mediate cellular immunity and can modify serologic immunity. The class includes CD4 (helper) cells and CD8 (suppressor) cells
Antigen-presenting cells (APCs)	Dendritic and Langerhans cells, macrophages, and B lymphocytes involved in the processing of antigens into cell-surface forms recognizable by lymphoid cells
Clusters of differentiation (CDs)	Specific cell surface constituents (characterized by monoclonal antibodies) identified by number (CD1, CD2, etc)
Major histocompatibility complex (MHC)	Cell surface molecules of antigen-presenting cells that bind antigen fragments for recognition by helper T cells
Cytokines	Polypeptide modulators of cellular functions; include interferons, interleukins, and growth-stimulating factors
Lymphokine	A cytokine capable of modulating lymphoid cell functions

CONCEPTS

The drugs used to alter immunologic processes comprise a wide variety of chemical and pharmacologic types (Figure 56–1).

IMMUNE MECHANISMS

A. Development of Immunity: The development of specific immunity requires the following steps: (1) antigen recognition and processing, (2) proliferation of lymphoid cells, (3) differentiation of lymphoid cells, and (4) immune effects. The critical initial step (antigen recognition and processing) involves **antigen-presenting cells (APCs),** including those derived from macrophages, which change antigens so that they become more recognizable to lymphoid cells.

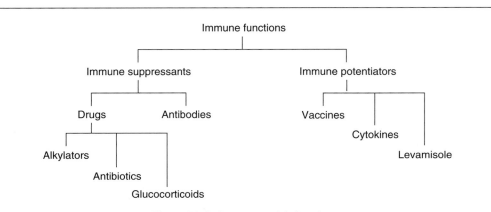

Figure 56–1. Immunomodulating drugs.

The cell types involved in the immune response can be identified by monoclonal antibodies to specific cell surface components designated **clusters of differentiation (CDs),** eg, CD4, CD8. Among the most important antigen-presenting cell surface molecules are the **major histocompatibility complex (MHC)** class II antigens (also called Ia antigens).

The **T (thymus) lymphoid cells** recognize and make contact with antigens on the surfaces of APCs. The clonal proliferation and differentiation of T cells leads to **cellular immunity** (Figure 56–2). Activated cytotoxic T cells kill virus-infected and neoplastic cells. Delayed hypersensitivity responses involve the release of lymphokines (endogenous immunomodulators) from T lymphocytes that activate macrophages and **natural killer (NK)** cells. NK cells play an important role in immune defense mechanisms, including tumor rejection and viral immunity, but their origin is unknown.

The **B (bone marrow) lymphoid cells,** which differentiate into specific antibody-forming cells, are responsible for **serologic immunity.** B cells respond to specific antigens by rapid proliferation, a process controlled by cytokines released from specific lymphocytes, the helper T cells (CD4) and the suppressor T cells (CD8).

Helper T cells are of two subtypes, designated TH1 and TH2. The TH1 helper T cell produces interferon gamma (IFN-γ), interleukin-2 (IL-2), and tumor necrosis factor-beta (TNF-β). These cytokines induce cell-mediated immunity by activating macrophages, cytotoxic T cells, and NK cells. The TH2 helper T cells produce other cytokines (IL-4, IL-5, IL-6) that induce B cell proliferation and differentiation into antibody-secreting cells.

Antibody-antigen interactions lead to precipitation of viruses, phagocytosis of bacteria, or lysis of red cells. The proliferation and differentiation of both B and T lymphocytes is under the control of a complex interplay between the cytokines (Table 56–2) and other endogenous molecules, including amines, leukotrienes, and prostaglandins.

B. Immunocompetence: Several techniques are used to assess immunologic competence and to measure drug effects on competence. These include, among others, delayed hypersensitivity testing with skin test antigens; assays of serum immunoglobulins, complement, and specific antibodies; measurement of antibody response to primary or secondary immunization; and absolute circulating lymphocyte count.

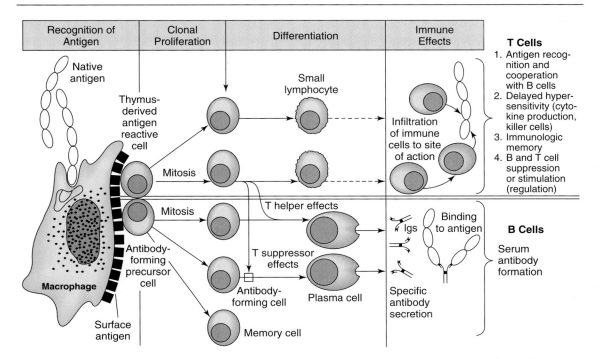

Figure 56–2. A simplified scheme of cellular and humoral immunity. (Modified and reproduced, with permission, from Katzung BG [editor]: *Basic & Clinical Pharmacology,* 7th ed. Appleton & Lange, 1998.)

Table 56–2. Cytokines modulating immune responses.*

Cytokine	Characteristic Properties
Interferon alpha	Activates NK cells; antiviral, oncostatic
Interferon beta	Activates NK cells; antiviral, oncostatic
Interferon gamma	Activates TH1, NK, cytotoxic T cells, and macrophages; antiviral, oncostatic
Interleukin-1	T cell activation, B cell proliferation
Interleukin-2	T cell proliferation, activation of TH1 and NK cells
Interleukin-4	Activates TH1 and cytotoxic T cells and B cell proliferation, including memory B cells
Interleukin-5	B cell proliferation and differentiation, including memory B cells
Interleukin-6	Proliferation of TH2 cells, cytotoxic T cells, and B cells
Interleukin-7	Proliferation of NK cells, cytotoxic T cells, and B cells
Interleukin-9	T cell proliferation
Interleukin-10	TH2 suppression, cytotoxic T cell activation, B cell proliferation
Interleukin-12	Proliferation and activation of TH1 and cytotoxic T cells
Interleukin-14	B cell proliferation and differentiation
Interleukin-15	Activation of TH1 cells, NK cells, and cytotoxic T cells
Interleukin-16	T cell chemotaxis; HIV suppression

*Modified and reproduced, with permission, from Katzung BG (editor): *Basic & Clinical Pharmacology,* 7th ed. Appleton & Lange, 1998.

C. Sites of Action of Immunosuppressant Agents: Sites of action of immunosuppressive agents are shown in Figure 56–3. Drugs that act at the step of antigen recognition are antibodies and include Rh$_o$(D) immune globulin, lymphocyte immune globulin (antithymocyte globulin, ATG), and a monoclonal antibody, muromonab-CD3. Lymphoid cell proliferation, a primary target of the cytotoxic drugs, is also inhibited by cyclosporine and tacrolimus, glucocorticoids, and antithymocyte globulin. The stages of differentiation of B and T cells are inhibited to some extent by cyclosporine and tacrolimus, dactinomycin, and lymphocyte immune globulin. Corticosteroids also modify tissue injury from immune responses via their anti-inflammatory properties.

D. Immunosuppression Compared With Cancer Chemotherapy: Since most cytotoxic drugs act on proliferating cells, there is a similarity between immunosuppressant agents and the drugs used in cancer chemotherapy. However, the therapeutic principles involved are not identical. In

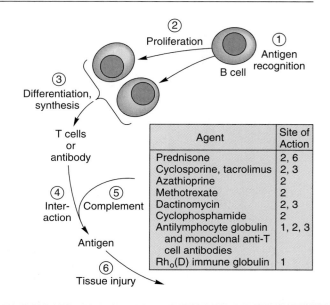

Figure 56–3. The sites of action of immunosuppressive agents on the immune response. (Reproduced, with permission, from Katzung BG [editor]: *Basic & Clinical Pharmacology,* 7th ed. Appleton & Lange, 1998.)

Agent	Site of Action
Prednisone	2, 6
Cyclosporine, tacrolimus	2, 3
Azathioprine	2
Methotrexate	2
Dactinomycin	2, 3
Cyclophosphamide	2
Antilymphocyte globulin and monoclonal anti-T cell antibodies	1, 2, 3
Rh$_o$(D) immune globulin	1

contrast to the random cell-cycle timing in most neoplasms, immune cell proliferation is *synchronized.* This permits a greater selective toxicity of anti-immune cytotoxic drugs if they are given at the time of initial antigen exposure. In addition, immunosuppressant drugs are usually given in *low doses, continuously,* whereas anticancer drug therapy is often given in *intermittent high-dose regimens.*

IMMUNOSUPPRESSANT DRUGS

A. Corticosteroids:

1. **Mechanism of action:** Glucocorticoids act at multiple cellular sites, leading to broad effects on inflammatory and immune processes (see Chapter 39). At the biochemical level, their actions on gene expression lead to decreases in the synthesis of prostaglandins, leukotrienes, and lymphokines (eg, interleukins, platelet activating factor). At the cellular level, the glucocorticoids inhibit the proliferation of T lymphocytes (suppressing cellular immunity), but B cells are less affected. At doses used for immunosuppression, the glucocorticoids are cytotoxic to certain subsets of T cells. Continuous therapy lowers IgG levels by increasing catabolism of this class of immunoglobulins.

2. **Clinical use:** Prednisone is the drug of choice in several autoimmune diseases, including idiopathic thrombocytopenic purpura, autoimmune hemolytic anemia, and acute glomerulonephritis. Corticosteroids are also used in combination with other agents as immunosuppressants in organ transplantation.

3. **Toxicity:** Predictable adverse effects include adrenal suppression, growth inhibition, muscle wasting, osteoporosis, salt retention, diabetogenesis, and possible psychoses (Chapter 39).

B. Cyclosporine:

1. **Mechanism of action:** This peptide antibiotic inhibits early stages of the differentiation of T cells and blocks their activation. Cyclosporine inhibits the synthesis of factors that stimulate the growth of T cells, including interleukins (IL-2, IL-3) and interferons (IFN-γ). The drug binds to the protein **cyclophilin,** and the complex inhibits a cytoplasmic phosphatase, **calcineurin,** that is needed for the activation of T cell-specific transcription factors. However, cyclosporine does not block the effects of such factors on primed T cells, nor does it block interaction with antigen.

2. **Clinical use:** Cyclosporine can be used orally, but since bioavailability is erratic, serum levels should be monitored. The drug undergoes slow hepatic metabolism and has a long half-life. Cyclosporine is the drug of choice for immunosuppression in organ transplantation and is used in the graft-versus-host syndrome in bone marrow transplants. Cyclosporine has been used in combination with glucocorticoids (and sometimes cytotoxic drugs) but may be equally effective when used alone. The drug may also be useful in autoimmune diseases, including the early treatment of type I diabetes, and possibly asthma.

3. **Toxicity:** The most frequent adverse effects are renal dysfunction, hypertension, hirsutism, and neurotoxicity. Cyclosporine may also cause hyperglycemia and hyperlipidemia. Transient liver dysfunction and an increase in viral infections may also occur. Cholelithiasis has occurred in children. One virtue of cyclosporine is its low incidence of bone marrow toxicity. Drugs that stimulate or inhibit liver microsomal drug-metabolizing enzymes may alter the plasma levels of cyclosporine.

C. Tacrolimus (FK 506):

1. **Mechanisms:** This immunosuppressive antibiotic has a mechanism of action similar to that of cyclosporine. While it binds to **FK-binding protein** (rather than cyclophilin), it still inhibits calcineurin and interferes with the synthesis of interleukins in activated T cells.

   Sirolimus is a new investigational immunosuppressive antibiotic with structural similarity to tacrolimus but a different mechanism of action.

2. **Clinical uses:** Tacrolimus is used in liver, kidney, pancreas, and heart transplantation. In terms of graft and patient survival in liver transplantation, tacrolimus is marginally more effective than cyclosporine.

3. **Toxicity:** The toxicity of tacrolimus may be greater than that of cyclosporine and includes nephrotoxicity, peripheral neuropathy, gastrointestinal distress, and hyperglycemia that usually requires insulin administration.

D. Azathioprine:
1. **Mechanism of action:** This prodrug is transformed in the body into the antimetabolite mercaptopurine, which upon further metabolic conversion inhibits enzymes involved in purine metabolism. Azathioprine is cytotoxic in the early phase of lymphoid cell proliferation and has a greater effect on the activity of T cells than B cells. The drug has minimal effects on established graft rejections.
2. **Clinical use:** Azathioprine is used in several autoimmune diseases, including lupus erythematosus and severe rheumatoid arthritis. It is also used for immunosuppression in renal homografts.
3. **Toxicity:** The major toxic effect is bone marrow suppression, but gastrointestinal irritation, skin rashes, and liver dysfunction also occur. The use of azathioprine is associated with an increased incidence of neoplasms. The active metabolite of azathioprine, mercaptopurine, is metabolized by xanthine oxidase, and toxic effects may be increased by allopurinol given for hyperuricemia.

E. Cyclophosphamide:
1. **Mechanism of action:** This orally active prodrug is transformed by liver enzymes into an alkylating agent that is cytotoxic to proliferating lymphoid cells. The drug has a greater effect on B cells than T lymphocytes and will inhibit an established immune response. Other cytotoxic drugs that act similarly—and are sometimes used as immunosuppressants—include **cytarabine, dactinomycin, methotrexate,** and **vincristine** (see Chapter 55).
2. **Clinical use:** Cyclophosphamide is effective in autoimmune diseases (including hemolytic anemia), antibody-induced red cell aplasia, bone marrow transplants, and possibly other organ transplants. Cyclophosphamide does not prevent the graft-versus-host (GVH) reaction in bone marrow transplantation.
3. **Toxicity:** Large doses of the drug (usually needed for immunosuppression) cause pancytopenia, gastrointestinal distress, hemorrhagic cystitis, and alopecia. Cyclophosphamide and other alkylating agents may cause sterility.

ANTIBODIES AS IMMUNOSUPPRESSANTS

A. Lymphocyte Immune Globulin:
1. **Mechanism of action:** Lymphocyte immune globulin (LIG), also known as antithymocyte globulin (ATG), is usually produced in horses by immunization against human thymus cells. Lymphocyte immune globulin binds to T cells involved in antigen recognition, initiating their destruction by serum complement. Lymphocyte immune globulin selectively blocks cellular immunity rather than antibody formation, which accounts for its clinical use to suppress organ graft rejection.
2. **Clinical use:** Lymphocyte immune globulin is used prior to bone marrow transplantation to prevent the graft-versus-host reaction. It is also used in combination with cyclosporine or cytotoxic drugs (or both) for maintenance following bone marrow, heart, and renal transplantations. Lymphocyte immune globulin has induced remissions in patients with aplastic anemia.
3. **Toxicity:** Since serologic immunity may remain intact, injection of lymphocyte immune globulin may cause hypersensitivity reactions, including serum sickness and anaphylaxis. Pain and erythema occur at injection sites, and histiocytic lymphoma has been noted as a late complication.

B. Muromonab-CD3 (OKT-3):
1. **Mechanism of action:** Muromonab-CD3 is a murine monoclonal antibody to the T3 (CD3) antigen on the surface of human thymocytes and mature T cells. The antibody blocks the killing action of cytotoxic T cells and probably interferes with other T cell functions.
2. **Clinical use:** Muromonab-CD3 is used intravenously to reverse the renal allograft rejection crisis.
3. **Toxicity:** First-dose effects include fever, chills, dyspnea, and pulmonary edema. Hypersensitivity reactions may also occur.

C. **$Rh_o(D)$ Immune Globulin:**
1. **Mechanism of action:** $Rh_o(D)$ immune globulin is a human IgG preparation that contains antibodies against red cell $Rh_o(D)$ antigens. Administration of this antibody to $Rh_o(D)$-negative, D^u-negative mothers at the time of antigen exposure (ie, birth of an $Rh_o(D)$-positive, D^u-positive child) blocks the primary immune response to the foreign cells. The mechanism probably involves "feedback immunosuppression."
2. **Clinical use:** $Rh_o(D)$ immune globulin is used for prevention of Rh hemolytic disease of the newborn. In women treated with $Rh_o(D)$, maternal antibodies to Rh-positive cells are not produced in subsequent pregnancies, and hemolytic disease of the neonate is thus averted.

IMMUNOMODULATING AGENTS

Agents that act as stimulators of immune responses represent a new area in immunopharmacology with the potential for important therapeutic uses, including the treatment of immune deficiency diseases, chronic infectious diseases, and cancer.

A. **Levamisole:** This antiparasitic drug can also act as an immunopotentiator. Levamisole stimulates the maturation and proliferation of T cells in patients with impaired immune function. The drug enhances T cell-mediated immune responses and restores delayed hypersensitivity. One of the actions of levamisole is to promote the oxidation of an endogenous molecule that is a precursor of **soluble immune response repressor substance (SIRS).** The drug has been used in the treatment of the nephrotic syndrome and adjunctively in cancer chemotherapy. Levamisole may also be useful in rheumatoid arthritis and in the immunodeficiency of Hodgkin's disease.

B. **Aldesleukin:** Aldesleukin is recombinant interleukin-2 (IL-2). It is an endogenous lymphokine that promotes the proliferation and differentiation of lymphocytes into cytotoxic cells and activates natural killer cells (Table 56–2). Aldesleukin is indicated for the adjunctive treatment of renal cell carcinoma. It is investigational for possible efficacy in restoring immune function in AIDS and other immune deficiency disorders.

C. **Colony-Stimulating Factors:** **Filgrastim** and **sargramostim** are recombinant forms of the human colony-stimulating factors G-CSF and GM-CSF (see Chapter 33). They are indicated for acceleration of marrow recovery in patients undergoing cytotoxic therapy for cancer.

D. **Interferons:** **Interferon alfa-2a** inhibits cell proliferation. It is used in hairy cell leukemia, chronic myelogenous leukemia, malignant melanoma, and Kaposi's sarcoma. It is also approved for use in hepatitis B and C. **Interferon beta-1b** has beneficial effects in relapsing multiple sclerosis. **Interferon gamma-1b** has greater immune-enhancing actions than the other interferons. It appears to act by increasing the synthesis of tumor necrosis factor (TNF). The recombinant form is used to decrease the incidence and severity of infections in patients with chronic granulomatous disease.

E. **BCG (Bacille Calmette-Guérin):** BCG has been used for immunization against tuberculosis and as an immunostimulant in cancer therapy. BCG activates macrophages and may enhance immune responses in patients with superficial bladder cancer.

F. **Thymosin:** Thymosin is a protein hormone from the thymus gland that stimulates the maturation of pre-T cells and promotes the formation of T cells from ordinary lymphoid stem cells. Thymosin-containing preparations have been used in DiGeorge's syndrome (thymic aplasia), but their efficacy in other immune deficiency states has not been established.

MECHANISMS OF DRUG ALLERGY

A. **Type I (Immediate) Drug Allergy:** Type I drug allergy involves **IgE-mediated** reactions to animal and plant stings as well as drugs. Such reactions include anaphylaxis, urticaria, and angioedema. Small drug molecules can act as haptens when linked to carrier proteins, initiating B cell proliferation and formation of IgE antibodies. These antibodies bind to tissue mast cells and blood basophils, which become sensitized. On subsequent exposure, the antigenic drug is bound to antibodies, triggering release of mediators of vascular responses and tissue injury, including histamine, kinins, prostaglandins, and leukotrienes. Drugs that commonly cause type I reactions include penicillins and sulfonamides.

B. Type II Drug Allergy: Type II allergy involves **IgG** or **IgM** antibodies, which bind to circulating blood cells. On reexposure to the antigen, complement-dependent cell lysis occurs. Type II reactions include autoimmune syndromes such as hemolytic anemia from methyldopa, systemic lupus erythematosus from hydralazine or procainamide, thrombocytopenic purpura from quinidine, and agranulocytosis from exposure to many drugs.

C. Type III Drug Allergy: Type III is a complex type of drug allergy reaction that involves complement-fixing **IgM** or **IgG** antibodies and—possibly—IgE antibodies. Drug-induced serum sickness and vasculitis are examples of type III reactions; Stevens-Johnson syndrome (associated with sulfonamide therapy) may also result from type III mechanisms.

D. Type IV Drug Allergy: Type IV allergy is a cell-mediated reaction that can occur from topical application of drugs. It results in contact dermatitis.

E. Modification of Drug Allergies: Drugs that modify allergic responses to other drugs or toxins may act at several steps of the immune mechanism. For example, corticosteroids inhibit lymphoid cell proliferation and reduce tissue injury and edema. However, most drugs that are useful in type I reactions (eg, isoproterenol, theophylline, epinephrine) block mediator release or act as physiologic antagonists of the mediators.

DRUG LIST

The following drugs are important members of the group discussed in this chapter. Prototypes should be learned in detail; features of the major variants should be known well enough so that the variants can be distinguished from prototypes and from each other; the other significant agents should be recognized as belonging to a specific subclass.

Subclass	Prototype	Major Variants	Other Significant Agents
Corticosteroids	Prednisone		
Antibiotics	Cyclosporine	Tacrolimus	Dactinomycin, rapamycin
Antimetabolites	Azathioprine	Mercaptopurine	Cytarabine, methotrexate
Alkylating agents	Cyclophosphamide		Chlorambucil
Antibodies	Lymphocytic immune globulin, muromonab-CD3, Rh_o(D) immune globulin		
Immunostimulants	Filgrastim, interferon-gamma, levamisole,		

QUESTIONS

DIRECTIONS: Each of the numbered items or incomplete statements in this section is followed by answers or by completions of the statement. Select the ONE lettered answer or completion that is BEST in each case.

  1. Cyclosporine is effective in organ transplantation. The immunosuppressant action of the drug appears to be due to
      (A)   Activation of natural killer (NK) cells

    (B) Blockade of tissue responses to inflammatory mediators
    (C) Increased catabolism of IgG antibodies
    (D) Inhibition of the gene transcription of interleukins
    (E) Interference with antigen recognition

2. Azathioprine
    (A) Blocks formation of tetrahydrofolic acid
    (B) Does not block cellular immune mechanisms
    (C) Is a precursor of cytarabine
    (D) Is markedly hematotoxic and has caused neoplasms
    (E) Is a metabolite of mercaptopurine

Items 3–4: A renal transplant recipient is given a combination of immunosuppressive agents to prevent allograft rejection. During the course of drug therapy, toxicity occurs.

3. If the toxicity includes fever, vomiting, cutaneous lesions, and lymphadenopathy, the most likely causative agent is
    (A) Cyclophosphamide
    (B) Cyclosporine
    (C) Dactinomycin
    (D) Lymphocyte immune globulin
    (E) $Rh_o(D)$ immune globulin

4. If the toxicity includes upper extremity tremor, limb paresthesias, and hallucinations, the most likely causative agent is
    (A) Azathioprine
    (B) Cyclosporine
    (C) Lymphocyte immune globulin
    (D) Methotrexate
    (E) Prednisone

5. Which of the following drugs is a widely used agent that suppresses cellular immunity, inhibits prostaglandin and leukotriene synthesis, and increases the catabolism of IgG antibodies?
    (A) Cyclophosphamide
    (B) Cyclosporine
    (C) Levamisole
    (D) Mercaptopurine
    (E) Prednisone

6. Which of the following agents activates "promiscuous killer" lymphocytes that are cytotoxic across MHC barriers and can kill cells that do not express MHC?
    (A) Aldesleukin
    (B) Cyclosporine
    (C) Levamisole
    (D) Macrophage colony-stimulating factor
    (E) Tumor necrosis factor

7. Which one of the following agents acts at the site of antigen recognition?
    (A) Cyclosporine
    (B) Cyclophosphamide
    (C) Methotrexate
    (D) $Rh_o(D)$ immune globulin
    (E) Tacrolimus

8. Which one of the following is NOT an action of lymphocytic immune globulin?
    (A) Facilitation of complement-mediated destruction of T cells
    (B) Development of lymphomas
    (C) Blockade of "antigen recognition"
    (D) Type III drug allergies
    (E) Stimulation of the release of lymphokines

9. Which one of the following statements about cyclosporine is LEAST accurate?
    (A) Mean blood pressure is more likely to be elevated than depressed
    (B) Viral infections can occur during treatment
    (C) Platelet and neutrophil counts must be performed weekly
    (D) Monitoring of blood levels may help in avoiding toxicity
    (E) Gingival hyperplasia and hirsutism may occur

Items 10–11: An immunosuppressed patient was treated for a bacterial infection with a parenteral penicillin. Within a few minutes after the penicillin injection, he developed severe bronchoconstriction, laryngeal edema, and hypotension. Because epinephrine was rapidly administered, the patient survived. A year later, he was treated with an antipsychotic drug and developed agranulocytosis.

10. The type of drug reaction caused by penicillin is
    (A) An autoimmune syndrome
    (B) A cell-mediated reaction
    (C) A type II drug allergy
    (D) Mediated by IgE
    (E) Serum sickness

11. The type of drug reaction caused by the antipsychotic drug is
    (A) A type III drug reaction
    (B) A type IV drug reaction
    (C) Delayed-type hypersensitivity
    (D) Mediated by IgG or IgM antibodies
    (E) The Stevens-Johnson syndrome

12. Which one of the following molecules is not a cytokine?
    (A) Granulocyte colony-stimulating factor
    (B) Interferon alpha
    (C) Interleukin-2
    (D) Muromonab-CD3
    (E) Tumor necrosis factor

DIRECTIONS (Items 13–15): Each set of matching questions in this section consists of a list of three to twenty-six lettered options (some of which may be figures) followed by several numbered items. For each numbered item, select the ONE lettered option that is most closely associated with it. Each lettered option may be selected once, more than once, or not at all.

    (A) Aldesleukin
    (B) Azathioprine
    (C) Cyclophosphamide
    (D) Cyclosporine
    (E) Interferon alpha
    (F) Interferon beta
    (G) Interferon gamma
    (H) Levamisole
    (I) Lymphocyte immune globulin
    (J) Methotrexate
    (K) Prednisone
    (L) Sargramostim
    (M) Tacrolimus
    (N) Thymosin

13. If administered prior to bone marrow transplantation, this agent is effective in preventing subsequent maculopapular rash, jaundice, hepatosplenomegaly, and diarrhea

14. This drug is the most likely (of the above agents) to be used in the management of patients with rheumatoid arthritis or systemic lupus erythematosus

15. In chronic granulomatous disease, this agent increases phagocytosis by macrophages

ANSWERS

1. Cyclosporine inhibits calcineurin, a serine phosphatase that is needed for activation of T cell-specific transcription factors. Gene transcription of IL-2, IL-3, and interferon gamma is inhibited. The answer is **(D)**.

2. Azathioprine blocks both cellular and serologic immunity. For azathioprine to exert its cytotoxic actions, it must first be metabolized to mercaptopurine. As is true for most purine antimetabolites, hematotoxicity is dose-limiting; the use of these agents as immunosuppressants is associated with an increase in cancer risk. The answer is **(D)**.

3. Lymphocyte immune globulin is produced mainly through the immunization of large animals. As a mixture of foreign proteins, the agent may cause a wide range of hypersensitivity reactions, including skin reactions, serum sickness, and even anaphylaxis. The symptoms described are typical of serum sickness. The answer is **(D)**.

4. Neurotoxic effects associated with the use of cyclosporine include limb paresthesias (incidence 50%), distal tremor (incidence 25%), hallucinations, and seizures. The answer is **(B)**.

5. The corticosteroid prednisone is used extensively as an immunosuppressant in autoimmune diseases and organ transplantation. Glucocorticoids have multiple actions, including those described. The answer is **(E)**.

6. Aldesleukin (IL-2) and several other interleukins activate natural killer cells (NK cells) and lymphokine-activated killer cells (LAK cells, "promiscuous killers"). The investigational use of aldesleukin in AIDS patients is partly based on the fact that lymphocytes from such individuals produce significantly less IL-2 than lymphocytes from healthy controls. The answer is **(A)**.

7. $Rh_o(D)$ immune globulin contains antibodies against $Rh_o(D)$ antigens. Administration to an Rh-negative mother within 72 hours after the birth of an Rh-positive baby prevents Rh hemolytic disease of the newborn (erythroblastosis fetalis) in subsequent pregnancies. The answer is **(D)**.

8. Lymphocyte immune globulin increases T cell destruction and blocks cellular immunity. However, the agent does not stimulate the release of cytokines. Since serologic immunity remains intact, the injection of lymphocyte immune globulin may cause hypersensitivity reactions. Histiocytic lymphomas have developed at the sites of injection. The answer is **(E)**.

9. Neurotoxicity and nephrotoxicity are the major adverse effects of cyclosporine, but the drug may also cause hyperglycemia, hyperlipidemia, hypertension, liver dysfunction, osteoporosis, hirsutism, and gum hyperplasia. Cyclosporine is relatively free of hematotoxicity, so weekly blood cell counts are not required. The answer is **(C)**.

10. The patient experienced an anaphylactic response to the penicillin. This is a type I (immediate) drug reaction, mediated by IgE antibodies. The answer is **(D)**.

11. Agranulocytosis (and systemic lupus erythematosus) are autoimmune syndromes that can be drug-induced. They are type II reactions involving IgM and IgG antibodies that bind to circulating blood cells. The patient was probably treated with clozapine for his psychosis (see clozapine toxicity, Chapter 29). The answer is **(D)**.

12. Cytokines are immunoregulatory proteins synthesized by lymphoreticular and other cells. They usually exert their effects via interaction with cell surface receptors. This class of endogenous compounds includes interferons, interleukins, colony-stimulating factors, and tumor necrosis factors. Muromonab-CD3 is a murine monoclonal *antibody* directed against a surface component of human lymphocytes and mature T cells. The answer is **(D)**.

13. The symptoms described (rash, liver dysfunction, diarrhea) are typical of the graft-versus-host reaction. Use of lymphocyte immune globulin (antithymocyte globulin) eliminates mature T cells from the graft. The answer is **(I)**.

14. The glucocorticoids are the most effective and the most widely used agents for management of patients with autoimmune diseases. In addition to rheumatoid arthritis and subacute lupus erythematosus, the therapeutic applications of glucocorticoids include acute glomerulonephritis, myasthenia gravis, insulin-resistant diabetes, Graves' disease, and idiopathic thrombocytopenic purpura (ITP). The answer is **(K)**.

15. Interferon gamma is approved for use in chronic granulomatous disease, a condition that results from phagocyte deficiency. The agent markedly reduces the frequency of recurrent infections. The answer is **(G)**.

57

Introduction to Toxicology

OBJECTIVES

You should be able to:

- List four major air pollutants and their clinical effects.
- Identify the major toxicities of common solvents and insecticides, including chlorinated hydrocarbons, inhibitors of cholinesterases, and botanicals.
- List two important herbicides and their major toxicities.
- Describe the toxicological significance of the environmental pollutants dioxins and polychlorinated biphenyls (PCBs).

Learn the definitions that follow.

Table 57–1. Definitions.[1]

Term	Definition
Toxicology	The area of pharmacology that deals with the adverse effects of chemicals on biologic systems
Occupational toxicology	The area that deals with the toxic effects of chemicals found in the workplace; regulated by the Occupational Safety & Health Agency (OSHA) in the USA
Environmental toxicology	The area that deals with the effects of agents found in the environment (air, water, etc); regulated by the Environmental Protection Agency (EPA) in the USA
Ecotoxicology	The area that deals with the untoward effects of agents found in the environment on whole populations as opposed to individuals
Risk	The expected frequency of occurrence of a particular toxic effect in response to a particular agent
Threshold limit value (TLV)	The amount of exposure to a given agent that is deemed safe for a stated time period. It is higher for shorter periods than for longer periods
Generally recognized as safe (GRAS)	An official list of substances that, through testing or experience, do not appear to have significant toxicity
Bioaccumulation	The increasing concentration of a substance in the environment as the result of environmental persistence and physical properties (eg, lipid solubility) that permit it to accumulate in the tissues of organisms
Biomagnification	The further concentration of chemicals within organisms that feed on other organisms and thereby concentrate the chemicals found in the tissues of the prey species
Acceptable daily intake (ADI)	Maximum daily intake of a chemical which, during an entire lifetime, is without appreciable risk

[1]Not all of the terms listed are used in this chapter, but knowledge of their definitions may be helpful.

CONCEPTS

Chemicals in the environment—home, workplace, atmosphere, etc—may be important health hazards. Some of these chemical groups are shown in Figure 57–1.

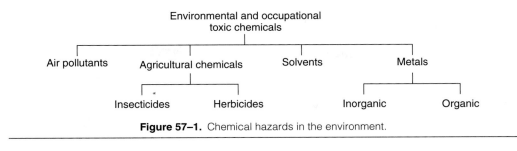

Environmental and occupational
toxic chemicals

Air pollutants   Agricultural chemicals   Solvents   Metals

Insecticides   Herbicides   Inorganic   Organic

Figure 57–1. Chemical hazards in the environment.

AIR POLLUTANTS

A. **Classification and Prototypes:** The major air pollutants in industrialized countries include carbon monoxide (about 50% of the total amount of air pollutants), sulfur oxides (18%), hydrocarbons (12%), particulate matter (eg, smoke particles, 10%), and nitrogen oxides (6%). Ambient air pollution appears to be a contributing factor in bronchitis, obstructive pulmonary disease, and lung cancer.

B. **Carbon Monoxide:** CO is an odorless, colorless gas that competes avidly with oxygen for hemoglobin. The affinity of CO for hemoglobin is more than 200-fold greater than that of oxygen. The threshold limit value (TLV) of CO for an 8-hour workday is 25 parts per million (ppm); in heavy traffic, the concentration of CO may exceed 100 ppm.
   1. **Effects:** Carbon monoxide causes tissue hypoxia. Headache is one of the first symptoms, followed by confusion, decreased visual acuity, tachycardia, syncope, coma, convulsions, and death. Collapse and syncope occur when approximately 40% of hemoglobin has been converted to carboxyhemoglobin. These adverse effects may be aggravated by high ambient temperature and high altitude.
   2. **Treatment:** Removal of the source of carbon monoxide and breathing pure oxygen are the major features of treatment. Hyperbaric oxygen accelerates the clearance of carbon monoxide.

C. **Sulfur Dioxide:** SO_2 is a colorless, irritating gas formed from the combustion of fossil fuels.
   1. **Effects:** SO_2 forms sulfurous acid on contact with moist mucous membranes; this acid is responsible for most of the pathologic effects. Conjunctival and bronchial irritation (especially in asthmatics) are the primary signs of exposure. Five to 10 ppm in the air is enough to cause severe bronchospasm. Heavy exposure may lead to delayed pulmonary edema. Chronic low-level exposure may aggravate cardiopulmonary disease.
   2. **Treatment:** Removal from exposure and relief of irritation and inflammation comprise the major treatment.

D. **Nitrogen Oxides:** Nitrogen dioxide (NO_2), a brownish irritant gas, is the principal member of this group. It is formed in fires and in silage on farms.
   1. **Effects:** NO_2 causes deep lung irritation and pulmonary edema. Farm workers exposed to high concentrations of the gas within enclosed silos may die rapidly of acute pulmonary edema. Irritation of the eyes, nose, and throat is also common.
   2. **Treatment:** No specific treatment is available. Measures to reduce inflammation and pulmonary edema are important.

E. **Ozone:** O_3 is a bluish irritant gas produced in air and water purification devices and in electrical fields.
   1. **Effects:** Exposure to 0.01–0.1 ppm may cause irritation and dryness of the mucous membranes. Pulmonary function may be impaired at higher concentrations. Chronic exposure leads to bronchitis, bronchiolitis, pulmonary fibrosis, and emphysema.
   2. **Treatment:** No specific treatment is available. Measures that reduce inflammation and pulmonary edema are emphasized.

SOLVENTS

Solvents used in industry and to clean clothing are a major source of direct exposure to hydrocarbons and also contribute to air pollution.

A. Aliphatic Hydrocarbons: This group includes halogenated solvents such as carbon tetrachloride, chloroform, and trichloroethylene.

    1. Effects: Solvents are potent CNS depressants. The acute effects of excessive exposure are nausea, vertigo, locomotor disturbance, headache, and coma. Chronic exposure to halogenated hydrocarbons leads to both hepatic dysfunction and nephrotoxicity. Long-term exposure to tetrachloroethylene—or to trichloroethane—has caused peripheral neuropathy.

    2. Treatment: Removal from exposure is the only specific treatment available. Serious CNS depression must be treated with support of vital signs (Chapter 60).

B. Aromatic Hydrocarbons: The aromatic hydrocarbons include benzene and toluene.

    1. Effects: Acute exposure leads to CNS depression with ataxia and coma. Long-term exposure to benzene is associated with hematotoxicity (thrombocytopenia, leukopenia, aplastic anemia), and the compound may be leukemogenic. Toluene is not a myelosuppressant.

    2. Treatment: Removal from exposure is the only specific way to reduce toxicity. CNS depression is managed by support of vital signs.

INSECTICIDES

A. Classification and Prototypes: The three major classes of insecticides are the chlorinated hydrocarbons (DDT and its analogs), acetylcholinesterase inhibitors (carbamates, organophosphates), and the botanical agents (nicotine, rotenone, pyrethrum alkaloids).

B. Chlorinated Hydrocarbons: These agents are persistent—very poorly metabolized—lipophilic chemicals that accumulate in body fat and thus are subject to both bioaccumulation and biomagnification (see Table 57–1).

    1. Effects: Chlorinated hydrocarbons block physiologic inactivation in the sodium channels of nerve membranes and cause uncontrolled firing of action potentials. Tremor is usually the first sign of acute toxicity and may progress to seizures. Chronic exposure of animals to these insecticides causes increased tumorigenesis. The toxicologic impact of long-term exposure in humans is unclear. No relationship has been shown in humans between risk of breast cancer and serum levels of DDT metabolites.

    2. Treatment: No specific treatment is available for the acute toxicity caused by chlorinated hydrocarbons. Because of their extremely long half-lives in organisms and in the environment (years), their use in North America and Europe has been curtailed to prevent more severe environmental toxicity.

C. Cholinesterase Inhibitors: The carbamates (eg, aldicarb, carbaryl) and organophosphates (eg, dichlorvos, malathion, parathion) are effective insecticides and have much shorter environmental half-lives than do the chlorinated hydrocarbons. The cholinesterase inhibitors are inexpensive and, unlike DDT and its analogs, are heavily used in agriculture in North America.

    1. Effects: As described in Chapter 7, these agents produce increased muscarinic and nicotinic stimulation; the effects include pinpoint pupils; sweating; salivation; bronchoconstriction; vomiting and diarrhea; CNS stimulation followed by depression; and muscle fasciculations, weakness, and paralysis. The most common cause of death is respiratory failure. Chronic exposure to some organophosphates (not carbamates) has resulted in delayed neurotoxicity with axonal degeneration. The toxic mechanism appears to involve phosphorylation of a neuropathy target esterase (NTE).

    2. Treatment: Atropine is used in large doses to control muscarinic excess; pralidoxime (2-PAM) is used to regenerate cholinesterase. Mechanical ventilation may be necessary.

D. Botanical Insecticides:

    1. Nicotine: Nicotine has the same effects on nicotinic cholinoceptors in insects as in mammals and probably kills by the same mechanism, ie, excitation followed by paralysis of ganglionic, CNS, and neuromuscular transmission. Treatment is supportive.

2. **Rotenone:** This plant alkaloid insecticide causes gastrointestinal distress when ingested and conjunctivitis and dermatitis following direct contact with exposed body surfaces. Treatment is symptomatic.

3. **Pyrethrum:** The most common toxic effect of this mixture of plant alkaloids is contact dermatitis. Ingestion or inhalation of large quantities may cause CNS excitation (including seizures) and peripheral neurotoxicity. Treatment is symptomatic, with anticonvulsants if necessary.

HERBICIDES

A. **Paraquat:** Paraquat is used extensively to kill weeds on farms and for highway maintenance.
1. **Effects:** The compound is relatively nontoxic unless ingested. After ingestion, the initial effect is gastrointestinal irritation with hematemesis and bloody stools. Within a few days, signs of pulmonary impairment occur and are usually progressive, resulting in severe pulmonary fibrosis and, in many cases, death.
2. **Treatment:** No antidote is available; the best supportive treatment, including gastric lavage and dialysis, still results in less than 50% survival after ingestion of as little as 5 mL.

B. **Phenoxyacetic Acids:** 2,4-Dichlorophenoxyacetic acid (2,4-D) and 2,4,5-trichlorophenoxy-acetic acid (2,4,5-T) are the most important members of this group. During the manufacturing process, dioxin contaminants are produced. (See below for dioxin toxicology.)
1. **Effects:** Large doses of 2,4-D or 2,4,5-T cause muscle hypotonia and coma. Long-term exposure has been associated with an increased risk of non-Hodgkin's lymphoma.

ENVIRONMENTAL POLLUTANTS

The chemical compounds that contribute to environmental pollution include the chlorinated hydrocarbons (see above), the dioxins, and the polychlorinated biphenyls.

A. **Dioxins:**
1. **Source:** The polychlorinated dibenzo-p-dioxins (PCDDs) are a large group of related compounds of which the most important is 2,3,7,8-tetrachlorodibenzo-p-dioxin (TCDD). The dioxins have no commercial uses. They have appeared in the environment as unwanted by-products of the chemical industry. PCDDs are chemically stable and highly resistant to environmental degradation
2. **Toxicology:** In certain laboratory animals, exposure to TCDD has caused teratogenic and carcinogenic effects. In humans, the most common signs of toxicity are dermatitis and chloracne. However, epidemiologic evidence suggests that the dioxins may have carcinogenic effects, perhaps increasing the risk of non-Hodgkin's lymphoma.

B. **Polychlorinated Biphenyls (PCBs):**
1. **Source:** The polychlorinated biphenyls (PCBs) were used extensively in manufacturing electrical equipment until their potential for environmental damage was recognized. PCBs constitute a large group of related compounds that are among the most stable organic compounds known. They are poorly metabolized and lipophilic. They are therefore highly persistent in the environment and accumulate in the food chain.
2. **Toxicology:** In workers exposed to PCBs, the most common effect is dermatotoxicity (acne, erythema, folliculitis, hyperkeratosis). Less frequently, mild increases in plasma triglycerides and elevated liver enzymes have been observed. Possible teratogenicity has been suggested following ingestion, for several months, of cooking oils containing PCBs.

QUESTIONS

DIRECTIONS: Each of the numbered items or incomplete statements in this section is followed by answers or by completions of the statement. Select the ONE lettered answer or completion that is BEST in each case.

1. The light-brownish color of smog often apparent in the Los Angeles area on a hot summer day is mainly due to
   (A) Carbon monoxide
   (B) Hydrocarbons
   (C) Ozone
   (D) Nitrogen dioxide
   (E) Sulfur dioxide

2. You are stuck in traffic in New York City in summer for 3 or 4 hours and you begin to get a headache, a feeling of tightness in the temporal region, and an increased pulse rate. The most likely cause of these effects is inhalation of
   (A) Carbon monoxide
   (B) Nicotine
   (C) Nitrogen dioxide
   (D) Ozone
   (E) Sulfur dioxide

3. An employee works all day in a storage facility that contains agricultural chemicals and solvents. Which one of the following statements about his possible exposure to toxic substances in the workplace is LEAST accurate?
   (A) Ambient air concentrations of such chemicals should be regularly monitored
   (B) He may experience fatigue and possibly become ataxic if he is exposed to halogenated hydrocarbon vapors
   (C) He may develop a delayed neuropathy if he is working in areas where organophosphates are stored
   (D) The worker may develop acne from exposure to chlorophenoxy herbicides
   (E) He may develop delayed pulmonary edema if he is exposed to chlorinated hydrocarbon insecticides

4. Correct pairings of toxic agent with the best method of treatment include all of the following EXCEPT
   (A) Carbon monoxide: 100% or hyperbaric oxygen
   (B) Carbon tetrachloride: Support of vital signs
   (C) Nitrogen dioxide: Nonspecific treatment of noncardiogenic pulmonary edema
   (D) Paraquat: Hemodialysis
   (E) Parathion: Atropine and pralidoxime

5. Which one of the following chemicals does NOT undergo bioaccumulation and biomagnification and is LEAST likely to be an environmental hazard?
   (A) DDT
   (B) Dichlorvos
   (C) Polychlorinated biphenyls
   (D) TCDD
   (E) Toxaphene

6. An employee of a company engaged in clearing vegetation from county roadsides accidentally ingested a small quantity of a herbicidal solution that contained paraquat. Within 2 hours he was admitted to the emergency room of a nearby hospital. Which of the following best describes his probable signs and symptoms?
   (A) Diarrhea, vomiting, sweating, and profound skeletal muscle weakness
   (B) Dizziness, nausea, agitation, and hyperreflexia
   (C) Dyspnea, pulmonary dysfunction, elevated body temperature
   (D) Gastrointestinal irritation with hematemesis and bloody stools
   (E) Hypotension, tachycardia, and respiratory impairment

7. Chemical warfare agents that had been manufactured in the 1950s were being stored at a military installation. Several civilian workers at the facility began to feel unwell, with symptoms that included dyspnea, abdominal cramps, and diarrhea. They also had copious nasal and tracheobronchial secretions. Which type of toxic compound is most likely to be the cause of these effects?
   (A) Aliphatic hydrocarbons
   (B) Botulinum toxin
   (C) Nitrogen mustards
   (D) Organophosphates
   (E) Rotenones

DIRECTIONS (Items 8–12): Each set of matching questions in this section consists of a list of three to twenty-six lettered options (some of which may be figures) followed by several numbered items. For each numbered item, select the ONE lettered option that is most closely associated with it. Each lettered option may be selected once, more than once, or not at all.

    (A) Aldicarb
    (B) Benzene
    (C) Carbon monoxide
    (D) Carbon dioxide
    (E) DDT
    (F) Dioxin
    (G) Malathion
    (H) Nitrogen dioxide
    (I) Paraquat
    (J) Pyrethrum
    (K) Rotenone
    (L) Sulfur dioxide
    (M) Tetrachloroethylene
    (N) Toluene

8. Asthma is often exacerbated in patients exposed to this reducing agent when concentrations in the air are as low as 1–2 ppm. It is formed mainly from combustion of fossil fuels

9. Acute exposure to this *aliphatic* hydrocarbon solvent causes CNS depression; chronic exposure has led to impairment of memory and peripheral neuropathy

10. This compound is a potential environmental hazard that is formed as a contaminating by-product in the manufacture of herbicides

11. Bone marrow cells in early stages of their development appear to be most sensitive to this agent, which has caused pancytopenia and aplastic anemia

12. This agent is derived from a botanical source. The most frequent adverse effect reported is contact dermatitis. Accidental oral ingestion causes CNS stimulation, including seizures

ANSWERS

1. Smog color is derived in part from suspended particulate matter. When smog is light brown, the color derives from nitrogen oxides. All of the other air pollutants listed are colorless. The answer is **(D).**

2. The symptoms described are those of carbon monoxide inhalation. The answer is **(A).**

3. Although DDT and related compounds are no longer used as insecticides in the USA, they continue to be manufactured here for foreign markets. Exposure to such compounds causes CNS excitation, not pulmonary dysfunction. The answer is **(E).**

4. Hemodialysis is of no value in paraquat poisoning. The answer is **(D).**

5. Dichlorvos, an organophosphate inhibitor of acetylcholinesterase, is rapidly biotransformed and subject to inactivation by hydrolysis. Carbamates and organophosphates do not accumulate in the environment. The chlorinated hydrocarbons (DDT, toxaphene), the polychlorinated biphenyls (PCBs), and the dioxins (TCDD) are persistent chemicals. The answer is **(B).**

6. Paraquat is highly corrosive to the gastrointestinal tract. Oral ingestion of the herbicide leads to marked gastrointestinal irritation, hematemesis, and usually blood in the stools. Gastric lavage with activated charcoal should be performed repeatedly to remove unabsorbed paraquat from the stomach. Signs of pulmonary impairment do not appear for several days and are usually progressive, resulting in severe pulmonary fibrosis and, often, death. The answer is **(D).** (See also the answer to Question 4.)

7. Too easy? Highly potent organophosphate inhibitors of acetylcholinesterase (eg, sarin, tabun) have been developed for chemical warfare purposes. Their storage represents a potential toxicologic hazard. It is important to recognize the signs and symptoms of excess acetylcholine (DUMBELS, Chapter 7), which include those described. The answer is **(D).**

8. Sulfur dioxide is a reducing agent that forms sulfurous acid on contact with moist surfaces. This is responsible for irritant effects on the mucous membranes of the eye, the oropharynx, and the respiratory tract. Asthmatics, patients with cardiac disease, and the elderly are especially sensitive to sulfur dioxide. Nitrogen dioxide causes similar problems, but it is an oxidizing agent formed from fires and in silage on farms. The answer is **(L).**

9. Three hydrocarbon solvents are listed: benzene, tetrachloroethylene, and toluene. Each may cause CNS effects such as headache, fatigue, and loss of appetite. Benzene and toluene are *aromatic* hydrocarbons. The answer is **(M)**.

10. Dioxin is a contaminant in the manufacture of 2,4-D and 2,4,5-T ("agent orange"). The answer is **(F)**.

11. Chronic exposure to benzene is markedly hematotoxic. Injury to bone marrow cells is characteristic of this aromatic hydrocarbon. Benzene has also been identified as a possible leukemogenic agent. The answer is **(B)**.

12. Rotenone and pyrethrum alkaloids are both derived from plants. Both agents may cause dermatitis through skin contact. Accidental oral ingestion of rotenone causes gastrointestinal irritation but no neurotoxic effects. The answer is **(J)**.

58

Chelators & Heavy Metals

OBJECTIVES

You should be able to:

- Describe the general mechanism of metal chelation.
- Identify the clinically useful chelators and know their indications and their adverse effects.
- Describe the major clinical features and treatment of acute and chronic lead poisoning.
- Describe the major clinical features and treatment of arsenic poisoning.
- Describe the major clinical features and treatment of inorganic and organic mercury poisoning.
- Describe the major clinical features and treatment of iron poisoning.

Learn the definitions that follow.

Table 58–1. Definitions.

Term	Definition
Chelating agent	A molecule with two or more electronegative groups that can form stable coordinate complexes with multivalent cationic metal atoms
Erethism	Syndrome resulting from mercury poisoning characterized by insomnia, memory loss, excitability, and delirium
Pica	The ingestion of nonfood substances; in the present context, pica refers to ingestion of lead-based paint fragments by small children
Plumbism	A range of toxic syndromes due to chronic lead poisoning that may vary as a function of blood or tissue levels and patient age

CONCEPTS

The metals discussed in this chapter—lead, arsenic, mercury, and iron—frequently cause significant toxicity in humans. The toxicity profiles of metals differ, but most of their effects appear to result from interaction with sulfhydryl groups of enzymes and regulatory proteins. Chelators are organic compounds with two or more electronegative groups that can form stable covalent-coordinate bonds with cationic metal atoms. As emphasized in this chapter, these stable complexes can often be excreted readily, thus reducing the toxicity of the metal.

CHELATORS

The most useful chelators for clinical purposes are dimercaprol (BAL), succimer, penicillamine, edetate (EDTA), and deferoxamine. Variations among these agents in their affinities for specific metals govern their clinical applications. Some of these applications are outlined in Table 58–2.

A. Dimercaprol: Dimercaprol (2,3-dimercaptopropanol, BAL [British anti-Lewisite]) is a *bidentate* chelator, ie, it forms two bonds with the metal ion, preventing the metal's binding to tissue proteins and permitting its rapid excretion.

1. Clinical use: Dimercaprol is approved for use in acute arsenic and mercury poisoning and for lead poisoning when used in conjunction with edetate. It is an oily liquid that must be given parenterally.

2. Toxicity: Dimercaprol causes a high incidence of adverse effects, perhaps because it is very lipophilic and readily enters cells. Its toxicity includes transient hypertension, tachycardia, headache, nausea, vomiting, paresthesias, and fever (especially in children). It may cause pain and hematomas at the injection site. Long-term use is associated with thrombocytopenia and decreased prothrombin time.

B. Succimer: Succimer (2,3-dimercaptosuccinic acid; DMSA) is a water-soluble bidentate congener of dimercaprol with reasonable oral bioavailability.

1. Clinical use: Succimer is currently approved for the oral treatment of lead toxicity in children, and it is as effective as parenteral EDTA in reducing blood lead concentration. Succimer also appears to be as effective as dimercaprol in arsenic and mercury poisoning.

2. Toxicity: While succimer appears to be less toxic than dimercaprol, gastrointestinal distress, CNS effects, skin rash, and elevation of liver enzymes may occur. This agent should not be administered with other chelating drugs.

C. Penicillamine: Penicillamine, a derivative of penicillin, is another bidentate chelator, forming two bonds with the metal ion.

1. Clinical use: The major uses of penicillamine are in the treatment of copper poisoning and of Wilson's disease. It is sometimes used as adjunctive therapy in gold, arsenic, and lead intoxication and in rheumatoid arthritis. The agent is water-soluble, well absorbed from the gastrointestinal tract, and excreted unchanged.

2. Toxicity: Adverse effects are common and may be severe. They include nephrotoxicity with proteinuria, pancytopenia, and autoimmune dysfunction, including lupus erythematosus and hemolytic anemia.

Table 58–2. Important characteristics of the toxicology of arsenic, iron, lead, and mercury.

Metal	Form Entering Body	Route of Absorption	Target Organs for Toxicity	Treatment[1]
Lead	Inorganic lead oxides and salts	Gastrointestinal tract, respiratory, skin (minor)	Hematopoietic system, CNS, kidneys	Dimercaprol, edetate, penicillamine, succimer
	Tetraethyl lead	Skin (major), gastrointestinal	CNS	Seizure control, supportive
Arsenic	Inorganic arsenic salts	All mucosal surfaces	Capillaries, gastrointestinal tract, hematopoietic system	Dimercaprol, succimer, penicillamine
	Arsine gas	Inhalation	Erythrocytes	Supportive
Mercury	Elemental	Inhalation	CNS, kidneys	Dimercaprol
	Inorganic salts	Gastrointestinal tract	Kidneys, gastrointestinal tract	Penicillamine, dimercaprol
	Organic mercurials	Gastrointestinal tract	CNS	Supportive
Iron	Ferrous sulfate	Gastrointestinal tract	Gastrointestinal tract, CNS, blood	Deferoxamine

[1]In all cases, removal from the source of toxicity is the first requirement of management.

D. Edetate: Edetate (EDTA) is a very efficient *polydentate* chelator of many divalent and trivalent cations (including calcium).

1. **Clinical use:** The primary use of EDTA is in the treatment of lead poisoning. Because the agent is very polar, it is given parenterally and does not enter cells. To prevent dangerous hypocalcemia, EDTA is given as the calcium disodium salt.

2. **Toxicity:** The most important adverse effect of the agent is nephrotoxicity, including renal tubular necrosis. This risk can be reduced by adequate hydration and by restricting treatment with EDTA to 5 days or less.

E. Deferoxamine: Deferoxamine is a polydentate bacterial product that has an extremely high and selective affinity for iron and a much lower affinity for aluminum. Fortunately, the drug competes poorly for heme iron in hemoglobin and cytochromes.

1. **Clinical use:** Deferoxamine is used parenterally in the treatment of acute iron intoxication.

2. **Toxicity:** Skin reactions (flushing, erythema, urticaria) may occur; with long-term use, neurotoxicity (eg, retinal degeneration), hepatic and renal dysfunction, and severe coagulopathies have been reported. Rapid intravenous administration may cause histamine release and hypotensive shock.

TOXICOLOGY OF HEAVY METALS

A. Lead: Lead serves no useful purpose in the body and may damage the hematopoietic tissues, liver, nervous system, kidneys, gastrointestinal tract, and reproductive system (Table 58–2). Lead represents a major environmental hazard since it is present in air and water throughout the world.

1. **Acute lead poisoning:** Acute inorganic lead poisoning is no longer common in the USA but may occur from industrial exposures (usually via inhalation of dust) and in children who have ingested a large quantity of chips or flakes from surfaces covered with lead-containing paint. The primary signs of this syndrome are acute abdominal colic and CNS changes. In children, the latter may take the form of acute encephalopathy. The mortality rate is high in lead encephalopathy, and prompt chelation therapy is mandatory.

2. **Chronic lead poisoning:** Chronic inorganic lead poisoning (plumbism) is much more common than the acute form. Signs include peripheral neuropathy (wrist-drop is characteristic), anorexia, anemia, tremor, weight loss, and gastrointestinal symptoms. Treatment includes removal from the source of exposure and chelation therapy, usually with edetate (severe cases), dimercaprol, or penicillamine. Chronic lead poisoning in children presents as growth retardation, neurocognitive deficits, and developmental delay. Succimer is also approved for use in such children. In workers exposed to lead, prophylaxis by means of oral chelating agents is contraindicated, since some evidence suggests that lead absorption may be enhanced by the presence of chelators. In contrast, high dietary calcium is indicated, since lead retention is reduced.

3. **Organic lead poisoning:** Poisoning by organic lead is usually due to tetraethyl lead or tetramethyl lead antiknock gasoline additives (no longer used in the USA). This form of lead is readily absorbed through the skin and lungs. The primary signs of intoxication occur in the CNS and may include hallucinations, headache, irritability, convulsions, and coma. Treatment consists of decontamination and seizure control.

B. Arsenic: Arsenic is widely used in industrial processes and is also an environmental pollutant released during the burning of coal. Although it exists in both trivalent and pentavalent forms, its toxicity is entirely due to the trivalent form.

1. **Acute arsenic poisoning:** Acute arsenic poisoning results in severe gastrointestinal discomfort, vomiting, rice-water stools, and capillary damage with dehydration and shock. A sweet, garlicky odor may be detected in the breath and the stools. Treatment consists of supportive therapy to replace water and electrolytes and chelation therapy with dimercaprol.

2. **Chronic arsenic poisoning:** Chronic arsenic intoxication is manifested by skin changes, hair loss, bone marrow depression and anemia, and chronic nausea and gastrointestinal disturbances. Dimercaprol therapy appears to be of value. Arsenic is a known human carcinogen.

3. **Arsine gas:** Arsine gas (AsH_3) is formed during the refinement and processing of certain metals and is used in the semiconductor industry; it is an occupational hazard. Arsine causes a unique form of toxicity characterized by massive hemolysis. Pigment overload from red cell breakdown may cause renal failure. Treatment is supportive.

C. **Mercury:** The main source of inorganic mercury as a toxic hazard is through the use of materials in dental laboratories and in the manufacture of wood preservatives, insecticides, and batteries. Organic mercury compounds are used as seed dressings and fungicides.

1. **Acute mercury poisoning:** Acute mercury poisoning usually occurs through inhalation of inorganic elemental mercury. It causes chest pain, shortness of breath, nausea and vomiting, kidney damage, gastroenteritis, and CNS damage. Chelation is effective with dimercaprol. Acute ingestion of mercuric chloride causes a severe (life-threatening) hemorrhagic gastroenteritis followed by renal failure.

2. **Chronic mercury poisoning:** Chronic mercury poisoning may occur with exposure to inorganic or organic mercury. Inorganic mercury poisoning in the chronic form usually presents as a diffuse syndrome involving the gums and teeth, gastrointestinal disturbances, and neurologic and behavioral changes. When mercury was used in the hat-making industry, the behavioral effects (erethism) were so common that they gave rise to the epithet "mad as a hatter." Chronic inorganic mercury intoxication has been treated with penicillamine and dimercaprol.

3. **Organic mercury poisoning:** Intoxication with organic mercury compounds was first recognized in connection with an epidemic of neurologic and psychiatric disease in the village of Minamata in Japan. The outbreak was found to be the result of consumption of fish containing a high content of methylmercury, which was produced by bacteria in sea water from mercury in the effluent of a nearby vinyl plastics manufacturing plant. Similar epidemics have resulted from the consumption of grain intended for use as seed and treated with fungicidal organic mercury compounds. Treatment with chelators has been tried, but the benefits are uncertain.

D. **Iron:** Acute poisoning from ingestion of ferrous sulfate tablets occurs in children as frequently as salicylate intoxication. The initial symptoms of iron poisoning include vomiting, gastrointestinal bleeding, lethargy, and gray cyanosis. This may be followed by signs of severe gastrointestinal necrosis, pneumonitis, jaundice, seizures, and coma. Deferoxamine is the chelating agent of choice (see Chapter 59). Chronic excessive intake of iron may lead to hemosiderosis or hemochromatosis.

QUESTIONS

DIRECTIONS: Each numbered item or incomplete statement in this section is followed by answers or by completions of the statement. Select the ONE lettered answer or completion that is BEST in each case.

Items 1–2: A small child is brought to a hospital emergency room suffering from severe gastrointestinal distress and abdominal colic.

1. The differential diagnosis will include all of the following EXCEPT
   (A) Acute inorganic lead poisoning
   (B) Appendicitis
   (C) Exposure to arsine gas
   (D) Pancreatitis
   (E) Peptic ulcer

2. If this patient has severe acute lead poisoning presenting as signs and symptoms of encephalopathy, treatment should be instituted immediately with
   (A) Acetylcysteine
   (B) Deferoxamine
   (C) EDTA
   (D) Penicillamine
   (E) Succimer

3. A young woman employed as a dental laboratory technician complains of conjunctivitis, skin irritation, and hair loss. On examination, she has perforation of the nasal septum and a "milk and roses" complexion. These signs and symptoms are most likely to be due to
   (A) Acute mercury poisoning
   (B) Chronic inorganic arsenic poisoning
   (C) Chronic mercury poisoning
   (D) Excessive use of supplementary iron tablets
   (E) Lead poisoning

4. A patient complains of chronic headache, fatigue, loss of appetite, and constipation. He has slight weakness of the extensor muscle in the upper limbs. The following data are obtained.

Test	Result in Patient	Normal
Hemoglobin	< 13 g/dL	> 14 g/dL
Urinary coproporphyrin	> 80 µg/100 mg creatinine	< 10 µg/100 mg creatinine
Urinary aminolevulinic acid	> 2 mg/100 mg creatinine	< 0.5 mg/100 mg creatinine

   The most reasonable diagnosis is that this patient is suffering from chronic poisoning due to
   (A) Arsenic
   (B) Hexane
   (C) Inorganic lead
   (D) Iron
   (E) Mercuric chloride

5. In the treatment of arsenic poisoning, removal of the source of arsenic exposure is the primary therapeutic objective, but if the patient is treated with an oral chelating agent, the drug most likely to be used is
   (A) Deferoxamine
   (B) Dimercaprol
   (C) EDTA
   (D) Penicillamine
   (E) Succimer

6. As a general rule, chelators used in lead poisoning are more effective if administered 48 *hours* after ingestion than if administered 48 *days* after a person has ingested the same quantity of lead. The main reason for this is that
   (A) Elimination of lead is 90% in the urine
   (B) The half-life of lead in the blood and soft tissues is only 24 days
   (C) Forty-eight days after ingestion, much of the absorbed lead is in the bone matrix
   (D) Only 5% of absorbed lead is retained in the body
   (E) Lead binding to erythrocytes is time-dependent

7. A 24-year-old man was employed in the supplies department of a company that manufactures semiconductors. Following an accident at the plant, he presented with nausea and vomiting, headache, hypotension, and shivering. Laboratory analyses showed hemoglobinuria and a plasma free hemoglobin level greater than 1.4 g/dL. This young man was probably exposed to
   (A) Arsine
   (B) Inorganic arsenic
   (C) Mercury vapor
   (D) Methylmercury
   (E) Tetraethyl lead

8. A 2-year-old child was brought to the emergency room 1 hour after ingestion of tablets he had managed to obtain from a bottle in the kitchen. His symptoms included marked gastrointestinal distress, vomiting (with hematemesis), and epigastric pain. Metabolic acidosis and leukocytosis were also present. This patient is most likely to have ingested tablets containing
   (A) Acetaminophen
   (B) Aspirin
   (C) Diphenhydramine
   (D) Iron
   (E) Vitamin C

DIRECTIONS (Items 9–12): Each set of matching questions in this section consists of a list of three to twenty-six lettered options (some of which may be figures) followed by several numbered items. For each numbered item, select the ONE lettered option that is most closely associated with it. Each lettered option may be selected once, more than once, or not at all.

(A) Arsine
(B) Deferoxamine
(C) Dimercaprol
(D) Edetate calcium disodium
(E) Inorganic mercury
(F) Iron
(G) Methylmercury
(H) Mercury vapor
(I) Penicillamine
(J) Succimer
(K) Tetraethyl lead
(L) Trivalent arsenic

9. Gingivitis, discolored gums, and loose teeth are common symptoms of chronic exposure to this agent
10. This compound may be produced in seawater by the action of bacteria and algae. It is also synthesized chemically for commercial use as a fungicide
11. This agent has been reported to cause lupus erythematosus and hemolytic anemia
12. High doses of this agent may cause histamine release and extreme vasodilation

ANSWERS

1. The diagnosis of acute lead poisoning may be difficult, since the symptoms may simulate a number of disorders of the gastrointestinal system, including acute appendicitis. In children with recent ingestion of lead-containing materials, radiopacities may be visible on abdominal x-ray. Exposure to arsine, an industrial gas, is highly unlikely in a small child, and the symptoms are those of acute hemolysis. The answer is **(C)**.

2. Encephalopathy in severe lead poisoning is a medical emergency. Of the drugs listed, intravenous EDTA is the most effective chelating agent. Dimercaprol (not listed) may also be used parenterally. Oral succimer is used in children with mild to moderate lead poisoning and may be initiated 4–5 days after the use of EDTA or dimercaprol in severe poisoning. The answer is **(C)**.

3. The "milk and roses" complexion, which results from vasodilation and anemia, is one characteristic of chronic inorganic arsenic poisoning, while patients with lead poisoning often have a gray pallor. Other signs and symptoms of arsenic poisoning include gastrointestinal distress, hyperpigmentation, and white lines on the nails. We hope you were not led astray by her employment. The answer is **(B)**.

4. Of the agents listed, lead is most likely to cause a decrease in heme biosynthesis. Exposure to inorganic arsenic may also cause anemia. The urinary concentrations of lead before and after EDTA treatment may confirm the diagnosis. The answer is **(C)**.

5. Only one of the agents listed is effective orally. Although it is more toxic, penicillamine is at present more likely to be used in an adult than the newer agent succimer. The answer is **(D)**.

6. Depending on patient age, from 10% to 40% of inorganic lead absorbed from the gastrointestinal tract is retained in the body, the balance being mostly eliminated in the urine. Of the fraction retained, over 90% is incorporated into the skeleton. By 2 months, a significant amount of the body burden of lead is present in the bone matrix. Chelating agents are much less able to penetrate into bone than into more vascular tissues and thus are less effective if they are not administered soon after lead exposure. The answer is **(C)**.

7. From the signs and symptoms alone, a diagnosis could not be made of arsine poisoning. However, clues to the etiology of poisoning can often be provided by knowing a patient's occupation. The lab reports suggest marked hemolysis. Arsine binds to hemoglobin and decreases erythrocyte glutathione levels, causing membrane fragility and resulting hemolysis. The answer is **(A)**.

8. This question emphasizes that the ingestion of iron tablets is a relatively common cause of accidental poisoning in young children. The signs and symptoms described usually occur in the

first 6 hours following ingestion. In a child of body weight 22 lb, the ingestion of 600 mg can cause severe, perhaps lethal toxicity. The answer is **(D).**

9. Oral and gastrointestinal complaints are common in chronic mercury poisoning, and tremor involving the fingers and arms is often present. The answer is **(E).**

10. Methylmercury continues to be used as a fungicide to prevent mold growth in seed grain. The answer is **(G).**

11. Autoimmune diseases have occurred during treatment of Wilson's disease with penicillamine. The answer is **(I).**

12. Deferoxamine may cause shock if given by rapid intravenous infusion. The answer is **(B).**

59 Management of the Poisoned Patient

OBJECTIVES

You should be able to list or describe the following:

- Steps involved in the management of the poisoned patient, including the emergency treatment of a comatose patient.
- Common toxic syndromes associated with major drug groups and individual agents frequently involved in poisoning.
- Methods for identification of toxic compounds, including physical findings and laboratory methods.
- Methods available for decontamination of poisoned patients and for increasing the elimination of toxic compounds.
- Specific antidotes available for management of poisoning.

CONCEPTS

Toxic substances include drugs usually used for therapeutic purposes as well as agricultural and industrial chemicals that have no medical applications. Most chemicals are capable of causing toxic effects when given in excessive dosage; even for therapeutic drugs, the difference between obtaining a therapeutic action and a toxic one is a matter of dose. Many toxic effects of therapeutic agents have been discussed in previous chapters. Common toxic syndromes associated with major drug groups are summarized below. Other chemicals commonly involved in poisonings are those readily accessible in the environment: solvents, corrosives, insecticides, heavy metals, and drugs of abuse. This unit reviews the principles of management of the poisoned patient.

TOXICOKINETICS, TOXICODYNAMICS, & CAUSE OF DEATH

A. Toxicokinetics: This term is used to describe the disposition of poisons in the body, ie, their pharmacokinetics. Knowledge of the absorption, distribution, and elimination permits assessment of the value of procedures designed to remove particular toxins from the skin or gastrointestinal tract. For example, drugs with large apparent volumes of distribution, such as antidepressants and antimalarials, are not amenable to dialysis procedures for drug removal. Drugs with low volumes of distribution, including lithium, phenytoin, and salicylates, are more readily removed by dialysis and diuresis procedures. In some cases, it is possible to accelerate renal elimination of weak acids by urinary alkalinization and weak bases by urinary acidification. The clearance of drugs may be different at toxic concentrations than at therapeutic concentrations. For example, in overdoses of phenytoin or salicylates, the capacity of the liver to metabolize the drugs may be exceeded and elimination will change from first-order (constant half-life) to zero-order (variable half-life) kinetics.

B. Toxicodynamics: Toxicodynamics is a term used to describe the injurious effects of toxins, ie, their pharmacodynamics. A knowledge of toxicodynamics can be useful in the diagnosis and management of poisoning. For example, hypertension and tachycardia are typically seen in overdoses with amphetamines, cocaine, and antimuscarinic drugs. Hypotension with bradycardia occurs with overdoses of calcium channel blockers, beta-blockers, and sedative-hypnotics. Hypotension with tachycardia occurs with tricyclic antidepressants, phenothiazines, and theophylline. Hyperthermia is most frequently a result of overdose of drugs with antimuscarinic actions, the salicylates, or sympathomimetics. Hypothermia is more likely with toxic doses of ethanol and other central nervous system depressants. Increased respiratory rate is often a feature of overdose with carbon monoxide, salicylates, and other drugs that cause metabolic acidosis or cellular asphyxia. Overdoses of agents that depress the heart are likely to affect the functions of all organ systems that are critically dependent on blood flow, including brain, liver, and kidney. Note that restoration of blood pressure after a period of hypotension may increase the tissue distribution of a toxin, which can result in a waxing and waning of signs and symptoms.

C. Cause of Death in Intoxicated Patients: The most common causes of death from drug overdose in the USA reflect the drug groups most often selected for abuse or for suicide. Sedative-hypnotics and narcotics cause respiratory depression, coma, aspiration of gastric contents, and other respiratory malfunctions. Drugs such as cocaine, PCP, tricyclic antidepressants, and theophylline cause seizures, which may lead to vomiting and aspiration of gastric contents and to postictal respiratory depression. Tricyclic antidepressants and cardiac glycosides cause dangerous and frequently lethal arrhythmias. Severe hypotension may occur with any of these drugs. A few intoxicants cause direct liver and kidney damage. These include acetaminophen, mushroom poisons of the *Amanita phalloides* type (amanitins), certain inhalants, and some heavy metals. The metals are discussed in Chapter 58.

MANAGEMENT OF THE POISONED PATIENT

Management of the poisoned patient consists of maintenance of vital functions, identification of the toxic substance, decontamination procedures, enhancement of elimination, and, in a few instances, the use of a specific antidote.

A. Vital Functions: The most important aspect of treatment of a poisoned patient is maintenance of vital functions, as indicated by the mnemonic **"ABCDs."** The most commonly endangered or impaired vital function is respiration. Therefore, an open and protected airway (the "A" of the mnemonic) must be established first, and effective ventilation ("B" for breathing) must be ensured. The circulation ("C") should be evaluated and supported as needed. The cardiac rhythm should be determined, and if ventricular fibrillation is present, it must be corrected at once. The blood pressure should be determined, but hypotension rarely needs immediate treatment except in cases of traumatic hemorrhage. Because of the danger of brain damage from hypoglycemia, intravenous 50% dextrose ("D" of the mnemonic) should be given to comatose patients immediately after blood has been drawn for laboratory tests and before laboratory results have been obtained. Similarly, thiamine should be given to prevent Wernicke's syndrome in the suspected alcoholic or malnourished patient. In patients with signs of respiratory or central nervous system depression, intravenous naloxone may be administered to offset possible toxic effects of opioid analgesic overdose.

B. Identification of Poisons: Many intoxicants cause a characteristic syndrome of clinical and laboratory changes. Table 59–1 summarizes toxic syndromes associated with major drug groups and the key interventions called for. The toxic features of selected individual agents are listed in Table 59–2. When the toxic agent responsible for a case of poisoning cannot be directly examined and identified, the clinician must rely on indirect means to identify the type of intoxication and the progress of therapy. In addition to the history and physical examination, certain laboratory examinations may be useful. A few intoxicants can be directly identified in

Table 59–1. Toxic syndromes caused by major drug groups.*

Drug Group	Clinical Features	Key Interventions
Antimuscarinic drugs (atropine, some antidepressants and antihistaminics, jimsonweed, etc)	Delirium, hallucinations, seizures, coma, tachycardia, hypertension, hyperthermia, mydriasis, decreased bowel sounds, urinary retention	Control hyperthermia. Physostigmine may be helpful but not for tricyclic overdose
Cholinomimetic drugs (carbamate and organophosphate inhibitors of acetyl-cholinesterase)	Anxiety, agitation, seizures, coma, bradycardia or tachycardia, pinpoint pupils, salivation, sweating, hyperactive bowel, muscle fasciculations, then paralysis	Support respiration. Treat with atropine and pralidoxime. Decontaminate
Opioids (heroin, morphine, methadone, etc)	Lethargy, sedation, coma, bradycardia, hypotension, hypoventilation, pinpoint pupils, cool skin, decreased bowel sounds, flaccid muscles	Provide airway and respiratory support. Give naloxone as required
Salicylates	Confusion, lethargy, coma, seizures, hyperventilation, hyperthermia, dehydration, hypokalemia, anion gap, metabolic acidosis	Correct acidosis and fluid and electrolyte imbalance. Alkaline diuresis or hemodialysis to aid elimination
Sedative-hypnotics (barbiturates, benzodiazepines, ethanol)	Disinhibition initially; later, lethargy, stupor, coma. Nystagmus is common. Decreased muscle tone, hypothermia. Small pupils, hypotension, and decreased bowel sounds in heavy overdose	Provide airway and respiratory support. Avoid fluid overload. Use flumazenil for benzodiazepine overdose
Stimulants (amphetamines, cocaine, phencyclidine)	Agitation, anxiety, seizures. Hypertension, tachycardia, arrhythmias. Mydriasis, vertical and horizontal nystagmus with PCP. Skin warm and sweaty. Hyperthermia, increased muscle tone, possible rhabdomyolysis	Control seizures. Treat hypertension and hyperthermia
Tricyclic antidepressants	Antimuscarinic effects (see above). The "three Cs" of coma, convulsions, cardiac toxicity (QRS prolongation, arrhythmias, hypotension)	Control seizures. Correct acidosis and cardiotoxicity with ventilation and bicarbonate. Control hyperthermia

*Modified and reproduced, with permission, from Katzung BG (editor): *Basic & Clinical Pharmacology,* 7th ed. Appleton & Lange, 1998.

the blood or urine, especially when information in the history helps to narrow the search. In the more common situation (a comatose patient unable to provide a history), general tests for replacement of anions or osmotic equivalents in the blood (anion gap, osmolar gap) may be useful. A few intoxicants can be identified or strongly suspected on the basis of electrocardiographic or radiologic findings.

1. **Osmolar gap:** The osmolar gap is the difference between the measured osmolality (measured by the freezing point depression method) and the predicted osmolality:

$$Gap = Osm\ (measured) - [(2 \times Na^+\ [meq/L]) + (Glucose\ [mg/dL] \div 18) + (BUN\ [mg/dL] \div 3)]$$

This gap is normally zero. A significant gap is produced by high serum concentrations of intoxicants of low molecular weight such as ethanol, methanol, and ethylene glycol.

2. **Anion gap:** The anion gap is the difference between the sum of the two primary cations, sodium and potassium, and the sum of the two primary anions, chloride and bicarbonate:

$$Gap = (Na^+ + K^+) - (HCO_3^- + Cl^-)$$

This gap is normally 12–16 meq/L. A significant increase may be produced by diabetic ketoacidosis, renal failure, or drug-induced metabolic acidosis. Drugs that may cause metabolic acidosis include ethanol, ethylene glycol, isoniazid, iron, methanol, phenelzine, salicylates, tranylcypromine, and verapamil.

3. **Serum potassium:** Myocardial function is critically dependent on the serum potassium level. Drugs that cause hyperkalemia include beta-adrenoceptor blockers, digitalis (in suici-

Table 59–2. Toxic features of specific agents.

Agent	Toxic Features
Acetaminophen	Mild anorexia, nausea, vomiting, delayed jaundice, hepatic and renal failure
Antifreeze (ethylene glycol)	Renal failure, crystals in urine, anion and osmolar gap, initial CNS excitation; eye examination normal
Botulism	Dysphagia, dysarthria, ptosis, ophthalmoplegia, muscle weakness; incubation period 12–36 hours
Carbon monoxide	Coma, metabolic acidosis, retinal hemorrhages
Cyanide	Bitter almond odor, seizures, coma, abnormal ECG
Gasoline	Distinctive odor, coughing, pulmonary infiltrates on x-ray
Iron	Bloody diarrhea, coma, radiopaque material in gut (seen on x-ray), high leukocyte count, hyperglycemia
Lead	Abdominal pain, hypertension, seizures, muscle weakness, metallic taste, anorexia, encephalopathy, delayed motor neuropathy, changes in renal and reproductive function
LSD	Hallucinations, dilated pupils, hypertension
Mercury	Acute renal failure, tremor, salivation, gingivitis, colitis, erethism (fits of crying, irrational behavior), nephrotic syndrome
Methanol	Rapid respiration, visual symptoms, osmolar gap, severe metabolic acidosis
Mushrooms (*Amanita phalloides* type)	Severe nausea and vomiting 8 hours after ingestion; delayed hepatic and renal failure
Paraquat	Oropharyngeal burning, headache, vomiting, delayed pulmonary fibrosis, and death
Phencyclidine (PCP)	Coma with eyes open, horizontal and vertical nystagmus, hyperacusis, myoclonic jerks, violent behavior
Plants	
Nightshade family, jimsonweed	Hallucinations, mydriasis, seizures (these plants contain atropine-like alkaloids)
Oleander and foxglove	Digitalis poisoning
Predatory bean (rosary pea)	Delayed severe gastrointestinal distress, seizures, hemolytic anemia, death

dal overdose), fluoride, and lithium. Drugs associated with hypokalemia include barium, beta-adrenoceptor agonists, methylxanthines, most diuretics, and toluene.

C. **Decontamination:** Decontamination consists of removing any unabsorbed poison from the patient's body. In the case of ingested noncorrosive toxins, this may involve inducing vomiting (emesis) by means of **syrup of ipecac** if the patient is conscious. (Apomorphine and *extract* of ipecac are dangerous emetics and should not be used.) In unconscious patients, emesis will lead to aspiration into the respiratory tree and must be avoided. **Gastric lavage** with a large-bore tube may be used to remove noncorrosive drugs from the stomach of a comatose patient if the airway has been protected with a cuffed endotracheal tube. Corrosives (strong acids and bases) may cause severe esophageal damage during emesis and should be diluted (not neutralized) in the stomach. **Activated charcoal,** given orally or by stomach tube, may be very effective in adsorbing any remaining drug. Toxins removed by multiple treatments with activated charcoal include amitriptyline, barbiturates, digitalis glycosides, phencyclidine, propoxyphene, theophylline, tricyclic antidepressants, and valproic acid. In the case of topical exposure (insecticides, solvents), the clothing should be removed and the patient washed to remove any chemical still present on the skin. Medical personnel must be careful not to contaminate themselves during this procedure.

D. **Enhancement of Elimination:** Enhancement of elimination is possible for a number of toxins, including manipulation of urine pH to accelerate renal excretion of weak acids and bases. For example, alkaline diuresis is effective in toxicity due to fluoride, isoniazid, fluoroquinolones, phenobarbital, and salicylates. Urinary acidification may be useful in toxicity due to weak bases, including amphetamines, nicotine, and phencyclidine, but care must be taken to avoid acidosis and renal failure in rhabdomyolysis. Hemodialysis or hemoperfusion enhances the elimination of many toxic compounds, including acetaminophen, ethylene glycol, formaldehyde, lithium, methanol, procainamide, quinidine, salicylates, and theophylline. Cathartics such as sorbitol (70%) may decrease absorption and hasten removal of toxins from the gastrointestinal tract.

E. Antidotes: Specific antidotes exist for only a few poisons (Table 59–3). Consideration must be given to the fact that the duration of action of most antidotes is shorter than that of the intoxicant, and the antidotes may need to be given repeatedly. The use of chelating agents for metal poisoning is discussed in Chapter 58. "Universal antidote" (burnt toast, magnesium oxide, tannic acid) is of no value and may be harmful.

F. Snakebite: The most common dangerous snake in the USA is the rattlesnake. Although snakebites are common (several thousand per year in the USA), severe envenomation is infrequent.

   1. Effects: Snake venom contains a large number of enzymes and tissue toxins. The most common effects of envenomation include local tissue necrosis, vascular damage, thrombosis, hemorrhage, and neural injury.

   2. Treatment: It is now well documented that once-popular remedies such as incision and suction, ice packs, and tourniquets are usually more dangerous than helpful. The most important prehospital therapy is to minimize movement of the bitten part to limit the spread of venom in the tissues. Effective therapy consists of adequate dosage with antivenin. Since antivenins are prepared in horses, serum sickness frequently follows and may also require therapy.

Table 59–3. Specific antidotes.*

Antidote	Poisons
Acetylcysteine	Acetaminophen; best given within 8–10 hours after overdose
Antivenin	Snakes, black widow spiders
Atropine	Cholinesterase inhibitors
Bicarbonate, sodium	Membrane-depressant cardiotoxic drugs, eg, quinidine, tricyclic antidepressants
Deferoxamine	Iron salts
Digoxin-specific Fab antibodies	Digoxin and related cardiac glycosides
Esmolol	Caffeine, theophylline, metaproterenol
Ethanol	Methanol, ethylene glycol
Flumazenil	Benzodiazepines, zolpidem
Glucagon	Beta-adrenoceptor blockers
Edetate	Lead
Dimercaprol	Lead, gold, arsenic
Hydroxocobalamin	Cyanide
Penicillamine	Copper, lead, arsenic, gold
Naloxone	Opioid analgesics
Oxygen	Carbon monoxide
Physostigmine	"Suggested" for muscarinic receptor blockers, *not* tricyclics
Pralidoxime	Organophosphate cholinesterase inhibitors
Sodium nitrite	Cyanide
Vitamin B_6	Isoniazid

*Modified and reproduced, with permission, from Katzung BG (editor): *Basic & Clinical Pharmacology*, 7th ed. Appleton & Lange, 1998.

QUESTIONS

DIRECTIONS: Each of the numbered items or incomplete statements in this section is followed by answers or by completions of the statement. Select the ONE lettered answer or completion that is BEST in each case.

Items 1–2: A patient has taken an overdose of aspirin that has caused metabolic acidosis. Serum electrolyte concentrations are Na^+, 147 meq/L; K^+, 6 meq/L; Cl^-, 100 meq/L; HCO_3^-, 15 meq/L.

1. The anion gap in this patient
   (A) Cannot be calculated from the data given
   (B) Is unchanged from normal
   (C) Is increased above normal
   (D) Is decreased below normal
   (E) Is reversed

2. Which of the following agents may cause an increase in anion gap?
   (A) Antifreeze solution
   (B) Iron tablets
   (C) Phenelzine
   (D) Verapamil
   (E) All of the above

3. Which one of the following drugs or toxins is LEAST likely to cause hyperthermia in overdosage?
   (A) Amphetamine
   (B) Aspirin
   (C) Heroin
   (D) Jimsonweed
   (E) Phencyclidine

4. A patient is brought to an emergency room suffering from nausea, vomiting, and abdominal pain. He has muscle weakness that seems to be progressing downward from the head and neck. The patient has difficulty talking clearly and has ptosis and ophthalmoplegia. The most likely cause of these symptoms is
   (A) Accidental ingestion of paraquat
   (B) An overdose of phenobarbital
   (C) Excessive consumption of ethanol
   (D) Food poisoning
   (E) Organophosphate poisoning

5. Which one of the following is LEAST likely to cause an osmolar gap when taken in overdose?
   (A) Digoxin
   (B) Ethanol
   (C) Ethylene glycol
   (D) Isopropanol
   (E) Methanol

6. A patient with congestive heart failure has accidentally taken an overdose of digitoxin. The blood concentration of the drug is four times the threshold for toxicity. Pharmacokinetic parameters for digitoxin include a clearance (hepatic) of 180 mL/h and an elimination half-life of 168 hours (1 week). If no procedures are instituted to decontaminate this patient, the time taken to reach a safe level of digitoxin will be approximately
   (A) 3.5 days
   (B) 7 days
   (C) 14 days
   (D) 28 days
   (E) 56 days

7. Regarding snakebite
   (A) A rattlesnake bite is almost always associated with significant tissue injury
   (B) A snakebite should be treated in the field with incision, suction, and a tourniquet before the victim is moved
   (C) The most common manifestation of serious envenomation is convulsions
   (D) When a victim of a serious envenomation reaches the hospital, the most effective therapy is prompt administration of snake antivenin
   (E) All of the above are correct

Items 8–9: A patient is brought to the emergency room having taken an overdose (unknown quantity) of a sustained-release preparation of theophylline by mouth 2 hours previously. He has marked gastrointestinal distress with vomiting, is agitated and hyperreflexic, and is hypotensive.

8. Regarding the management of this patient, which one of the following interventions is LEAST likely to be employed?
   (A) Activated charcoal orally
   (B) Hemoperfusion
   (C) Intravenous normal saline
   (D) Ipecac extract
   (E) Whole bowel irrigation

9. The plasma level of theophylline is measured immediately upon hospitalization of this patient. The peak plasma level is 80 mg/L. If the oral bioavailability of theophylline is 98%, the clearance is 50 mL/min, volume of distribution is 35 L, and the elimination half-life is 7.5 hours, the amount ingested must have been at least
   (A) 0.3 g
   (B) 0.6 g
   (C) 1.6 g
   (D) 2.8 g
   (E) 8.0 g

10. Intoxicants correctly associated with their effects include
   (A) All of the following
   (B) Carbon monoxide: Carboxyhemoglobinemia
   (C) Cyanide: Cytochrome oxidase inactivation
   (D) Paraquat: Pulmonary fibrosis
   (E) Sodium nitrite: Methemoglobinemia

DIRECTIONS (Items 11–16): Each set of matching questions in this section consists of a list of three to twenty-six lettered options (some of which may be figures) followed by several numbered items. For each numbered item, select the ONE lettered option that is most closely associated with it. Each lettered option may be selected once, more than once, or not at all.
   (A) Acetaminophen
   (B) Aspirin
   (C) Benzene
   (D) Carbon monoxide
   (E) Heroin
   (F) Hydrogen sulfide
   (G) Iron
   (H) Malathion
   (I) Methanol
   (J) Paraquat
   (K) Sodium cyanide
   (L) Theophylline
   (M) Triazolam

11. The best antidote for overdose of this substance is atropine
12. The most likely drug to be needed in an overdose due to this substance is an anticonvulsant, but beta-blockers are appropriate when cardiac arrhythmias are present
13. Acetylcysteine should be administered to a patient who overdoses on this drug
14. The ingestion of this chemical is best managed by intravenous ethanol
15. The standard antidote for this substance is sodium nitrite followed by sodium thiosulfate
16. Intravenous flumazenil will reverse the effects of this drug in overdose

ANSWERS

1. Anion gap is calculated by subtracting measured serum anions (bicarbonate plus chloride) from cations (potassium plus sodium). Increases in anion gap above normal are due to the presence of unmeasured anions that accompany acidosis. The gap in this case (38 meq/L) is well in excess of the normal gap (12–16 meq/L). The answer is **(C)**.

2. The ingestion of ethylene glycol (antifreeze), iron tablets, monoamine oxidase inhibitors used for depressive disorders (eg, phenelzine), or verapamil can result in metabolic acidosis, with an increase in anion gap. The answer is **(E)**.

3. Aspirin, sympathomimetics, agents with muscarinic blocking actions, and drugs that cause muscle rigidity or seizures are all likely to cause hyperthermia at toxic doses. Hypothermia is more typical of overdoses with opioids or sedative-hypnotics. The answer is **(C)**.

4. Food-borne botulism (due to *C botulinum*) may lead to a symmetric descending paralysis that results in respiratory failure. Patients are initially alert but may suffer from dysarthria and dysphagia. Ptosis and ophthalmoplegia are also characteristic symptoms. The answer is **(D)**.

5. Digoxin is lethal at levels much too low to be detected by the osmolar gap method. This method is useful only for poisoning with low-potency substances of low molecular weight, eg, methanol and ethylene glycol. The answer is **(A)**.

6. Estimations of the time required for drug or toxin elimination may be of value in the management of the poisoned patient. If no procedures were used to hasten the elimination of digitoxin in this patient, the time taken to reach a safe plasma level of the drug (25% of the measured level) is two half-lives, or approximately 2 weeks. The answer is **(C)**.

7. Only about 20% of rattlesnake bites involve significant envenomation. Incision, suction, and tourniquets are usually more damaging than helpful. Ice packs are contraindicated. Serious envenomation causes primarily local tissue damage. Antivenin is by far the most effective therapy for serious envenomation. The answer is **(D)**.

8. Activated charcoal is effective in decreasing theophylline absorption from the gastrointestinal tract, and whole bowel irrigation is especially useful for decontamination of orally administered sustained-release formulations of the drug. Hypotension is often managed by saline infusion, though vasopressors may be required. The blood levels of theophylline are decreased by charcoal hemoperfusion or by hemodialysis. Ipecac *extract* contains cardiotoxic alkaloids and should never be used as an emetic. The answer is **(D)**.

9. Estimations of the quantity of a drug or toxin ingested may be of value in management of the poisoned patient. Applying toxicokinetic principles, a rough estimate of the ingested dose of theophylline could be made by multiplying the peak plasma level of the drug (80 mg/L) by its volume of distribution (35 L) to give a value of 2800 mg or 2.8 g. Because only about one-fourth of a half-life has passed since ingestion, the amount eliminated since that time will be rather small. The answer is **(D)**.

10. All are correct. The answer is **(A)**.

11. Atropine is the primary antidote for poisoning due to inhibitors of acetylcholinesterase, including carbamate and organophosphate insecticides (eg, malathion). Pralidoxime may be administered to regenerate the enzyme. The answer is **(H)**.

12. The most dangerous toxic effect of theophylline is convulsions. The cardiovascular toxicity of theophylline (eg, arrhythmias) often responds to beta-blockers. The answer is **(L)**.

13. Hepatotoxicity due to overdose of acetaminophen (more likely in alcoholic patients) is due to the formation of a toxic metabolite. Early administration of acetylcysteine can be protective. The answer is **(A)**.

14. Ethanol competes with methanol for alcohol dehydrogenase, preventing its conversion to the toxic compounds formaldehyde and formic acid. The answer is **(I)**.

15. Mitochondrial cytochrome oxidase is inactivated by the binding of cyanide to the iron in heme. Sodium nitrite converts hemoglobin to methemoglobin, which competes effectively for the cyanide ion to form cyanmethemoglobin. Administration of sodium thiosulfate releases methemoglobin with the formation of thiocyanate. The answer is **(K)**.

16. Flumazenil displaces benzodiazepines from their binding sites on the GABA receptor-chloride ion channel macromolecular complex in neural membranes. The answer is **(M)**.

60

Drugs Used
in Gastrointestinal Disorders

OBJECTIVES

You should be able to:

- Name five different drug groups used in the treatment of peptic ulcer and describe their mechanisms.
- Name four drugs used in the prevention of chemotherapy-induced vomiting.
- Name three laxative drugs and describe their mechanisms.
- Name the two most important antidiarrheal drugs.

CONCEPTS

The gastrointestinal tract serves several functions: digestive, excretory, endocrine, exocrine, etc. These functions provide numerous important drug targets, and many of the drugs used in gastrointestinal disease have been discussed in earlier chapters of this book. However, several important drugs used in common gastrointestinal diseases are not members of the drug groups discussed earlier. These drugs are described in this chapter.

A. **Drugs Used in Acid-Peptic Disease:** Ulceration and erosion of the lining of the GI tract are common problems, and several drug groups used in these diseases have been discussed in previous chapters (H_2 blockers, antimuscarinic drugs, misoprostol). Other drugs used in peptic disease include the antacids, sucralfate, omeprazole, and antibiotics. Figure 60–1 summarizes the actions of these drugs.
  1. **Antacids:** Antacids are simple physical agents that react with protons in the lumen of the gut. Some antacids (eg, aluminum-containing antacids) may also stimulate the protective functions of the gastric mucosa. The antacids effectively reduce the recurrence rate of peptic ulcers when used regularly in doses that significantly raise the stomach pH.

     The antacids differ mainly in their absorption and effects on stool consistency. The most popular antacids in use in the USA are **magnesium hydroxide** ($Mg[OH]_2$) and **aluminum hydroxide** ($Al[OH]_3$). Neither of these weak bases is absorbed from the bowel. Magnesium hydroxide has strong laxative effects, while aluminum hydroxide has constipating actions. These drugs are available as single-ingredient products and as combined preparations. Calcium carbonate and sodium bicarbonate are also weak bases, but they differ from aluminum and magnesium hydroxides in being absorbed from the gut. Because of their systemic effects, calcium and bicarbonate salts are less popular as antacids than the magnesium and aluminum compounds listed.
  2. **Sucralfate:** Sucralfate is aluminum sucrose sulfate, a small, poorly soluble molecule that polymerizes in the acid environment of the stomach. This polymer binds to injured tissue and forms a protective coating over ulcer beds. The drug has been shown to accelerate the healing of peptic ulcers and to reduce the recurrence rate. Sucralfate is too insoluble to have significant systemic effects when taken by the oral route.
  3. **Omeprazole:** Omeprazole is the prototype of a class of inhibitors of the proton pump of gastric parietal cells. This pump, an H^+/K^+ ATPase located in the luminal membrane of parietal cells, binds omeprazole irreversibly; inhibition of acid secretion persists for 48

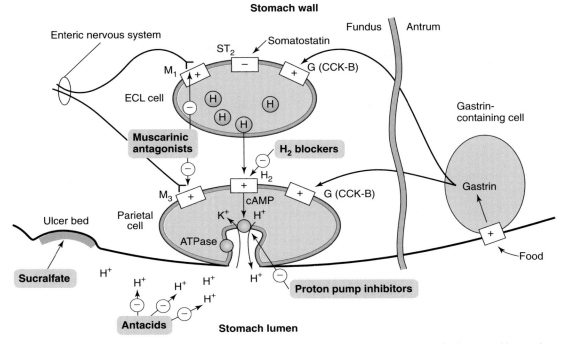

Figure 60–1. Sites of action of some drugs used in peptic ulcer disease. The site of action of misoprostol is not shown; it is thought to reduce acid secretion and increase secretion of protective factors such as mucus and bicarbonate. ECL cell, enterochromaffin-like cell; G(CCK-B), gastrin-cholecystokinin-B receptor; H, histamine; H_2, histamine H_2 receptor; M_1, M_3, muscarinic receptors; ST_2, somatostatin$_2$ receptor; ATPase, K^+/H^+ ATPase proton pump. (Modified and reproduced, with permission, from Katzung BG [editor]: *Basic & Clinical Pharmacology,* 7th ed. Appleton & Lange, 1998.)

hours or longer. Omeprazole is particularly useful in the treatment of Zollinger-Ellison syndrome (usually associated with a gastrin-secreting tumor) and gastroesophageal reflux, conditions in which the H_2 blockers are not completely satisfactory.

4. **Antibiotics:** Chronic infection with *Helicobacter pylori* occurs in a large proportion of patients with recurrent peptic ulcers, and eradication of this organism reduces the rate of recurrence of ulcer. The antibiotic regimens of choice consist of a course of bismuth (Pepto-Bismol), tetracycline, and metronidazole or a course of amoxicillin plus clarithromycin. Omeprazole should accompany either antibiotic regimen.

B. **Drugs That Promote Upper GI Motility:** Diabetes and other diseases that damage nerves to the viscera frequently cause a marked loss of motility in the esophagus and stomach (gastric paralysis or gastroparesis). This loss of motility is often associated with delayed emptying, nausea, and severe bloating. **Metoclopramide** and **cisapride** are able to stimulate motility in this condition, probably by acting as acetylcholine facilitators or as dopamine receptor antagonists in the enteric nervous system. This "prokinetic" action is also of some value in preventing emesis from surgical anesthesia and emesis induced by cancer chemotherapeutic drugs. Adverse effects include induction of parkinsonism and other extrapyramidal effects.

C. **Drugs With Antiemetic Actions:** A variety of drugs have been found to be of some value in the prevention and treatment of vomiting, especially cancer chemotherapy-induced vomiting. In addition to **metoclopramide** and **cisapride,** useful antiemetic drugs include the following: **dexamethasone,** some H_1 **antihistamines,** several **phenothiazines,** the 5-HT$_3$ inhibitors (eg, **ondansetron**), and **dronabinol,** the active ingredient in marijuana. The 5-HT$_3$ inhibitors, ondansetron and granisetron, are extremely useful in preventing nausea and vomiting in patients receiving cancer chemotherapy.

D. **Pancreatic Enzyme Replacements:** Steatorrhea, a condition of decreased fat absorption coupled with an increase in stool fat excretion, results from inadequate pancreatic secretion of li-

Table 60–1. The major laxative mechanisms and some representative laxative drugs.

Mechanism	Examples
Irritant	Castor oil, cascara, senna, phenolphthalein
Bulk-forming	Saline cathartics (eg, Mg[OH]$_2$), psyllium
Stool-softening	Dioctyl sodium sulfosuccinate (docusate)
Lubricating	Mineral oil, glycerin

pase. The abnormality of fat absorption can be significantly relieved by oral administration of pancreatic lipase (**pancrelipase**) obtained from pigs. Pancreatic lipase is inactivated at a pH below 4.0; thus, up to 90% of an administered dose will be destroyed in the stomach, unless the pH is raised with antacids or drugs that reduce acid secretion.

E. Laxatives: Laxatives increase the probability of a bowel movement by several mechanisms: an irritant or stimulant action on the bowel wall; a bulk-forming action on the stool that evokes reflex contraction of the bowel; a softening action on hard or impacted stool; and a lubricating action that eases passage of stool through the rectum and anus. Examples of drugs that act by these mechanisms are set forth in Table 60–1.

F. Antidiarrheal Agents: The most effective antidiarrheal drugs are the opioids and derivatives of opioids that have been selected for maximal antidiarrheal and minimal CNS effect. Of the latter group, the most important are **diphenoxylate** and **loperamide,** meperidine analogs with very weak analgesic effects. Diphenoxylate is formulated with atropine to reduce the already minimal likelihood of abuse; loperamide is formulated alone and sold as such.

QUESTIONS

DIRECTIONS: Each numbered item or incomplete statement in this section is followed by answers or by completions of the statement. Select the ONE lettered answer or completion that is BEST in each case.

1. A 55-year-old woman with insulin-dependent diabetes of 40 years' duration complains of severe bloating and abdominal distress, especially after meals. Evaluation is consistent with diabetic gastroparesis. The drug you would be most likely to recommend is
   (A) Docusate
   (B) Dopamine
   (C) Loperamide
   (D) Metoclopramide
   (E) Sucralfate

2. A patient who must take verapamil for hypertension and angina has become severely constipated. Which of the following drugs would be most suitable as a cathartic?
   (A) Aluminum hydroxide
   (B) Diphenoxylate
   (C) Magnesium hydroxide
   (D) Metoclopramide
   (E) Mineral oil

3. Your cousin is planning a 3-week trip overseas and asks your advice regarding medications for traveler's diarrhea. A drug suitable for noninfectious diarrhea is
   (A) Aluminum hydroxide
   (B) Diphenoxylate
   (C) Magnesium hydroxide
   (D) Metoclopramide
   (E) Mineral oil

4. Which of the following drugs or drug groups is NOT useful in the prevention of nausea and vomiting induced by cancer chemotherapy:
   (A) Dexamethasone
   (B) Dronabinol
   (C) Ketanserin
   (D) Ondansetron
   (E) Phenothiazines

DIRECTIONS (Items 5–10): The following section consists of a list of three to twenty-six lettered options followed by several numbered items. For each numbered item, select the ONE option that is most closely associated with it. Each answer may be selected once, more than once, or not at all.
   (A) Aluminum hydroxide
   (B) Castor oil
   (C) Dexamethasone
   (D) Diphenoxylate
   (E) Loperamide
   (F) Magnesium hydroxide
   (G) Metoclopramide
   (H) Metronidazole
   (I) Mineral oil
   (J) Omeprazole
   (K) Ondansetron
   (L) Sucralfate

5. A drug that irreversibly inhibits the H^+/K^+ ATPase in gastric parietal cells
6. A drug with antacid and laxative properties
7. An antidiarrheal drug related to meperidine; it is formulated without any admixed drug
8. An antibiotic used in the treatment of recurrent peptic ulcer
9. A glucocorticoid used in preventing chemotherapy-induced vomiting
10. A lubricating laxative; not very effective if bowel tone is severely reduced or absent

ANSWERS

1. Of the drugs listed, only metoclopramide is considered a prokinetic agent, ie, one that increases propulsive motility in the gut. The answer is **(D)**.
2. A cathartic that mildly stimulates the gut would be most suitable in a patient taking a smooth muscle relaxant drug such as verapamil. Magnesium hydroxide, by holding water in the intestine, provides additional bulk and stimulates increased contractions. The answer is **(C)**.
3. Diphenoxylate and loperamide are the traditional drugs used for traveler's diarrhea. Diphenoxylate requires a prescription in the USA but is much less expensive than loperamide. The answer is **(B)**.
4. Ketanserin is an inhibitor of 5-HT$_2$ receptors (Chapter 16) and has no antiemetic action. All of the other drugs listed are useful in preventing chemotherapy-induced nausea and vomiting. The answer is **(C)**.
5. Omeprazole irreversibly inhibits the proton pump. The answer is **(J)**.
6. Magnesium hydroxide has both antacid and laxative effects. The answer is **(F)**.
7. Loperamide is formulated alone; diphenoxylate is mixed with atropine alkaloids. The answer is **(E)**.
8. Metronidazole is part of the antibiotic therapy used to eradicate *H pylori*. The answer is **(H)**.
9. Dexamethasone is a useful antiemetic in cancer chemotherapy. The answer is **(C)**.
10. Mineral oil is a lubricant. It has no irritant or bulk-forming properties. The answer is **(I)**.

61

Drug Interactions

OBJECTIVES

You should be able to:

- Describe the primary pharmacokinetic mechanisms that underlie drug interactions.
- Describe how the pharmacodynamic characteristics of different drugs administered concomitantly may lead to additive, synergistic, or antagonistic effects.
- Identify specific drug interactions that occur commonly in clinical practice.

Learn the definitions that follow.

Table 61–1. Definitions.

Term	Definition
Pharmacokinetic interaction	A change in the pharmacokinetics of one drug caused by the interacting drug, eg, an inducer of hepatic enzymes
Pharmacodynamic interaction	A change in the pharmacodynamics of one drug caused by the interacting drug, eg, additive action of two drugs having similar effects
Addition	The effect of two drugs given together is equal to the sum of the responses to the same doses given separately
Antagonism	The effect of two drugs given together is less than the sum of the responses to the same doses given separately

CONCEPTS

"Drug interactions" are actions of a drug in the body that are the result of another drug or affect the actions of another drug. Such actions are usually quantitative—ie, an increase or a decrease in the magnitude of an expected response. Drug interactions may be the result of pharmacokinetic alterations, pharmacodynamic changes, or a combination of both. Interactions between drugs in vitro (eg, precipitation when mixed in solutions for intravenous administration) are usually classified as **drug incompatibilities.**

Although hundreds of drug interactions have been documented, only a few are of clinical significance and constitute a contraindication to simultaneous use or require a change in dosage. Some of these are listed in Table 61–2. In patients taking many drugs, however, the likelihood of significant drug interactions is increased. This is especially true in elderly patients, who often have age-related changes in drug clearance.

PHARMACOKINETIC INTERACTIONS

A. Interactions Based on Absorption: Absorption from the gastrointestinal tract may be influenced by agents that bind drugs (eg, resins, antacids, calcium-containing foods) and by agents that increase or decrease gastrointestinal motility (eg, metoclopramide or antimuscarinics, respectively). Problems caused by slowed gastric emptying may be unexpected because the antimuscarinic action of a particular agent is often not a desired one but an unwanted side effect. Concomitant use of antacids has resulted in decreased gut absorption of digoxin, ketoconazole, quinolone antibiotics, and tetracyclines. On the other hand, erythromycin appears to increase oral bioavailability of digoxin in some patients, probably by reducing gut flora that degrades digoxin. Absorption from subcutaneous sites may be slowed predictably by vasoconstrictors given simultaneously (eg, local anesthetics and epinephrine) and by cardiac depressants that decrease tissue perfusion (eg, beta-blockers).

Table 61–2. Some important drug interactions.

Drug Causing the Interaction	Drugs Affected	Comment
Alcohol	Sedative-hypnotics, opioid analgesics, tricyclic antidepressants, antihistamines	Additive CNS depression, sedation, ataxia, increased risk of accidents
Aminoglycosides	Loop diuretics	Enhanced ototoxicity
Antacids	Iron supplements, fluoroquinolones, ketoconazole, tetracyclines	Decreased gut absorption due either to reaction with the drug affected or to reduced gut acidity
Antibiotics	Estrogens, including oral contraceptives	Many antibiotics lower estrogen levels and reduce contraceptive effectiveness
Antihistamines (H$_1$ blockers)	Antimuscarinics, sedatives	Additive effects with the drugs affected
Antimuscarinic drugs	Drugs absorbed from the small intestine	Slowed onset of effect because stomach emptying is delayed
Barbiturates, especially phenobarbital	Azoles, calcium channel blockers, propranolol, quinidine, corticosteroids, warfarin, and many other drugs metabolized in the liver	Increased clearance of the affected drugs due to enzyme induction, possibly leading to decreases in drug effectiveness
Beta-blockers	Insulin	Masking of symptoms of hypoglycemia
	Prazosin	Increased "first-dose" syncope
Bile acid-binding resins	Acetaminophen, digitalis, thiazides, thyroxine	Reduced absorption of the affected drug
Carbamazepine	Doxycycline, estrogen, haloperidol, theophylline, warfarin	Reduced effect because of induction of metabolism
Cimetidine	Benzodiazepines, lidocaine, phenytoin, quinidine, theophylline, warfarin	Increased effect due to inhibition of hepatic metabolism
Disulfiram, metronidazole, certain cephalosporins	Ethanol	Increased hangover effect of ethanol because aldehyde dehydrogenase is blocked
Erythromycin	Astemizole, cisapride, terfenadine, theophylline	Risk of toxicity due to inhibition of metabolism of these drugs
Ketoconazole	Astemizole, cisapride, terfenadine	Risk of cardiac arrhythmia due to inhibition of metabolism of these drugs
	Cyclosporine, lovastatin, warfarin	Decreased clearance due to inhibition of hepatic metabolism
MAO inhibitors	Catecholamine releasers (amphetamine, ephedrine)	Increased norepinephrine in sympathetic nerve endings released by the interacting drugs
	Tyramine-containing foods and beverages	Hypertensive crisis
Nonsteriodal anti-inflammatory drugs	Anticoagulants	Increased bleeding tendency because of reduced platelet aggregation
	ACE inhibitors	Decreased efficacy of ACE inhibitor
	Furosemide	Reduced diuretic efficacy
Phenytoin	Doxycycline, methadone, quinidine, steroids, verapamil	Increased metabolism due to enzyme induction
Quinidine	Digoxin	Increased digoxin levels due to decreased clearance; displacement may play a role
Rifampin	Azole antifungal drugs, corticosteroids, methadone, theophylline, tolbutamide	Decreased efficacy of these drugs due to induction of hepatic P450 isozymes
Salicylates	Corticosteroids	Additive toxicity to gastric mucosa
	Heparin, warfarin	Increased bleeding tendency
	Methotrexate	Decreased clearance causing greater methotrexate toxicity
	Sulfinpyrazone	Decreased uricosuric effect

(continued)

Table 61–2. Some important drug interactions (continued).

Drug Causing the Interaction	Drugs Affected	Comment
Selective serotonin reuptake inhibitors	MAO inhibitors	"Serotonin syndrome"—hypertension, tachycardia, muscle rigidity, hyperthermia, seizures
Thiazides	Digitalis	Increased risk of digitalis toxicity because thiazides diminish potassium stores
	Lithium	Increased plasma levels of lithium due to decreased total body water
Warfarin	Cimetidine, erythromycin, lovastatin, metronidazole	Increased anticoagulant effect via inhibition of warfarin metabolism
	Anabolic steroids, aspirin, NSAIDs, quinidine, thyroxine	Increased anticoagulant effects via pharmacodynamic mechanisms
	Barbiturates, carbamazepine, phenytoin, rifampin	Decreased anticoagulant effects due to increased clearance of warfarin via induction of hepatic P450 isozymes

B. **Interactions Based on Distribution and Binding:** Distribution of a drug may be altered by other drugs that compete for binding sites on plasma proteins. For example, antibacterial sulfonamides can displace methotrexate, phenytoin, sulfonylureas, and warfarin from binding sites on albumin. However, it is difficult to document many clinically significant interactions of this type, and they seem to be the exception rather than the rule. The ability of quinidine to raise the blood levels of digoxin was originally attributed to displacement from tissue binding sites but probably involves a reduction in the clearance of digoxin. Changes in drug distribution can occur if one agent alters the size of the physical compartment in which another drug is distributed. For example, diuretics, by reducing total body water, can increase plasma levels of aminoglycosides and of lithium, possibly enhancing drug toxicities.

C. **Interactions Based on Metabolic Clearance:** Interactions of this type have well-documented clinical significance. The metabolism of many drugs can be increased by other agents that induce hepatic drug-metabolizing enzymes, especially cytochrome P450 isozymes. Induction of drug-metabolizing enzymes occurs predictably with the chronic administration of **barbiturates, carbamazepine, ethanol, phenytoin,** or **rifampin.** Conversely, the metabolism of some drugs may be decreased by other drugs that inhibit drug-metabolizing enzymes. Such inhibitors of drug-metabolizing enzymes include **cimetidine, disulfiram, erythromycin, ketoconazole, propoxyphene, quinidine,** and **sulfonamides.** The CYP3A4 isozyme of cytochrome P450—the dominant form in the human liver—is particularly sensitive to such inhibitory actions.

Drugs that reduce hepatic blood flow, eg, **propranolol,** may also reduce the clearance of other drugs metabolized in the liver, eg, theophylline.

A modified form of an interaction based on metabolic clearance results from the ability of some drugs to increase the stores of endogenous substances by blocking their metabolism. These endogenous drugs may subsequently be released by other exogenous drugs, resulting in an unexpected action. The best-documented reaction of this type is the sensitization of patients taking **MAO inhibitors** to indirectly acting sympathomimetics (amphetamine, phenylpropanolamine, etc). Such patients may suffer a severe hypertensive reaction in response to ordinary doses of cold remedies, decongestants, and appetite suppressants.

D. **Interactions Based on Renal Function:** Excretion of drugs by the kidney may be changed by drugs that reduce renal blood flow (eg, beta-blockers) or inhibit specific renal transport mechanisms (eg, the action of aspirin on uric acid secretion in the S_2 segment of the proximal tubule). Drugs that alter urinary pH may change the ionization state of drugs that are weak acids or weak bases, leading to changes in renal tubular reabsorption.

PHARMACODYNAMIC INTERACTIONS

A.   Interactions Based on Opposing Actions or Effects: Antagonism, the simplest type of drug interaction, is often predictable. For example, antagonism of the bronchodilating effects of beta$_2$-adrenoceptor activators used in asthma is to be anticipated if a beta-blocker is given for another condition. Likewise, the action of a catecholamine on heart rate (via beta-adrenoceptor activation) is antagonized by an inhibitor of acetylcholinesterase that acts through acetylcholine (via muscarinic receptors). Antagonism by mixed agonist-antagonist drugs (eg, pentazocine) or by partial agonists (eg, pindolol) are not as easily predicted but should be expected when such drugs are used with pure agonists. Some drug antagonisms do not appear to be based on receptor interactions. For example, nonsteroidal anti-inflammatory drugs may decrease the antihypertensive action of ACE inhibitors by reducing renal elimination of sodium.

B.   Interactions Based on Additive Effects: Additive interaction is the result of arithmetic summing of the effects of two drugs. The two drugs may or may not act on the same receptor to produce such effects. The combined use of tricyclic antidepressants with diphenhydramine or promethazine is predicted to cause excessive atropine-like effects since each of these drugs has marked muscarinic receptor-blocking actions. Tricyclic antidepressants may increase the pressor responses to sympathomimetics by interference with amine transporter systems.

One of the most common drug interactions in medicine is the additive depression of central nervous system function caused by concomitant administration of sedatives, hypnotics, and opioids with each other or with the consumption of ethanol. In such cases, multiple receptor systems in the brain are presumed to be involved. The patient with moderate to severe hypertension maintained on several drugs with different sites of action to lower blood pressure is at risk for excessive actions of such agents. Additive effects of anticoagulant drugs can lead to bleeding complications. In the case of warfarin, the potential for such adverse effects is enhanced by aspirin (via an antiplatelet action), quinidine (additive hypoprothrombinemia), thrombolytics (via plasminogen activation), and the thyroid hormones (via enhanced clotting factor catabolism).

QUESTIONS

DIRECTIONS: Each of the numbered items or incomplete statements in this section is followed by answers or by completions of the statement. Select the ONE lettered answer or completion that is BEST in each case.

1.   Which one of the following drugs enhances digitalis toxicity by pharmacokinetic mechanisms?
   (A) Captopril
   (B) Hydrochlorothiazide
   (C) Lidocaine
   (D) Quinidine
   (E) Sulfasalazine

2.   Thiazides are known to reduce the excretion of
   (A) Diazepam
   (B) Fluoxetine
   (C) Imipramine
   (D) Lithium
   (E) Potassium

3.   A hypertensive patient has been using nifedipine for some time without untoward effects. If he experiences a rapidly developing enhancement of the antihypertensive effect of the drug, it is probably due to
   (A) Concomitant use of antacids
   (B) Foods containing tyramine
   (C) Grapefruit juice
   (D) Induction of drug metabolism
   (E) Over-the-counter decongestants

4.   Which one of the following agents is LEAST likely to enhance the anticoagulant effects of warfarin?
   (A) Aspirin

     (B)   Cholestyramine
     (C)   Cimetidine
     (D)   Quinidine
     (E)   Thyroxine

5. Patients should be cautioned not to consume alcoholic beverages when given a prescription for any of the following drugs EXCEPT
     (A)   Cefixime
     (B)   Chloral hydrate
     (C)   Chlorpropamide
     (D)   Glipizide
     (E)   Metronidazole

6. A patient suffering from a depressive disorder is being treated with imipramine. If he uses diphenhydramine for allergic rhinitis, a drug interaction is likely to occur because
     (A)   Diphenhydramine inhibits imipramine metabolism
     (B)   Both drugs block reuptake of norepinephrine released from sympathetic nerve endings
     (C)   Imipramine inhibits the metabolism of diphenhydramine
     (D)   Both drugs block muscarinic receptors
     (E)   The drugs compete with each other for renal elimination

7. If tranylcypromine is administered to a patient taking fluoxetine, the most likely result is
     (A)   Antagonism of the antidepressant action of fluoxetine
     (B)   Decrease in the plasma levels of fluoxetine
     (C)   Hypertensive crisis
     (D)   Priapism
     (E)   Agitation, muscle rigidity, hyperthermia, seizures

8. Following organ transplantation, a patient is being maintained on cyclosporine. Which one of the following drugs is LEAST likely to enhance the nephrotoxicity of cyclosporine?
     (A)   Carbamazepine
     (B)   Diltiazem
     (C)   Gentamicin
     (D)   Ketoconazole
     (E)   Verapamil

DIRECTIONS (Items 9–14):   The following section consists of a list of three to twenty-six lettered options (some of which may be figures) followed by several numbered items. For each numbered item, select the ONE option that is most closely associated with it. Each answer may be selected once, more than once, or not at all.

     (A)   Allopurinol
     (B)   Astemizole
     (C)   Carbamazepine
     (D)   Cholestyramine
     (E)   Cimetidine
     (F)   Cyclosporine
     (G)   Digoxin
     (H)   Erythromycin
     (I)   Ethinyl estradiol
     (J)   Lithium
     (K)   Phenelzine
     (L)   Rifampin
     (M)   Sodium salicylate
     (N)   Tetracycline
     (O)   Theophylline
     (P)   Warfarin

9. This antibiotic is a potent inducer of hepatic drug-metabolizing enzymes

10. This drug interferes with the antihypertensive action of captopril and enalapril

11. This drug has no effect on platelets but increases the likelihood of bleeding in patients who are also taking aspirin

12. This drug increases the hematotoxicity of azathioprine

13. A meal with a high content of fermented foods would be dangerous in a person taking this drug

14. This drug is capable of blocking potassium channels in cardiac cell membranes; inhibition of its metabolism has led to cardiac arrhythmias

ANSWERS

1. Quinidine and thiazide diuretics both enhance the toxicity of digitalis. The action of quinidine is attributed to pharmacokinetic mechanisms, including competition with digoxin for tissue-binding sites and inhibition of its clearance. The enhancement of digitalis toxicity by thiazides is a pharmacodynamic mechanism resulting from the action of these diuretics to reduce extracellular potassium. Sulfasalazine decreases plasma levels of digitalis by interfering with gut absorption of the drug. The answer is **(D)**.

2. Thiazides reduce the clearance of lithium by about 25%. They do not alter the clearance of the other agents mentioned except for potassium, the clearance of which is increased. The answer is **(D)**.

3. Naringenin in grapefruit juice can increase the rate and extent of bioavailability of several dihydropyridine calcium channel blockers, including felodipine and nifedipine. This interaction may be due to inhibition of the presystemic (first-pass) metabolism of the dihydropyridines. The answer is **(C)**.

4. Cholestyramine interferes with the oral absorption of many drugs (including warfarin), resulting in decreased effectiveness. Aspirin and thyroid hormones enhance the action of warfarin via pharmacodynamic mechanisms. Increased anticoagulant effects with cimetidine or quinidine result from the inhibition of metabolism of warfarin. The answer is **(B)**.

5. Only a few cephalosporins (eg, cefoperazone, cefotetan, moxalactam) cause disulfiram-like reactions with ethanol. Sulfonylureas used in type II diabetes may cause such reactions, and ethanol may enhance their hypoglycemic actions, especially in fasting patients. The answer is **(A)**.

6. This is a good example of an additive drug interaction resulting from two drugs acting on the same type of receptor. Most tricyclic antidepressants, phenothiazines, and older antihistaminic drugs (those available without prescription) are blockers of muscarinic receptors. Used concomitantly, any pair of these drugs will predictably increase atropine-like adverse effects. The answer is **(D)**.

7. The drug interaction between the inhibitors of monoamine oxidase used for depression and the drugs that selectively block serotonin reuptake (SSRIs) is called the "serotonin syndrome." Key interventions include control of hyperthermia and seizures. The answer is **(E)**.

8. Concomitant use of nephrotoxic drugs (eg, aminoglycosides, amphotericin B, vancomycin) with cyclosporine leads to enhanced nephrotoxicity. Diltiazem, ketoconazole, and verapamil inhibit the metabolism of cyclosporine, enhancing its toxic effects unless the dosage is reduced. Carbamazepine induces cytochrome P450 and reduces both the therapeutic and the toxic effects of the immunosuppressant drug. The answer is **(A)**.

9. Rifampin is an effective inducer of hepatic P450 isozymes. Cyclosporine and tetracycline, the other antibiotics listed, have no such effect. The answer is **(L)**.

10. Salicylates and other NSAIDs may interfere with the antihypertensive action of angiotensin-converting enzyme inhibitors. The answer is **(M)**.

11. Warfarin, the oral anticoagulant, reduces the synthesis of prothrombin and several other clotting factors. An interaction occurs with antiplatelet drugs such as aspirin. The answer is **(P)**.

12. Azathioprine is converted to 6-mercaptopurine, which is responsible for both its immunosuppressant action and its hematotoxicity. Allopurinol inhibits xanthine oxidase, the enzyme that metabolizes 6-mercaptopurine. The answer is **(A)**.

13. Monoamine oxidase inhibitors used in depressive disorders (phenelzine, isocarboxazid, tranylcypromine) increase the stores of norepinephrine in sympathetic nerve endings. They also inhibit the metabolism of tyramine, which at high levels in the blood can act as an indirect sympathomimetic to release norepinephrine. The answer is **(K)**.

14. Astemizole is metabolized by a cytochrome P450 isozyme that is inhibited by erythromycin and by ketoconazole. Decreased clearance of the antihistaminic drug may result in cardiotoxicity. The answer is **(B)**.

62

Vaccines, Immune Globulins, & Other Complex Biologic Products

OBJECTIVES

You should be able to:

- Describe the principles of active and passive immunization, and know the differences between them.
- List the types of materials available for passive immunization and the special uses of immune globulin.
- List the types of materials available for active immunization and describe the relative merits and disadvantages of live versus dead immunogens.
- List the vaccines recommended for the active immunization of children.

CONCEPTS

A. Passive Immunization: In passive immunization, **preformed antibodies** of human or animal origin are used to transfer immunity to the host. Such materials, usually **immunoglobulins,** may contain high titers of specific or relatively nonspecific antibodies (eg, **immune globulin; IG**). Their clinical uses include prevention or amelioration of diseases after exposure (eg, hepatitis, measles, poliomyelitis), treatment of certain snake and insect bites, and management of hypogammaglobulinemias. The most commonly used preparation is IG, a 25-fold concentration of gamma globulins (95% IgG) from human plasma, available in formulations for intramuscular and intravenous use. The biologic half-life of IG is about 23 days, and hypersensitivity reactions are rare. IG is used for passive immunization to hepatitis A, measles, poliomyelitis, and rubella and for hypogammaglobulinemia and idiopathic thrombocytopenic purpura (ITP). More specific products include diphtheria antitoxin, snake and spider antivenins, $Rh_o(D)$ immune globulin, and immune globulins for hepatitis B, pertussis, rabies, tetanus, vaccinia, and varicella. Such antibodies usually have a half-life of only 5–7 days. Because animal antibodies can act as antigens in humans, allergic reactions to antibodies from nonhuman sources are more common and severe than those from human sources. Examples of materials used in passive immunization are shown in Table 62–1.

B. Active Immunization: In active immunization, **antigens** are used to stimulate antibody formation and host cell-mediated immunity, giving protection against disease vectors. The major advantage of active over passive immunization is that it confers stronger host resistance by stimulating higher antibody levels. Immunization can be produced by live (attenuated) or dead (inactivated) immunogens. Live attenuated products stimulate natural resistance and confer longer-lasting immunity than dead immunogens; however, the risk of disease is greater. Examples of the use of live attenuated immunogens include the vaccines for measles, mumps, rubella, and poliovirus. Materials utilizing dead immunogehs include diphtheria and tetanus toxoids, rabies vaccine, and both hepatitis A and B viruses. *Haemophilus influenzae,* type b conjugate (Hib-conjugate), derived from a bacterial polysaccharide, is used in children and in selected high-risk persons. Similar polysaccharide vaccines are also available for active immunization of individuals at high risk of infection from meningococci and pneumococci. Selected examples of products used in active immunization are shown in Table 62–2.

C. Active Immunization of Children: Recommended schedules for active immunization of children are presented in Table 62–3. They include hepatitis B vaccine, DTP (toxoids of diphtheria and tetanus with pertussis antigen), Hib-conjugate vaccine, oral poliovaccine, and MMR (measles, mumps, and rubella) vaccines.

Table 62–1. Materials used for passive immunization.*

Indication	Product	Comments
Black widow spider (BWS) bite	BWS antivenin (equine)	Treatment; use only in children less than 15 kg
Botulism	ABE polyvalent antitoxin (equine)	Treatment
Hepatitis A (infectious)	Immune globulin (ISG)	Prophylaxis; postexposure and chronic exposure
Hepatitis B (serum)	Hepatitis B immune globulin (HBIG)	Prophylaxis; postexposure
Hepatitis E (formerly non-A, non-B)	Immune globulin (ISG)	Prophylaxis
Hypogammaglobulinemia	Immune globulin (ISG)	Treatment
Organ transplant	Lymphocyte immune globulin (equine)	Adjunctive immunosuppressant
Rabies	Rabies immune globulin (equine)	Give as soon as possible; also need rabies vaccine
Rh isoimmunization	$Rh_o(D)$ immune globulin	To suppress formation of anti-$Rh_o(D)$ in $Rh_o(D)$-negative, D^u-negative women exposed to Rh-positive blood during delivery
Snakebite	Coral snake antivenin; crotalid antivenin (equine)	Treatment; also need antitetanus therapy
Tetanus	Tetanus immune globulin	Only for major or contaminated wounds
Vaccinia	Vaccinia immune globulin	Treatment; generalized, ocular, skin infections
Varicella	Varicella-zoster immune globulin	Immunosuppressed children in contact with the index case

*Adapted, with permission, from Katzung BG (editor): *Basic & Clinical Pharmacology,* 7th ed. Appleton & Lange, 1998.

Table 62–2. Materials for active immunization.*

Pathogen or Disease	Product	Comments
Haemophilus influenzae type b conjugate	Bacterial polysaccharide conjugate	For all children, asplenics, and others at risk
Hepatitis A	Inactivated virus	Give 2–4 weeks prior to travel to endemic areas
Hepatitis B	Inactive hepatitis B viral antigen (human or from recombinant DNA technology)	Give (before exposure) to infants and high-risk individuals (> 90% effective). Duration: years
Influenza	Influenza virus vaccine (chick embryo)	Annually for the elderly, those with chronic disease, and other high-risk individuals
Meningococci	Meningococcal polysaccharide vaccine	Epidemic situations
Pneumococci	Pneumococcal polysaccharide vaccine	High-risk individuals (asplenia, hemoglobinopathies, cardiovascular disease)
Rabies	Rabies vaccine (human)	Prophylaxis for individuals at risk; postexposure after bites (plus rabies immune globulin)
Rubella	Rubella virus vaccine (human)	Avoid during pregnancy. Duration of protection: permanent
Tetanus	DTP (diphtheria and tetanus toxoids, pertussis antigen)	Recommended every 7–10 years
Typhoid	Typhoid vaccine	Exposure from travel, epidemic, or household contact (> 70% effective). Duration: 3 years

*Adapted, with permission, from Katzung BG (editor): *Basic & Clinical Pharmacology,* 7th ed. Appleton & Lange, 1998.

Table 62–3. Recommended schedule for active immunization of children.*

Age	Product Administered
Birth to 4 days	HBV (hepatitis B vaccine)
2 months	DTP (toxoids of diphtheria and tetanus, pertussis bacterial antigen); HBV; oral poliovaccine (OPV); *Haemophilus influenzae* type b conjugate (Hib)
4 months	DTP; HBV; Hib; OPV
6 months	DTP; Hib
6–18 months	HBV; OPV
12–18 months	DTP; Hib; measles, mumps, rubella vaccines (MMR)
4–6 years	DTP; MMR (or at 11–12 years); OPV
14–16 years	TD (tetanus and diphtheria toxoids)

*Adapted, with permission, from Katzung BG (editor): *Basic & Clinical Pharmacology,* 7th ed. Appleton & Lange, 1998.

QUESTIONS

DIRECTIONS: Each of the numbered items or incomplete statements in this section is followed by answers or by completions of the statement. Select the ONE lettered answer or completion that is BEST in each case.

1. Which one of the following antibodies has the longest half-life?
    (A) Black widow spider antivenin
    (B) Botulinum antitoxin
    (C) Diphtheria antitoxin
    (D) Hepatitis B immune globulin
    (E) Snake bite antivenin

2. Passive immunization involves
    (A) Live immunogens
    (B) Polysaccharide vaccines
    (C) Stimulation of antibody formation
    (D) Use of antigens
    (E) Use of preformed antibodies

3. A businessman intends to travel abroad in a geographic region where several diseases are endemic. He would NOT be able to be vaccinated against
    (A) Cholera
    (B) Malaria
    (C) Meningococcal infections
    (D) Typhoid fever
    (E) Yellow fever

4. Which one of the following statements about passive immunization is LEAST accurate?
    (A) Rabies immune globulin is recommended only in patients who demonstrate an antibody response from preexposure prophylaxis
    (B) Patients with IgA deficiency may develop hypersensitivity reactions to IG
    (C) Equine-derived antivenins are used in the treatment of snakebite
    (D) Passive immunization is useful in the treatment of certain diseases that are normally prevented by active immunization (eg, tetanus)
    (E) Cytomegalovirus immune globulin is useful in bone marrow transplantation

5. Which one of the following statements about active immunization is LEAST accurate?
    (A) Immunization against hepatitis B involves the use of a purified and inactivated virus coat protein
    (B) Poliovirus vaccine containing live virus can be administered orally
    (C) The vaccine against *Haemophilus influenzae* type b is a polysaccharide conjugate
    (D) Some protective factors may not be stimulated with the use of inactivated (killed) products
    (E) Active immunization results in permanent protection

6. Which of the following is used in active immunization of children and combines bacterial toxoids with a bacterial antigen?
   (A) BCG
   (B) BSA
   (C) DTP
   (D) IG
   (E) $Rh_o(D)$

7. Which of the following is a polysaccharide used for active immunization in patients with chronic cardiorespiratory ailments?
   (A) Antilymphocyte immune serum
   (B) BCG vaccine
   (C) Mumps virus vaccine
   (D) Pertussis immune globulin
   (E) Pneumococcal vaccine

8. Which one of the following statements about the administration of $Rh_o(D)$ immune globulin is LEAST accurate?
   (A) It provides Rh isoimmunization from fetal-maternal transfusion
   (B) Its administration more than 48 hours after exposure is not effective
   (C) It is used for nonimmune females only
   (D) Its use is a form of passive immunization
   (E) It has been used for transfusion of Rh-positive blood to an Rh-negative woman

9. A needle stick injury occurs to a health care worker and the blood is known to contain HBV surface antigens. The health care worker should be given
   (A) Nothing
   (B) Immune globulin (IG)
   (C) Hepatitis B immune globulin (HBIG)
   (D) Hepatitis B vaccine
   (E) Hepatitis B vaccine and hepatitis B immune globulin

10. Hepatitis B vaccine is LEAST likely to be recommended for use in
    (A) Dialysis patients
    (B) IV drug abusers
    (C) Newborns
    (D) Raw oyster eaters
    (E) Surgeons

ANSWERS

1. Antibodies derived from human serum not only diminish the risk of hypersensitivity, but also have much longer half-lives than those from animal sources. For example, human IgG antibodies have a half-life of more than 20 days, compared to 5–7 days for the antibodies derived from animals. Smaller doses of human antibodies can be administered to provide therapeutic levels for several weeks. The answer is **(D)**.

2. Passive immunization utilizes preformed immunologic products (immunoglobulins) of human or animal origin to transfer immunity to the host. Other products of the cellular immune system, including interferons, have clinical uses in hematological, infectious, and neoplastic diseases. The answer is **(E)**.

3. Vaccines are available for the active immunization against all of the diseases listed except malaria. Drug prophylaxis against malaria is described in Chapter 53. A vaccine is also available for travelers to hepatitis A-endemic geographical regions. The answer is **(B)**.

4. Rabies immune globulin should be given as soon as possible after exposure and must be combined with immunization using human diploid cell-derived rabies vaccine. Passive immunization is not recommended for individuals with demonstrated antibody response to preexposure prophylaxis with rabies vaccine. The answer is **(A)**.

5. Active immunization does not always result in permanent protection. Primary immunization against measles, mumps, poliomyelitis, and rubella appears to be permanent, and in each case live viruses are used. However, the duration of effect of active immunization with killed virus products is about 6 months for cholera, 1–3 years for influenza, and more than 3 years for tetanus. The answer is **(E)**.

6. DTP contains diphtheria and tetanus toxoids and pertussis antigen. The answer is **(C)**.

7. The pertussis and antilymphocyte preparations are used in passive immunization. Both the mumps vaccine and BCG (used for tuberculosis) are used in active immunization, but they are live viruses. Pneumococcal vaccine is a polysaccharide recommended for individuals at high risk for pneumococcal disease. The *Haemophilus* and meningococcal vaccines (not listed) are also polysaccharides. The answer is **(E)**.

8. Ideally, $Rh_o(D)$ should be administered to an Rh(D)-negative woman within 72 hours of abortion, amniocentesis, obstetric delivery of an Rh-positive child, or transfusion of Rh-positive blood. However, the product may be effective at much greater postexposure intervals, and should be given even if more than 72 hours has elapsed. The answer is **(B)**.

9. The HBV needle stick situation is best handled by a combination passive-active immunization approach. Immediate and long-term protection is afforded by the administration of hepatitis B vaccine and hepatitis B immune globulin at different intramuscular sites. The answer is **(E)**.

10. Too easy? Hepatitis A commonly arises from fecally contaminated water, or foods grown in such water and consumed raw. The administration of hepatitis B vaccine is recommended in all of the other situations. The answer is **(D)**.

Appendix I

Key Words for Key Drugs

The following list is a compilation of the drugs that are most likely to appear on examinations. The brief descriptions serve as a rapid review. Use the list in two ways: First, cover the column of properties and test your ability to provide some descriptive information about drugs picked at random from the left column; second, cover the left column and attempt to name a drug that fits the properties described.

Abbreviations: ACE, angiotensin-converting enzyme; ANS, autonomic nervous system; AV, atrioventricular; BP, blood pressure; BPH, benign prostatic hyperplasia; CHF, congestive heart failure; CNS, central nervous system; CV, cardiovascular system; ECG, electrocardiogram; ENS, enteric nervous system; EPS, extrapyramidal system; GI, gastrointestinal; HR, heart rate; HTN, hypertension; MI, myocardial infarction; NM, neuromuscular; PANS, parasympathetic autonomic nervous system; SANS, sympathetic autonomic nervous system; Tox, toxicity; WBC, white blood cells.

Drug	Properties
Abciximab	Monoclonal antibody to fibrin receptor (glycoprotein IIb/IIIa) on platelets: used to prevent clotting after coronary angioplasty.
Acetaminophen	Antipyretic analgesic: very weak cyclooxygenase inhibitor; not anti-inflammatory. Less toxic than aspirin but more dangerous in overdose. *Tox:* hepatic necrosis. *Antidote:* acetylcysteine.
Acetazolamide	Carbonic anhydrase inhibitor diuretic: produces an $NaHCO_3$ diuresis, results in bicarbonate depletion, and therefore has self-limited action. Used in glaucoma and mountain sickness. Dorzolamide is a topical analog for glaucoma.
Acetylcholine	Cholinomimetic prototype: transmitter in CNS, ENS, all ANS ganglia, parasympathetic postganglionic synapses, sympathetic postganglionic fibers to sweat glands, and skeletal muscle end plate synapses.
Acyclovir	Antiviral: inhibits DNA synthesis in herpes simplex and varicella-zoster. Requires activation by viral thymidine kinase (TK^- strains are resistant). *Tox:* behavioral effects and nephrotoxicity (crystalluria) but not myelosuppression.
Adenosine	Antiarrhythmic: unclassified ("group V"); parenteral only. Hyperpolarizes AV nodal tissue, blocks conduction for 10–15 seconds. Used for nodal reentry arrhythmias.
Albuterol, metaproterenol, terbutaline	Important β_2 agonists; used mainly for asthma.
Allopurinol	Antigout: inhibitor of xanthine oxidase; reduces production of uric acid.
Alprazolam	Benzodiazepine sedative-hypnotic: widely used in anxiety states, selectivity for panic attacks and phobias; possible antidepressant actions. *Tox:* psychologic and physical dependence, additive effects with other CNS depressants.
Alteplase (rt-PA)	Thrombolytic: human recombinant tissue plasminogen activator. Used in acute MI to recanalize the occluded coronary. Occasionally used in pulmonary embolism, stroke. *Tox:* bleeding.
Amiloride	K^+-sparing diuretic: blocks Na^+ channels in cortical collecting tubules.

Aminoglutethimide	Nonsteroidal inhibitor of steroid synthesis: reduces conversion of cholesterol to the hormone precursor pregnenolone. Used in metastatic breast cancer.
Amiodarone	Group IA and III antiarrhythmic: broad spectrum; blocks sodium, potassium, calcium channels, beta receptors. High efficacy and very long half-life (weeks–months). *Tox:* deposits in tissues; hypo- or hyperthyroidism; pulmonary fibrosis.
Amitriptyline	Tricyclic antidepressant: blocks reuptake of norepinephrine and serotonin. *Tox:* atropine-like, postural hypotension, sedation; cardiac arrhythmias in overdose, additive effects with other CNS depressants.
Amoxicillin	Penicillin: wider spectrum than pen G with activity similar to ampicillin but greater oral bioavailability; less adverse effects on GI tract than ampicillin. Susceptible to penicillinases unless used with clavulanic acid. *Tox:* penicillin allergy.
Amphetamine	Indirectly acting sympathomimetic: displaces stored catecholamines in nerve endings. Marked CNS stimulant actions; high abuse liability. *Tox:* psychosis, HTN, MI, seizures.
Amphotericin B	Antifungal: polyene drug of choice for most systemic mycoses; binds to ergosterol to disrupt fungal cell membrane permeability. *Tox:* chills and fever, hypokalemia, hypotension, nephrotoxicity (dose-limiting, possibly less with liposomal forms).
Ampicillin	Penicillin: wider spectrum than pen G, susceptible to penicillinases unless used with sulbactam. Activity similar to pen G, plus *E coli, H influenzae, P mirabilis, Shigella.* Synergy with aminoglycosides versus enterococci and *Listeria. Tox:* penicillin allergy; more adverse effects on GI tract than other penicillins; maculopapular skin rash.
Anistreplase (APSAC)	Thrombolytic: bacterial streptokinase complexed with human plasminogen. Longer-acting in body than other thrombolytics (rt-PA, streptokinase, urokinase). *Tox:* bleeding, allergy to streptococcal protein.
Aspirin	NSAID prototype: inhibits cyclooxygenase (COX) I and II irreversibly. Potent antiplatelet agent as well as antipyretic analgesic and anti-inflammatory drug.
Astemizole	Antihistamine H_1 blocker: newer, less sedating, used in hay fever. *Tox:* arrhythmias, especially if used with P450 inhibitors, eg, ketoconazole, erythromycin.
Atenolol	Beta$_1$-selective blocker: low lipid solubility, less CNS effect; used for HTN. (Note mnemonic for beta$_1$-selective blockers: their names start with A through M [exceptions: carteolol and labetolol are not selective].)
Atropine	Muscarinic cholinoceptor blocker prototype: lipid soluble, CNS effects. *Tox:* "red as a beet, dry as a bone, blind as a bat, mad as a hatter," urinary retention, mydriasis.
Azithromycin	Antibiotic: similar to erythromycin but greater activity versus chlamydiae and streptococci; long half-life due to tissue accumulation. *Tox:* GI distress but no inhibition of drug metabolism.
Baclofen	GABA analog, orally active: spasmolytic; activates GABA$_B$ receptors in the spinal cord.
Benztropine	Centrally acting antimuscarinic prototype for parkinsonism.
Bethanechol	Muscarinic agonist: choline ester with good resistance to cholinesterase; used for atonic bowel or bladder.
Botulinum	Toxin: produced by *Clostridium botulinum;* interacts with synaptobrevin to block release of acetylcholine vesicles.
Bromocriptine	Ergot derivative: dopamine agonist in CNS; inhibits prolactin release. Used in parkinsonism and hyperprolactinemia. *Tox:* CNS, dyskinesias, hypotension.

Bupivacaine	Long-acting amide, local anesthetic prototype: greater CV toxicity than most local anesthetics.
Buspirone	Anxiolytic: atypical drug that interacts with 5-HT$_{1A}$ receptors; slow onset. Minimal potentiation of CNS depressants, including ethanol; negligible abuse liability.
Captopril	ACE inhibitor prototype: used in HTN, diabetic renal disease, and CHF. *Tox:* hyperkalemia, fetal renal damage, cough ("sore throat").
Carbachol	Nonselective muscarinic and nicotinic agonist: choline ester with good resistance to cholinesterase; used for glaucoma (not a first-line drug).
Carbamazepine	Anticonvulsant: tricyclic derivative used for tonic-clonic and partial seizures; blocks Na$^+$ channels in neuronal membranes. Drug of choice for trigeminal neuralgia; backup drug in mania. *Tox:* CNS depression, hematotoxic, induces liver drug-metabolizing enzymes.
Cefazolin	First-generation cephalosporin prototype: bactericidal beta-lactam inhibitor of cell wall synthesis. Active against gram-positive cocci, *E coli, K pneumoniae,* but does not enter CSF. *Tox:* potential allergy; partial cross-reactivity with penicillins.
Cefoxitin	Second-generation cephalosporin: active against a wide spectrum of gram-negative bacteria, including anaerobes *(B fragilis).* Does not enter the CNS.
Ceftriaxone	Third-generation cephalosporin: active against resistant bacteria, including gonococci, *H influenzae,* and other gram-negative organisms. Crosses the blood-brain barrier.
Chloramphenicol	Antibiotic: broad-spectrum agent; inhibits protein synthesis (50S); uses restricted to backup drug for bacterial meningitis, infections due to anaerobes, *Salmonella. Tox:* reversible myelosuppression, aplastic anemia, gray baby syndrome.
Chloroquine	Antimalarial: blood schizonticide used for treatment and as a chemosuppressant where *P falciparum* is susceptible. *Tox:* GI distress and skin rash at low doses; peripheral neuropathy, skin lesions, auditory and visual impairment, quinidine-like myocardial depression at high doses.
Chlorpheniramine	Antihistamine H$_1$ blocker prototype: *Tox:* mild sedation, antimuscarinic.
Chlorpromazine	Phenothiazine antipsychotic drug prototype: blocks most dopamine receptors in the CNS. *Tox:* atropine-like, EPS dysfunction, hyperprolactinemia, postural hypotension, sedation, seizures (in overdose), additive effects with other CNS depressants.
Cholestyramine, colestipol	Bile acid-binding resins: sequester bile acids in gut and divert more cholesterol from the liver to bile acids instead of circulating lipoproteins. *Tox:* constipation, bloating; interfere with absorption of some drugs.
Cimetidine	H$_2$ blocker prototype: used in acid-peptic disease. *Tox:* inhibits hepatic drug metabolism; antiandrogen effects. Less toxic analogs: ranitidine, famotidine, nizatidine.
Ciprofloxacin	Fluoroquinolone antibiotic: bactericidal inhibitor of topoisomerases; active against many gram-negative rods, including *E coli, H influenzae, Campylobacter, Enterobacter, Pseudomonas, Shigella. Tox:* CNS dysfunction, GI distress, superinfection, collagen damage (avoid in children and pregnant women). *Interactions:* caffeine, theophylline, warfarin.
Cisplatin	Platinum-containing alkylating cancer chemotherapeutic agent: used for solid tumors (eg, testes, lung). Carboplatin is similar. Oto- and nephrotoxic.
Clindamycin	Lincosamide antibiotic: bacteriostatic inhibitor of protein synthesis (50S); active against gram-positive cocci, *B fragilis. Tox:* GI distress, pseudomembranous colitis.

Clomiphene	Estrogen partial agonist: synthetic used in infertility to induce ovulation.
Clonidine	Alpha$_2$ agonist: acts centrally to reduce SANS outflow, lowers BP. *Tox:* rebound HTN if stopped suddenly.
Clozapine	Atypical antipsychotic: low affinity for dopamine D$_2$ receptors, higher for D$_4$ and 5-HT$_{2A}$ receptors; less EPS adverse effects than other antipsychotic drugs. *Tox:* ANS effects, agranulocytosis (infrequent but significant).
Cocaine	Indirectly acting sympathomimetic: blocks amine reuptake into nerve endings. Local anesthetic (ester type). Marked CNS stimulation, euphoria; high abuse liability. *Tox:* psychosis, cardiac arrhythmias, seizures.
Colchicine	Microtubule assembly inhibitor: reduces mobility and phagocytosis by WBCs in gout-inflamed joints; useful in acute (not chronic) gout. *Tox:* GI, hepatic, renal damage.
Cyclopentolate, tropicamide	Antimuscarinics for ophthalmology: shorter duration than atropine (a few hours or less); cause cycloplegia and mydriasis.
Cyclophosphamide	Antineoplastic, immunosuppressive: cell cycle-nonspecific alkylating agent. *Tox:* alopecia, gastrointestinal distress, hemorrhagic cystitis, myelosuppression.
Cyclosporine	Immunosuppressant: antibiotic; inhibits interleukin-2 synthesis, suppresses T cells. *Tox:* HTN, hirsutism, nephrotoxicity (dose-limiting), seizures (in overdose). Not a myelosuppressant.
Dantrolene	Blocks Ca^{2+} release from sarcoplasmic reticulum of skeletal muscle: used in muscle spasm (cerebral palsy, multiple sclerosis, cord injury) and in emergency treatment of hyperthermia caused by malignant hyperthermia, malignant neuroleptic syndrome, and serotonin syndrome.
DDAVP	ADH analog: synthetic peptide used for pituitary diabetes insipidus.
DDT	Insecticide: prevents inactivation of sodium channels, causes uncontrolled neuronal activity. Stored for years in body fat in mammals, birds, fish.
Deferoxamine	Chelator: bacterial product; chelates iron very avidly, aluminum less so.
Dexamethasone	Glucocorticoid: very potent, long-acting; no mineralocorticoid activity.
Dexfenfluramine	5-HT reuptake inhibitor and receptor agonist: used as anorexic. *Tox:* produces cardiac valve damage when used in combination with phentermine.
Diazepam	Benzodiazepine prototype: binds to BZ receptors of the GABA$_A$ receptor-chloride ion channel complex; facilitates the inhibitory actions of GABA by increasing *frequency* of channel opening. Uses: anxiety states, ethanol detoxification, muscle spasticity, status epilepticus. *Tox:* psychologic and physical dependence, additive effects with other CNS depressants.
Didanosine (ddI)	Antiviral: nucleoside inhibitor of HIV reverse transcriptase: *Tox:* peripheral neuropathy, pancreatitis.
Digitoxin	Cardiac glycoside: half-life 168 hours, excreted in the bile (partially as digoxin); subject to enterohepatic circulation. See Digoxin.
Digoxin	Cardiac glycoside prototype: positive inotropic drug for CHF, half-life 40 hours; renal excretion; inhibits Na$^+$/K$^+$ ATPase, also a cardiac parasympathomimetic. *Tox:* calcium overload arrhythmias, GI upset.
Diltiazem	Calcium channel (L-type) blocker prototype: like verapamil, has more depressant effect on heart than dihydropyridines (eg, nifedipine). *Tox:* AV block, CHF, edema, constipation.
Dimercaprol (BAL)	Chelator (British anti-Lewisite): used for arsenic, lead, and mercury poisoning.
Dioxin (TCDD)	Toxin: byproduct of the manufacture of herbicides 2,4-D and 2,4,5-T. *Tox:* extremely potent carcinogen in guinea pigs; poorly documented in humans except for chloracne, a skin disorder that occurs acutely upon exposure.

Diphenhydramine	Antihistamine H_1 blocker prototype: used in hay fever, motion sickness, dystonias. *Tox:* antimuscarinic, alpha-adrenoceptor blocker, sedative.
Disopyramide	Group IA antiarrhythmic: used for ventricular arrhythmias. *Tox:* strong antimuscarinic; may cause CHF.
Dopamine	Neurotransmitter and agonist drug at dopamine receptors: used in shock to increase renal blood flow, stimulate heart.
Doxorubicin	Antineoplastic: anthracycline drug (cell cycle-nonspecific); intercalates between base pairs to disrupt DNA functions and forms cytotoxic free radicals. *Tox:* cardiotoxicity, myelosuppression.
Doxycycline	Tetracycline antibiotic: protein synthesis inhibitor (30S), more effective than other tetracyclines against bacillary dysentery. Unlike other tetracyclines, it is eliminated mainly in the feces. *Tox:* see Tetracycline.
Echothiophate	Organophosphate cholinesterase inhibitor: less lipid-soluble than most organophosphates; used in glaucoma.
Edetate (EDTA)	Chelating agent: used in lead poisoning. *Tox:* renal tubular necrosis.
Edrophonium	Cholinesterase inhibitor: very short duration of action (15 minutes). Used to reverse NM blockade and as diagnostic test for myasthenia gravis.
Enoxaparin	Low-molecular-weight heparin: primary effect is anti-factor X. Other LMW heparin-like products: dalteparin, danaparoid. *Tox:* bleeding.
Ephedrine	Indirectly acting sympathomimetic: like amphetamine but less CNS stimulation, more smooth muscle effects.
Epinephrine	Adrenoceptor agonist prototype: product of adrenal medulla, some CNS neurons. Affinity for all alpha and all beta receptors. Used in asthma; as hemostatic and adjunct with local anesthetics; drug of choice in anaphylaxis.
Ergonovine	Ergot alkaloid: uterine effect prototype, causes prolonged uterine contraction. Used in postpartum bleeding.
Ergotamine	Ergot alkaloid: vascular effect prototype, causes prolonged vasoconstriction, uterine contraction. Used in migraine, obstetrics.
Erythromycin	Macrolide antibiotic: inhibitor of protein synthesis (50S); activity includes gram-positive cocci and bacilli, *M pneumoniae, Legionella pneumophila, C trachomatis.* *Tox:* cholestatic jaundice, inhibits liver drug-metabolizing enzymes, interactions with astemizole, theophylline, terfenadine, warfarin.
Ethacrynic acid	Loop diuretic: not a sulfonamide derivative. *Tox:* like furosemide but does not increase serum uric acid.
Ethanol	Sedative-hypnotic: acute actions include impaired judgment, ataxia, loss of consciousness, vasodilation, and cardiovascular and respiratory depression. Chronic use leads to dependence and liver, cardiovascular, endocrine, gastrointestinal, hepatic, and nervous system disease. *Note:* zero-order elimination kinetics.
Ethosuximide	Anticonvulsant: used in absence seizures; may block T-type Ca^{2+} channels in thalamic neurons. *Tox:* GI distress but safe in pregnancy.
Etidronate, pamidronate, alendronate	Bisphosphonates: reduce turnover of bone calcium. Used in Paget's disease, osteoporosis; alendronate increases bone formation. *Tox:* severe esophageal ulceration.
Finasteride	Steroid inhibitor of 5α-reductase: inhibits synthesis of dihydrotesterone, the active androgen in prostate. Used in BPH.
Flecainide	Group IC antiarrhythmic prototype: used in ventricular tachycardia and rapid atrial arrhythmias with Wolff-Parkinson-White syndrome. *Tox:* arrhythmogenic, CNS excitation.

Fluconazole	Imidazole antifungal: used for esophageal candidiasis and in coccidioidomycosis; high CSF levels provide prophylaxis against fungal meningitis in immunosuppressed patients.
Fludrocortisone	Synthetic corticosteroid: high mineralocorticoid and moderate glucocorticoid activity; long duration of action.
Flumazenil	Benzodiazepine receptor antagonist: used to reverse CNS depressant effects of benzodiazepines (overdose or when used in anesthesia).
Fluorouracil	Antineoplastic: pyrimidine antimetabolite (cell cycle-specific), causes "thymineless" cell death; used mainly for solid or superficial tumors. *Tox:* GI distress, myelosuppression.
Fluoxetine	Antidepressant: selective serotonin reuptake inhibitor (SSRI) prototype. Less ANS adverse effects and cardiotoxic potential than tricyclics. *Tox:* CNS stimulation, seizures in overdose.
Flutamide	Androgen receptor inhibitor: nonsteroid used in prostatic carcinoma.
Foscarnet	Antiviral: effective against CMV and HSV (including TK^- strains); *Tox:* electrolyte imbalance, nephrotoxicity.
Furosemide	Loop diuretic prototype: blocks $Na^+/K^+/2Cl^-$ transporter; high efficacy; used in acute pulmonary edema, refractory edematous states, hypercalcemia. *Tox:* ototoxicity, K^+ wasting, hypovolemia, increased serum uric acid.
Ganciclovir	Antiviral: effective against CMV; requires bioactivation via viral phosphotransferase. *Tox:* myelosuppression, nephrotoxicity.
Gemfibrozil, clofibrate	Antilipemics: stimulate lipoprotein lipase in peripheral tissues. Used in hypertriglyceridemias and mixed triglyceridemia/hypercholesterolemia.
Gentamicin	Aminoglycoside prototype: bactericidal inhibitor of protein synthesis (30S); active against many aerobic gram-negative bacteria. Narrow therapeutic window; dose reduction required in renal impairment. *Tox:* renal dysfunction, ototoxicity; once-daily dosing is effective (postantibiotic effect) and less toxic.
Glipizide, glyburide	Oral hypoglycemics: second generation, very potent. Like other sulfonylureas, act by closing K channels in pancreatic B cells, causing depolarization and release of insulin. *Tox:* hypoglycemia.
Glucagon	Hormone product of pancreatic A cells: increases blood sugar via increased cAMP.
Guanethidine	Postganglionic sympathetic neuron blocker: enters nerve ending by means of uptake-1 and is stored in the ending (effect reversed by TCAs, cocaine). *Tox:* severe orthostatic hypotension, sexual dysfunction.
Haloperidol	Antipsychotic butyrophenone: blocks brain dopamine D_2 receptors. *Tox:* marked EPS dysfunction, hyperprolactinemia; less ANS adverse effects than phenothiazines.
Halothane	General anesthetic prototype: inhaled halogenated hydrocarbon. Causes cardiovascular and respiratory depression and relaxes skeletal and smooth muscle. Use has decreased owing to sensitization of heart to catecholamines and occurrence (rare) of hepatitis and malignant hyperthermia.
Heparin	Anticoagulant: large polymeric molecule with antithrombin and anti-factor X activity. Primary rapid onset, in vitro and in vivo anticoagulation. *Antidote:* protamine. See also Enoxaparin.
Hydralazine	Antihypertensive: arteriolar vasodilator, orally active; used in HTN, CHF. *Tox:* tachycardia, salt and water retention, lupus-like syndrome.
Hydrochlorothiazide	Thiazide diuretic prototype: acts in distal convoluted tubule; blocks Na^+/Cl^- transporter; used in HTN, CHF, chronic renal stone syndrome. *Tox:* increased serum lipids, uric acid, glucose; K^+ wasting.

Ibuprofen	NSAID prototype: short duration. Inhibits cyclooxygenase (both I and II) reversibly. Used in arthritis, dysmenorrhea, muscle inflammation. *Tox:* peptic ulcer, renal damage.
Imipenem	Antibiotic: carbapenem beta-lactam active against many aerobic and anaerobic bacteria, including penicillinase-producing organisms; a bactericidal inhibitor of cell wall synthesis. Used with cilastatin (which inhibits metabolism by renal dehydropeptidases). *Tox:* allergy (partial cross-reactivity with penicillins), seizures (overdose).
Imipramine	Tricyclic antidepressant prototype: blocks reuptake of norepinephrine and serotonin. *Tox:* ANS (alpha and muscarinic) blockade, cardiac arrhythmias.
Indinavir	Antiviral HIV protease inhibitor: used as component of combination regimens in AIDS. *Tox:* anemia, nephrolithiasis, inhibits P450 drug metabolism reactions. Other protease inhibitors: ritonavir, saquinavir.
Indomethacin	NSAID prototype: highly potent. Usually reserved for acute inflammation (eg, acute gout), not chronic; neonatal patent ductus arteriosus. *Tox:* GI (bleeding), renal damage.
Insulin	Hypoglycemic peptide hormone of B (beta) cells of the pancreas: stimulates transport of glucose into cells and glycogen formation; inhibits lipolysis and protein catabolism.
Ipodate	Antithyroid: iodine-containing radiocontrast medium; also used in thyrotoxicosis. Reduces peripheral conversion of T_4 to T_3; may also reduce release of hormone from thyroid.
Ipratropium	Antimuscarinic agent: aerosol for asthma, COPD. Good bronchodilator in 20–30% of patients. Not as effective as $beta_2$ agonists.
Isoniazid	Antimycobacterial: primary drug in combination regimens for tuberculosis; used as sole agent in prophylaxis. Metabolic clearance via *N*-acetyltransferases (genetic variability). *Tox:* hepatotoxicity (age-dependent), peripheral neuropathy (reversed by pyridoxine), hemolysis (in G6PD deficiency).
Isoproterenol	$Beta_1$, $beta_2$ agonist catecholamine prototype: bronchodilator, cardiac stimulant. Always causes tachycardia because both direct and reflex actions increase HR. *Tox:* arrhythmias, angina.
Ketoconazole	Antifungal azole prototype: active systemically; inhibits the synthesis of ergosterol. Used for *C albicans,* dermatophytosis and non-life-threatening systemic mycoses. *Tox:* hepatic dysfunction, inhibits steroid synthesis and P450-dependent drug metabolism.
Labetalol	Alpha- and beta-blocker: used in HTN. *Tox:* AV block, hypotension.
Leuprolide	GnRH analog: synthetic peptide used in pulse therapy to stimulate gonadal steroid synthesis (infertility); used in continuous or depot therapy to shut off steroid synthesis, especially in prostate carcinoma.
Levodopa	Dopamine precursor: used in parkinsonism, usually combined with carbidopa (a peripheral inhibitor of dopamine metabolism). *Tox:* dyskinesias, hypotension, on-off phenomena, behavioral changes.
Lidocaine	Local anesthetic, medium-duration amide prototype: highly selective use-dependent group IB antiarrhythmic; used for nerve block and post-MI ischemic ventricular arrhythmias. *Tox:* CNS excitation.
Lithium	Antimanic prototype: drug of choice in mania and bipolar affective disorders; blocks recycling of the phosphatidylinositol second messenger system. *Tox:* tremor, diabetes insipidus, goiter, seizures (in overdose), teratogenic potential (Ebstein's malformations).
Lovastatin	Antilipemic HMG-CoA reductase inhibitor prototype: acts in liver to reduce synthesis of cholesterol. Other "statins": atorvastatin, fluvastatin, pravastatin, simvastatin. *Tox:* liver damage (elevated enzymes), muscle damage.

LSD	Lysergic acid diethylamide, "Acid": semisynthetic ergot derivative; orally active; hallucinogen.
Malathion	Organophosphate insecticide cholinesterase inhibitor: prodrug converted to malaoxon. Less toxic in mammals and birds because metabolized to inactive products.
Meperidine	Opioid analgesic: synthetic, equivalent to morphine in efficacy but orally bioavailable. Strong agonist at mu opioid receptors; blocks muscarinic receptors. *Tox:* see Morphine.
Mestranol	Synthetic estrogen: used in many oral contraceptives.
Metformin, phenformin	Oral biguanide hypoglycemics: mechanism not understood, different from sulfonylurea oral hypoglycemics. Some efficacy in the *absence* of functioning pancreatic B cells.
Methadone	Opioid analgesic: synthetic mu agonist, equivalent to morphine in efficacy but orally bioavailable with longer half-life (used to suppress withdrawal symptoms and in maintenance programs). *Tox:* see Morphine.
Methotrexate	Antineoplastic, immunosuppressant: cell cycle-specific drug that inhibits dihydrofolate reductase. Major dose reduction required in renal impairment. *Tox:* gastrointestinal distress, myelosuppression. Leucovorin rescue used to reduce toxicity after very high doses.
Methyldopa	Antihypertensive: prodrug of methylnorepinephrine, a CNS-active α_2 agonist. Reduces SANS outflow from vasomotor center. *Tox:* positive Coombs test, hemolysis, sedation.
Methysergide	Ergot alkaloid: used as prophylactic in migraine. *Tox:* retroperitoneal and subendocardial fibroplasia.
Metoprolol	Beta$_1$-selective blocker: used in HTN and for prevention of post-MI sudden death arrhythmias.
Metronidazole	Antiprotozoal antibiotic: drug of choice in extraluminal amebiasis and trichomoniasis; active against bacterial anaerobes, including *B fragilis* and in antibiotic-induced colitis due to *C difficile*. *Tox:* peripheral neuropathy, gastrointestinal distress, ethanol intolerance, mutagenic potential.
Mexiletine	Group IB antiarrhythmic drug: like lidocaine but orally active.
Mibefradil	Newer Ca^{2+} channel blocker: blocks T-type as well as L-type channels. Used in HTN.
Mifepristone (RU 486)	Progesterone, glucocorticoid inhibitor: abortifacient, antineoplastic.
Minoxidil	Antihypertensive: prodrug of minoxidil sulfate, a high-efficacy arteriolar vasodilator. Used in HTN; topically for baldness. *Tox:* tachycardia, salt and water retention, pericardial effusion.
Misoprostol	PGE_1 derivative: orally active prostaglandin used to prevent peptic ulcers in patients taking NSAIDs for arthritis. *Tox:* diarrhea.
Morphine	Opioid analgesic prototype: strong mu receptor agonist. Poor oral bioavailability. Effects include analgesia, constipation, emesis, sedation, respiratory depression, miosis, and urinary retention. Tolerance may be marked; high potential for psychologic and physical dependence. Additive effects with other CNS depressants.
Nafcillin	Penicillinase-resistant penicillin prototype: used for suspected or known staphylococcal infections; not active against methicillin-resistant staphylococci. *Tox:* penicillin allergy.
Nalbuphine	Opioid: mixed agonist-antagonist analgesic that activates kappa and weakly blocks mu receptors. Effective analgesic, but with lower abuse liability and less respiratory depressant effects than most strong opioid analgesics.

Naloxone	Opioid mu receptor antagonist: used to reverse CNS depressant effects of opioid analgesics (overdose or when used in anesthesia).
Neostigmine	Cholinesterase inhibitor prototype: quaternary nitrogen carbamate with little CNS effect.
Niacin	Antilipemic: reduces release of VLDL from liver into circulation. *Tox:* flushing.
Nifedipine	Calcium channel blocker prototype: vasoselective (less cardiac depression); used in angina, HTN. *Tox:* constipation, headache.
Nitroglycerin	Antianginal vasodilator prototype: releases NO in smooth muscle of veins, less in arteries, and causes relaxation. Standard of therapy in angina (both atherosclerotic and variant). *Tox:* tachycardia, orthostatic hypotension, headache.
Norepinephrine	Adrenoceptor agonist prototype: acts at $beta_1$ and all alpha adrenoceptors; used as vasoconstrictor. Causes reflex bradycardia. *Tox:* ischemia, arrhythmias, HTN.
Norfloxacin	Fluoroquinolone antibiotic: inhibits bacterial DNA gyrase; active against many urinary pathogens, including *E coli, H influenzae, Klebsiella, Enterobacter, Pseudomonas, Serratia. Tox:* See Ciprofloxacin.
Norgestrel	Progestin: used in many oral contraceptives and Norplant implantable contraceptive.
Olanzapine	Atypical antipsychotic: high-affinity antagonist at $5\text{-}HT_{2A}$ with minimal extrapyramidal side effects; improves both positive and negative symptoms of schizophrenia.
Omeprazole	Antiulcer: irreversible blocker of H^+/K^+ ATPase proton pump in parietal cells of stomach. Used in Zollinger-Ellison syndrome, gastroesophageal reflux disease (GERD).
Ondansetron, granisetron	$5\text{-}HT_3$ receptor blockers: very important antiemetics for cancer chemotherapy; also used postoperatively to reduce vomiting.
Paraquat	Toxic herbicide: very small oral (but not inhaled) doses cause lethal pulmonary fibrosis.
Parathion	Organophosphate acetylcholinesterase inhibitor prototype: used as insecticide. Prodrug: converted in body to paraoxon. Other organophosphates: DFP, soman, tabun, echothiophate. *Tox:* "DUMBELS" mnemonic (Chapter 7).
Penicillamine	Chelator, immunomodulator: copper and sometimes lead, mercury, arsenic. Used in Wilson's disease and rheumatoid arthritis.
Penicillin G	Penicillin prototype: active against common streptococci, gram-positive bacilli, gram-negative cocci, spirochetes, and enterococci (if used with an aminoglycoside); penicillinase-susceptible. *Tox:* penicillin allergy.
Phenobarbital	Long-acting barbiturate prototype: used as a sedative and for tonic-clonic seizures. Facilitates GABA-mediated neuronal inhibition (by increasing *duration* of channel opening) and may block excitatory neurotransmitters. Partial renal clearance that can be increased by urinary alkalinization. Chronic use leads to induction of liver drug-metabolizing enzymes and ALA synthase. *Tox:* psychologic and physical dependence liability; additive effects with other CNS depressants.
Phenoxybenzamine	Alpha-blocker prototype: irreversible action. Used in pheochromocytoma.
Phentolamine	Alpha-blocker prototype: reversible action. Used in pheochromocytoma.
Phenytoin	Anticonvulsant: used for tonic-clonic and partial seizures; blocks Na^+ channels in neuronal membranes. Serum levels variable due to first-pass metabolism and dose-dependent nonlinear elimination kinetics. *Tox:* sedation, diplopia, gingival hyperplasia, hirsutism, respiratory depression in overdose, teratogenic potential. Drug interactions via effects on plasma protein binding or induction of hepatic metabolism.

Physostigmine	Cholinesterase inhibitor prototype: alkaloid tertiary amine carbamate, enters eye and CNS readily. Used in glaucoma.
Pilocarpine	Muscarinic agonist prototype: tertiary amine alkaloid. May cause paradoxic hypertension by activating excitatory muscarinic EPSP receptors in postganglionic sympathetic neurons. Used in glaucoma. *Tox:* muscarinic excess.
Piroxicam	NSAID with longest duration of action ($t_{1/2}$ about 40 hours).
Pralidoxime	Acetylcholinesterase regenerator: very high affinity for phosphorus in organophosphates.
Prazosin, terazosin, doxazosin	Alpha$_1$-selective blockers: used in HTN. *Tox:* first-dose orthostatic hypotension.
Prednisone	Glucocorticoid prototype: potent, short-acting; much less mineralocorticoid activity than cortisol but more than dexamethasone or triamcinolone.
Probenecid	Uricosuric: inhibitor of renal weak acid secretion and reabsorption in S$_2$ segment of proximal tubule; prolongs half-life of penicillin, accelerates clearance of uric acid. Used in gout.
Probucol	Antilipemic: unknown mechanism; recently withdrawn but new evidence suggests efficacy in preventing restenosis of coronary arteries after angioplasty. *Tox:* causes arrhythmias.
Procainamide	Group IA antiarrhythmic drug: short half-life; similar to quinidine but may cause lupus erythematosus.
Propranolol	Nonselective beta-blocker prototype: local anesthetic action but no partial agonist effect. Used in HTN, angina, arrhythmias, migraine, hyperthyroidism, tremor. *Tox:* asthma, AV block, CHF.
Propylthiouracil	Antithyroid drug prototype: reduces iodination of tyrosine and coupling of MIT and DIT in the thyroid; orally active. *Tox:* rash, agranulocytosis (rare).
Prostacyclin	PGI$_2$: prostaglandin vasodilator and inhibitor of platelet aggregation.
Pyridostigmine	Cholinesterase inhibitor: long-acting (8 hours) quaternary carbamate; used in myasthenia gravis.
Quinidine	Group IA antiarrhythmic prototype: used in atrial and ventricular arrhythmias. *Tox:* cinchonism, GI upset, thrombocytopenic purpura, arrhythmogenic.
Quinine	Antimalarial: blood schizonticide; no effect on liver stages. Isomer of quinidine, same toxicity.
Ranitidine	H$_2$ blocker: like cimetidine but less inhibition of hepatic drug metabolism; no antiandrogenic effects.
Reserpine	Antihypertensive: selective inhibitor of vesicle catecholamine/H$^+$ antiporter; used in HTN, causes depletion of catecholamines and 5-HT from their stores. *Tox:* severe depression, suicide, ulcers.
Rifampin	Antimicrobial: inhibitor of DNA-dependent RNA polymerase used in drug regimens for tuberculosis and the meningococcal carrier state. *Tox:* hepatic dysfunction, induction of liver drug-metabolizing enzymes (drug interactions), flu-like syndrome with intermittent dosing.
Selegiline	MAO-B inhibitor: selective inhibitor of the enzyme that metabolizes dopamine (no tyramine interactions). Used in parkinsonism as adjunct.
Streptokinase	Thrombolytic: protein from streptococci that accelerates plasminogen-to-plasmin conversion. *Tox:* bleeding, allergy.
Succimer (DMSA)	Chelator: dimercaptosuccinic acid; used to chelate lead and arsenic.
Succinylcholine	Depolarizing neuromuscular relaxant prototype: short duration (5 minutes) if patient has normal plasma cholinesterase (genetically determined). No antidote (compare with tubocurarine).

Sumatriptan	5-HT$_{1D}$ receptor agonist: used to abort migraine attacks.
Tamoxifen	Estrogen partial agonist: used in breast carcinoma.
Terfenadine	Antihistamine, H$_1$ blocker: withdrawn, less sedating drug. Was used in hayfever. *Tox:* like astemizole.
Tetracaine	Local anesthetic: long-acting ester prototype.
Tetracycline	Antibiotic: tetracycline prototype; bacteriostatic inhibitor of protein synthesis (30S). Broad spectrum, but many resistant organisms. Used for Lyme disease, mycoplasmal, chlamydial, rickettsial infections, chronic bronchitis, acne, cholera; a backup drug in syphilis. *Tox:* GI upset and superinfections (*Candida,* staphylococci), antianabolic actions, Fanconi's syndrome (outdated drug), photosensitivity, dental enamel dysplasia.
Tetrodotoxin	Toxin: very potent sodium channel blocker; blocks action potential propagation in nerve, heart, and skeletal muscle. From puffer fish, California newt. *Tox:* paresthesias, paralysis.
Thiazides	Diuretic prototype: block Na$^+$/Cl$^-$ transporter in distal convoluted tubule; used in HTN, CHF, chronic stone formers. *Tox:* K$^+$ wasting; increased serum lipids, uric acid, and glucose.
Thioridazine	Antipsychotic phenothiazine: blocks most dopamine receptors in the CNS. *Tox:* atropine-like effects (marked), ECG abnormalities, postural hypotension, retinal pigmentation, sedation, additive effects with other CNS depressants (but less EPS dysfunction than other phenothiazines).
Thyroxine, triiodothyronine	Major hormones produced by the thyroid: stimulate metabolism, growth, and development.
Ticarcillin	Extended-spectrum penicillin: active against selected gram-negative bacteria, including *Pseudomonas aeruginosa* (synergistic with aminoglycosides). Susceptible to penicillinases unless used with clavulanic acid. *Tox:* penicillin allergy.
Ticlopidine	Antiplatelet agent with uncertain mechanism: irreversible inhibitor of fibrin binding to platelets. Used to prevent strokes.
Tolbutamide, tolazamide, chlorpropamide, acetohexamide	Oral hypoglycemics: older sulfonylurea group. See Glipizide. Chlorpropamide has longest duration of action.
Trimethaphan	Ganglion blocker (antinicotinic agent) prototype: recently discontinued. Was used in malignant HTN and for controlled hypotension (in neurosurgery).
Trimethoprim-sulfamethoxazole	Antimicrobial drug combination: causes synergistic sequential blockade of folic acid synthesis. Active against many gram-negative bacteria, including *Aeromonas, Enterobacter, H influenzae, Klebsiella, Moraxella, Salmonella, Serratia, Shigella.* Possible backup agent for methicillin-resistant staphylococci. *Tox:* mainly due to sulfonamide; includes hypersensitivity, hematotoxicity, kernicterus, and drug interactions due to competition for plasma protein binding.
Tubocurarine	Nondepolarizing neuromuscular blocking agent prototype: competitive nicotinic blocker. Releases histamine and may cause hypotension. Analogs: pancuronium, atracurium, vecuronium, and other "-curiums" and "-curoniums." *Antidote:* cholinesterase inhibitor, eg, neostigmine.
Tyramine	Indirectly acting sympathomimetic prototype: releases or displaces norepinephrine from stores in nerve endings. Usually inactive by the oral route because of high first-pass effect but will cause potentially lethal hypertensive responses in patients taking MAO inhibitors.
Valproic acid	Anticonvulsant: used in absence, clonic-tonic and myoclonic seizure states. *Tox:* GI distress, hepatic necrosis (rare), teratogenic (spina bifida); inhibits drug metabolism.

Vancomycin

Glycopeptide bactericidal antibiotic: inhibits synthesis of cell wall precursor molecules. Drug of choice for methicillin-resistant staphylococci and effective in antibiotic-induced colitis. Dose reduction required in renal impairment (or hemodialysis). *Tox:* ototoxicity, hypersensitivity, renal dysfunction (rare).

Verapamil

Calcium channel blocker prototype: blocks "L-type" channels; cardiac depressant and vasodilator; used in HTN, angina, and arrhythmias. *Tox:* AV block, CHF, constipation.

Vesamicol

Inhibitor of vesicle ACh/H^+ antiporter in cholinergic nerve endings: prevents storage of ACh. No clinical application.

Vincristine

Antineoplastic plant alkaloid: cell cycle (M phase)-specific agent; inhibits mitotic spindle formation. *Tox:* peripheral neuropathy. Compare with vinblastine, a congener that causes myelosuppression.

Warfarin

Oral anticoagulant prototype: causes synthesis of nonfunctional versions of the vitamin K-dependent clotting factors (II, VII, IX, X). *Tox:* bleeding, teratogenic. *Antidote:* vitamin K, fresh plasma.

Zidovudine (AZT)

Antiviral: prototype nucleoside inhibitor of HIV reverse transcriptase. *Tox:* severe myelosuppression.

Zolpidem

Nonbenzodiazepine hypnotic: acts via the BZ_1 (omega$_1$) receptor subtype and is reversed by flumazenil; less amnesia and muscle relaxation; lower dependence liability.

Appendix II

Examination 1

The following examination consists of 120 questions in the two formats ("single best answer" and "matching") used in the actual United States Medical Licensing Examination (USMLE). As in an actual examination, clinical descriptions, tables, or graphs are provided in many of the questions.

It is suggested that you time yourself in taking this examination—in a USMLE examination you are allowed 1 minute per question; thus, 2 hours would be appropriate for this examination.

DIRECTIONS: Each numbered item or incomplete statement in this section is followed by answers or by completions of the statement. Select the ONE lettered answer or completion that is BEST in each case.

1. Phase II clinical trials typically involve
   (A) Measurement of the pharmacokinetics of the new drug in normal volunteers
   (B) Double-blind evaluation of the new drug in thousands of patients with the target disease
   (C) Evaluation of late effects of depolarizing neuromuscular blockers in humans
   (D) Evaluation of the new drug in 50 to several hundred patients with the target disease
   (E) Collection of late toxicity data from patients previously studied in phase I trials

2. A patient is admitted to the emergency department for treatment of a drug overdose. The identity of the drug is unknown, but it is observed that when the urine pH is acidic, the renal clearance of the drug is less than the glomerular filtration rate and that when the urine pH is alkaline, the clearance is greater than the glomerular filtration rate. The drug is probably
   (A) A strong acid
   (B) A weak acid
   (C) A nonelectrolyte
   (D) A weak base
   (E) A strong base

3. A 45-year-old patient is to have reconstructive surgery on a hand that was recently injured in an accident. The anesthesiologist plans to use regional anesthesia of the arm for a fairly long procedure. The amide-type local anesthetic with the longest duration of action is
   (A) Cocaine
   (B) Bupivacaine
   (C) Lidocaine
   (D) Procaine
   (E) Tetracaine

4. A 60-year-old woman is in the coronary care unit following an acute myocardial infarction. She has developed signs of pulmonary edema of rapidly increasing severity. Aminophylline, dobutamine, and digoxin can each
   (A) Increase the amount of cAMP in cells
   (B) Increase cardiac contractile force
   (C) Decrease conduction velocity in the atrioventricular node
   (D) Increase peripheral vascular resistance
   (E) Decrease venous return

5. The peptide agent with the strongest vasodilator properties is
   (A) Angiotensin II
   (B) Bradykinin

      (C) Glucagon
      (D) Nitroprusside
      (E) Prostacyclin

6. A patient with Zollinger-Ellison syndrome has been receiving high doses of cimetidine for 7 weeks. A frequent adverse effect of cimetidine is
      (A) Agranulocytosis
      (B) Systemic lupus erythematosus
      (C) Inhibition of hepatic metabolism of other drugs
      (D) Antiestrogenic effects
      (E) Hypertension

7. A 67-year-old patient has recovered from the acute phase of a myocardial infarction but requires an antiarrhythmic drug for ventricular tachycardia. One property of quinidine not associated with procainamide is its
      (A) Ability to control atrial as well as ventricular arrhythmias
      (B) Activity by the oral route
      (C) Prolongation of the PR interval
      (D) Prolongation of the QRS interval
      (E) Tendency to produce cinchonism

8. A patient discharged from the hospital after a myocardial infarction had been receiving small doses of quinidine to suppress a ventricular tachycardia. One month later, his local physician prescribed high-dose hydrochlorothiazide therapy for ankle edema, which was ascribed to congestive heart failure. Three weeks after beginning thiazide therapy, the patient was readmitted to the hospital with a rapid multifocal ventricular tachycardia. The most probable cause of this arrhythmia is
      (A) Quinidine toxicity caused by inhibition of quinidine metabolism by the thiazide
      (B) Direct effects of hydrochlorothiazide on the pacemaker of the heart
      (C) Thiazide toxicity caused by the effects of quinidine on the kidneys
      (D) Reduction of serum sodium caused by the diuretic action of hydrochlorothiazide
      (E) Reduction of serum potassium caused by the diuretic action of hydrochlorothiazide

9. An important therapeutic or toxic effect of loop diuretics is
      (A) Decreased heart rate
      (B) Decreased blood volume
      (C) Increased total body potassium
      (D) Metabolic acidosis
      (E) Increased serum sodium

10. The most useful drug for reversing myasthenic crisis in a patient who is experiencing diplopia, dysarthria, and difficulty swallowing is
      (A) Neostigmine
      (B) Pilocarpine
      (C) Physostigmine
      (D) Succinylcholine
      (E) Tubocurarine

11. Soon after being put to bed for a nap, a 4-year-old child is found convulsing. Diarrhea and sweating are apparent. The heart rate is 70/min, and the pupils are markedly constricted. Drug intoxication is suspected. The most probable cause is
      (A) An organophosphate-containing insecticide
      (B) A nicotine-containing insecticide
      (C) Amphetamine-containing diet pills
      (D) Phenylephrine-containing eye drops
      (E) An atropine-containing medication

12. A patient is admitted to the emergency room 2 hours after taking an overdose of phenobarbital. The plasma level of the drug at time of admission is 100 mg/L, and the apparent volume of distribution, half-life, and clearance of phenobarbital are 35 L, 4 days, and 6.1 L/d, respectively. The ingested dose was approximately
      (A) 1 g
      (B) 3.5 g
      (C) 6.1 g
      (D) 40 g
      (E) 70 g

13. Most weak acid drugs as well as weak base drugs are absorbed primarily from the small intestine after oral administration because
    (A) Both types are more ionized in the small intestine
    (B) Both types are less ionized in the small intestine
    (C) The blood flow is greater in the small intestine than in other parts of the gut
    (D) The surface area of the small intestine is greater than that of most other parts of the gut
    (E) The small intestine has nonspecific carriers for most drugs

14. The primary site of action of tyramine is
    (A) Preganglionic sympathetic nerve terminals
    (B) Ganglionic receptors
    (C) Postganglionic sympathetic nerve terminals
    (D) Vascular smooth muscle cell receptors
    (E) Gut and liver catechol-O-methyltransferase

15. A semiconscious patient in the intensive care unit is being artificially ventilated. Random spontaneous respiratory movements are rendering the mechanical ventilation ineffective. A useful drug to reduce the patient's ineffective spontaneous respiratory activity is
    (A) Baclofen
    (B) Dantrolene
    (C) Pancuronium
    (D) Pyridostigmine
    (E) Succinylcholine

16. A drug suitable for producing mydriasis and cycloplegia lasting more than 24 hours is
    (A) Atropine
    (B) Echothiophate
    (C) Edrophonium
    (D) Ephedrine
    (E) Tropicamide

17. A 45-year-old surgeon has developed symmetric early morning stiffness in her hands. She wishes to take a nonsteroidal anti-inflammatory drug to relieve these symptoms. Which of the following would provide the longest duration of action?
    (A) Aspirin
    (B) Ibuprofen
    (C) Indomethacin
    (D) Naproxen
    (E) Piroxicam

18. A 59-year-old woman with a 60-pack-year smoking history was diagnosed with lung cancer 2 months ago. She now enters the hospital in coma. Her serum calcium is 16 mg/dL. Which of the following (given with IV fluids) would be most useful to reduce serum calcium rapidly in this patient?
    (A) Acetazolamide
    (B) Furosemide
    (C) Hydrochlorothiazide
    (D) Mannitol
    (E) Spironolactone

19. A 50-year-old man has a macrocytic anemia and early signs of neurologic abnormality. The drug that will probably be required in this case is
    (A) Erythropoietin
    (B) Filgrastim
    (C) Folic acid
    (D) Iron dextran
    (E) Vitamin B_{12}

20. A patient in the coronary care unit has been receiving warfarin for 2 weeks. As a result of this therapy, she will probably have
    (A) Reduced plasma Factor II
    (B) Reduced plasma Factor VIII
    (C) Reduced plasma plasminogen
    (D) Increased tissue plasminogen activator
    (E) Increased platelet adenosine stores

Items 21–22: A 55-year-old man with a strong family history of cardiovascular disease has moderate hypertension and angina pectoris. Blood pressure is 160/109 mm Hg, and the ECG shows left ventricular hypertrophy. The rest of his physical examination and laboratory results are normal. His angina is precipitated by exercise. You have been asked to recommend a drug regimen for both conditions.

21. The antihypertensive drug most likely to aggravate angina pectoris is
    (A) Clonidine
    (B) Guanethidine
    (C) Hydralazine
    (D) Methyldopa
    (E) Propranolol

22. A drug lacking vasodilator properties that is useful in angina is
    (A) Isosorbide dinitrate
    (B) Metoprolol
    (C) Nifedipine
    (D) Nitroglycerin
    (E) Verapamil

23. A substance that reduces arterial clotting of blood (thrombi) is
    (A) Leukotriene B_4
    (B) Prostacyclin
    (C) Prostaglandin E_2
    (D) Prostaglandin $F_{2\alpha}$
    (E) Thromboxane A_2

24. A potent facilitator of platelet aggregation is
    (A) Leukotriene B_4
    (B) Prostacyclin
    (C) Prostaglandin E_2
    (D) Prostaglandin $F_{2\alpha}$
    (E) Thromboxane A_2

25. A drug useful in the treatment of asthma but lacking bronchodilator action is
    (A) Cromolyn
    (B) Ephedrine
    (C) Isoproterenol
    (D) Metaproterenol
    (E) Metoprolol

26. The toxicity of aspirin involves all of the following EXCEPT
    (A) Increased prothrombin levels
    (B) Metabolic acidosis
    (C) Respiratory alkalosis
    (D) Increased risk of peptic ulcers
    (E) Increased risk of hepatic damage and encephalopathy in children with viral infections

27. Although it does not act at any histamine receptor, epinephrine reverses many effects of histamine. Epinephrine is a
    (A) Competitive inhibitor of histamine
    (B) Noncompetitive antagonist of histamine
    (C) Physiologic antagonist of histamine
    (D) Chemical antagonist of histamine
    (E) Metabolic inhibitor of histamine

28. Most drug receptors are
    (A) Small molecules with a molecular weight between 100 and 1000
    (B) Lipids arranged in a bilayer configuration
    (C) Proteins located on cell membranes or in the cytosol
    (D) DNA molecules
    (E) RNA molecules

29. After an intravenous bolus injection of lidocaine, the major factors determining the initial plasma concentration are
    (A) Dose and clearance
    (B) Dose and apparent volume of distribution
    (C) Apparent volume of distribution and clearance

    (D)   Clearance and half-life

    (E)   Half-life and dose

30. The shortest-acting insulin preparation is

    (A)   Human lente

    (B)   Human ultralente

    (C)   Insulin lispro

    (D)   Pork lente

    (E)   Regular crystalline insulin

31. Intravenous administration of norepinephrine in a patient already taking an effective dose of atropine will often

    (A)   Increase heart rate

    (B)   Decrease total peripheral resistance

    (C)   Decrease blood sugar

    (D)   Increase skin temperature

    (E)   Reduce pupil size

32. A 26-year-old woman comes to the outpatient clinic with a complaint of rapid heart rate and easy fatigability. Laboratory workup reveals low hemoglobin and microcytic red cells. The most suitable therapy will be

    (A)   Ferrous sulfate

    (B)   Folic acid

    (C)   Iron dextran

    (D)   Pyridoxine

    (E)   Vitamin B_{12}

33. Which of the following statements is most correct?

    (A)   Maximum efficacy of a drug is directly correlated with its potency

    (B)   The therapeutic index is the LD50 (or TD50) divided by the ED50

    (C)   A partial agonist has no effect on its receptors unless another drug is present

    (D)   Graded dose-response data provide information about the standard deviation of sensitivity to the drug in the population studied

34. The heart rate response to the infusion of a moderate dose of phenylephrine in conscious patients is NOT blocked by

    (A)   Atropine

    (B)   Hexamethonium

    (C)   Phenoxybenzamine

    (D)   Reserpine

    (E)   Scopolamine

35. All of the following statements about scopolamine are correct EXCEPT

    (A)   It has depressant actions on the CNS

    (B)   It may cause hallucinations

    (C)   It is poorly distributed across the placenta to the fetus

    (D)   It may prevent motion sickness when applied as a patch to the skin

    (E)   It is similar to atropine in reducing gastrointestinal motility

36. Which of the following statements about antiplatelet drugs is LEAST correct?

    (A)   Abciximab is an antibody that binds to the platelet fibrin receptor

    (B)   Aspirin inhibits thromboxane synthesis more than it inhibits prostacyclin synthesis

    (C)   Ibuprofen reversibly inhibits cyclooxygenase in platelets

    (D)   Ticlopidine is an inhibitor of the platelet thromboxane receptor

    (E)   Dipyridamole is occasionally used with warfarin in patients with artificial heart valves

37. A 70-year-old man has severe urinary hesitancy associated with benign prostatic hyperplasia. A drug that blocks 5α-reductase in the prostate and other tissues is

    (A)   Cyproterone

    (B)   Finasteride

    (C)   Flutamide

    (D)   Ketoconazole

    (E)   Leuprolide

38. The increase in heart rate and force of cardiac contraction normally induced by electrical stimulation of sympathetic nerves can be blocked by which of the following?

    (A)   Atropine

    (B)   Clonidine

     (C) Hydralazine
     (D) Neostigmine
     (E) Propranolol

39. A treatment of angina that consistently decreases the heart rate and that can prevent vasospastic angina attacks is
     (A) Isosorbide dinitrate
     (B) Nifedipine
     (C) Nitroglycerin
     (D) Propranolol
     (E) Verapamil

40. Verapamil and diltiazem diminish the symptoms of angina pectoris by causing all of the following EXCEPT
     (A) Reduction in blood pressure
     (B) Reduction in heart rate
     (C) Reduction in cardiac contractile force
     (D) Increase in heart size
     (E) Increase in diastolic interval

41. In a study of diuretics, a new drug was given twice daily for 8 days. The following data were obtained.

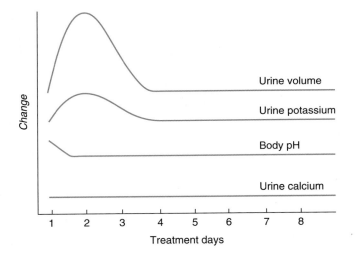

    Which of the following mechanisms best explains the effects shown on the graph?
     (A) Carbonic anhydrase inhibition
     (B) Blockade of a $Na^+/K^+/2Cl^-$ transporter in the ascending limb of the loop of Henle
     (C) Blockade of an NaCl transporter in the distal convoluted tubule
     (D) Osmotic diuresis
     (E) Block of aldosterone in the cortical collecting tubule

42. Diuretics that increase the delivery of poorly absorbed solute to the thick ascending limb of the nephron include
     (A) Furosemide
     (B) Indapamide
     (C) Mannitol
     (D) Spironolactone
     (E) All of the above

Items 43–44: A 65-year-old man with cardiomyopathy has recurrent congestive heart failure. Addition of digitalis to his regimen is being considered.

43. In a patient receiving digoxin for congestive heart failure, conditions that may facilitate the appearance of toxicity include

(A) Hyperkalemia
(B) Hypernatremia
(C) Hypocalcemia
(D) Hypomagnesemia
(E) All of the above

44. Causes of digitalis toxicity include
    (A) Intracellular calcium overload
    (B) Intracellular potassium overload
    (C) Increased parasympathetic activity
    (D) Increased adrenocorticosteroid levels
    (E) All of the above

45. Methylxanthine drugs such as aminophylline cause all of the following EXCEPT
    (A) Vasodilation in many vascular beds
    (B) Increase in the amount of cAMP in mast cells
    (C) Bronchodilation
    (D) Activation of the enzyme phosphodiesterase

46. Drugs used in asthma that often cause tachycardia and tremor include
    (A) Beclomethasone
    (B) Cromolyn sodium
    (C) Ipratropium
    (D) Isoproterenol
    (E) All of the above

47. Drugs with potentially useful effects in the treatment of inoperable metastatic pheochromocytoma include all of the following EXCEPT
    (A) Phenoxybenzamine
    (B) Phentolamine
    (C) Propranolol
    (D) Reserpine
    (E) Metyrosine

48. Agents that can readily cause edema if released or injected near capillaries include
    (A) Angiotensin II
    (B) Epinephrine
    (C) Histamine
    (D) Norepinephrine
    (E) Serotonin

49. Typical results of beta-receptor activation include all of the following EXCEPT
    (A) Hyperglycemia
    (B) Lipolysis
    (C) Glycogenolysis
    (D) Decreased skeletal muscle tremor
    (E) Increased renin secretion

50. A patient has been taking aspirin for rheumatoid arthritis for 8 years. Exacerbations are becoming worse, and she asks the physician about drugs that might stop the progression of the disease. All of the following are disease-modifying (slow-acting) antirheumatic drugs EXCEPT
    (A) Auranofin
    (B) Hydroxychloroquine
    (C) Ibuprofen
    (D) Methotrexate
    (E) Penicillamine

51. A neuronal cell body is located in the locus ceruleus, with fine axonal projections to most brain levels. The neurotransmitter that it releases, which can be either excitatory or inhibitory, is most likely to be
    (A) Acetylcholine
    (B) Dopamine
    (C) Glutamic acid
    (D) Norepinephrine
    (E) Serotonin

Items 52–53: A 40-year-old man had been consuming alcoholic beverages at lunch and in the evenings all his adult life. During the last 2 years, his alcohol consumption had steadily increased, continuing throughout the day. In response to family pressures, he abruptly stopped drinking alcohol, and within a few hours he became increasingly anxious and agitated and showed symptoms of autonomic hyperexcitability. He developed a hand tremor and the following day had delusions and visual hallucinations. At this point, he was brought to the hospital.

52. Which of the following statements about the chronic consumption of alcohol in this patient is most accurate?

(A) Because of his gender, he is more susceptible to hepatotoxicity than a female in the same situation

(B) Intravenous thiamine will reverse the symptoms he is experiencing

(C) The rate of his metabolism of ethanol is dependent on its blood level

(D) He is probably tolerant to ethanol as a result of an increase in the activity of liver alcohol dehydrogenase

(E) Delirium tremens would be an appropriate preliminary diagnosis of his present condition

53. In the emergency room, the symptoms increased in severity, with hyperreflexia progressing to seizures. He was given an intravenous injection of a drug that controlled the seizure activity and was then hospitalized. During the recovery period, the same agent was used in oral form with gradual dose-tapering. The drug most likely to have been used is

(A) Clonidine

(B) Diazepam

(C) Haloperidol

(D) Phenytoin

(E) Propranolol

54. The pharmacokinetic characteristics of several hydantoin derivatives, each with anticonvulsant activity equivalent to that of phenytoin, were examined in phase I clinical trials. The rationale was to identify a drug with more desirable kinetic properties than those of phenytoin.

Drug	Oral Bioavailability (%)	Plasma Protein Binding (%)	Elimination Kinetics	Cytochrome P450 Induction
ABC	10	90	First order	++
DEF	90	50	First order	++
GHI	50	98	Zero order	None
JKL	85	10	First order	None
MNO	95	10	First order	++

Based on the data shown in the table above, which drug has the optimal pharmacokinetic properties for oral use in the management of patients with seizure disorders?

(A) ABC

(B) DEF

(C) GHI

(D) JKL

(E) MNO

55. Which of the following statements concerning anesthetic agents is most accurate?

(A) Anesthetic potency is quantitated by the minimum alveolar concentration (MAC) that causes 50% of subjects to fail to respond to a standardized painful stimulus

(B) General anesthesia is associated with increased blood pressure and total peripheral resistance

(C) If an anesthetic agent is very soluble in the blood, it will have a relatively fast onset of action

(D) Inhalational agents are used for long procedures because intravenous anesthetics are too toxic to use for more than a few minutes

(E) The state of surgical anesthesia is associated with complete muscle paralysis

56. A patient is to undergo day surgery for a short procedure, and intravenous anesthesia will be used. Which of the following statements about the intravenous anesthetic agents is most accurate?
    (A) Emesis is more likely to occur with propofol than with other agents
    (B) Hypotension is the major limitation to the use of ketamine
    (C) Postoperative respiratory depression due to midazolam may be attenuated by flumazenil
    (D) The main value of fentanyl is its ability to cause muscle relaxation
    (E) Thiopental is likely to increase cerebral blood flow

57. A patient with terminal cancer is suffering from pain that is gradually increasing in intensity. In the management of pain in such a patient
    (A) Addiction occurs universally in the later stages of the disease because of the very large opioid doses required
    (B) To delay the development of addiction, opioid analgesics should never be given for initial management of chronic pain
    (C) Meperidine is more effective than morphine in cancer pain states
    (D) Nonsteroidal anti-inflammatory drugs may control symptoms during a significant portion of the course of the disease
    (E) The placebo effect is absent

58. Which one of the following effects of the opioid analgesics is mediated via activation of mu receptors?
    (A) Decreased gastrointestinal peristalsis
    (B) Elevation of arterial P_{CO_2}
    (C) Emesis
    (D) Miosis
    (E) Vasodilation

59. Recreational use of drugs sometimes leads to dependence. Which of the following is LEAST likely to lead to dependence?
    (A) Amphetamine
    (B) Cocaine
    (C) Heroin
    (D) Mescaline
    (E) Secobarbital

60. This agent is currently a first-choice drug in the management of absence seizures and partial, primary generalized, and tonic-clonic seizures.
    (A) Carbamazepine
    (B) Clonazepam
    (C) Ethosuximide
    (D) Phenytoin
    (E) Valproic acid

61. If one patient is taking amitriptyline and another is taking chlorpromazine, they are BOTH likely to experience
    (A) Amnesia
    (B) Extrapyramidal dysfunction
    (C) Gynecomastia
    (D) Increased gastrointestinal motility
    (E) Postural hypotension

62. The following data concern the relative activities of hypothetical investigational drugs as blockers of the membrane transporters (reuptake systems) for three CNS neurotransmitters.

| Drug | Blocking Actions on CNS Transporters for | | |
	Dopamine	Serotonin	Norepinephrine
UCSF 1	+++	None	None
UCSF 2	+++	++++	++
UCSF 3	None	++	++
UCSF 4	None	+++	++
UCSF 5	+	+	None

Number of + signs denotes intensity of blocking actions.

Which one of the drugs is likely to be effective in the treatment of major depressive disorders but may also cause marked adverse effects, including thought disorders, delusions, hallucinations, and paranoia?

(A) UCSF 1

(B) UCSF 2

(C) UCSF 3

(D) UCSF 4

(E) UCSF 5

63. A 38-year-old divorced woman who lived alone visited a psychiatrist because she was depressed. Her symptoms included low self-esteem, with frequent ruminations on her worthlessness, and hypersomnia. She was hyperphagic as well and complained that her limbs felt heavy. An initial diagnosis was made of major depressive disorder with atypical symptoms. Treatment was initiated with amitriptyline, but after 2 months the patient had not improved significantly. Since this depressed patient had atypical symptoms, amitriptyline was terminated. Treatment should be started now with

(A) Buspirone

(B) Doxepin

(C) Phenelzine

(D) Methylphenidate

(E) Risperidone

64. Psychiatric evaluation of a patient after 6 weeks of treatment with a monoamine oxidase (MAO) inhibitor shows no improvement. The psychiatrist now writes a prescription for fluoxetine, which the patient starts 2 days after her final dose of the MAO inhibitor. Since the MAO inhibitors used as antidepressants continue to exert effects for 2 or more weeks after discontinuance, the most likely result of the administration of fluoxetine will now be to cause

(A) A rapid amelioration of her depressive symptoms

(B) ECG abnormalities

(C) Extrapyramidal dysfunction

(D) The serotonin syndrome

(E) Weight gain

65. The phenothiazines have a variety of actions at different receptor types. Which of the following receptor types are they LEAST likely to act on?

(A) Dopamine receptors

(B) Histamine receptors

(C) Nicotine receptors

(D) Norepinephrine receptors

(E) Muscarine receptors

66. Which of the following statements about tardive dyskinesias is most accurate?

(A) Symptoms may be temporarily alleviated by raising antipsychotic drug dosage

(B) Their severity can be reduced by muscarinic receptor blocking drugs

(C) They occur during the first few weeks of treatment with antipsychotic drugs

(D) Clozapine is likely to exacerbate the symptoms

(E) They are parkinsonism-like movement disorders

67. A psychiatric patient on medication develops a tremor, thyroid enlargement, and leukocytosis. The drug he is taking is most likely to be

(A) Clomipramine

(B) Haloperidol

(C) Isocarboxazid

(D) Lithium

(E) Sertraline

68. The mechanism of action of benzodiazepines is

(A) Activation of $GABA_B$ receptors

(B) Antagonism of glycine receptors in the spinal cord

(C) Blockade of the action of glutamic acid

(D) Increased GABA-mediated chloride ion conductance

(E) Inhibition of GABA transaminase

69. A drug that is used in the treatment of parkinsonism and that will also attenuate reversible extrapyramidal side effects of neuroleptics is

(A) Amantadine

    (B) Levodopa
    (C) Pergolide
    (D) Selegiline
    (E) Trihexyphenidyl

70. Following a very large overdose of a benzodiazepine, a patient is admitted to the hospital. Subsequent management of this patient is LEAST likely to include
    (A) Administration of naloxone
    (B) Gastric lavage if an endotracheal tube is in place
    (C) Intravenous flumazenil
    (D) Protection of the airway
    (E) Ventilatory support

71. A 65-year-old man with bacteremia is to be treated with a combination of antibiotics. The amikacin included in the drug regimen is LEAST likely to be effective against
    (A) *B fragilis*
    (B) *E coli*
    (C) *Enterobacter* species
    (D) *K pneumoniae*
    (E) *Serratia marcescens*

72. If an aerobic gram-negative rod causing bacteremia proves to be resistant to amikacin, the mechanism of resistance is most likely due to
    (A) Changed pathway of bacterial folate synthesis
    (B) Decreased intracellular accumulation of the drug
    (C) Drug inactivation by bacterial group transferases
    (D) Induced synthesis of beta-lactamases
    (E) Production of drug-trapping thiol compounds

73. The characteristics of once-daily dosing with aminoglycosides compared with conventional dosing protocols (every 6–12 hours) include
    (A) Decreased drug uptake into the renal cortex
    (B) Higher peak serum drug levels to MIC ratios
    (C) Postantibiotic actions
    (D) All of the above
    (E) None of the above

74. Beta-lactamase production by strains of *Haemophilus influenzae, Moraxella catarrhalis,* and *Neisseria gonorrhoeae* confers resistance against penicillin G. Which one of the following antibiotics is most likely to be effective against all strains of each of the above organisms?
    (A) Ampicillin
    (B) Ceftriaxone
    (C) Clindamycin
    (D) Gentamicin
    (E) Piperacillin

Items 75–76: A 36-year-old patient is hospitalized following injuries sustained in an automobile accident. After several days, he develops a urinary tract infection due to *Pseudomonas aeruginosa.* Current drug treatment of the patient is limited to opioid analgesics and ibuprofen for pain. Past drug history of the patient includes a mild skin rash following treatment of otitis media with cefaclor. The following data show the antimicrobial sensitivity of aerobic isolates from urine sources in the hospital.

Organism	Percentage of Isolates From Urine Sources Susceptible to				
	Ampicillin	**Ciprofloxacin**	**Gentamicin**	**Ceftazidime**	**Piperacillin**
E coli	50	99	98	100	50
K pneumoniae	5	100	99	100	50
P mirabilis	90	98	98	100	90
P aeruginosa	0	76	81	94	92
S marcescens	8	70	80	85	82
S aureus	13	87	0	0	13
S epidermidis	14	67	0	0	12

75. If a single drug is to be administered to this patient, the most appropriate choice in terms of efficacy and safety is
   (A) Ampicillin
   (B) Ceftazidime
   (C) Ciprofloxacin
   (D) Gentamicin
   (E) Piperacillin

76. Since the mortality rate approaches 50% in patients who develop sepsis due to *Pseudomonas aeruginosa,* it may be advisable to treat the patient with a combination of antibiotics known to have synergistic activity against this microorganism. The best regimen would be the combination of
   (A) Ampicillin and gentamicin
   (B) Ceftazidime and piperacillin
   (C) Ciprofloxacin and ampicillin
   (D) Gentamicin and piperacillin
   (E) Piperacillin and vancomycin

77. A 24-year-old woman with a young infant is to be treated with ciprofloxacin for a urinary tract infection. In providing the patient with information about the ciprofloxacin, which of the following would be LEAST correct?
   (A) Antacids taken concomitantly may interfere with oral absorption of ciprofloxacin
   (B) Ciprofloxacin will also be effective against an accompanying yeast infection
   (C) If she is breast-feeding, she should stop while taking ciprofloxacin
   (D) Ciprofloxacin has caused tendonitis in some patients
   (E) Ciprofloxacin may make her light-headed, dizzy, or drowsy

78. A 19-year-old woman with recurrent sinusitis has been treated with different antibiotics on several occasions. During the course of one such treatment, she developed severe diarrhea and was hospitalized. Sigmoidoscopy revealed colitis, and pseudomembranes were confirmed histologically. Which of the following drugs, administered orally, is LEAST likely to be effective in the treatment of colitis due to *C difficile?*
   (A) Bacitracin
   (B) Cefotetan
   (C) Metronidazole
   (D) Vancomycin
   (E) All of the above drugs will be effective

79. In the management of patients with AIDS, the sulfonamides are often used in combination with inhibitors of folate reductase. However, such combinations have minimal activity against
   (A) Methicillin-resistant staphylococcal species
   (B) *Nocardia* species
   (C) *Pneumocystis carinii*
   (D) *Toxoplasma gondii*
   (E) *Treponema pallidum*

Items 80–81: A patient with metastatic choriocarcinoma was treated first with methotrexate plus dactinomycin and subsequently with a combination of cisplatin and vincristine. In both regimens, drug dosage was maximized to a toxicity limit of a 2-log decrease in blood platelets. The effects of chemotherapy were monitored by urinary chorionic gonadotropin (UCG, units/24 h), as shown in the data below.

Drug Regimen	Urinary Chorionic Gonadotropin (units per 24 h)	
	Initial	After Treatment
Methotrexate plus dactinomycin	10^8	10^5
Cisplatin plus vincristine	10^7	10^3

80. Which one of the following statements about the data is most accurate?
    (A) The maximal effect of methotrexate plus dactinomycin was a 2-log decrease in UCG
    (B) The drug-induced changes in UCG are directly proportional to decreases in platelet count
    (C) The maximal effect of the cisplatin plus vincristine regimen was a 4-log decrease in UCG
    (D) The effects of the anticancer drugs on UCG have a direct relationship to cell kill
    (E) The final UCG demonstrates that the patient was cured
81. All of the following statements about the drugs used in this case are accurate EXCEPT
    (A) Cardiotoxicity is the dose-limiting toxicity of dactinomycin
    (B) Leucovorin rescue should be employed during and after treatment with methotrexate
    (C) Methotrexate and vincristine are both cell cycle–specific drugs
    (D) Saline hydration will be employed during treatment with cisplatin to reduce its nephrotoxicity
    (E) The cisplatin plus vincristine regimen is likely to be neurotoxic
82. A 20-year-old foreign exchange student attending college in California is to be treated for pulmonary tuberculosis contracted while he was living in Southeast Asia. Since drug resistance is anticipated, the proposed antibiotic regimen for treatment includes ethambutol, isoniazid (with supplementary vitamin B_6), pyrazinamide, and rifampin. Provided that his disease responds well to the drug regimen, it would be appropriate after 2 months to
    (A) Change his drug regimen to prophylaxis with isoniazid
    (B) Discontinue pyrazinamide
    (C) Establish baseline ocular function
    (D) Monitor amylase activity
    (E) Stop the supplementary vitamin B_6
83. Which one of the following statements about the pharmacodynamics of antifungal drugs is most accurate?
    (A) Amphotericin B blocks the conversion of lanosterol to ergosterol
    (B) Flucytosine is currently the drug of choice for esophageal candidiasis
    (C) Griseofulvin inhibits hepatic cytochrome P450
    (D) Ketoconazole binds to ergosterol to form artificial pores in fungal cell membranes
    (E) Oral fluconazole is prophylactic against fungal meningitis

Items 84–85: A 20-year-old college student is brought to the emergency room after taking an overdose of a nonprescription drug. The patient is confused and lethargic. He has been hyperventilating and is now dehydrated, with an elevated temperature. Serum analyses demonstrate that the patient has an anion gap metabolic acidosis.

84. The most likely cause of these signs and symptoms is overdosage of
    (A) Aspirin
    (B) Acetaminophen
    (C) Dextromethorphan
    (D) Diphenhydramine
    (E) Ethanol
85. In the management of this patient, which one of the following procedures is LEAST appropriate?
    (A) Alkalinization of the urine
    (B) Correction of metabolic acidosis and electrolyte imbalance
    (C) Gastric lavage with endotracheal tube in place
    (D) Hemodialysis, if pH or CNS signs are not readily controlled
    (E) Universal antidote administration
86. A young mother is breast-feeding her 2-month-old infant. Which one of the following drug situations involving the mother is most likely to be safe for the nursing infant?
    (A) Doxycycline, for Lyme disease
    (B) Metronidazole, for trichomoniasis
    (C) Nystatin, for a yeast infection
    (D) Phentermine, used for weight reduction
    (E) Triazolam, used as a sleeping pill
87. Chemoprophylaxis for travelers to geographic regions where *P falciparum* is endemic is best provided by
    (A) Chloroquine
    (B) Mefloquine

    (C) Primaquine
    (D) Pyrimethamine plus sulfadoxine
    (E) Quinine

88. Which one of the following statements about mebendazole is LEAST accurate?
    (A) It is the drug of choice for hookworm and pinworm infections
    (B) It causes the Mazzotti reaction, which is due to toxic products from dying worms
    (C) It should be avoided in pregnancy
    (D) It inhibits microtubule aggregation
    (E) It has a high therapeutic index

89. In patients with chronic granulomatous disease, which of the following agents increases the synthesis of tumor necrosis factor, leading to activation of phagocytosis?
    (A) Aldesleukin
    (B) Cyclosporine
    (C) Filgrastim
    (D) Interferon gamma-1b
    (E) Levamisole

90. A 43-year-old woman was brought to a hospital emergency room by her brother. Visiting the halfway house in which she lived, he had found her to be lethargic, with slurred speech. The patient had a long history of treatment of psychiatric problems, and the brother feared that she might have overdosed on one or more of the several drugs that had been prescribed for her. Physical examination revealed tachycardia with irregular heart rate, shallow respiration, decreased bowel sounds, dilated pupils, and hyperthermia. ECG revealed a widened QRS complex with diffuse T wave changes. If this patient had taken a drug overdose, the most likely causative agent was
    (A) Clozapine
    (B) Fluoxetine
    (C) Lithium
    (D) Thioridazine
    (E) Zolpidem

91. Cocaine intoxication has become a common problem in hospital emergency rooms. All of the following drugs have proved useful in the management of cocaine overdose EXCEPT
    (A) Dantrolene
    (B) Diazepam
    (C) Lidocaine
    (D) Naltrexone
    (E) Nitroprusside

Items 92–93: A 30-year-old hospitalized AIDS patient has a CD4 cell count of 50/μL. He is being treated with an anti-HIV drug "cocktail" composed of zidovudine (ZDV), lamivudine (3TC), and indinavir. Other drugs being administered include acyclovir, clarithromycin, foscarnet, rifabutin, and trimethoprim-sulfamethoxazole.

92. Which one of the following statements about the drug management of this patient is most accurate?
    (A) Acyclovir is highly effective in CMV infections
    (B) Foscarnet has activity against TK⁻ strains of HSV
    (C) Indinavir induces the formation of liver drug-metabolizing enzymes
    (D) Pancreatitis is the dose-limiting toxicity of zidovudine
    (E) Viral RNA will be undetectable in the blood of this patient

93. None of the drugs being administered to this patient are useful for prophylaxis against, or treatment of, opportunistic infections due to
    (A) *Candida albicans*
    (B) Cytomegalovirus
    (C) *M avium-intracellulare*
    (D) *Pneumocystis carinii*
    (E) *Toxoplasma gondii*

94. After an all-night party, a 38-year-old man is brought to the emergency room at 5 AM by friends. In the early morning hours, the patient had become very happy, excited, and talkative. An hour later, he had become dizzy and quite pale and then vomited. Subsequently, his friends noticed that his lips and fingers were twitching and that he seemed to be hallucinating. In the

hospital, the physical examination reveals a well-dressed, apparently affluent young man who is agitated and incoherent. His blood pressure is 180/110 mm Hg, heart rate 100/min, and respiratory rate 20/min. Other signs and symptoms include pale and dry mucous membranes, mydriasis, hyperthermia, and increased deep tendon reflexes. The most reasonable preliminary diagnosis in this case is that the patient is intoxicated by

- (A) Cocaine
- (B) Ethanol
- (C) Flunitrazepam
- (D) Hashish
- (E) Heroin

95. Which one of the following is LEAST characteristic of chronic lead poisoning?
- (A) Acute tubular necrosis
- (B) Specific x-ray findings
- (C) Hemorrhagic pulmonary edema
- (D) Microcytic hypochromic anemia
- (E) Radial nerve palsy

DIRECTIONS: The following section consists of lists of three to twenty-six lettered options followed by several numbered items. For each numbered item, select the ONE option that is most closely associated with it. Each answer may be selected once, more than once, or not at all.

Items 96–100:
- (A) 3-Methoxy-4-hydroxy mandelic acid
- (B) Botulinum toxin
- (C) Captopril
- (D) Cocaine
- (E) Guanethidine
- (F) Methyldopa
- (G) Prazosin
- (H) Reserpine
- (I) Saxitoxin
- (J) Tetrodotoxin

96. A drug that blocks a carrier mechanism located in the membrane of synaptic transmitter storage vesicles
97. A prodrug that is converted into the active form in the brain
98. A substance that inhibits reuptake of norepinephrine into sympathetic nerve terminals
99. A toxic substance that is synthesized in protozoans and concentrated in shellfish
100. A substance that prevents release of transmitter from cholinergic nerve endings

Items 101–105:

(A)	Amitriptyline	(J)	Ketamine	(R)	Risperidone
(B)	Benztropine	(K)	Levorphanol	(S)	Selegiline
(C)	Carbamazepine	(L)	Methadone	(T)	Trifluoperazine
(D)	Chlorpromazine	(M)	MPTP (*N*-methyl-4-phe-	(U)	Valproic acid
(E)	Disulfiram		nyltetrahydropyridine)	(V)	XTC (MDMA;
(F)	Fentanyl	(N)	Naltrexone		methylene-
(G)	GHB (gamma hydro-	(O)	NMDA (*N*-methyl-D-		dioxymetham-
	xybutyric acid)		aspartic acid)		phetamine)
(H)	Haloperidol	(P)	Paroxetine	(W)	Zolpidem
(I)	Imipramine	(Q)	Pentazocine		

101. A 35-year-old woman who has never been pregnant suffers from pain, discomfort, and mood depression every month at the time of menses. She may benefit from the use of this selective inhibitor of the reuptake of serotonin, which was recently approved for the management of premenstrual tension.

102. A 23-year-old heroin addict was brought to a hospital suffering from marked bradykinesia, muscle rigidity, and tremor at rest. Unfortunately, the extrapyramidal dysfunction was permanent in this patient, since he had used this home-synthesized agent that is cytotoxic to nigro-striatal dopaminergic neurons.

103. This drug is moderately effective for the relief of pain, but if administered prior to morphine, it may temporarily interfere with the actions of the stronger analgesic. Based on its interactions with different types of opioid receptors, this drug is classified as a mixed agonist-antagonist.

104. A 24-year-old schizophrenic man has been treated for several years with standard antipsychotic drugs, but extrapyramidal effects are worsening and are not alleviated by concomitant use of muscarinic receptor blocking agents. This drug would be potentially useful since it reduces many of the positive symptoms of schizophrenia without causing marked extrapyramidal dysfunction; it has a greater affinity for serotonin receptors than for dopamine receptors in the CNS.

105. A 44-year-old patient suffering from alcoholism enters a residential treatment program that emphasizes group therapy but uses pharmacologic agents adjunctively. In this patient, this drug appears to decrease the craving for alcohol, possibly by interference with the neuroregulatory functions of opioid peptides.

Items 106–110:

(A)	Amphotericin B	**(I)**	Doxycycline	**(Q)**	Nafcillin
(B)	Ampicillin	**(J)**	Erythromycin	**(R)**	Norfloxacin
(C)	Bleomycin	**(K)**	Fluorouracil	**(S)**	Procarbazine
(D)	Busulfan	**(L)**	Ganciclovir	**(T)**	Rifampin
(E)	Cefoxitin	**(M)**	Isoniazid	**(U)**	Ritonavir
(F)	Cyclophosphamide	**(N)**	Methotrexate	**(V)**	Vancomycin
(G)	Cyclosporine	**(O)**	Mechlorethamine	**(W)**	Vincristine
(H)	Doxorubicin	**(P)**	Methicillin	**(X)**	Zidovudine

106. A 32-year-old woman presents with left lower quadrant abdominal pain and a purulent vaginal discharge, which on Gram's stain revealed gram-negative rods. The preliminary diagnosis is pelvic inflammatory disease, and bacteriologic tests subsequently identify *Bacteroides fragilis*. This cell wall synthesis inhibitor is normally considered a drug of first choice in pelvic inflammatory disease caused by anaerobic gram-negative rods.

107. This agent, which is used in the chemotherapy of Hodgkin's lymphoma, is potentially leukemogenic.

108. The most effective drug combination regimens used for Hodgkin's disease and in the chemotherapy of testicular carcinoma include this antineoplastic agent. Side effects of the drug commonly involve pulmonary dysfunction and blisters on the palms of the hands or the soles of the feet.

109. A high school student presents with headache, fever, and cough of 2 days' duration. Sputum is scant and nonpurulent, and Gram's stain reveals many white cells but no organisms. Since this patient appears to have an atypical pneumonia, you should initiate treatment with this drug.

110. This bactericidal drug is representative of a class of antibiotics that interfere with nucleic acid functions. Their overuse in the last decade has led to the emergence of resistant strains of gram-positive cocci, including pneumococci and staphylococci. The drug is not recommended for use in patients under 18 years of age.

Items 111–113:

(A) Etidronate
(B) Glyburide
(C) Norgestrel
(D) Oxandrolone
(E) Tamoxifen

111. A drug that is used for Paget's disease and has been shown to reduce fractures in patients with osteoporosis

112. A drug that closes potassium channels, depolarizing its target cells and causing the release of a peptide hormone

113. A modified androgenic steroid used for increasing muscle mass

Items 114–115: An anesthetized subject was given an IV bolus dose of a drug **(Drug 1)** while blood pressure (color) and heart rate were recorded, as shown on the left side of the graph below. While the recorder was stopped, **Drug 2** was given (center). **Drug 1** was then administered again, as shown on the right side of the graph.

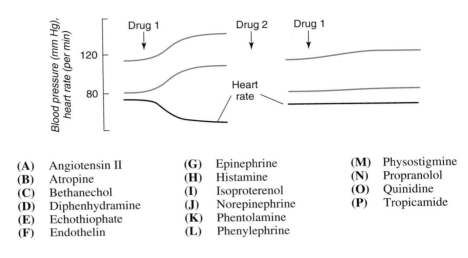

(A) Angiotensin II	**(G)** Epinephrine	**(M)** Physostigmine
(B) Atropine	**(H)** Histamine	**(N)** Propranolol
(C) Bethanechol	**(I)** Isoproterenol	**(O)** Quinidine
(D) Diphenhydramine	**(J)** Norepinephrine	**(P)** Tropicamide
(E) Echothiophate	**(K)** Phentolamine	
(F) Endothelin	**(L)** Phenylephrine	

114. Identify Drug 1 from the above list
115. Identify Drug 2 from the above list

Item 116:
- **(A)** Atropine
- **(B)** Bretylium
- **(C)** Epinephrine
- **(D)** Flecainide
- **(E)** Fluoxetine
- **(F)** Lidocaine
- **(G)** Nitroglycerin
- **(H)** Prazosin
- **(I)** Propranolol
- **(J)** Quinine

116. A cardiac Purkinje fiber was isolated from an animal heart and placed in a recording chamber. One of the Purkinje cells was impaled with a microelectrode, and action potentials were recorded while the preparation was stimulated at one stimulus per second. A representative control action potential is shown in black in the graph. After equilibration, a drug was added to the perfusate while recording continued. A representative action potential obtained at the peak of drug action is shown as the superimposed action potential (color). Identify the drug from the above list.

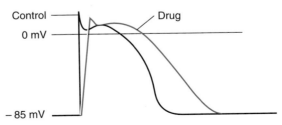

Items 117–120:
- **(A)** Calcitonin
- **(B)** Diazoxide

(C) Glucagon
(D) Metformin
(E) Nitric oxide
(F) Pamidronate
(G) Propylthiouracil
(H) Thyroxine
(I) Tolbutamide
(J) Troglitazone

117. A drug used in hyperthyroidism that inhibits the organification of iodine (the coupling of iodine to tyrosine)

118. A nonprotein drug used in non-insulin-dependent diabetes that increases tissue sensitivity to insulin and reduces hyperinsulinemia

119. A drug that opens potassium channels in cells that secrete insulin-like peptides and reduces insulin concentration in the blood

120. A biguanide oral hypoglycemic agent; effective even in the absence of insulin-secreting pancreatic cells

Answer Key for Examination 1*

1. D (5)	34. D (9)	71. A (45, 51)	
2. B (1)	35. C (8)	72. C (45)	
3. B (26)	36. D (34)	73. D (45)	
4. B (9, 13, 20)	37. B (40)	74. B (43, 51)	
5. B (17)	38. E (10)	75. E (43, 51)	
6. C (16)	39. E (12)	76. D (43, 45)	
7. E (14)	40. D (12)	77. B (46)	
8. E (14, 15)	41. A (15)	78. B (43, 51)	
9. B (11, 15)	42. C (15)	79. E (46, 53)	
10. A (7)	43. D (13)	80. C (55)	
11. A (7)	44. A (13)	81. A (55)	
12. B (3)	45. D (20)	82. B (47)	
13. D (1)	46. D (20)	83. E (48)	
14. C (6, 9)	47. D (10, 11)	84. A (36, 59)	
15. C (27)	48. C (16)	85. E (59)	
16. A (8)	49. D (9)	86. C (48)	
17. E (36)	50. C (36)	87. B (53)	
18. B (15)	51. D (21)	88. B (54)	
19. E (33)	52. E (23, 32)	89. D (56)	
20. A (33)	53. B (22, 23, 59)	90. D (30, 59)	
21. C (11, 12)	54. D (3, 24)	91. D (58)	
22. B (12)	55. A (25)	92. B (49)	
23. B (18)	56. C (22, 25)	93. A (48, 49)	
24. E (18)	57. D (31, 36)	94. A (32, 59)	
25. A (20)	58. B (31)	95. C (32, 59)	
26. A (36)	59. D (32)	96. H (11)	
27. C (2)	60. E (24)	97. F (11)	
28. C (1)	61. E (29, 30)	98. D (6)	
29. B (3)	62. B (29, 30)	99. I (6)	
30. C (41)	63. C (30)	100. B (6)	
31. A (6, 8, 9)	64. D (30)	101. P (30)	
32. A (33)	65. C (29)	102. M (28, 32)	
33. B (2)	66. A (29)	103. Q (31)	
	67. D (29)	104. R (29)	
	68. D (21, 22)	105. N (23, 31)	
	69. E (28, 29)	106. E (43, 51)	
	70. A (22, 59)	107. S (55)	

*Numbers in parentheses are chapters in which answers may be found.

108. C (55)
109. J (44, 51)
110. R (46)
111. A (42)
112. B (41)

113. D (40)
114. L (9)
115. K (10)
116. J (14)
117. G (38)

118. J (41)
119. B (41)
120. D (41)

DIRECTIONS: Each numbered item or incomplete statement in this section is followed by answers or by completions of the statement. Select the ONE lettered answer or completion that is BEST in each case.

1. Common effects of muscarinic stimulant drugs include all of the following EXCEPT
    (A)   Increased secretion by salivary glands
    (B)   Increased peristalsis
    (C)   Mydriasis
    (D)   Stimulation of sweat glands
    (E)   Tachycardia

2. Which of the following statements about nitric oxide is LEAST accurate?
    (A)   Nitric oxide is synthesized in vascular endothelium and the brain.
    (B)   Nitric oxide is released from storage vesicles by acetylcholine
    (C)   Nitric oxide is released from exogenous molecules, eg, nitrates and nitroprusside
    (D)   Nitric oxide synthase is stimulated by histamine
    (E)   Nitric oxide synthase exists in both inducible and constitutive forms

3. With regard to distribution of a drug from the blood into tissues
    (A)   Blood flow to the tissue is an important determinant
    (B)   Solubility of the drug in the tissue is an important determinant
    (C)   Concentration of the drug in the blood is an important determinant
    (D)   Size (volume) of the tissue is an important determinant
    (E)   All of the above are important determinants

4. Receptors that communicate their activation by turning on an integral intracellular tyrosine kinase are typically
    (A)   Acetylcholine or GABA channels
    (B)   G protein-coupled
    (C)   Insulin or epidermal growth factor receptors
    (D)   Steroid receptors
    (E)   Vitamin D receptors

5. A patient with an arrhythmia is to receive lidocaine by constant IV infusion. The target plasma concentration is 3 mg/L. The pharmacokinetic parameters for lidocaine in the general population are: V_d 70 L, CL 35 L/h, and $t_{1/2}$ 1.4 hours. An infusion is begun. The plasma concentration of lidocaine is measured 2.8 hours later and reported to be 1.5 mg/L. This indicates that the final steady state plasma concentration in this patient will be
    (A)   1.5 mg/L
    (B)   2.0 mg/L
    (C)   3.0 mg/L
    (D)   6.0 mg/L
    (E)   Insufficient data to answer

6. A new drug is to be evaluated. Before human trials are begun, FDA regulations require that
    (A)   The drug be studied in three mammalian species
    (B)   All acute and chronic animal toxicity data be submitted to the FDA
    (C)   The drug must be shown to be safe in animals with the target disease
    (D)   The drug must be shown to be free of carcinogenic effects
    (E)   The effect of the drug on reproduction must be studied in at least two animal species

7. A drug that blocks the heart rate effect of a slow IV infusion of phenylephrine is
   (A) Atropine
   (B) Haloperidol
   (C) Physostigmine
   (D) Pilocarpine
   (E) Propranolol

8. A patient is admitted to the emergency room with orthostatic hypotension and evidence of marked GI bleeding. Which of the following most accurately describes the probable autonomic response to this bleeding?
   (A) Slow heart rate, dilated pupils, damp skin
   (B) Rapid heart rate, dilated pupils, damp skin
   (C) Slow heart rate, dry skin, increased bowel sounds
   (D) Rapid heart rate, dry skin, constricted pupils, increased bowel sounds
   (E) Rapid heart rate, constricted pupils, warm skin

9. A patient has open-angle glaucoma. The LEAST likely drug for this condition is
   (A) Acetazolamide
   (B) Epinephrine
   (C) Isoproterenol
   (D) Pilocarpine
   (E) Timolol

10. A new drug was administered to a group of normal volunteers. Intravenous bolus doses produced the changes in blood pressure and heart rate shown in the graph below. The most probable receptor affinities of this new drug are
    (A) Alpha$_1$, alpha$_2$, and beta$_1$
    (B) Alpha$_1$ and alpha$_2$ only
    (C) Beta$_1$ and beta$_2$ only
    (D) Muscarinic M$_3$ only
    (E) Nicotinic N$_N$ only

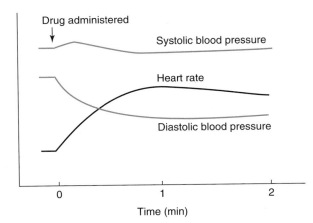

Time (min)

11. A 14-year-old boy is developing signs of anaphylaxis after an injection of penicillin in the doctor's office. Probable effects of an IM injection of epinephrine include all of the following EXCEPT
    (A) Hypoglycemia
    (B) Leukocytosis
    (C) Hyperkalemia
    (D) Tachycardia
    (E) Bronchodilation

12. Infusion of phentolamine into the cerebrospinal fluid of an experimental animal will prevent the blood pressure-lowering action of
    (A) Clonidine
    (B) Enalapril
    (C) Guanethidine
    (D) Reserpine
    (E) Trimethaphan

Items 13–14: A 52-year-old plumber comes to the office with a complaint of periodic onset of chest pain—described as a sensation of heavy pressure over the sternum—that comes on when he exercises and disappears within 15 minutes when he stops exerting himself. After a full physical examination and further evaluation, you make the diagnosis of angina of effort.

13. In considering medical therapy for this patient, which of the following correctly describes the beneficial action of nitroglycerin in this condition?
    (A) Dilation of systemic veins results in decreased diastolic cardiac size
    (B) Dilation of coronary arterioles reduces resistance and increases coronary flow through ischemic tissue
    (C) Increased sympathetic outflow increases coronary flow
    (D) Dilation of peripheral arterioles increases cardiac work
    (E) Tachycardia increases diastolic coronary flow

14. A drug that is used in angina but causes constipation, edema, and increased cardiac size is
    (A) Diltiazem
    (B) Hydralazine
    (C) Isosorbide dinitrate
    (D) Nitroglycerin
    (E) Propranolol

15. A drug suitable for producing a brief increase (5–15 minutes) in cardiac vagal tone is
    (A) Digoxin
    (B) Edrophonium
    (C) Ergotamine
    (D) Pralidoxime
    (E) Pyridostigmine

16. A patient with a 30-year history of insulin-dependent diabetes comes to you with a complaint of bloating and sour belching after meals. On several occasions, vomiting has occurred after a meal. Evaluation reveals delayed emptying of the stomach, and you diagnose diabetic gastroparesis. Which of the following drugs would be most useful in this patient?
    (A) Famotidine
    (B) Metoclopramide
    (C) Misoprostol
    (D) Omeprazole
    (E) Ondansetron

17. Drugs that block the alpha receptor on effector cells at adrenergic synapses cause
    (A) Reversal of the effects of isoproterenol on the heart rate
    (B) Reversal of the effects of epinephrine on the blood pressure
    (C) Reversal of the effects of epinephrine on adenylyl cyclase
    (D) A decrease in blood glucose levels
    (E) Mydriasis

Items 18–19: A 47-year-old salesperson has developed cardiomyopathy with severe congestive heart failure. In addition to the signs and symptoms of heart failure, he has become very depressed about his poor prognosis.

18. The most accurate description of digitalis's mechanism of action in congestive heart failure is
    (A) Reduction of the inward sodium gradient results in increased calcium stores in sarcoplasmic reticulum
    (B) Blockade of the sodium pump results in increased calcium entry through calcium channels
    (C) Blockade of potassium transport results in increased intracellular potassium
    (D) Sensitization of actin-myosin filaments to calcium
    (E) Increased inward trigger calcium influx causes increased release of calcium from the sarcoplasmic reticulum

19. Six months after starting digoxin therapy, the patient attempts suicide by swallowing 75 digoxin tablets (0.25 mg each). He is discovered by his wife and brought to the emergency room by paramedics. His blood pressure is 100/50 mm Hg, heart rate 40/min, and respirations 15/min. Toxicity caused by suicidal digoxin overdose should be treated by
    (A) Administration of phenytoin IV
    (B) Raising the serum potassium to 7 meq/L
    (C) Lowering serum magnesium

    (D)   Administration of digoxin antibodies

    (E)   Administration of sodium bicarbonate

20. When treating hypertension, orthostatic hypotension is greatest with

    (A)   Clonidine

    (B)   Guanethidine

    (C)   Hydralazine

    (D)   Methyldopa

    (E)   Propranolol

21. An elderly man comes to the clinic with a chief complaint of chronic constipation. The history indicates that he is sedentary, lives alone, and prepares his own meals, mostly from canned food. He has non-insulin-dependent diabetes that is well controlled with an oral hypoglycemic agent, but he is otherwise in good health. Physical examination reveals no obvious physical explanation for his bowel complaint. Which of the following recommendations is LEAST appropriate for this patient?

    (A)   He should exercise by walking at least 30 minutes a day

    (B)   His diet should include fresh fruit and vegetables at least twice a day

    (C)   He should take a phenolphthalein laxative whenever his bowels have not moved in 24 hours

    (D)   He should designate a specific time of day, preferably after a meal, when he can regularly spend 15 minutes without interruption on the toilet

22. Agents that have been shown to protect the upper gastrointestinal tract from ulcer formation include all of the following EXCEPT

    (A)   Antacids

    (B)   Cimetidine

    (C)   Ibuprofen

    (D)   Misoprostol

    (E)   Sucralfate

Items 23–24: A 52-year-old woman is admitted to the emergency room with a history of drug treatment for several conditions. Her serum electrolytes and pH are found to be as follows: Na^+ 140 meq/L, K^+ 3.0 meq/L, Cl^- 100 meq/L, pH 7.50.

23. This patient has probably been taking

    (A)   Acetazolamide

    (B)   Amiloride

    (C)   Digoxin

    (D)   Furosemide

    (E)   Quinidine

24. In view of the electrolyte panel shown (and regardless of its cause), which of the following is most correct?

    (A)   The patient will be more sensitive to the toxic actions of quinidine

    (B)   The patient will be more sensitive to the toxic actions of digoxin

    (C)   The patient will be more sensitive to the toxic actions of warfarin

    (D)   The patient will be more sensitive to the toxic actions of imipramine

    (E)   The patient will be more sensitive to the toxic actions of propranolol

25. A drug that is used to decrease blood pressure and has analgesic and spasmolytic effects when given intrathecally is

    (A)   Atenolol

    (B)   Clonidine

    (C)   Morphine

    (D)   Nitroprusside

    (E)   Prazosin

26. The most common route of drug entry into cells is

    (A)   Uptake by special carrier

    (B)   Diffusion through the lipid phase

    (C)   Pinocytosis after combining with coated pit receptors

    (D)   Aqueous diffusion

    (E)   Transport by amino acid carriers

27. Propranolol and hydralazine have which of the following effects in common?

    (A)   Tachycardia

    (B)   Decreased cardiac force

    (C) Increased systemic vascular resistance
    (D) Decreased mean arterial blood pressure
    (E) Decreased cardiac output

28. A 54-year-old farmer has a 5-year history of frequent, recurrent, and very painful kidney stones. Appropriate chronic therapy for this man is
    (A) Furosemide
    (B) Hydrochlorothiazide
    (C) Morphine
    (D) Spironolactone
    (E) Triamterene

29. The mechanism of action of furosemide is best described as
    (A) Interference with H^+/HCO_3^- exchange
    (B) Blockade of a $Na^+/K^+/2Cl^-$ transporter
    (C) Blockade of a Na^+/Cl^- cotransporter
    (D) Blockade of carbonic anhydrase
    (E) Inhibition of genetic expression of DNA in the kidney

30. All of the following are vasodilator peptides EXCEPT
    (A) Atrial natriuretic factor
    (B) Calcitonin gene-related peptide
    (C) Endothelin
    (D) Substance P
    (E) Vasoactive intestinal peptide

31. Cyclooxygenase I and II are responsible for
    (A) The synthesis of prostaglandins from arachidonate
    (B) The synthesis of leukotrienes from arachidonate
    (C) The synthesis of cAMP
    (D) The metabolic degradation of cAMP
    (E) The conversion of GTP to cGMP

Items 32–33: A 16-year-old student has had asthma for 5 years. The number of episodes of severe bronchospasm has increased recently, and you have been asked to review the therapeutic plan.

32. Bronchodilators useful in ordinary bronchospastic attacks include all of the following EXCEPT
    (A) Albuterol
    (B) Ipratropium
    (C) Metaproterenol
    (D) Nedocromil
    (E) Theophylline

33. The toxicities of theophylline in asthma include all of the following EXCEPT
    (A) Tachycardia
    (B) Tremor
    (C) Hypertension
    (D) Insomnia
    (E) Convulsions

34. Local anesthetic toxicities include all of the following EXCEPT
    (A) Cardiovascular arrhythmias and collapse (bupivacaine)
    (B) Convulsions (lidocaine)
    (C) Dizziness, sedation (lidocaine)
    (D) Hypertensive emergencies, strokes (procaine)
    (E) Methemoglobinemia (prilocaine)

35. A patient who has been taking fluoxetine for depression is talked into trying one of her friend's antidepressants. She develops signs and symptoms of rigidity, hypertension, and hyperthermia. The diagnosis of serotonin syndrome is made. The most appropriate therapy for the hyperthermia in this case would be
    (A) Baclofen
    (B) Cyclobenzaprine
    (C) Dantrolene
    (D) Diazepam
    (E) Succinylcholine

36. A 56-year-old man is admitted to the coronary care unit with myocardial infarction. You would like to attempt dissolution of the coronary occlusion with a thrombolytic agent. The patient's recent medical history includes streptococcal throat infection (1 month previously) and hemorrhage from a tooth socket following a difficult extraction (6 months previously). His problem list includes renal parenchymal disease. He has been taking aspirin, one tablet daily, for the last 6 years. Which of the following is most correct?
  (A) Because of his history of bleeding, all thrombolytics are contraindicated
  (B) Because of his history of strep infection, anistreplase carries a high risk of anaphylaxis
  (C) Because of his history of strep infection, streptokinase will be less effective than would otherwise be expected
  (D) Alteplase would be hazardous in this patient because of his recent consumption of aspirin
  (E) Urokinase should not be used in a patient with a history of renal disease

37. Which of the following drugs is correctly associated with its clinical application?
  (A) Erythropoietin: Macrocytic anemia
  (B) Filgrastim: Thrombocytopenia due to myelocytic leukemia
  (C) Iron dextran: Severe macrocytic anemia
  (D) Ferrous sulfate: Microcytic anemia of pregnancy
  (E) Folic acid: Hemochromatosis

38. Regarding trimethoprim-sulfamethoxazole (TMP-SMZ), which one of the following statements is LEAST accurate?
  (A) Active against some strains of MRSA
  (B) Bactericidal actions occur through sequential blockade of folic acid synthesis
  (C) Folinic acid will reduce hematologic side effects
  (D) Respiratory tract infections often respond since TMP-SMZ has activity against pneumococci, *H influenzae,* and *M catarrhalis*
  (E) The trimethoprim component of TMP-SMZ is responsible for the enhanced hypoglycemia seen with certain sulfonylureas used in diabetes

39. Which one of the following matches of antifungal agent with a characteristic feature is LEAST accurate?
  (A) Amphotericin B: Dose-limiting nephrotoxicity
  (B) Flucytosine: Causes "thymine-less" death of fungal cells
  (C) Ketoconazole: Inhibition of cytochromes P-450
  (D) Itraconazole: Binds to ergosterol to form artificial membrane "pores"
  (E) Terbinafine: Effective treatment of onychomycosis

40. The CD4 count of an AIDS patient drops below 200/μL, and prophylaxis is initiated to prevent *Pneumocystis* pneumonia. Which one of the following is LEAST likely to be effective?
  (A) Atovaquone
  (B) Pentamidine
  (C) Primaquine
  (D) Pyrimethamine plus sulfadiazine
  (E) Trimethoprim plus sulfamethoxazole

41. Regarding antiparasitic drugs, which one of the following statements is NOT accurate?
  (A) Common tapeworm infections are usually responsive to praziquantel
  (B) Diethylcarbamazine is effective in filariasis
  (C) Ivermectin has been used for the mass treatment of onchocerciasis
  (D) Metrifonate is the drug of choice for intestinal nematode infections
  (E) Pinworm and whipworm infections respond well to mebendazole

42. This agent is the drug of choice in severe amebic disease and for hepatic abscess. It is activated to toxic intermediates by the pyruvate-ferredoxin oxidoreductase enzyme system present in the parasite.
  (A) Diloxanide furoate
  (B) Emetine
  (C) Iodoquinol
  (D) Metronidazole
  (E) Paromomycin

43. A 14-year-old girl is brought to the emergency room of a hospital by her friends after being thrown from a horse and hitting a fence. She does not appear to be seriously hurt, but she does have dirty abrasions and scratches over her arms and face. The teenager does not recall any immunizations she might have received in early childhood but states that none have been given since she was 4 or 5 years old. This patient should be treated with

    (A)   A broad spectrum antibiotic
    (B)   Tetanus-diphtheria toxin
    (C)   Tetanus immune globulin
    (D)   Tetanus-diphtheria toxin and a broad spectrum antibiotic
    (E)   Tetanus-diphtheria toxin and tetanus immune globulin

44. A young patient with end-stage renal disease receives a kidney transplant from a living related donor who is HLA-identical and red blood cell ABO-matched. To prevent rejection, the transplant recipient is treated with cyclosporine. Which one of the following statements about this immunosuppressant drug is LEAST accurate?
    (A)   Binding to cyclophilin decreases activation of transcription factor for interleukin-2
    (B)   Cyclosporine has no direct actions on B cell-mediated immune responses
    (C)   Myelosuppression is dose-limiting
    (D)   Nephrotoxicity occurs in more than 10% of patients
    (E)   Seizures may occur in overdosage

45. Blizzard weather conditions have forced a family living on welfare to stay in their poorly ventilated apartment for several days. During this time, all family members have developed slight nausea, headache, and dizziness. When the youngest member of the family becomes confused, starts breathing rapidly, and then faints, she is brought to the emergency room of the local hospital. The condition of this patient is most likely due to
    (A)   Glue sniffing
    (B)   Ingestion of lead-based paints (pica)
    (C)   Inhalation of carbon monoxide
    (D)   Malnutrition
    (E)   Sulfur dioxide poisoning

46. A young woman using an oral contraceptive is to be treated for pulmonary tuberculosis. She is advised to use an additional method of contraception since the efficacy of the oral agents is commonly decreased if her drug regimen includes
    (A)   Amikacin
    (B)   Ethambutol
    (C)   Isoniazid
    (D)   Pyrazinamide
    (E)   Rifampin

47. All of the following statements about heavy metal poisoning are accurate EXCEPT
    (A)   Acute necrotizing gastroenteritis may occur with ingestion of iron tablets
    (B)   Chelation with succimer is the standard management of copper poisoning
    (C)   Ingestion of flaking paint is a major source of lead poisoning in young children
    (D)   An odor of garlic on the breath and rice-water stools are signs of poisoning due to inorganic arsenic
    (E)   Pneumonitis may occur following inhalation of mercury vapor

48. Poisoning due to inhalation of carbon monoxide remains one of the leading causes of poisoning deaths in the United States. Which one of the following statements about such poisoning and its management is LEAST accurate?
    (A)   Administration of oxygen (100%) via a tight-fitting nonrebreather mask should be instituted immediately
    (B)   A preliminary diagnosis would be confirmed by determination of the carboxyhemoglobin blood level
    (C)   Hyperbaric oxygen (2–3 atm) is usually recommended if the patient has ECG abnormalities, is unconscious, or is pregnant
    (D)   Permanent neurologic deficits may occur in survivors of severe poisoning
    (E)   Red mucous membranes and nail bed lunulae are present in over 90% of cases

49. Which one of the following statements about the fluoroquinolone group of antibiotics is LEAST accurate?
    (A)   Antibacterial spectrum includes common pathogens of the urogenital system and the gastrointestinal tract
    (B)   Fluoroquinolones may interfere with collagen metabolism
    (C)   Oral absorption is decreased by antacids
    (D)   Resistance mechanisms include point mutations in the gene for DNA-dependent RNA polymerase
    (E)   Strains of resistant gram-positive cocci are increasing in frequency

50. This neurotransmitter, located in the spinal cord, is inhibitory to motor neurons via an increase in chloride ion conductance.
    (A) Acetylcholine
    (B) Dopamine
    (C) Glycine
    (D) Serotonin
    (E) Substance P

Items 51–52: The research division of a pharmaceutical corporation has characterized the receptor blocking actions of five new drugs, each of which may have potential therapeutic value. The relative intensities of their blocking actions are shown in the following table. Since each of these drugs is lipophilic and can cross the blood-brain barrier, they are expected to have CNS effects.

Drug	Blocking Action on CNS Receptors			
	Adrenergic (beta)	Cholinergic (M)	Dopaminergic (D$_2$)	GABAergic (A)
A	++	+++	+++	None
B	None	None	None	++++
C	None	++++	+	None
D	+	None	+++	+
E	None	+	+	+

Number of + signs denotes intensity of blocking actions.

51. Based on the data shown in the table above, which drug is most likely to exacerbate the symptoms of Parkinson's disease?
    (A) Drug A
    (B) Drug B
    (C) Drug C
    (D) Drug D
    (E) Drug E

52. Based on the data shown in the table above, which drug is most likely to lower the threshold to seizures?
    (A) A
    (B) B
    (C) C
    (D) D
    (E) E

53. A 20-year-old man who had become physically dependent following illicit use of secobarbital ("reds") is undergoing severe withdrawal symptoms, including nausea, vomiting, delirium, and periodic seizures. Which one of the following drugs is LEAST likely to be effective in alleviating these symptoms?
    (A) Buspirone
    (B) Chlordiazepoxide
    (C) Diazepam
    (D) Midazolam
    (E) Phenobarbital

54. Benzodiazepines are LEAST effective in
    (A) Alcohol withdrawal syndromes
    (B) Balanced anesthesia regimens
    (C) Initial management of phencyclidine overdose
    (D) Obsessive-compulsive disorders
    (E) Social phobias

55. An individual has ingested an antifreeze solution containing ethylene glycol and is brought to a hospital emergency room. Which one of the following statements about his case is LEAST accurate?
    (A) Dialysis is indicated in the treatment

(B) Ethanol is likely to be administered in management

(C) Metabolic acidosis is very likely

(D) Oxalate crystals may be present in the urine

(E) Visual function of the patient will be impaired by flickering white spots "like a snowstorm"

56. Which one of the following drugs is thought to exert its anticonvulsant effects by blocking sodium channels in neuronal membranes?

(A) Acetazolamide

(B) Carbamazepine

(C) Diazepam

(D) Gabapentin

(E) Valproic acid

57. A young woman suffering from myoclonic seizures was receiving effective single drug therapy with valproic acid. Since she was planning a pregnancy, her physician switched her to an alternative medication with less potential for teratogenicity. Which one of the following drugs is effective in myoclonic seizures but often makes the patient extremely drowsy at the dose level required for effective seizure control?

(A) Carbamazepine

(B) Clonazepam

(C) Ethosuximide

(D) Lamotrigine

(E) Topiramate

58. Regarding the pharmacodynamic actions of local anesthetics, which one of the following statements is most accurate?

(A) All local anesthetics with ester bonds are vasodilators

(B) Amides cause a high incidence of hypersensitivity reactions

(C) Protonated forms of such drugs readily penetrate biomembranes

(D) The ionized forms of local anesthetics cause a use-dependent blockade of sodium ion channels

(E) Type A alpha nerve fibers are highly sensitive to blockade

59. A patient is brought to an emergency room suffering from an overdose of an illicit drug. She is agitated, has disordered thought processes, suffers from paranoia, and "hears voices." The drug most likely to be responsible for her condition is

(A) Gamma-hydroxybutyrate (GHB)

(B) Hashish

(C) Heroin

(D) Methamphetamine

(E) Methylphenyltetrahydropyridine (MPTP)

60. A patient undergoing surgery is given a drug for muscle relaxation. The anesthesiologist notes a marked drop in blood pressure and an increase in airway resistance immediately after the injection. Intravenous administration of diphenhydramine quickly restores the patient's blood pressure and airway diameter. The muscle relaxant used was probably

(A) Atracurium

(B) Baclofen

(C) Diazepam

(D) Tubocurarine

(E) Vecuronium

61. The following table contains data on two properties of different compounds under study for use as inhalation anesthetics.

Properties of Inhalation Anesthetics		
Anesthetic	Blood-Gas Partition Coefficient	Minimal Alveolar Anesthetic Concentration (%)
A	0.8	9.7
B	1.4	1.4
C	9.8	0.6
D	2.3	0.8
E	1.8	1.7

The agent most likely to have the slowest rate of recovery from its anesthetic action is
(A) Anesthetic A
(B) Anesthetic B
(C) Anesthetic C
(D) Anesthetic D
(E) Anesthetic E

62. Which one of the following properties is most characteristic of opioid analgesics?
(A) The ratio of maximal efficacy to addiction liability is a constant
(B) Tolerance to ocular and gastrointestinal effects develops rapidly during chronic use
(C) Mixed agonist-antagonists are more likely to depress respiratory function than pure agonist drugs
(D) They have many effects in common with a group of endogenous polypeptides
(E) All opioid analgesics have good oral bioavailability

63. Retarded body growth, poor coordination, microcephaly, and underdevelopment of the mid face region in an infant are associated with chronic maternal abuse of
(A) Amphetamine
(B) Cocaine
(C) Ethanol
(D) Mescaline
(E) Phencyclidine

64. After the ingestion of a meal that included sardines, cheese, and red wine, a patient under treatment for depression experiences a hypertensive crisis. The drug most likely to be responsible is
(A) Bupropion
(B) Fluoxetine
(C) Imipramine
(D) Isocarboxazid
(E) Trazodone

65. Following a stroke, a 54-year-old man develops marked muscle spasticity. A number of spasmolytics could be used to reduce muscle spasm without significant loss of muscle strength. Which one of the following drugs would NOT be effective in this patient?
(A) Baclofen
(B) Cyclobenzaprine
(C) Dantrolene
(D) Diazepam
(E) Tizanidine

66. A 48-year-old surgical patient was anesthetized with an intravenous bolus dose of propofol, then maintained on isoflurane with vecuronium as the skeletal muscle relaxant. At the end of the surgical procedure, she was administered pyridostigmine and glycopyrrolate. Postoperative pain was managed by parenteral morphine. Which of the following statements about the drugs used in this case is most accurate?
(A) Continuous infusion of propofol is contraindicated owing to its emetic effects
(B) Glycopyrrolate protects against the potential cardiovascular effects of pyridostigmine
(C) Muscle fasciculation due to vecuronium causes postoperative pain
(D) Pyridostigmine is likely to cause CNS effects
(E) Isoflurane has less skeletal muscle-relaxing effects than other inhalation anesthetics

67. A woman taking haloperidol develops a spectrum of adverse effects that include the amenorrhea-galactorrhea syndrome and extrapyramidal dysfunction, including bradykinesia, muscle rigidity, and tremor at rest. Her psychiatrist prescribes a newer antipsychotic drug that improves both positive and negative symptoms of schizophrenia with few of the side effects that result from dopamine receptor blockade. Since weekly blood tests are not deemed necessary, the drug prescribed by the psychiatrist is probably
(A) Bupropion
(B) Clozapine
(C) Nefazodone
(D) Olanzapine
(E) Pimozide

68. Naloxone is LEAST likely to antagonize or reverse
(A) Analgesic effects of morphine in a cancer patient
(B) Drug actions resulting from activation of mu opioid receptors

(C) Opioid-analgesic overdose in a patient on methadone maintenance
(D) Pupillary constriction caused by levorphanol
(E) Respiratory depression caused by overdose of nefazodone

69. Which one of the following statements about the use of carbidopa with levodopa in the treatment of parkinsonism is LEAST accurate?
(A) Carbidopa inhibits L-aromatic amino acid decarboxylase
(B) CNS side effects are reduced when the drugs are used together
(C) Lower doses of levodopa are effective when used with carbidopa
(D) Nausea and hypotension occur less frequently than with levodopa alone
(E) The physicochemical properties of carbidopa limit its CNS penetration

70. Five patients are scheduled for a short surgical procedure during which succinylcholine will be used for muscle relaxation. Selected blood laboratory values for each patient are shown in the table.

Patient Number	Aspartate Aminotransferase Normal Range 8–20 units/L	Urinary Nitrogen (BUN) Normal Range 7–18 mg/dL	Dibucaine Number (% inhibition) Normal 20%
1	28 units/L	12 mg/dL	18%
2	16 units/L	30 mg/dL	23%
3	13 units/L	14 mg/dL	82%
4	26 units/L	25 mg/dL	20%
5	18 units/L	15 mg/dL	34%

Which patient is most likely to experience a prolonged respiratory paralysis following the administration of a bolus dose of succinylcholine?
(A) Patient 1
(B) Patient 2
(C) Patient 3
(D) Patient 4
(E) Patient 5

Items 71–72: A young man comes to a community clinic with a urogenital infection that, based on the Gram stain, appears to be due to *Neisseria gonorrhoeae*. Upon questioning, it appears that the patient acquired the infection while vacationing in a Pacific Rim country. The physician is concerned about drug resistance of the gonococcus infecting this patient and also about his drug compliance. He notes that the patient had an anaphylactic reaction to penicillin G administered intramuscularly 6 months earlier.

71. Which one of the following drugs is most likely to be effective and safe to use in the treatment of gonorrhea in this patient?
(A) Amoxicillin-clavulanate
(B) Ceftriaxone
(C) Clarithromycin
(D) Spectinomycin
(E) Tetracycline

72. The physician is also concerned about the possibility of nongonococcal urethritis in this patient. Such infections are usually eradicated by the administration of a single dose of
(A) Azithromycin
(B) Doxycycline
(C) Erythromycin
(D) Tetracycline
(E) Trimethoprim-sulfamethoxazole

73. Which one of the following statements about the mechanisms of action of antibiotics is most accurate?
(A) Aminoglycosides bind to receptors on the 50S ribosomal subunit to prevent attachment of aminoacyl-tRNA
(B) Cephalosporins inhibit the synthesis of precursors of the linear peptidoglycan chains of the cell wall

(C) Fluoroquinolones inhibit DNA-dependent RNA polymerase
(D) The bactericidal action of penicillins is partly due to their activation of autolytic enzymes
(E) Vancomycin inhibits peptidyltransferases involved in protein synthesis
74. A 26-year-old woman with chronic bronchitis lives in a region of the country with harsh winter conditions. Her physician recommends the prophylactic use of oral tetracycline during the winter season. Which one of the following statements about the drug is LEAST accurate?
(A) Absorption from the GI tract may be decreased by milk products
(B) Decreased intracellular accumulation is a mechanism of bacterial resistance
(C) Elimination is predominantly via biliary excretion
(D) The patient should discontinue the tetracycline if she becomes pregnant
(E) Vaginal candidiasis may occur during treatment

Items 75–76: A 52-year-old insurance agent receiving chemotherapy for leukemia is given intramuscular cefazolin (500 mg) for treatment of pneumococcal pneumonia. Within a few minutes, he is wheezing, he develops an urticarial rash, and his systolic blood pressure falls markedly. The patient recovers following the administration of epinephrine, dexamethasone, and fluids.
75. Which one of the following statements regarding the use of cefazolin in this case is most accurate?
(A) A first-generation cephalosporin should not be used in a patient who is likely to be immunosuppressed
(B) Gentamicin would be more effective in an immunosuppressed patient
(C) It would have been preferable to use nafcillin in this patient
(D) Penicillin G is a more appropriate drug for pneumococcal pneumonia, though resistant strains do occur
(E) The reaction could have been avoided with a lower dose of the drug
76. Regarding the drug reaction in this case, which one of the following statements is LEAST accurate?
(A) It is likely that the reaction would have been less severe if a test dose (50 mg) of cefazolin was administered initially
(B) Reactions of this type are more frequent after use of the penicillins than with the cephalosporins
(C) Skin testing with a dilute solution of cefazolin is routinely used to detect hypersensitivity
(D) The reaction was IgE-mediated
(E) This was a type I allergic reaction
77. Which one of the following statements about the macrolide group of antibiotics is LEAST accurate?
(A) Cholestatic hepatitis, which can occur with the use of erythromycin, is age-dependent
(B) Clarithromycin has activity against *M avium-intracellulare*
(C) High tissue levels and prolonged half-life are distinctive features of azithromycin
(D) Organisms sensitive to macrolides include gram-positive cocci, *Mycoplasma,* and *Chlamydia*
(E) Stimulation of the activity of hepatic drug-metabolizing enzymes commonly occurs during erythromycin treatment
78. A 30-year-old man who is HIV-positive has a CD4 count of 450/μL and a viral RNA load of 11,000/mL. His treatment involves a three-drug regimen consisting of zidovudine, didanosine, and ritonavir. Nystatin had been used for oral candidiasis, but for the past week the patient has been taking ketoconazole. Because of weight loss, he has just started using dronabinol. Which one of the following statements about this case is LEAST accurate?
(A) Bitter taste and GI distress with ritonavir interfere with patient compliance
(B) Ketoconazole may increase blood levels of ritonavir
(C) Ritonavir decreases the blood levels of dronabinol
(D) Serum amylase activity should be monitored
(E) The anti-HIV "cocktail" of multiple drugs should slow progression of the disease

Items 79–80: A 73-year-old patient has chronic pulmonary dysfunction requiring daily hospital visits for respiratory therapy. She is hospitalized with pneumonia, and it is not clear whether the infection is community- or hospital-acquired. Assume that the data in the table on the next page concerning the antimicrobial drug sensitivity of bacterial isolates are appropriate in either case.

Antimicrobial Sensitivity of Aerobic Isolates From Nonurine Sources

Organism	% of Isolates Susceptible to				
	Ampicillin	Ceftriaxone	Ciprofloxacin	Erythromycin	TMP-SMZ
E coli	50	99	98	20	70
H influenzae	5	95	97	23	87
K pneumoniae	90	98	98	98	90
M catarrhalis	20	76	76	91	96
L pneumophila	8	20	48	100	88
S pneumoniae	13	87	85	90	90
S aureus	14	87	65	50	50

79. If she has a community-acquired pneumonia, coverage must be provided for atypical pathogens. In such a case, the most appropriate drug treatment in this elderly patient with pulmonary disease is
    (A) Ampicillin and erythromycin
    (B) Ceftriaxone
    (C) Ceftriaxone and erythromycin
    (D) Ciprofloxacin
    (E) TMP-SMZ

80. If she has a hospital-acquired pneumonia, coverage must be provided for gram-negative rods and staphylococci. In such a case, empiric treatment is likely to include
    (A) Ampicillin and ceftriaxone
    (B) Ceftriaxone and TMP-SMZ
    (C) Ceftriaxone, erythromycin, and nafcillin
    (D) Ciprofloxacin and erythromycin
    (E) Erythromycin, nafcillin, and ticarcillin

81. Which one of the following statements about mechanisms of antiviral drug resistance is LEAST accurate?
    (A) CMV resistance to ganciclovir can involve decreased expression of the viral phosphotransferase
    (B) Famciclovir is active against TK⁻ strains of HSV
    (C) Point mutations in the *pol* gene lead to zidovudine resistance
    (D) Resistance to cidofovir results from changes in viral DNA polymerase
    (E) There is limited cross-resistance between saquinavir and other protease inhibitors

82. A male patient with AIDS has a CD4 count of 50/μL. He is being maintained on a multidrug regimen composed of acyclovir, clarithromycin, fluconazole, lamivudine, ritonavir, trimethoprim-sulfamethoxazole, and zidovudine. The drug most likely to provide prophylaxis against cryptococcal infections of the meninges is
    (A) Acyclovir
    (B) Clarithromycin
    (C) Fluconazole
    (D) Ritonavir
    (E) Trimethoprim-sulfamethoxazole

Items 83–84: A patient with diffuse non-Hodgkin's lymphoma is treated with a combination drug regimen (BACOP) that includes bleomycin, doxorubicin, cyclophosphamide, vincristine, and prednisone.

83. Concerning the adverse effects of these drugs, which one of the following is LEAST likely to occur?
    (A) Cardiotoxicity
    (B) Liver dysfunction
    (C) Osteoporosis
    (D) Peripheral neuropathy
    (E) Pulmonary fibrosis

84. Which one of the drugs employed in this case acts primarily in the G_2 stage of the cell cycle?

(A) Bleomycin
(B) Cyclophosphamide
(C) Doxorubicin
(D) Prednisone
(E) Vincristine

DIRECTIONS: The following section consists of lists of lettered options followed by several numbered items. For each numbered item, select the ONE option that is most closely associated with it. Each answer may be used once, more than once, or not at all.

Items 85–88:
(A) Cimetidine
(B) Diphenhydramine
(C) Ergotamine tartrate
(D) Ranitidine
(E) Terfenadine

85. A prodrug that may cause serious cardiac arrhythmias if coadministered with ketoconazole
86. A drug with significant efficacy against motion sickness
87. A drug that decreases gastric acid secretion and has antiandrogenic effects
88. A drug with partial agonist effects at serotonin receptors and alpha receptors

Items 89–92:
(A) Digoxin
(B) Lidocaine
(C) Propranolol
(D) Quinidine
(E) Verapamil

89. A drug that predictably prolongs the PR interval and increases cardiac contractility
90. A drug that is useful in supraventricular tachycardias and angina pectoris and is not contraindicated in asthma
91. A drug that is useful in ventricular and atrial arrhythmias and may cause tinnitus
92. A drug that is very useful in early post-myocardial infarction ventricular arrhythmias but not very effective in atrial arrhythmias

Items 93–95:
(A) Abciximab
(B) Epoetin alfa (erythropoietin)
(C) Sargramostim
(D) Omeprazole
(E) Misoprostol

93. Used to prevent recurrence of peptic ulcers in patients taking high-dose anti-inflammatory drugs for rheumatoid arthritis
94. Used to reduce restenosis due to platelet aggregation in patients undergoing coronary angioplasty
95. Used to accelerate recovery of neutrophils and other white blood cells in patients receiving marrow-depressing doses of cancer chemotherapy drugs

Items 96–99:
(A) Alteplase
(B) Aspirin
(C) Heparin
(D) Ticlopidine
(E) Warfarin

96. A drug that acts immediately in vitro to prevent blood from clotting
97. This drug is manufactured by recombinant DNA technology and must be used in the first few hours after myocardial infarction
98. A new drug that prevents platelet aggregation without altering prostaglandin synthesis
99. The anticoagulant of choice in pregnant women

Items 100–104:

(A)	Amphetamine	**(J)**	Dronabinol	**(S)**	Olanzapine
(B)	Bromocriptine	**(K)**	Donepezil	**(T)**	Phenytoin
(C)	Bupropion	**(L)**	Fentanyl	**(U)**	Propofol
(D)	Buspirone	**(M)**	Fluoxetine	**(V)**	Propoxyphene
(E)	Carbamazepine	**(N)**	Lamotrigine	**(W)**	Pyridostigmine
(F)	Clomipramine	**(O)**	Meperidine	**(X)**	Selegiline
(G)	Clonazepam	**(P)**	Methadone	**(Y)**	Sertraline
(H)	Clozapine	**(Q)**	Mirtazapine	**(Z)**	Triazolam
(I)	Cocaine	**(R)**	Nalbuphine		

100. A 24-year-old man with a history of partial seizures has been treated with standard anticonvulsants for several years. He is currently taking valproic acid, which is not fully effective, and his neurologist prescribes a new drug approved for adjunctive use in partial seizures. Unfortunately, the combination of the two drugs leads to a life-threatening rash with toxic epidermal necrolysis. The new drug prescribed was which of the above?

101. The introduction of this drug may represent a novel approach to the treatment of major depressive disorders since it appears to act as an antagonist at alpha$_2$-adrenoceptors in the central nervous system.

102. A patient suffering from the pain of terminal cancer is likely to require administration of a powerful analgesic. If this drug is prescribed, miosis is UNLIKELY to occur.

103. A patient with Alzheimer's disease may benefit from the use of this drug, which appears to inhibit acetylcholinesterase in the CNS.

104. This drug, together with behavioral psychotherapy, has proved helpful in patients who suffer from obsessive-compulsive disorder. While it blocks the reuptake of serotonin, the drug is a tricyclic structure and is therefore potentially cardiotoxic.

Items 105–109:

(A)	Amoxicillin	**(J)**	Etoposide	**(S)**	Quinine
(B)	Azathioprine	**(K)**	Flucytosine	**(T)**	Rifabutin
(C)	Azithromycin	**(L)**	Ganciclovir	**(U)**	Ritonavir
(D)	Busulfan	**(M)**	Ketoconazole	**(V)**	Sargramostim
(E)	Ciprofloxacin	**(N)**	Leuprolide	**(W)**	Spectinomycin
(F)	Chloroquine	**(O)**	Mebendazole	**(X)**	Trimethoprim
(G)	Cyclophosphamide	**(P)**	Meropenem	**(Y)**	Vinblastine
(H)	Daunorubicin	**(Q)**	Niclosamide	**(Z)**	Zidovudine
(I)	Ethambutol	**(R)**	Paclitaxel		

105. This cell cycle-nonspecific agent is commonly used as a component of cancer chemotherapy regimens, including those for non-Hodgkin's lymphoma and for breast cancers. Concomitant administration of mercaptoethanesulfonate, which traps acrolein, decreases the risk of hematuria caused by this drug.

106. This drug may be used in HIV patients and is a potent inhibitor of the CYP3A isoform of hepatic cytochrome P450. The drug blocks the enzymatic cleavage of protein precursors needed for the formation of mature virions.

107. Adverse effects of this antiprotozoal drug include flushed and sweaty skin, tinnitus, impaired vision and hearing, gastrointestinal upset, and disturbances in cardiac rhythm and conduction. Intravascular hemolysis is a rare hypersensitivity reaction to this drug.

108. This cytotoxic agent acts in the M phase of the cell cycle and has been approved for use in advanced breast and endometrial cancers. While it is a myelosuppressant, the most distinctive toxicity of the drug is peripheral neuropathy, which occurs in over 50% of patients.

109. This immunosuppressive agent forms a prodrug, which in turn is bioactivated to a nucleotide inhibitor of DNA polymerases. While myelosuppression is dose-limiting, the drug also causes dose-dependent hepatotoxicity.

Items 110–113:

    (A) Aspirin
    (B) Gold salts
    (C) Ibuprofen

      (D) Indomethacin
      (E) Methotrexate
      (F) Misoprostol
      (G) Penicillamine

110. Used exclusively in rheumatoid arthritis; has a very slow onset of action (months); efficacy is disputed

111. Used in all forms of arthritis except gouty arthritis; onset of maximum effect is hours to days, but GI toxicity is limiting

112. A drug used in cancer chemotherapy and in rheumatoid arthritis

113. Nonsteroidal anti-inflammatory drug with less GI toxicity and short duration of action; good efficacy in dysmenorrhea

Items 114–117:
      (A) Danazol
      (B) Ipodate
      (C) Mestranol
      (D) Norethindrone
      (E) Norgestrel
      (F) Potassium iodide solution
      (G) Propylthiouracil
      (H) Thyroxine
      (I) Triiodothyronine
      (J) Ultralente insulin

114. Drug of choice for maintenance therapy of hypothyroid patients

115. Blocks the synthesis of thyroid hormone by preventing coupling of iodotyrosine molecules; agranulocytosis is a rare toxicity

116. Inhibits iodination of tyrosine in the thyroid gland; also reduces size and vascularity of a hyperplastic thyroid gland

117. A partial agonist progestin and androgen; used in endometriosis

Items 118–120:
      (A) Angiotensin
      (B) Endothelin
      (C) Epinephrine
      (D) Guanethidine
      (E) Hexamethonium
      (F) Isoproterenol
      (G) Norepinephrine
      (H) Phenylephrine
      (I) Prazosin
      (J) Propranolol

118. A drug was given as an IV bolus to an anesthetized subject while the blood pressure was recorded. The results are shown in the graph below. Systolic and diastolic pressures in response to the injection of **Drug X** are shown. Identify **Drug X** from the above list.

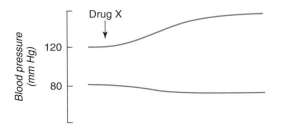

Items 119–120: A drug (**Drug 1**) was given as an IV bolus to another anesthetized subject while blood pressure and heart rate were recorded as shown on the left side of the graph on the next page.

After recovery from the effects of **Drug 1,** a long-acting dose of **Drug 2** was given. After the recorder was turned back on, **Drug 1** was repeated with the results shown on the right side of the graph.

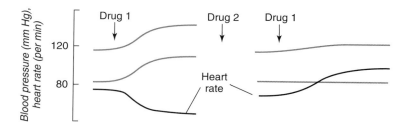

119. Identify Drug 1 from the above list.
120. Identify Drug 2 from the above list.

Answer Key for Examination 2*

1. C (7)	**39.** D (48)	**80.** C (43, 44, 46)
2. B (19)	**40.** C (53)	**81.** B (49)
3. E (1)	**41.** D (53, 54)	**82.** C (48)
4. C (2)	**42.** D (53)	**83.** B (55)
5. B (3)	**43.** E (62)	**84.** A (55)
6. E (5)	**44.** C (56)	**85.** E (16)
7. A (6, 8, 9)	**45.** C (57)	**86.** B (16)
8. B (6)	**46.** E (47, 61)	**87.** A (16)
9. C (10)	**47.** B (58)	**88.** C (16)
10. C (9)	**48.** E (57, 59)	**89.** A (13, 14)
11. A (9)	**49.** D (46)	**90.** E (12, 14)
12. A (11)	**50.** C (21)	**91.** D (14)
13. A (12)	**51.** D (21, 28)	**92.** B (14)
14. A (12)	**52.** B (21, 24)	**93.** E (18, 36, 60)
15. B (7)	**53.** A (22)	**94.** A (34)
16. B (60)	**54.** D (22)	**95.** C (33)
17. B (10)	**55.** E (23)	**96.** C (34)
18. A (13)	**56.** B (24)	**97.** A (34)
19. D (13)	**57.** B (24)	**98.** D (34)
20. B (11)	**58.** D (26)	**99.** C (34)
21. C (60)	**59.** D (32)	**100.** N (24)
22. C (60)	**60.** D (27)	**101.** Q (30)
23. D (15)	**61.** C (25)	**102.** O (31)
24. B (13)	**62.** D (31)	**103.** K (7, 21)
25. B (11)	**63.** C (23)	**104.** F (30)
26. B (1, 3)	**64.** D (30, 61)	**105.** G (55)
27. D (10, 11)	**65.** B (27)	**106.** U (49)
28. B (15)	**66.** B (7, 8, 27)	**107.** S (53)
29. B (15)	**67.** D (29)	**108.** R (55)
30. C (17)	**68.** E (31)	**109.** B (55, 56)
31. A (18)	**69.** B (28)	**110.** B (36)
32. D (20)	**70.** C (27)	**111.** A (36)
33. C (20)	**71.** D (45)	**112.** E (36)
34. D (26)	**72.** A (44)	**113.** C (36)
35. C (27)	**73.** D (43–46)	**114.** H (38)
36. C (34)	**74.** C (44)	**115.** G (38)
37. D (33)	**75.** D (43)	**116.** F (38)
38. E (46)	**76.** C (43, 56)	**117.** A (40)
	77. E (44)	**118.** C (9)
	78. C (49)	**119.** G (9, 10)
	79. C (43, 44, 46)	**120.** I (10)

*Numbers in parentheses are chapters in which answers may be found.

Appendix IV

Case Histories

This Appendix contains case histories that illustrate selected aspects of pharmacologic management of clinical problems.* Each case is followed by general self-evaluation questions. Answers will be found at the end of this Appendix.

Note: Ranges of numbers in parentheses or brackets are the ranges of normal values at the institution where the patient was studied.

CASE 1. THE GARDENER†

A 55-year-old man was found unconscious by his wife in the greenhouse behind their home. During the past week, he had been complaining of abdominal discomfort and frequent stools. His medical history was restricted to mild hypertension controlled by salt restriction (about 5 years) and non-insulin-dependent diabetes controlled by diet (about 10 years). He had no history of mental illness or of alcohol or tobacco use, and he was not taking any medication. His last trip outside the country had been to Mexico 5 years earlier. He and his wife operated a small flower shop, and he was an enthusiastic home gardener.

Upon arrival at the emergency room, the patient was unconscious, salivating profusely, and breathing shallowly. His skin was warm and moist. Blood pressure was 140/90 mm Hg, pulse 72/min and regular, respirations 30/min, and temperature normal. There was no evidence of trauma. Both pupils were constricted and did not respond to light. Auscultation of the chest revealed moderate wheezing and numerous rhonchi. The heart was normal. Examination of the abdomen revealed no abnormalities other than hyperactive bowel sounds. The extremities showed subcutaneous muscle fasciculations at the time of admission. These disappeared during the course of the examination, but muscle tone decreased and breathing became shallower during this time. The neurologic examination revealed coma with no response to painful stimuli, no localizing signs, and no abnormal reflexes.

Questions, Case 1
1. What are the possible toxic causes of the patient's signs and symptoms?
2. What immediate steps must be taken?
3. What drugs may be considered for the treatment of this patient? What are the risks and benefits of their use?

CASE 2. THE SUICIDAL CARDIAC PATIENT‡

A 39-year-old man with a long history of mitral stenosis ingested 90 digoxin tablets (0.25 mg each) in a suicide attempt approximately 2 hours before admission. Upon admission, the blood pressure

---

*These case histories are *not* meant to typify the "clinical vignette" questions found in Step I of the USMLE examination—such questions are to be found at the end of each chapter. Rather, the cases in this Appendix should be used to test one's preparation for pharmacologic questions that occur in Steps 2 and 3 of the USMLE.

†Modified and reproduced, with permission, from Goldfrank L, Kirstein R: SLUD. Hosp Physician 1976;12:20.

‡Modified and reproduced, with permission, from Smith TW et al: Reversal of advanced digoxin intoxication with Fab fragments of digoxin-specific antibodies. N Engl J Med 1976;294:797.

was 110/70 mm Hg and the pulse 40–60/min and irregular. The rest of the examination was normal.

Initial laboratory data included a blood ethanol of 190 mg/dL, but electrolytes were normal. An electrocardiogram revealed atrial fibrillation with a high degree of atrioventricular block and periods of atrioventricular junctional and atrial tachycardias. Ventricular rate did not exceed 50/min. Atropine had no effect on ventricular rate; therefore, a transvenous pacing catheter was inserted, with ventricular pacing instituted at 60/min.

During the next 8 hours, the spontaneous ventricular rate (determined by briefly halting the transvenous pacemaker) progressively decreased to 33 and then to 13/min. No atrial activity could be detected on the ECG. The QRS duration reached a maximum of 0.33 s (normal: 0.1 s). Serum potassium increased to 8.7 meq/L (3.5–5). An antidote was administered. Serum potassium rapidly fell to the normal range and the patient made a complete recovery.

Questions, Case 2
1. What was the mechanism and the primary source of the elevated serum potassium?
2. Describe the probable basis for the cardiac rhythm and electrocardiographic abnormalities.
3. Outline the conventional therapy for less severe digitalis intoxication, and explain why it was not used in this case. What antidote was used?
4. What treatment is available for severe intoxication with digitoxin?

CASE 3. A SEED EATER*

A 15-year-old boy was brought to the emergency room by the police because he "had a flushed face and was acting crazy." He had been found nude, incoherent, and wandering about aimlessly.

Physical examination showed blood pressure 170/100 mm Hg, respirations 44/min, pulse 144/min, and temperature 38 °C. He was comatose, unresponsive to verbal stimuli, and minimally responsive to deep painful stimuli. Sporadic decerebrate posturing was noted. The skin was flushed, dry, and hot to the touch. The pupils were widely dilated and equal, with a minimal response to light. Rectal temperature was 39.8 °C.

Physostigmine salicylate, 2 mg, was given intravenously under electrocardiographic, electroencephalographic, and temperature monitoring. Within 15 minutes, the rectal temperature had fallen to 38.8 °C, while blood pressure, respirations, and pulse were 160/68 mm Hg, 40/min, and 112/min, respectively. The patient became more alert and responsive to verbal commands but remained agitated. When questioned about ingestion of a toxic agent, the patient said that he had eaten "loco seeds," small black seeds of a weed that grew freely in the area. Remote memory was intact, but recent memory was grossly impaired.

Six hours later, the rectal temperature was 37 °C, and other vital signs were stable. The patient was talking spontaneously in a rapid and garbled manner. Although completely oriented, he continued to speak of imaginary objects and voices.

The patient improved rapidly and was discharged on the eighth hospital day without neurologic deficit.

Questions, Case 3
1. Identify the probable drug or drug group contained in "loco seeds."
2. What is the most life-threatening effect of the intoxicant in this case?
3. What are the dangers of physostigmine therapy? What are the risks of other treatments?

CASE 4. IATROGENIC SHOCK†

A 61-year-old patient had suffered from severe chronic asthmatic bronchitis with episodes of respiratory failure in the past and was admitted on this occasion with bronchopneumonia. In spite of therapy with antibiotics and bronchodilators, he deteriorated and became confused. His arterial blood pH

---

*Modified and reproduced, with permission, from Mikolich JR, Paulson GW, Cross CJ: Acute anticholinergic syndrome due to Jimson seed ingestion: Clinical and laboratory observation in six cases. Ann Intern Med 1975;83:321.

†Modified and reproduced, with permission, from Spoerel WE, Seleny FL, Williamson RD: Shock caused by continuous infusion of metaraminol bitartrate (Aramine). Can Med Assoc J 1964;90:349.

was 7.29 (7.35–7.45), and the P_{CO_2} was 73 mm Hg (35–45). A tracheostomy was performed under general anesthesia, and he was admitted to the intensive care unit.

Thirty minutes later, his pH was 7.41 and his P_{CO_2} was 59 mm Hg, but his O_2 saturation remained very low at 64% (94–100%). Intermittent positive-pressure breathing was begun, and his condition transiently improved. Two hours later, however, his systolic blood pressure had fallen to 60 mm Hg, and an infusion of metaraminol (a sympathomimetic drug with both direct and indirect actions) was started. His blood pressure rose, and the heart rate promptly decreased from 120 to 75/min. During the next 36 hours, he received an average of 7 mg of metaraminol per hour, but he developed manifestations of shock, with a falling urine output. His heart rate gradually increased to 90/min. An attempt to overcome these changes by increasing the dosage of metaraminol (up to 50 mg/h) did not influence the progressive deterioration. He had cold extremities and peripheral cyanosis in spite of adequate respiratory exchange on 100% oxygen. His arterial hematocrit was markedly elevated to 70% (40–52).

In an attempt to correct the severe hemoconcentration, the patient was given 1500 mL of dextran solution over the next 18 hours, and blood pressure was maintained with norepinephrine infusion. With this treatment, urine output rose, extremities became warmer, and his color improved. His blood pressure was stable for about 48 hours, requiring only occasional support with norepinephrine in small doses. Two days after initiation of this treatment, his hematocrit was 47% and norepinephrine was no longer needed.

Questions, Case 4
1. What is the mechanism by which metaraminol reduced the heart rate?
2. Why did the patient's hematocrit rise?
3. What was the cause of the patient's deteriorating renal function, cold extremities, and cyanosis?
4. What effects (if any) of the dextran and norepinephrine infusions led to the improvement in the patient's condition?

CASE 5. AN ASTHMATIC BUSINESSWOMAN*

A businesswoman with a history of mild asthma attacks had onset of symptoms of bronchoconstriction in a restaurant during a business luncheon. Repeated self-administration of a drug from an inhaler did not provide relief, and symptoms progressed until she became cyanotic. Paramedics were called, and they administered a subcutaneous drug upon arrival. She was admitted to the hospital emergency room in severe respiratory distress. Her pulse was 100/min, respiratory rate 32/min, and blood pressure 140/90 mm Hg. Severe wheezing was present.

After this evaluation, she was given another subcutaneous dose of the same medication that had been administered by the paramedics. Fifteen minutes later, her symptoms had decreased markedly, but she still had some respiratory wheezing. Use of a bronchodilator administered by handheld nebulizer abolished the wheezing, and she was discharged 3 hours later.

Questions, Case 5
1. What are the probable mediators of the bronchoconstriction noted in this woman's asthma attack?
2. What medications are commonly used for the outpatient treatment of mild to moderate asthma? What are their mechanisms of action?
3. What drug was administered subcutaneously by the paramedics and later in the emergency room? Which agents are suitable for nebulizer use?

CASE 6. ERGOTAMINE TOXICITY†

A 44-year-old woman with a history of moderate intake of ergotamine for migraine was admitted to hospital because of 3 days of increasingly cold and painful legs. Upon examination, the legs were

---

*Modified and reproduced, with permission, from Simon RA: Management of severe asthma in relapse: Case discussion. Chapter 28, p 241 in: *The Practical Management of Asthma*. Grune & Stratton, 1984.

†Modified and reproduced, with permission, from Christensen KN et al: Sodium nitroprusside and epidural blockade in the treatment of ergotism. N Engl J Med 1977;296:1271.

found to be cyanotic and cold, with no detectable pulses distal to the femoral arteries. Transfemoral aortography showed normal aortic and pelvic vessels. However, the external iliac and femoral arteries were severely constricted, as were the smaller arteries of both legs.

Continuous epidural blockade with bupivacaine was started but had no effect. A continuous infusion of nitroprusside was then begun, starting at 25 μg/min and increasing by 25 μg/min every 15 minutes. When the infusion rate reached 100 μg/min, the skin temperature of the great toe suddenly rose from 21.8 to 31.0 °C, the cyanosis cleared, and a normal pulse was felt in the peripheral vessels. Over a period of several hours, the skin temperature of the toe rose to 36 °C. Thirty-six hours after admission, the infusion was withdrawn without recurrence of vasoconstriction.

Questions, Case 6
1. What is the mechanism of ergot-induced vasospasm?
2. What is the safe limit of ergot consumption?
3. What is the mechanism of action of nitroprusside?
4. What medications should this patient receive to reduce her dependence on ergotamine for migraine relief?

CASE 7. ABSENCE SEIZURES*

An 18-year-old woman was admitted for evaluation of therapy for frequent epileptic absence attacks associated with minor automatisms. The patient had a history of unsuccessful treatment with ethosuximide. The electroencephalogram showed generalized 3/s spike and wave complexes and intermittent left temporal discharges.

Therapy was restarted using sodium valproate and carbamazepine. A 24-hour electroencephalographic study revealed 71 absence attacks. Increasing the valproate dosage from 1200 to 2400 mg/d was associated with a significant but transient decline in absence frequency. Mean serum levels of valproic acid at that time were 81 mg/L (109 mg/L peak, 36 mg/L trough) on a twice-daily dosage regimen. Slow withdrawal of carbamazepine resulted in a decrease in the number of clinical or electroencephalographic attacks. The addition of ethosuximide, 1000 mg/d, resulted in disappearance of all seizure activity. The mean serum ethosuximide level was 70 mg/L.

Six months later, an attempt was made to reduce the dosage of valproate. On a twice-daily dose of 300 mg (600 mg/d total), mean serum levels dropped to 34 mg/L. There was a prompt recurrence of seizures, but they declined again when valproate dosage was returned to 2400 mg/d. A follow-up study 8 months later demonstrated a continuing favorable response.

Questions, Case 7
1. What was the rationale for the initial treatment with carbamazepine? Why was the drug subsequently withdrawn, and why did the frequency of the seizures decrease?
2. Why were blood levels of the drugs measured several times during the day?
3. What are the hazards of therapy with ethosuximide? With sodium valproate?
4. What alternative drugs are possible for the management of absence seizures? What are the side effects of such backup drugs?

CASE 8. THE TIRED PATIENT†

A 47-year-old man visited an outpatient clinic with initial complaints of chronic tiredness, frequent bouts of stomach upset, and weight loss. Physical examination and laboratory studies were within normal limits. A psychiatric evaluation revealed that the patient had come to the clinic at the request of his wife, who thought that he was "depressed." He had been waking during the early morning hours and could not get back to sleep. The patient acknowledged that over the past year, he had lost interest in his work and had started to worry about providing for his family. He admitted to having also lost interest in sex. A diagnosis of major depression was made.

---

*Modified and reproduced, with permission, from Rowan AJ et al: Valproate-ethosuximide combination therapy for refractory absence seizures. Arch Neurol 1983;40:797.

†Modified and reproduced, with permission, from Coleman JH, Johnston JA: Affective disorders. Page 1021 in: *Applied Therapeutics,* 3rd ed. Katcher BS, Young LY, Koda-Kimble MA (editors). Applied Therapeutics, 1983.

Amitriptyline, 50 mg daily, was prescribed, to be taken at bedtime for 3 nights and 100 mg daily thereafter, also taken at bedtime. Two weeks later, an interview indicated that the patient was sleeping better but that his appetite remained poor and his mood was unimproved. The dosage of amitriptyline was increased to 200 mg/d.

Eight weeks after the initial visit, the patient had regained most of his lost weight and no longer had insomnia. However, he was not feeling much better. The side effects of the drug were bothersome, and he was becoming increasingly worried about his job and his family life. His feelings of inadequacy seemed to be increasing, and he had begun questioning what use he was to anybody. The psychiatrist initiated dose-tapering of amitriptyline and prescribed paroxetine (5 mg daily), with weekly increments of 5 mg up to a maximum dose of 20 mg/d.

Evaluation of the patient after 4 weeks of treatment with paroxetine revealed a major improvement in mood. He had a renewed interest in his job and in the activities of his family. His sex life had improved overall, though he was occasionally anorgasmic. Dry mouth, constipation, and occasional "jitteriness" were his only complaints about the drug he was taking.

Questions, Case 8
1. What are the major drug groups available for the treatment of major depression?
2. What considerations would support the initial choice of amitriptyline in this patient?
3. What reasons can you offer for the change to paroxetine?
4. What side effects and potential drug interactions must be dealt with during treatment of depressions with SSRIs?

CASE 9. THYROID DISEASE*

A 27-year-old woman was referred for evaluation of thyroid disease. She had a 3-month history of intermittent heat intolerance, sweats, tremor, tachycardia, and muscle weakness. She had lost weight in spite of a marked increase in appetite. She denied taking any medications before seeing her family physician. She had been taking iodide drops since seeing her doctor and initially noted a decrease in symptoms. For the past month, however, they had worsened.

Physical examination revealed blood pressure 180/90 mm Hg, heart rate 110/min, minimal proptosis, and an enlarged thyroid gland. Laboratory tests showed elevated thyroxine, resin T_3 uptake, radioactive iodine uptake, and antimicrosomal antibodies. A diagnosis of hyperimmune hyperthyroidism (Graves' disease) was made.

Questions, Case 9
1. What therapeutic measures should be considered in this case? Why did the iodide drops the patient was taking reduce symptoms at first and then lose their effectiveness?
2. What are the benefits and hazards of pharmacologic therapy in hyperthyroidism?
3. What therapy should be considered if thyrotoxic crisis (thyroid storm) occurs?

CASE 10. A DIABETIC STUDENT†

An 18-year-old college student was referred to the endocrine clinic at her student health service because a routine urinalysis revealed glycosuria, and a subsequently measured random plasma glucose was 250 mg/dL.

The history disclosed that this was the student's first time away from home and that she had had a number of symptoms she attributed to anxiety associated with the move to college. These symptoms included weight loss (5 kg), polydipsia, nocturia, fatigue, and three episodes of vaginal yeast infections in the past 3 months. Before coming to college, she had experienced a series of upper respiratory tract infections. The family history was negative for diabetes, and she was taking no medications.

---

*Modified and reproduced, with permission, from Dong BJ: Thyroid diseases. Page 1313 in: *Applied Therapeutics,* 3rd ed. Katcher BS, Young LY, Koda-Kimble MA (editors). Applied Therapeutics, 1983.

†Modified and reproduced, with permission, from Koda-Kimble MA, Rotblatt MD: Diabetes mellitus. Page 1357 in: *Applied Therapeutics,* 3rd ed. Katcher BS, Young LY, Koda-Kimble MA (editors). Applied Therapeutics, 1983.

The physical examination was within normal limits. Her weight was 50 kg, which is in the 20th percentile for her height. The laboratory results were as follows: fasting plasma glucose 280 mg/dL (< 115), urine glucose and ketones strongly positive. On the basis of these and other findings, a diagnosis of type I diabetes was made.

Questions, Case 10
1. What are the primary therapeutic strategies available in this case?
2. What are the complications and hazards of the major therapies for diabetes?
3. What methods of monitoring and adjusting therapy are available to the patient?

CASE 11. SEVERE RHEUMATOID ARTHRITIS*

A 60-year-old woman was referred for management of severe rheumatoid arthritis. She had had the disease for 15 years and had been treated until age 55 with aspirin. She was then switched to ibuprofen, which diminished the gastrointestinal adverse effects she had developed from aspirin. One year before referral, she started to complain of increased joint pain and stiffness, and laboratory studies confirmed that the disease had become more active. Several attempts to control her symptoms with an increased dosage of ibuprofen and with a trial of another NSAID were not successful, and the decision was made to add corticosteroids to the regimen.

Prednisone was started in a dosage of 5 mg daily, given in the morning. After a period of evaluation, the dosage was increased to 10 mg and then to 15 mg daily. At this dosage, the patient's symptoms were tolerable.

Questions, Case 11
1. What are the relative advantages and disadvantages of corticosteroids versus NSAIDs in the treatment of inflammatory disease?
2. Why was prednisone given to this patient in the morning?
3. What is the advantage of alternate-day therapy with corticosteroids? Which steroids are unsuitable for alternate-day therapy?

CASE 12. A PRESCHOOLER WITH FEVER†

A 42-month-old child was brought to a hospital emergency room with fever and signs suggestive of bacterial meningitis. Two months earlier, she had been treated for otitis media with cefaclor and had developed an urticarial rash. There was no record of vaccination against *Haemophilus influenzae* type b. On hospitalization, the child was treated with ampicillin and chloramphenicol for 72 hours and then placed on chloramphenicol alone on the basis of the results of microbiologic laboratory tests.

After 10 days of antibiotic treatment, the patient was afebrile and cerebrospinal fluid was sterile, with normal protein and glucose levels. Drug treatment was discontinued, but after 2 days she developed vomiting and fever to 40.5 °C. Cerebrospinal fluid culture was sterile, but counterimmunoelectrophoresis was positive for *Haemophilus influenzae* type b polyribosylribitol phosphate antigen.

The patient was treated for 10 days with ceftriaxone and remained afebrile after the second day. At completion of therapy, cerebrospinal fluid was sterile, counterimmunoelectrophoresis was negative, and the white cell count and protein levels were returning toward the normal range.

Questions, Case 12
1. Why was antibiotic treatment started before microbiologic laboratory examinations were completed?
2. What was the basis for the initial choice of ampicillin and chloramphenicol?
3. Why was ampicillin therapy stopped after 3 days?
4. What is the most likely cause of the apparent relapse after discontinuance of chloramphenicol?
5. What was the basis for the use of ceftriaxone?
6. What prophylaxis (if any) should be given to the close contacts of this child?

---

*Modified and reproduced, with permission, from Kishi DT: Disorders of the adrenals. Page 1279 in: *Applied Therapeutics,* 3rd ed. Katcher BS, Young LY, Koda-Kimble MA (editors). Applied Therapeutics, 1983.

†Adapted from Ampicillin and chloramphenicol resistance in systemic *Haemophilus influenzae* disease. Morb Mortal Wkly Rep 1984;33:35.

CASE 13. A DRUG REACTION*

A 64-year-old man was hospitalized for evaluation and treatment of carcinoma of the tongue. Following a course of chemotherapy, the patient was brought to the operating room for radical neck dissection. He was intubated and given 2 g of cefoxitin intravenously. Ten minutes later, he had developed severe hypotension with a systolic blood pressure of 40–50 mm Hg, wheezing over both lung fields, and urticaria.

The operation was postponed, and the patient was given intravenous epinephrine, dexamethasone, diphenhydramine, and fluids over the next 2 hours. Blood pressure was restored and maintained by intravenous infusion of dopamine. In the intensive care unit, electrocardiography suggested acute cardiac injury; the patient had no history of angina pectoris or heart disease. Subsequent chest x-ray revealed a normal heart size with bilateral pulmonary edema.

Questions, Case 13
1. Why was cefoxitin given at the time of surgery?
2. What type of drug allergy did the patient experience?
3. Why were epinephrine, diphenhydramine, and a corticosteroid administered?

CASE 14. DIARRHEA FOLLOWING ANTIBIOTICS†

A 10-year-old girl received erythromycin for a prolonged respiratory tract infection. She continued to have headaches and a stuffy nose; a facial x-ray suggested maxillary sinusitis, but the diagnosis could not be confirmed following sinus puncture. Erythromycin was stopped, and she was given amoxicillin (250 mg three times a day) for 10 days.

On the last day of amoxicillin treatment, she developed diarrhea with some abdominal pain but no vomiting. Initially, the stools were alternately watery and solid, but later they became mucoid with some blood. After 11 days of these symptoms, she was given loperamide for her diarrhea, and a stool culture was positive for *Clostridium difficile*.

She was hospitalized, and sigmoidoscopy revealed colitis with pseudomembranes, confirmed histologically. Stool culture was positive for *C difficile* and negative for *Salmonella, Shigella, Yersinia,* and *Campylobacter*. The girl was treated with oral vancomycin, 250 mg four times daily for 7 days, and was discharged following proctoscopic examination that proved normal and a negative *C difficile* stool culture.

Questions, Case 14
1. What was the rationale for the treatment of the upper respiratory tract infections with erythromycin?
2. Why was amoxicillin used to treat the suspected sinusitis?
3. What was the most likely cause of the diarrhea and the overgrowth of *C difficile* in the gastrointestinal tract?
4. Why was oral vancomycin used in this case? What alternative drug treatment should have been employed?

CASE 15. DIARRHEA FOLLOWING A TRIP‡

After returning from a trip to Mexico, a 41-year-old woman had a week-long bout of diarrhea that resolved spontaneously. She did not feel well for the succeeding 4 months, and then abdominal discomfort became severe and fever (but no bowel symptoms) occurred. There was no history of jaundice, gallstones, or hepatitis, but acute cholecystitis was suspected. The patient was admitted to the hospital for what proved to be a normal oral cholecystogram.

---

*Adapted and reproduced, with permission, from Austin SM, Barooah B, Chung SK: Reversible acute cardiac injury during cefoxitin-induced anaphylaxis in a patient with normal coronary arteries. Am J Med 1984;77:729.

†Adapted and reproduced, with permission, from Vesikari T et al: Pseudomembranous colitis with recurring diarrhea and prolonged persistence of *Clostridium difficile* in a 10-year-old girl. Acta Paediatr Scand 1984;73:135.

‡Modified and reproduced, with permission, from Strum WB: Persistent pain, fever after a trip to Mexico. Hosp Pract 1984;19:86.

Following the x-ray studies, diarrhea reappeared. She was referred to another institution and was initially treated with metronidazole, ampicillin, and gentamicin for presumed amebic liver abscesses or acute cholecystitis with liver abscesses. Subsequently, a serologic test for amebic infection was positive, and liver and spleen scans confirmed the presence of abscesses. Based on these findings, gentamicin and ampicillin were discontinued.

The patient's symptoms improved with a 10-day course of oral metronidazole and tetracycline. She became afebrile, and serologic tests for amebic infection reverted to negative. Oral iodoquinol was given for 3 weeks, and follow-up examinations showed resolution of the abscess cavities and no recurrence of symptoms.

Questions, Case 15

1. What are the most likely causes of diarrhea in a tourist following a trip to Mexico? Should such cases of traveler's diarrhea be routinely treated with antibiotics?
2. What antimicrobial activity is anticipated for ampicillin and gentamicin used in this case?
3. Why was metronidazole treatment continued after discontinuance of the above antibiotics? What does tetracycline add to the therapeutic regimen?
4. What was the rationale for the 3 weeks of oral treatment with iodoquinol?

CASE 16. POLYPHARMACY AND THE AIDS PATIENT

A 28-year-old male patient with HIV infection who was being treated as an outpatient with zidovudine and didanosine came to an AIDS clinic with complaints of abdominal pain, nausea, and vomiting. At his last visit, the CD4 count was > 500/μL and viral load was < 500 RNA copies/mL. Current laboratory data included amylase 240 units/L, creatinine 1 mg/dL, CD4 < 400/μL, viral load > 5000 RNA copies/mL. At this point, the drug regimen was changed to zidovudine plus lamivudine.

The patient's gastrointestinal symptoms resolved, but several months later he complained of feeling weak and presented with symptoms of thrush. At this time his CD4 count was 300/μL, the viral load was 11,000 copies/mL, and a tuberculin skin test was positive. The attending physician prescribed clotrimazole troches, isoniazid plus pyridoxine, and indinavir to supplement the combination of zidovudine and lamivudine.

During the next few months, the viral load declined to 6000 RNA copies/mL and then stabilized, but the CD4 count dropped to 150/μL, at which point two more agents were added to his drug regimen to prevent opportunistic infections. Unfortunately, the patient developed a gastric ulcer and had to be treated with bismuth subsalicylate, metronidazole, and tetracycline for *Helicobacter pylori*.

Ultimately, the patient's viral load began to increase, and when the CD4 count decreased to 40/μL, three more drugs were prescribed. By this time, a total of 11 drugs were being administered to slow disease progression and to prevent opportunistic infections.

Questions, Case 16

1. Why was didanosine discontinued and replaced by lamivudine when the patient complained of abdominal pain? What drug class do these anti-HIV agents represent?
2. Why was treatment with indinavir initiated? What type of drug is indinavir? What are its anticipated adverse effects?
3. Which two (or three) prophylactic drugs were most likely to have been administered when the CD4 count dropped below 200/μL, and what infections will they prevent?
4. Which three prophylactic drugs were most likely to have been administered when the CD4 count dropped below 50/μL, and what infections will they prevent?

CASE 17. THE AFRICAN TRAVELER*

A 20-year-old woman in good health planned to visit Kenya in a travel and study program. She was immunized against tetanus, typhoid, cholera, and yellow fever; received immune globulin; and in Kenya took chloroquine and Fansidar (pyrimethamine-sulfadoxine) for malaria prophylaxis. After

---

*Adapted from Acute schistosomiasis with transverse myelitis in American students returning from Kenya. Morb Mortal Wkly Rep 1984;33:445.

10 weeks, she was one of 15 students (of 18 in the original group) to become ill with fever, abdominal pain, and nonbloody diarrhea. Five days later, she developed severe back pain and then rapidly lost the ability to walk. Stool examination showed ova of *Schistosoma mansoni,* and she was diagnosed as having schistosomiasis with transverse myelitis.

She was treated with oxamniquine and transported to the USA, where evaluation showed flaccid paralysis and decreased sensation of touch and temperature over the skin of the legs. Cerebrospinal fluid examination showed pleocytosis and protein elevation. Serologic tests for *Mycoplasma* and viral agents were negative. A myelogram showed no masses amenable to surgical removal.

The patient was treated with praziquantel and large doses of dexamethasone. Her motor function and sensation improved with treatment, and within a month she was ambulating with assistance in a rehabilitation center.

Questions, Case 17

1. Why was this patient taking both chloroquine and pyrimethamine-sulfadoxine for malaria prophylaxis?
2. Why was oxamniquine used for the initial treatment of schistosomiasis in this case? What are its anticipated adverse effects?
3. How does praziquantel differ from other drugs used in schistosomiasis? What is known about its mechanism of action?
4. What are the anticipated adverse effects of praziquantel? Is there any reason to believe that praziquantel (or oxamniquine) might have been contraindicated in this patient?
5. Why was dexamethasone administered?

ANSWERS: CASE HISTORIES

Answers, Case 1

1. The most probable chemical intoxicants in the case of the 55-year-old gardener are insecticides. The most common constituents of currently available insecticides that produce acute poisoning are the cholinesterase inhibitors and nicotine. This patient's signs of muscarinic excess (abdominal discomfort and diarrhea) developed over a week, suggesting that a long-acting drug was gradually accumulating to a toxic level. The symptoms of cholinergic toxicity are described in Chapter 7. Miosis and perspiration are common signs of cholinesterase inhibition. Nicotine toxicity rarely has such a slow onset and usually includes signs of sympathetic as well as parasympathetic discharge. The diagnosis can be confirmed by measuring the patient's blood cholinesterase level and by identifying a carbamate- or organophosphate-containing insecticide among the patient's stock of garden supplies.
2. Immediate measures must be taken to maintain vital signs and to make certain that exposure to the intoxicant has ceased. Because the patient is unconscious, induction of emesis is contraindicated, and gastric lavage should not be attempted unless a cuffed endotracheal tube is in place. Since the patient's symptoms developed over a 1-week period, it is unlikely that the present stomach contents are contributing much to his intoxication. Since the organophosphates can be absorbed across the skin, the clothing should be removed and the skin cleansed (with care to avoid contamination of medical personnel). With an endotracheal tube in place, mechanical respiratory assistance can be applied as required to maintain normal blood gases, and gastric lavage may be done if there is any chance that the intoxicant was ingested. An intravenous line should be placed for the administration of drugs and fluids for maintenance of good hydration.
3. Drugs to be considered for this patient include (a) atropine for control of muscarinic effects; (b) pralidoxime for regeneration of cholinesterase, especially at the neuromuscular junction; and (c) cardiovascular stimulants, but only if required to maintain a normal tissue perfusion. (Cardiovascular stimulants are rarely required.)

Answers, Case 2

1. The cause of the dramatic rise in serum potassium was the poisoning of membrane Na^+/K^+ ATPase (the sodium pump)—in the entire body, not just the heart. The serum potassium concentration can be used as an index of the severity of poisoning and may be more accurate as a prognostic tool than the blood level of digoxin. The source of the potassium is the intracellular space, particularly that of skeletal muscle (because of the large mass of this organ system).

2. Digitalis has the well-deserved reputation of causing any and all types of cardiac arrhythmias. The most common are junctional tachycardia (originating in the atrioventricular node) and ventricular tachycardia. The atrial fibrillation detected on admission of this patient was probably a chronic condition related to his mitral stenosis. The high degree of atrioventricular block, with the slow ventricular rate, could reflect the strong vagal effects of the cardiac glycoside, but in view of this patient's resistance to atropine, the AV block probably represents direct depression by the drug or by the elevated potassium. The widened QRS complex and the very slow spontaneous rate when pacing was interrupted reflect severe depression of Purkinje and ventricular cell automaticity and excitability. Such depression was probably caused by depolarization by the high extracellular potassium level. Under these circumstances, administration of antiarrhythmic agents, which are also cardiac depressants, was clearly contraindicated.

   The effects noted in this patient were unusually severe. At the levels of toxicity commonly observed in nonsuicidal patients, automaticity is usually increased, not decreased. In such patients, depressant interventions such as administration of potassium or antiarrhythmic drugs are often successful in controlling arrhythmias.

3. Conventional therapy of mild to moderate cardiac glycoside intoxication consists of: (a) Normalization of low serum K^+. In the present case and in most cases of gross overdosage, the serum K^+ is high. However, in many cases of mild to moderate toxicity, the serum K^+ is low or normal. In some cases (usually involving vomiting or diarrhea), low serum magnesium is found, and correction of this deficiency corrects the arrhythmia. (b) Use of antiarrhythmic drugs. Lidocaine is usually tried first. (c) Avoidance of DC cardioversion unless ventricular fibrillation occurs.

   The first two of these approaches were clearly not suitable for this severely intoxicated patient.

4. Severe intoxication is less common with digitoxin than with digoxin because digitoxin is rarely used. Anti-digoxin Fab fragments cross-react sufficiently to be useful in reversing digitoxin effects. Lavage of the small intestine with steroid-binding resins (eg, cholestyramine) has been of value in some cases. The success of such treatment reflects the importance of enterohepatic circulation of digitoxin. Anti-digoxin Fab fragments have been used successfully in cases of poisoning with oleander cardiac glycoside as well.

Answers, Case 3

1. The case description is typical of antimuscarinic drug poisoning. A common source of such agents in nature is jimsonweed *(Datura stramonium)*. The patient had ingested several of the 2- to 3-mm round black seeds from the pods of this plant.

2. The most life-threatening effect of the antimuscarinic agents in many patients, especially small children and infants, is hyperthermia. Unsupervised hallucinating patients may fall and injure themselves. Convulsions and arrhythmias may occur. Other effects of these drugs, though uncomfortable, are not life-threatening.

3. The chief danger of physostigmine is its central stimulant effect, which may lead to convulsions. Because of this hazard, many emergency departments prefer to treat antimuscarinic poisoning symptomatically. Other anticholinesterase drugs, such as neostigmine, do not enter the CNS as readily as physostigmine; they are less dangerous but also less effective in reversing the central effects of the intoxicant. Symptomatic treatment includes cooling fans or cooling blankets and IV fluids. Cardiac arrhythmias may occasionally require treatment with antiarrhythmic drugs.

Answers, Case 4

1. Because metaraminol is an alpha-adrenoceptor agonist, it causes marked vasoconstriction, which can be accompanied by reflex bradycardia. This patient rapidly became dependent upon the exogenous stimulant for maintenance of cardiac output, and attempts to stop the infusion resulted in hypotension.

2. The hematocrit increased because of hemoconcentration. Marked vasoconstriction results in increased Starling forces acting outward across the capillary wall, and increased capillary permeability caused by local ischemia facilitates the movement of plasma water out of the vascular compartment and into the tissues and the urine.

3. The patient went into shock because of the loss of blood volume described in Answer 2 and because the increased cardiac work (caused by vasoconstriction) was causing heart failure. The result was a form of hypotension that responds well to volume replacement and renal vasodilators.

4. As noted in Answer 3, volume replacement (eg, with dextran solution) is the most important aspect of therapy in this situation. Because the patient's cardiovascular system had become dependent upon exogenous sympathomimetics, norepinephrine was necessary for a short time. However, rapid removal of this stimulus was indicated and successfully accomplished in this case.

Answers, Case 5

1. The mediators most important in causing asthmatic bronchoconstriction are leukotrienes LTC_4 and LTD_4. Another leukotriene (LTB_4), prostaglandins, peptides, and histamine probably also play a role (Chapter 20).
2. The most commonly used bronchodilators are the beta-adrenoceptor agonists and the methylxanthines. In some patients, a muscarinic blocking drug (eg, ipratropium) has a useful bronchodilating effect. Cromolyn and nedocromil inhibit the degranulation of mast cells and are useful as prophylactic agents in some patients. They are not useful in an acute attack. Systemic corticosteroids are reserved for patients with severe asthma who do not respond adequately to other agents, but inhaled steroids (eg, beclomethasone) are appropriate prophylactic therapy for all individuals with moderate or severe recurrent asthma.
3. The drug administered by the paramedics and by the personnel in the emergency room was epinephrine. This agent is extremely effective and has a rapid onset of action. However, it is probably no more effective than inhaled β_2-selective agonists (albuterol, terbutaline, metaproterenol). The drugs commonly used in nebulizers include epinephrine, isoproterenol, and the β_2-selective agonists. Note that nebulized drug is less efficacious than canister aerosols because the latter consist of smaller particles of drug-containing liquid that reach farther down into the airways.

Answers, Case 6

1. Ergot causes vasoconstriction through the activation of several receptors, including alpha-adrenoceptors and serotonin receptors. The alkaloids are partial agonists but have an extremely high affinity for the receptors. The high affinity results in inability of alpha blockers (eg, phentolamine) to displace the partial agonist molecules and an extremely long duration of effect. Additional receptors may be involved, since blockade of both adrenoceptors and serotonin receptors is often ineffective in reversing ergot-induced vasospasm.
2. The recommended limits of ergotamine consumption are 2–6 mg of ergotamine tartrate per episode of migraine and not more than 10 tablets (10 mg) per week. For severe migraine, intravenous administration of dihydroergotamine mesylate is sometimes effective. A maximum of 2 mg per dose of this drug is recommended, with a limit of 6 mg per week.
3. Nitroprusside breaks down spontaneously to release nitric oxide. Nitric oxide stimulates the production of cGMP in vascular smooth muscle, which causes relaxation (Chapter 12).
4. If the patient has frequent attacks of migraine, prophylactic medication is indicated. Ergonovine and methysergide, a semisynthetic ergot derivative, have been used with partial success in many patients. Propranolol, amitriptyline, some calcium channel blockers, and cyproheptadine have also been effective. Note that sumatriptan, a 5-HT_{1D} agonist, is very useful in treating acute migraine attacks but not in preventing recurrences.

Answers, Case 7

1. Carbamazepine was probably used at the start of treatment to prevent the automatisms (complex partial seizures) that were reportedly part of the patient's seizure repertoire. Carbamazepine is considered the drug of choice for this seizure type. When it became apparent that such seizures were actually infrequent in this patient, the drug was withdrawn. Carbamazepine has been reported to make absence (or myoclonic) seizures worse.
2. Monitoring of blood levels can be important in the management of epilepsy because the therapeutic window of most antiepileptic drugs is narrow. The effective levels for valproate and ethosuximide are 50–100 mg/L. Thus, the levels measured in this patient while she was receiving the high dose of valproate were within the effective range for both agents. When the dose of valproate was reduced to 600 mg/d, the plasma levels dropped below the minimum effective range, and seizures recurred.
3. Ethosuximide is associated with a very low incidence of serious adverse effects. Gastric irritation and lethargy, fatigue, and other CNS effects are reported. In contrast, valproate carries with it a low but significant risk of serious hepatic injury; liver function should be moni-

tored. Valproic acid is contraindicated in pregnant women because it has been shown to cause spina bifida in infants born to mothers taking the drug. Valproic acid may inhibit the hepatic metabolism of other anticonvulsant drugs, including carbamazepine, lamotrigine, and phenytoin.

4. Alternative drugs for the management of absence seizures include clonazepam and lamotrigine. Clonazepam is less effective than ethosuximide or valproic acid; tolerance develops rapidly; and the doses used cause drowsiness, drooling, and ataxia. Lamotrigine is a recently introduced anticonvulsant drug with activity in absence seizures as well as in both generalized and partial seizures. The most distinctive toxicity of lamotrigine is life-threatening rashes, which can include Stevens-Johnson syndrome and toxic epidermal necrolysis.

Answers, Case 8

1. Several drug groups are available for the treatment of major (endogenous) depression. These include the selective serotonin reuptake inhibitors (SSRIs), the tricyclic agents (TCAs), a group of heterocyclic "second-generation" antidepressants, and the monoamine oxidase inhibitors (MAOIs).

2. While the SSRIs are the drugs most frequently used for treatment of major depressions, the tricyclics remain valuable alternatives. In some patients, a tricyclic may be the first choice, especially if the past history indicates a positive therapeutic response to such drugs. The sedative actions of tricyclics may be of value in depressed patients, with insomnia or weight loss, since SSRIs tend to exacerbate such symptoms. *Generic* formulations of the tricyclics are much less costly than any other antidepressant drugs. For example, the cost to the pharmacist for a 30-day supply of generic amitriptyline is less than $3, while the cost of a similar supply of paroxetine is 60 dollars or more.

3. Limited effectiveness and toxicity are the major reasons for switching a patient from one antidepressant drug to another. SSRIs are often superior to tricyclics in their clinical efficacy, and in this case amitriptyline had not proved effective after a reasonable trial (8 weeks). At that time, the depressive symptoms in this patient included feelings of worthlessness and possibly suicidal ideation. Tricyclic overdose is especially dangerous in depressed patients, who often use medications close at hand in attempting suicide. Ingestion of just a 2-week supply of amitriptyline can cause severe hypotension, cardiac arrhythmias, seizures, coma, and death.

4. The most common adverse effects associated with the SSRIs are nausea, headache, jitteriness, and insomnia. The SSRIs are less likely than tricyclics to cause weight gain, hypotension, and anticholinergic side effects, though paroxetine does have mild atropine-like side effects. The selective serotonin reuptake inhibitors are relatively free of life-threatening toxicities but may cause seizures in overdose. Concomitant use of MAO inhibitors with SSRIs may cause a **serotonin syndrome,** which is characterized by muscle rigidity, hyperpyrexia, hypotension, coma, and death. The SSRIs are inhibitors of hepatic cytochrome P450 and may enhance the actions of other drugs including tricyclic antidepressants and warfarin.

Answers, Case 9

1. The major therapies available for Graves' disease are surgery, thyroid-suppressant drugs, and radioactive iodine in sufficient dosage to destroy the gland. Ipodate, an iodine-containing x-ray contrast material, and beta-blockers are of value in severe thyrotoxicosis.

   Iodide therapy (usually saturated solution of potassium iodide) is useful in reducing thyroid hormone release and in decreasing the vascularity of the gland prior to surgery. However, escape from the inhibitory effect of iodide often occurs in Graves' disease, and the increased iodine substrate made available by the therapy may actually accentuate the disease.

2. Radioactive iodine is often the treatment of choice for young adult patients. This treatment provides a permanent cure. (In fact, hypothyroidism is common after treatment and is managed with levothyroxine replacement therapy.) There is no evidence that the exposure to this radioactivity increases the incidence of cancer, even after 35 years of follow-up. However, radioactive iodine should not be used in pregnant women because it crosses the placenta and will damage the fetal thyroid as well as that of the mother.

   Antithyroid drugs include iodide (discussed above) and the thioamides. The principal thioamides are propylthiouracil and methimazole. Almost all patients respond promptly to these agents. However, immunologic complications are not rare. Skin rashes are the most common. Agranulocytosis, cholestatic jaundice, hepatocellular damage, and exfoliative dermatitis are uncommon.

Surgical thyroidectomy is the treatment of choice for patients with very large or multinodular glands. Patients are treated preoperatively with antithyroid drugs until they are euthyroid, and they receive iodine for 2 weeks prior to surgery to reduce vascularity of the gland.

3. Patients in thyrotoxic crisis usually have multiple system involvement. The cardiovascular system is particularly susceptible, and severe tachycardia, arrhythmias, and heart failure are common. The sympathetic nervous system is hyperactive, and this is one of the major causes of the cardiovascular effects. The CNS is also affected, and signs may include severe agitation, delirium, and coma.

Ipodate, which inhibits the conversion of thyroxine to triiodothyronine, is very useful in reducing the intensity of thyroid storm. Sympathoplegic drugs are also very useful, and propranolol is the one most commonly used. Further release of hormone from the gland is blocked by intravenous administration of sodium iodide supplemented by oral potassium iodide. Synthesis is inhibited by oral or, if necessary, parenteral antithyroid drugs. Corticosteroids are sometimes used.

Answers, Case 10

1. In a young diabetic of low or normal weight with a history of viral infections preceding onset of hyperglycemia, it is likely that the disease is due to loss of functioning pancreatic islet B cells. The diagnosis of insulin deficiency (type I) diabetes was made in this case. The oral hypoglycemic agents are not useful in type I diabetes, but they are used in non-insulin-dependent (type II) diabetes. The strategies available in this case are dietary management and insulin.

2. The most important acute toxicity of insulin therapy is hypoglycemia. This is an emergency that the patient and family must be prepared to deal with, since it may occur suddenly or insidiously and can result in brain damage or death if not treated promptly and effectively. Treatment is by administration of glucose or glucagon.

The long-term complications of insulin therapy include immunologic problems, such as insulin allergy and insulin resistance caused by formation of antibodies to the insulin used. These effects can be minimized by the use of purified preparations that contain lower concentrations of noninsulin protein or by the use of human insulin preparations.

Another complication of insulin therapy is lipodystrophy at the site of injection. This consists of atrophy of the subcutaneous lipid tissue. It has become much less common since the advent of improved methods of purifying insulin, and even the standard preparations are now relatively free of the effect. In fact, lipid hypertrophy may occur.

The toxicities of the oral hypoglycemic drugs (not suitable in this case) are more varied than those of insulin therapy. Tolbutamide is associated with a low incidence of skin rashes and interactions with other drugs that result in prolonged hypoglycemia. Chlorpropamide causes prolonged hypoglycemia more often than tolbutamide, as well as jaundice and an antidiuretic effect. The latter action may cause dilutional hyponatremia. The second-generation agents (glipizide, glyburide) are so much more potent than the older sulfonylureas that care must be exercised to avoid significant hypoglycemia.

3. Most patients should monitor their blood glucose as an aid to adjustment of insulin dosage. The major reason for daily (or even more often) adjustment of dosage is that insulin requirement is altered by many factors: diet, exercise, disease, etc. Considerable evidence indicates that close control of blood glucose is associated with a lower incidence of long-term complications of diabetes.

The major adjustments made by most patients are the total number of units of insulin injected and the proportions of rapid-acting and intermediate- or long-acting preparations used.

Answers, Case 11

1. Corticosteroids are more effective than NSAIDs in controlling acute severe flare-ups of joint inflammation. However, the severe toxicities of corticosteroids (adrenocortical suppression, weight gain, buffalo hump, striae, osteoporosis, diabetes, peptic ulcers, cataracts, glaucoma, and psychoses) preclude their use for chronic therapy in most patients.

2. The normal diurnal variation of glucocorticoid release includes a peak in the morning hours and a trough late at night. Therefore, a single morning dose of an intermediate-acting (12–24 hours) agent such as prednisone mimics the normal variation and reduces the degree of suppression of the pituitary.

3. Alternate-day therapy permits maintenance of a greater degree of pituitary-adrenal interaction and also allows temporary recovery of peripheral tissues from stimulation by high levels of

glucocorticoid. This is particularly valuable in growing children. The longest-acting cortico-steroids are not suitable for alternate-day regimens because the duration of pituitary suppression extends over 48 hours, and nothing is gained. Such long-acting agents include paramethasone, dexamethasone, and betamethasone.

Answers, Case 12

1. The principal justification for empiric, presumptive antimicrobial therapy is that the infection is best treated early to avoid serious morbidity or death. Suspected bacterial meningitis is a classic example of the need to initiate therapy immediately—after relevant samples have been taken for culture and sensitivity determination—on the basis of the clinical diagnosis and the initial microbiologic diagnosis. The latter should include history, physical signs, and Gram's stain.

2. The most likely pathogens involved in bacterial meningitis in children from age 3 months to 7 years are *S pneumoniae,* meningococci, and *Haemophilus influenzae* type b. The latter organism has become a less common cause of bacterial meningitis in infants and young children since the introduction of protein-conjugated vaccines. Most infectious disease specialists would now *start* treatment of suspected bacterial meningitis in children with a third-generation cephalosporin such as ceftriaxone or cefotaxime. However, some practitioners may initiate treatment with chloramphenicol and ampicillin until microbiologic laboratory results identify the infecting organism and document its susceptibility to antimicrobial drugs.

3. The microbiology laboratory confirmed *H influenzae* type b and demonstrated that the isolate was beta-lactamase-positive. Ampicillin is inactivated by penicillinases unless used in combination with an inhibitor of such enzymes. Beta-lactamase-producing isolates of *H influenzae* type b are not resistant to chloramphenicol or to third-generation cephalosporins.

4. Although the cerebrospinal fluid was apparently sterile, the counterimmunoelectrophoresis analysis suggests a relapse caused by *H influenzae* type b owing to inadequate treatment with chloramphenicol or development of resistance.

5. The third-generation cephalosporins cefotaxime and ceftriaxone are effective in the empiric treatment of bacterial meningitis caused by most strains of meningococci, pneumococci, and *H influenzae.* However, the prevalence of drug-resistant *S pneumoniae* can influence empiric therapy and may necessitate the addition of vancomycin. Note that many isolates of *H influenzae* are now resistant to both ampicillin and chloramphenicol.

6. Rifampin is recommended for household or day care contacts of the index case with meningitis due to *H influenzae* type b, and the drug would also be prophylactic against meningococcal meningitis.

Answers, Case 13

1. Chemoprophylaxis is indicated when the wound infection rate for surgical procedures under optimal conditions is 5% or more. This patient had been treated for cancer, possibly with immuno-suppressive agents, and may have been at particular risk for infection. The cephalosporins are the most commonly used antimicrobial agents for surgical prophylaxis because they have activity against gram-positive cocci and selected gram-negative bacilli that are likely pathogens. Most commonly, a first-generation drug (eg, cefazolin) should be used, but under some circumstances a second-generation cephalosporin such as cefoxitin may be appropriate.

2. The patient experienced a classic type I (immediate) IgE-mediated allergic reaction, which often includes anaphylaxis, urticaria, and angioedema. Antimicrobial drugs, particularly the beta-lactams and sulfonamides, can cause type I reactions. The degree of cross-allergenicity between penicillins and cephalosporins is probably less than 10%. Skin testing with a dilute solution of drug may reveal drug sensitivity but often gives false-negative results.

3. Epinephrine and isoproterenol (via cAMP mechanisms) and theophylline (via cAMP or block of adenosine receptors) inhibit the release of mediators from mast cells and basophils and cause bronchodilation. Diphenhydramine competitively blocks histamine actions at H_1 receptors, actions that would otherwise cause bronchoconstriction and increased capillary permeability. Dexamethasone has multiple cellular effects, including inhibition of IgE-producing clone proliferation, block of T helper cell function, and anti-inflammatory actions. Most of the actions of glucocorticoids result from decreases in the synthesis of cytokines (eg, interleukins, platelet-activating factor) or eicosanoids (leukotrienes, prostaglandins).

Answers, Case 14

1. There is no information in the history of the original upper respiratory tract infection regarding possible or confirmed pathogens or their susceptibility to antimicrobial drugs. Erythromycin has activity against common streptococci, staphylococci (including penicillinase-producing strains), and *Mycoplasma pneumoniae;* this presumably underlies the choice of the drug in this case. Erythromycin may cause gastrointestinal irritation, occasional cholestasis (rare in children), and drug interactions via its inhibition of hepatic cytochrome P450. There is no cross-allergenicity with the penicillin group.

2. The suspected sinusitis had not responded to erythromycin. Since attempts to confirm bacterial infection had failed, amoxicillin therapy was started on empiric grounds. Amoxicillin has activity against many streptococci and some *H influenzae* strains as well as selected gram-negative rods. The drug is not active against penicillinase-producing organisms or *M pneumoniae.* However, these organisms should have been eradicated by the prior treatment with erythromycin.

3. Ampicillin is more likely to cause diarrhea than most other penicillins, partly by direct gastrointestinal irritation and partly by disturbing the normal gut flora. In this case, its close congener, amoxicillin, resulted in diarrhea that persisted more than a week after drug discontinuance, suggesting the possibility of microbial superinfection. This was confirmed by culture of *Clostridium difficile.* This organism causes colitis following therapy with a variety of antibiotics, including clindamycin, the tetracyclines, and beta-lactam agents.

4. When given orally, vancomycin has been effective in the treatment of colitis caused by toxin-producing bacteria, including *C difficile.* However, most infectious disease specialists advocate treatment of pseudomembranous colitis with metronidazole. Oral metronidazole is equally effective, and the cost of treatment is only one third that of vancomycin. Most importantly, because of the increasing incidence of vancomycin-resistant enterococci and staphylococci, this drug should not be used if an alternative agent is readily available. Bacitracin has also been used successfully in the treatment of pseudomembranous colitis.

Answers, Case 15

1. The most common causes of traveler's diarrhea are infections due to coliform bacteria and viruses. Most such infections are self-limiting, and fluid and electrolyte replacement is usually adequate treatment. Antibiotics (eg, doxycycline, trimethoprim-sulfamethoxazole) are useful prophylactic agents against coliforms but are ineffective in gastrointestinal infections due to viruses and only minimally effective against intestinal protozoans.

2. Ampicillin and gentamicin were included in the drug regimen on the basis of a possible bacterial involvement in acute cholecystitis, a component of the initial clinical diagnosis. Neither drug is active against amebic infection. Ampicillin would provide coverage for streptococci (including enterococci) and selected gram-negative enteric organisms, and gentamicin is active against aerobic gram-negative rods. Neither drug has good activity against gram-negative anaerobes, and anaerobic bacteria are a major cause of bacterial liver abscess.

3. The confirmed diagnosis of amebic disease justified therapy with metronidazole, which is effective in most cases of extraluminal amebiasis, though it is not a luminal amebicide. Metronidazole also has antibacterial actions, including activity against gram-negative anaerobes. Oral tetracycline is an inhibitor of bacteria that associate with *Entamoeba histolytica* in the gut, and the drug may indirectly affect luminal amebas by such an action.

4. Iodoquinol and diloxanide furoate are not effective in severe intestinal amebiasis or in amebic hepatic abscess. These drugs are used in asymptomatic intestinal amebiasis to treat concurrent intestinal infection and to totally eradicate the protozoan to prevent disease recurrence.

Answers, Case 16

1. In the initial management of this patient, two nucleoside reverse transcriptase inhibitors were administered, presumably for additive anti-HIV effects. Hematologic suppression is a major adverse effect of zidovudine, while peripheral neuropathy and pancreatitis are important toxicities of didanosine. The gastrointestinal symptoms, together with the elevated amylase levels, were the reasons for discontinuance of didanosine and the substitution of another nucleoside reverse transcriptase inhibitor (lamivudine) in the drug regimen.

2. The availability of quantitative measures of viral RNA now permits direct measurement and monitoring of antiviral drug effects. Since the viral load was increasing despite the administration of two reverse transcriptase inhibitors, a protease inhibitor (indinavir) was added to the

anti-HIV drug regimen. The adverse effects of indinavir include kidney stones (which may be diminished by full hydration), hyperbilirubinemia, and drug interactions due to inhibition of hepatic cytochrome P450.

3. When the CD4 count of an HIV patient falls below 200/μL, prophylaxis against pneumocystis pneumonia is instituted, usually with trimethoprim-sulfamethoxazole plus dapsone. Alternative prophylactic regimens include aerosol pentamidine plus dapsone. Trimethoprim-sulfamethoxazole plus dapsone is also prophylactic against toxoplasmosis.

4. When the CD4 count of an HIV patient falls below 50/μL, prophylaxis is recommended against *M avium-intracellulare* with azithromycin or clarithromycin. To prevent fungal infections due to *C albicans* or *Cryptococcus,* oral fluconazole is recommended. In addition, ganciclovir (or foscarnet) may be given prophylactically if the patient is seropositive for CMV.

Answers, Case 17

1. Chloroquine-resistant *P falciparum* is endemic in many regions of Africa, including Kenya, and the prophylactic use of chloroquine as a sole agent will not prevent infection. While pyrimethamine-sulfadoxine has been used prophylactically, it is not the drug of choice. Weekly doses of mefloquine 1 week before entering an endemic area, during the stay, and for 4 weeks after leaving, is the preferred method.

2. Oxamniquine is active against mature and immature forms of *Schistosoma mansoni* (but not other schistosomes), though resistance can occur. The initial use of the drug was presumably based on identification of the parasite ova in stools, this drug's ease of administration (it is orally effective), and—possibly—its availability. Adverse effects of oxamniquine include dizziness, headache, drowsiness, gastrointestinal irritation, and pruritus. Effects probably due to dying parasites include eosinophilia, pulmonary infiltrates, and urticaria. At high doses, oxamniquine may cause hallucinations and seizures.

3. Praziquantel is the drug of choice for infections caused by all species of schistosomes. The agent increases the permeability of the parasite cell membrane to calcium, causing initial contraction and then paralysis of its musculature. The tegmen becomes vacuolized and disintegrates, causing parasite death.

4. The most common toxic effects of praziquantel are malaise, headache, dizziness, gastrointestinal irritation, urticaria, and fever. Some of these effects may be caused by dying parasites.

5. Corticosteroids are used to suppress host immune responses and inflammation, including reactions to eggs deposited in the venules in and around the spinal cord.

Appendix V

Strategies for Improving Test Performance

There are many strategies for studying and exam taking, and decisions about which ones to use are partly a function of individual habit and preference. However, basic study rules may be applied to any learning exercise; test-taking strategies depend upon the type of examination. For those interested in *test-writing* strategies, the Case and Swanson reference is strongly recommended (see References).

FIVE BASIC STUDY RULES

1. Never read more than a few pages of dense textual material without stopping to write out the gist of it from memory. This is a universal rule for effective study. If necessary, refer to the material just read. After finishing a chapter, make up your own tables of the major drugs, receptor types, mechanisms, etc, and fill in as many of the blanks as you can. Refer to tables and figures in the book as needed to amplify your own notes. Make up and write down your own mnemonics if possible. Look up other mnemonics in books if you can't think of one yourself.* This is active learning; just reading is passive and far less effective unless you happen to have a photographic memory. Notes should be legible and saved for ready access when reviewing before exams.

2. Experiment with additional study methods until you find out what works for you. This may involve solo study or group study, flash cards, or text reading. You won't know how effective these techniques are until you have tried them.

3. Don't scorn "cramming," but don't rely on it either. Some steady, day-by-day reading and digestion of conceptual material is usually needed to avoid last-minute indigestion. Similarly, don't substitute memorization of lists (eg, the Key Words list, Appendix I) for more substantive understanding.

4. If you are preparing for a course examination, make every effort to attend all the lectures. The lecturer's view of what is important may be very different from that of the author of the textbook, and the chances are good that exam questions will be based on the instructor's own lecture notes.

5. If old test questions are legitimately available (as they are for the USMLE and courses in most medical schools), be sure to make use of these guides to study. By definition, they are a strong indicator of what the examination writers have considered core information in the recent past (also see 4, above).

STRATEGIES APPLICABLE TO ALL EXAMINATIONS

Three general rules apply to all examinations.
1. When starting the examination, scan the entire question set before answering any. If the examination has several parts, allot time to each part in proportion to its length. Within each part, answer the easy questions first, placing a mark in the margin by the questions to which you will return.

---

*This book contains many mnemonics. Another good source is Bhushan V, et al: *First Aid for the USMLE Step 1*. Appleton & Lange. An annual publication.

Practice saving enough time for the more difficult questions by scheduling one minute or less for each question on practice examinations such as those in Appendices II and III in this book. (The time available in the USMLE examination is approximately one minute per question.)

2. When answering multiple-choice questions such as those on the USMLE, don't change your first guess unless you find a convincing reason for doing so.

3. Understand the method for scoring wrong answers. The USMLE does not penalize for wrong answers; it scores only the total number of correct answers. Therefore, even if you have no idea what the correct answer may be, make a guess anyway since there is no penalty for an incorrect answer. In other words, *do not leave any blanks on a USMLE answer sheet*. Note that this may not be true for some local examinations; some scoring algorithms do penalize for incorrect answers. Make sure you understand the rules for such local examinations.

STRATEGIES FOR SPECIFIC QUESTION FORMATS

A certain group of students—often characterized as "good test-takers"—may not know every detail about the subject matter being tested but seem to perform extremely well most of the time. The strategy used by these people is not a secret, though few instructors seem to realize how easy it is to break down their questions into much simpler ones. Lists of these strategies are widely available, eg, in the descriptive material distributed by the National Board of Medical Examiners to its candidates. A paraphrased compendium of this advice is presented below.

A. Strategies for the "Choose the One Best Answer" Type Question:

1. Many of the newer "clinical correlation" questions on the USMLE have an extremely long stem that provides a great deal of clinical data. Much of the data presented may be irrelevant. The challenge becomes one of *finding out what is being asked*. One method for rapidly narrowing the search is to scan the answer list *first* when confronted with a very long stem. The nature of the answers will provide a clue to the parts of the stem that are relevant and those that are not.

2. If two statements are contradictory (ie, only one can be correct), chances are good that one of the two is the correct answer, ie, the other three choices may be distracters. For example, consider the following:

    In treating quinidine overdose, the best strategy would be to
    (A) Alkalinize the urine
    (B) Acidify the urine
    (C) Give procainamide
    (D) Give potassium chloride
    (E) Administer a calcium chelator such as EDTA

    The correct answer is **(B)**, acidify the urine. The instructor revealed what was being tested in the first pair of choices and used the last three as "filler." Therefore, if you don't know the answer, you are better off guessing (A) or (B) (a 50% success probability) than (A) or (B) or (C) or (D) or (E) (a 20% success probability). Note that this strategy is valid only if you **must** guess; many instructors now introduce contradictory pairs as distracters. Another "rule" that should only be used if you must guess is the "longest choice" rule. When all the answers in a multiple-choice question are relatively long, the correct answer is often the longest one. Note again that sophisticated question writers may introduce especially long **incorrect** choices to defeat this strategy.

3. Statements that contain the words "always," "never," "must," etc, are usually false. For example:

    Acetylcholine always increases the heart rate when given intravenously because it lowers blood pressure and evokes a strong baroreceptor-mediated reflex tachycardia.

    The statement is false because although acetylcholine often increases the heart rate, it can also cause bradycardia. (When given as a bolus, it may reach the sinus node in high enough concentration to cause initial bradycardia.) The use of "trigger" words such as "always" and "must" suggests that the instructor had some exception in mind. However, be aware that there are a few situations in which the statement with a trigger word is correct.

4. Choices that do not grammatically fit the stem are usually wrong. For example:

    A drug that acts on a beta receptor and produces a maximal effect that is equal to one-half the effect of a large dose of isoproterenol is called a

    (A)   Agonist
    (B)   Partial agonist
    (C)   Antagonist
    (D)   Analog of isoproterenol
        The use of the article *a* rather than *an* at the end of the stem implies that the answer must start with a consonant, ie, choice **(B).** Similar use may be made of disagreements in number. Note that careful question writers will avoid this problem by placing the articles in the choice list, not in the stem.

    5.   A statement is not false just because changing a few words will make it somewhat more true than you think it is now. "Choose the one best answer" does not mean "Choose the only correct statement."

B. Strategies for Matching Type Questions: Matching questions usually test name recognition, and the most efficient approach consists of reading each stem item and then scanning the list of choices from the start and picking the first clear "hit." This is especially important on extended matching questions in which just reading the list can be time-consuming. (It should be noted, however, that the strategy suggested by the National Board of Medical Examiners for the USMLE differs from the above; see its *General Instructions* publication.) Occasionally, the strategies described above for "the single best answer" type question can be applied to the matching and extended matching types.

C. Strategies for the "Answer A if 1, 2, and 3 Are Correct" Type Question: This type of question, known as the "K type," has been dropped from the USMLE and therefore is no longer represented among the practice questions provided in this review. However, it is still used in many local examinations.

    For this type of question, one rarely must know the truth about all four statements to arrive at the correct answer. The instructions are to select

    (A)   if only (1), (2), and (3) are correct;
    (B)   if only (1) and (3) are correct;
    (C)   if only (2) and (4) are correct;
    (D)   if only (4) is correct;
    (E)   if all are correct.

Useful strategies include the following:

    1.   If statement (1) is correct and (2) is wrong, the answer must be **(B),** ie, (1) and (3) are correct. You don't need to know anything about (3) or (4).
    2.   If statement (1) is wrong, then answers **(A), (B),** and **(E)** are automatically excluded. Concentrate on statements (2) and (4).
    3.   The converse of 1 above: If choice (1) is wrong and (2) is correct, the answer must be **(C),** ie, (2) and (4) are correct.
    4.   If statement (2) is correct and (4) is wrong, the answer is **(A),** ie, (1) and (3) must be correct and you need not even look at them. (See example below.)
    5.   If statements (1), (2), and (4) are correct, the answer must be **(E).** You need not know anything about (3).
    6.   Similarly, if statements (2) and (3) are correct and (4) is wrong, the answer must be **(A),** and statement (1) must be correct.
    7.   If statements (2), (3), and (4) are correct, then the answer must be **(E),** and statement (1) must be correct.

    No doubt more of these rules exist. In general, if you know whether two or three of the four statements in each question are right or wrong (ie, 50–75% of the material), you should achieve a perfect score on this kind of question. The best way to learn these rules is to apply them to practice questions until the principles are firmly ingrained.

    Consider the following question. Using the above rules, you should be able to answer it correctly even though there is no reason why you should know anything about the information contained in two of the four statements. The answer follows.

    Which of the following statements is (are) correct?
      1.   The "struck bushel" is equal to 2150.42 cubic inches
      2.   Medicine is one of the health sciences

3. The fresh meat of the Atlantic salmon contains 220 IU of vitamin A per 100 g edible portion
4. Hippocrates was the founder of modern psychoanalysis

The answer is **(A).** Since statement (2) is clearly correct, and (4) is just as patently incorrect (let's give Freud the credit), the answer can only be **(A),** and statements (1) and (3) must be correct. (The data in [1] and [3] are from Lentner C [editor]: *Geigy Scientific Tables,* 8th ed. Vol 1. Ciba-Geigy, 1981.)

REFERENCES

Bhushan V, et al: *1997 First Aid for the USMLE STEP 1.* Appleton & Lange, 1997.

Case SM, Swanson DB: Constructing written test questions for the basic and clinical sciences. National Board of Medical Examiners, 1996. Available from the World Wide Web (www.nbme.org; Guide for Writing Test Items).

1997 Step 1 General Instructions, Content Outline, and Sample Items. National Board of Medical Examiners, 1997. See also the USMLE World Wide Web page at www.usmle.org.

Index

NOTE: A *t* following a page number indicates tabular material and an *f* following a page number indicates an illustration. Drugs are listed under their generic names.

Medical Epidemiology, 2/e
Greenberg, Daniels, Flanders, Eley, & Boring
1996, ISBN 0-8385-6206-X, A6206-5

Basic & Clinical Endocrinology, 5/e
Greenspan & Strewler
1997, ISBN 0-8385-0588-0, A0588-2

Occupational & Environmental Medicine, 2/e
LaDou
1997, ISBN 0-8385-7216-2, A7216-3

Primary Care of Women
Lemcke, Marshall, Pattison, & Cowley
1995, ISBN 0-8385-9813-7, A9813-5

Clinical Anesthesiology, 2/e
Morgan & Mikhail
1996, ISBN 0-8385-1381-6, A1381-1

Fundamentals of Surgery
Niederhuber
1998, ISBN 0-8385-0509-0, A0509-8

Dermatology
Orkin, Maibach, & Dahl
1991, ISBN 0-8385-1288-7, A1288-8

Rudolph's Fundamentals of Pediatrics, 2/e
Rudolph & Kamei
1998, ISBN 0-8385-8236-2, A8236-0

Genetics in Primary Care & Clinical Medicine
Seashore
1995, ISBN 0-8385-3128-8, A3128-4

The Principles and Practice of Medicine, 23/e
Stobo, Hellman, Ladenson, Petty, & Traill
1996, ISBN 0-8385-7963-9, A7963-0

Smith's General Urology, 14/e
Tanagho & McAninch
1995, ISBN 0-8385-8612-0, A8612-2

General Ophthalmology, 14/e
Vaughan, Asbury, & Riordan-Eva
1995, ISBN 0-8385-3127-X, A3127-6

Clinical Oncology
Weiss
1993, ISBN 0-8385-1325-5, A1325-8

CURRENT Clinical References

CURRENT Critical Care Diagnosis & Treatment, 2/e
Bongard & Sue
1999, ISBN 0-8385-1454-5, A1454-6

CURRENT Diagnosis & Treatment in Cardiology
Crawford
1995, ISBN 0-8385-1444-8, A1444-7

CURRENT Diagnosis & Treatment in Vascular Surgery
Dean, Yao, & Brewster
1995, ISBN 0-8385-1351-4, A1351-4

CURRENT Obstetric & Gynecologic Diagnosis & Treatment, 9/e
DeCherney
1999, ISBN 0-8385-1401-4, A1401-7

CURRENT Diagnosis and Treatment in Psychiatry
Ebert, Loosen, & Nurcombe
1999, ISBN 0-8385-1462-6, A1462-9

CURRENT Diagnosis & Treatment in Gastroenterology
Grendell, McQuaid, & Friedman
1996, ISBN 0-8385-1448-0, A1448-8

CURRENT Pediatric Diagnosis & Treatment, 13/e
Hay, Groothius, Hayward, & Levin
1997, ISBN 0-8385-1400-6, A1400-9

CURRENT Emergency Diagnosis & Treatment, 4/e
Saunders & Ho
1992, ISBN 0-8385-1347-6, A1347-2

CURRENT Diagnosis & Treatment in Orthopedics
Skinner
1995, ISBN 0-8385-1009-4, A1009-8

CURRENT Medical Diagnosis & Treatment 1998, 37/e
Tierney, McPhee, & Papadakis
1998, ISBN 0-8385-1524-X, A1524-6

CURRENT Surgical Diagnosis & Treatment, 11/e
Way
1999, ISBN 0-8385-1456-1, A1456-1

LANGE Clinical Manuals

Dermatology
Diagnosis and Therapy
Bondi, Jegasothy, & Lazarus
1991, ISBN 0-8385-1274-7, A1274-8

Manual for Human Dissection
Callas
1994, ISBN 0-8385-6133-0, A6133-1

Practical Oncology
Cameron
1994, ISBN 0-8385-1326-3, A1326-6

Office & Bedside Procedures
Chesnutt, Dewar, & Locksley
1993, ISBN 0-8385-1095-7, A1095-7

Psychiatry
Diagnosis & Treatment, 2/e
Flaherty, Davis, & Janicak
1993, ISBN 0-8385-1267-4, A1267-2

Practical Gynecology
Jacobs & Gast
1991, ISBN 0-8385-1336-0, A1336-5

Geriatrics
Lonergan
1996, ISBN 0-8385-1094-9, A1094-0

Ambulatory Medicine
The Primary Care of Families, 2/e
Mengel & Schwiebert
1996, ISBN 0-8385-1466-9, A1466-0

Poisoning & Drug Overdose, 3/e
Olson
1999, ISBN 0-8385-0260-1, A0260-8

Internal Medicine
Diagnosis and Therapy, 3/e
Stein
1993, ISBN 0-8385-1112-0, A1112-0

Surgery
Diagnosis and Therapy
Stillman
1989, ISBN 0-8385-1283-6, A1283-9

Medical Perioperative Management
Wolfsthal
1989, ISBN 0-8385-1298-4, A1298-7

LANGE Handbooks

Handbook of Gynecology & Obstetrics
Brown & Crombleholme
1993, ISBN 0-8385-3608-5, A3608-5

HIV/AIDS Primary Care Handbook, 2/e
Carmichael, Carmichael, & Fischl
1999, ISBN 0-8385-3777-4, A3777-8

Clinician's Pocket Reference, 8/e
Gomella
1997, ISBN 0-8385-1476-6, A1476-9

Neonatology
Management, Procedures, On-Call Problems, Diseases, and Drugs, 3/e
Gomella
1995, ISBN 0-8385-1331-X, A1331-6

Surgery on Call, 2/e
Gomella & Lefor
1996, ISBN 0-8385-8746-1, A8746-8

Internal Medicine On Call, 2/e
Haist, Robbins, & Gomella
1997, ISBN 0-8385-4056-2, A4056-6

Obstetrics & Gynecology On Call
Horowitz & Gomella
1993, ISBN 0-8385-7174-3, A7174-4

Pocket Guide to Commonly Prescribed Drugs, 2/e
Levine
1996, ISBN 0-8385-8099-8, A8099-2

Handbook of Pediatrics, 18/e
Merenstein, Kaplan, & Rosenberg
1997, ISBN 0-8385-3625-5, A3625-9

Pocket Guide to Diagnostic Tests, 2/e
Nicoll, McPhee, Chou, & Detmer
1997, ISBN 0-8385-8100-5, A8100-8

Quick Medical Spanish, 2/e
Rogers
1997, ISBN 0-8385-8258-3, A8258-4

How to Examine the Nervous System, 3/e
Ross
1998, ISBN 0-8385-3852-5, A3852-9

Pocket Guide to the Essentials of Diagnosis & Treatment
Tierney
1997, ISBN 0-8385-3605-0, A3605-1

Appleton & Lange • P.O. Box 120041 • Stamford, CT • 06912-0041 • 1-800-423-1359